TEXTBOOK OF IMMUNOLOGY

AN INTRODUCTION TO IMMUNOCHEMISTRY AND IMMUNOBIOLOGY

TEXTBOOK OF IMMUNOLOGY

AN INTRODUCTION TO IMMUNOCHEMISTRY AND IMMUNOBIOLOGY

JAMES T. BARRETT, Ph.D.

Professor of Microbiology
University of Missouri School of Medicine
Columbia, Missouri

FOURTH EDITION

With **194** illustrations

The C. V. Mosby Company

ST. LOUIS • TORONTO • LONDON   1983

MOSBY

A TRADITION OF PUBLISHING EXCELLENCE

Editor: Samuel E. Harshberger
Assistant editor: Anne Gunter
Manuscript editor: Susan K. Hume
Book design: Jeanne Bush
Production: Judy England, Barbara Merritt

FOURTH EDITION

The C.V. Mosby Company
11830 Westline Industrial Drive, St. Louis, Missouri 63141

Library of Congress Cataloging in Publication Data

Barrett, James T., 1927-
   Textbook of immunology.

   Bibliography: p.
   Includes index.
   1. Immunology. I. Title. |DNLM: 1. Immunity.
2. Immunochemistry. 3. Serology. QW 504 B274t|
QR181.B28   1983   616.07'9   82-8286
ISBN 0-8016-0504-0

GW/VH/VH 9 8 7 6 5 4 3   02/B/247

To
my former students

They who are not in the habit of conducting experiments
may not be aware of the coincidence of circumstances necessary
for their being managed so as to prove perfectly decisive;
nor how often men engaged in professional pursuits are liable
to interruptions which disappoint them almost at the instant
of their being accomplished: however, I feel no room for hesitation. . . .

Edward Jenner, 1798

PREFACE to fourth edition

In reviewing the literature during the preparation of this volume, I was impressed by two things: the breadth of subject matter to be included and its recency. Both of these tend to make instruction of immunology more difficult, whether it be in the lecture hall or in the development of a text. Present day immunologists are expected to show competence in basic genetics (the inheritance of transplantation antigens, blood group antigens, and the relationship of these to immunity and autoimmunity), to understand genetic engineering and molecular cloning (the techniques used to locate the genes used in immunoglobulin synthesis and interferon production), to demonstrate biochemical expertise (immunoglobulin structure, the mode of action of immunosuppressive drugs, the chemistry of the inorganic forms of oxygen used by phagocytic cells, and the place of lipids and arachidonic acid derivatives in chemotaxis and anaphylaxis), to understand the structure and behavior of several cell types, and, of course, to be expert immunologists. This required versatility illustrates the impact immunology has on its sister sciences, and vice versa—a matter of pride for all immunologists but a difficult task to master.

Instructors of immunology are simultaneously faced with this broad subject to impart and a broad audience of students from numerous disciplines, most of whom are only partially informed about the biochemical, genetic, cytologic, or other disciplines aside from their own that they need to understand before they can master the subject of their primary interest: immunology. This challenge and the success of most instructors in meeting it in company with the application of immunology to so many different sciences have sustained immunology as a topic of wide interest.

In addition, whereas a decade ago one could write a text and use fully viable references that were themselves a decade old, this is no longer possible. The dynamic pace and expansion of immunologic research now make it inadvisable in many instances to use references published more than 5 years previously. Consequently many instructors rely more on texts now than they did before, trusting that the text will present the vastness of modern-day immunology in an intelligible manner.

It has been the central idea in the design of this text since its first edition to provide a complete coverage of immunology. Rather than present cellular immunology and omit allergy, present immunochemistry and omit serology, or establish other arbitrary limits, it was the goal to generate an introductory text that fairly presents the scope of immunology in a style that a student with a limited background can still comprehend and appreciate. And although in each edition the factual base of this science has been updated and expanded, it seldom has been done so extensively as in this edition.

In this process I have had considerable assistance from a number of my colleagues who have provided beautiful illustrative material. Of those, Professor Edward Adelstein of our Department of Pathology should be mentioned for his contribution of many electron micrographs. Additional illustrations by my wife, Barbro, and by commercial artists have improved this edition. Karen Ehlert did virtually all the typing, and an excellent job it was. Now the pages are in the hands of The C.V. Mosby Company staff. I have always admired their ability to create a good product, but perhaps even more I appreciate their continued friendship, their cooperation, and their encouragement.

J.T.B.

PREFACE to first edition

In its most recent growth, immunology has expanded from its origins in the medical sciences to permeate all of biology. The recognition by biologists of immunologic methods as important and sensitive research weapons has been responsible in a large measure for this rebirth of immunology. At the same time the utilization of modern biochemical knowledge and technology has given immunologists a new insight into their own science. These developments have presented additional problems to both students and teachers of immunology. On the one hand, undergraduate students who have had little opportunity to master complex chemical and biologic problems are drawn early to immunology as an exciting and "new" science. On the other hand, students who might have been content to continue in their chosen specialty now see a need to include immunology in their curriculum. The teacher is thus presented with a more varied audience than ever before. A partial solution to this dilemma is a textbook of immunology that will be equally useful to undergraduate and graduate students. This does not necessarily mean that the interests of students in the health sciences have been ignored, as is pointed out below.

To meet the demands of a broad audience the contents of this book have been tailored in several ways. First, the book is intended as a general textbook of immunology—one that overemphasizes neither immunochemistry nor immunobiology.

Consequently complementary sections on the chemistry of the immunoglobulins and immunochemistry are balanced by sections on the phylogeny of the immune response and cellular aspects of the immunoglobulin response. A similar balance has been attempted in other sections. For example, the chapters on immunity and hypersensitivity, subjects of considerable interest to students in the medical and paramedical sciences, have been developed from the viewpoint that the fundamentals of these topics are essential to all students of immunology. Second, the references have been limited and chosen to emphasize reviews and specialty books. Several excellent immunologic review series are now available. These provide extended discussions of various items and lengthy bibliographies. In this way a broad base of additional readings has been provided without the necessity of a voluminous and, all too soon, outdated bibliography in this volume. Only a few students have the time for extensive outside reading during their course work in any case. Third, a brief appendix, which summarizes the highlights of macromolecular biochemistry, is included for those who are as yet uninitiated or need a quick refresher on the subject. Fourth, a genuine effort has been made to use a concise and intelligible writing style.

Introspection is an unreliable witness to the origin of ideas, and this is no more evident than in authorship. Many of the concepts incorporated

ix

here were derived from my past professors, current colleagues, and perhaps, most vitally, interested students. To this legion, I give a salute of gratitude, with the hope that my efforts have in some small measure been worthy of them. Of those persons whom I wish to name, that of my wife, Barbro, must come first, both for her many hours of silent support and her active participation as an artist. To those wonderful girls at the typewriters, especially Anne, Carol, Linda, and Vera, I give my thanks for a job well done.

J.T.B.

CONTENTS

FOUNDATION
OF IMMUNOLOGY

THE HISTORY OF IMMUNOLOGY

Within the last 15 years immunology has emerged as an individual science, and, like all modern sciences, it draws from and contributes to many other closely related biologic and chemical sciences, including microbiology, biochemistry, genetics, medicine, zoology, and pathology. The recent outburst of advances in immunology has followed very closely and in some instances has been responsible for notable progress in these other sciences. Virtually the entire history of immunology has been recorded in the past 100 years; even if we calculate the origin of immunology from the time of the introduction of smallpox vaccination into the western world, immunology has existed for only about 150 years. During that time the development of immunology and the sciences on which it has depended has been gradual and uneven. Consequently it is only within the past century that the growth of subdisciplines within the area of immunology has become apparent.

The first of the subdivisions of immunology to emerge was *immunity*. In its infancy immunology was devoted almost exclusively to the prevention of infectious diseases by vaccination and immunization. In the 1880s immunology and immunity were synonymous, but this is no longer true. Even though considerable effort still is being directed toward the improvement of old and the development of new vaccines and toward the improvement of immunizing techniques, new subjects of study such as autoimmunity, tumor immunity, interferon induction, transplantation immunity, and the fantastic recent advances in cell-mediated immunity, the mechanism of phagocytosis, and the role of complement have magnified immunity as a distinct discipline within the broader subject of immunology. This health-related component of immunology is closely bonded to the subjects of virology, genetics, immunochemistry, and serology, sometimes clouding immunity as the principal subject under study.

Serology, then, also could be thought of as a subdivision of immunity, but it is such a vast subject that it deserves an equal status. Like immunity, serology has obvious practical implications for human and veterinary medicine, but as a diagnostic rather than a preventive aid. Today's serologists seek not only to discover new specific serologic tests for disease, such as those employing fluorescent or electron microscopy, but also to improve existing serologic techniques, identify new immunoglobulins, analyze the behavior of serum complement, purify and improve antigen and antiserum preparations, and clarify the mechanisms of serologic reactions through fundamental studies.

A third subdivision of immunology emerged with the others at the turn of the twentieth century. It attempted to view immunologic phenomena primarily as macromolecular phenomena, as expressions of complex chemical reactions between antigens and haptens with immunoglobulins and complement. In the beginning this new area of *immunochemistry* was almost totally dominated by Landsteiner and his studies with haptens. Gradually, as biochemical and biophysical procedures became more sophisticated, macromolecular antigens, antibodies, and complement became subjects of truer chemical investigation. Already vast rewards have been harvested, including a knowledge of the chemical basis of antigenic determinants, the structure and chemistry—including amino acid sequence—of immunoglobulins, the chemistry of complement, the means by which the components of the complement system influence chemotaxis and anaphylaxis, and the chemistry of immunosuppression.

In contrast to immunochemistry, a fourth area, perhaps poorly described as *immunobiology* but certainly based on broad biologic principles, has evolved. Many aspects of immunobiology are primarily immunologically oriented; theories of antibody formation, how allergies and hypersensitivities develop, immunologic tolerance, and the origin of autoimmune disease are examples, but these and subjects such as the phylogeny and ontogeny of the immune response, the genetics of the immune response, the cellular biology of immunology, and transplantation and tumor immunity all have obvious ramifications into other biologic sciences.

These four subdivisions (*immunity, serology, immunochemistry,* and *immunobiology*) encompass the field of immunology as it exists today. The dividing lines between these areas of immunology are all but invisible and in fact make subdivision rather artificial. Consideration of these four entities as individual units is intended only as an organizational convenience. After all, if one is studying the chemistry of the transplantation antigens involved in serologic tests for tissue rejection, it is clear he is working in all four of the subdisciplines of immunology. Indeed several immunologists have made important contributions that have been of nearly equal importance in two or more areas of immunology, although they have been categorized somewhat arbitrarily in the following pages. The Nobel Prize in Physiology and Medicine has been awarded to several of these scientists whose discoveries were of paramount importance to science as a whole (Table 1-1).

IMMUNITY

The first exciting area of study for immunologists and the foundation from which the whole of immunology sprang was that of immunity to infectious diseases. Many unrecorded observers must have noted that the contraction of and recovery from certain diseases resulted in a permanent resistance to recurrence of the same illness. Despite such knowledge among the lay population, it was not until the early eighteenth century that the purposeful contraction of a disease with the intent of creating immunity came under study. The disease was smallpox.

Although ancient Chinese and Arabic writings referred to the deliberate transmission of smallpox to healthy persons by inhalation of powdered smallpox crusts from diseased persons, immunization against smallpox was not practiced in the western world until 1721. Even so, this followed by several years correspondence to the Royal Society by physicians traveling to China and Turkey that the custom was widespread there. Credit is given to Lady Mary Wortley Montagu, wife of the British Ambassador to Turkey, for introducing variolization to England and Europe.

Table 1-1. Nobel Prize winners in immunology and closely related subjects

1901	Emil von Behring	Antiserum therapy
1905	Robert Koch	Tuberculosis research
1908	Paul Ehrlich	Theories of immunity
	Elie Metchnikoff	Phagocytosis
1912	Alexis Carrell	Organ grafting
1913	Charles Richet	Anaphylaxis
1919	Jules Bordet	Complement and theories of immunity
1930	Karl Landsteiner	Human blood groups
1951	Max Theiler	Yellow fever vaccine
1957	Daniel Bovet	Antihistamine research
1960	Macfarlane Burnet and Peter Medawar	Immunologic tolerance
1972	Rodney R. Porter and Gerald M. Edelman	Structure of immunoglobulins
1977	Rosalyn Yalow	Radioimmunoassay
1980	Baruj Benacerraf, Jean Dausset, and George Snell	Immunogenetics and histocompatibility

Shortly after her arrival in Turkey in 1717 Lady Montagu wrote to a friend in England*:

> The small-pox, so fatal, and so general amongst us, is here entirely harmless. . . . People send to one another to know if any of their family has a mind to have the small-pox: they make parties for this purpose, and when they are met (commonly 15 or 16 together), the old woman comes with a nutshell of the matter of the best sort of small-pox, and asks what vein you please to have opened. She immediately rips open that you offer her, with a large needle (which gives you no more pain than a common scratch) and puts into the vein, as much matter as can lie upon the head of her needle. . . . There is no example of anyone that had died in it: and you may believe I am well satisfied of the safety of this experiment, since I intend to try it on my dear little son. I am patriot enough to take pains to bring this useful invention into fashion in England.

Lady Montagu was faithful to this proclamation and had her son inoculated in March of 1718. Three years later her daughter became the first person to be so immunized in England.

*From Dixon, C.W.: Smallpox, London, 1962, J. & A. Churchill, Ltd.

Despite the favorable claims for variolization (smallpox was then known as variola), it was not without hazard. The disease did not always take the mild course seen in the donor, and occasional infections of other types such as leprosy or syphilis were transmitted. Still the risk was less than that from acquiring ''wild smallpox,'' which was extremely disfiguring, if not fatal. Variolization became widespread in England and in the American colonies and by the middle of the eighteenth century was common in central Europe.

Shortly after this time a more scientific and far safer approach to smallpox immunization was developed by Jenner, a country physician in England (Fig. 1-1). Jenner (1749-1823) was a vicar's son and was born in May of 1749. By the time he was 13 years old he exhibited an intense interest in nature and was apprenticed to a physician. He was later a student in London but returned to his hometown to practice medicine; he also continued an interest in zoology, music, and poetry. His observations on cowpox and smallpox spanned a quarter of a century before he performed his famous experiment. Jenner became impressed, first by rumor and later by his own observations,

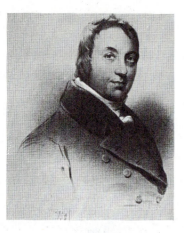

Fig. 1-1. Edward Jenner (1749-1823). From his objective observations that milkmaids who contracted cowpox were thereafter resistant to smallpox, Jenner transformed rumor into a scientific procedure that saved millions of lives. Jenner's announcement in 1798 of a new method of vaccination was at first rebuked, but since it was based on sound scientific fact, it was soon accepted as the great immunologic discovery that it truly was. (From Smith, A.L.: Principles of microbiology, ed. 6, St. Louis, 1969, The C.V. Mosby Co.)

that persons who acquired cowpox were thereafter protected against smallpox. Cowpox is a mild viral pox of cattle that is easily transmitted to herdsmen and dairy maids. Jenner's experiments with cowpox and smallpox are said to have begun on May 14, 1796, when he transferred matter from a cowpox lesion on the hand of Sarah Nelmes to the arm of a lad named James Phipps. Nearly 6 weeks later he subjected young Master Phipps to an inoculation of pus taken directly from a smallpox pustule. No infection followed. By 1798 Jenner had published a booklet on the nature of cowpox and how it prevented variola. After an initial few years of resistance and neglect, jennerian vaccination became accepted and is still the preferred method of vaccination against smallpox. This practice apparently has eliminated smallpox from the advanced parts of the world.

For almost a century no further advances in immunity followed Jenner's discovery. This is not really surprising, since the infectious agents were just then being described, and it was still uncertain which organisms caused a specific disease. Pure culture techniques were just being developed, and many uncertainties surrounded the sparse understanding of microorganisms. In addition, smallpox was a very exceptional case. Smallpox is one of the few diseases that is entirely preventable by recovery from another closely related illness. Cross-immunity of this sort now can be explained in exact chemical terms, but its discovery 185 years ago, and in its most absolute form, must have been confusing.

The next great discoveries in immunity were made by Pasteur (1822-1895), a French chemist turned biologist, who by accident hit on two different methods of reducing the virulence of pathogenetic microbes (Fig. 1-2). Pasteur found that aged cultures of the chicken cholera bacillus would not cause disease in chickens. Subsequent injections of young cultures, which ordinarily killed normal chickens, had no effect on the birds previously inoculated with the impotent culture. Aged cultures of the chicken cholera organisms thus became the first attenuated vaccine. Pasteur noted that a similar type of protection against anthrax resulted when sheep were inoculated with cultures of *Bacillus anthracis* that had been cultivated at 42° C. At their usual growth temperature of 37° C these organisms are fully pathogenic for sheep, but this virulence is lost on cultivation at the higher temperature. However, animals first inoculated with the 42° C culture were immune to subsequent inoculations with the 37° C culture. Attenuation (virulence reduction) of a pathogen by these or other means such as radiation or genetic selection has been the key to the development of vaccines against tuberculosis, yellow fever, poliomyelitis, rabies, measles, mumps, and other infectious diseases. Incidentally, Pasteur coined the term *vaccination* for these immunization procedures in honor of Jenner's initial discoveries with cowpox (Latin *vacca,* cow). In its present usage vaccination generally refers to immunization with cellular vaccines and does not include

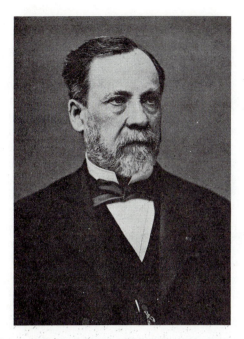

Fig. 1-2. Louis Pasteur (1822-1895). The genius of Pasteur, first evidenced by his discovery that polarization of light could be related to the structure of crystals, carried him to the solution of many problems: the spoilage of beers and wines, with the accompanying pasteurization process; the discovery of anaerobic bacteria, virus vaccines, and attenuation of virulence; and studies of spontaneous generation. His studies in immunology have rightly earned him the position as father of the science. (From Carpenter, P.L.: Microbiology, ed. 2, Philadelphia, 1967, W.B. Saunders Co.)

immunization with toxoids or purely fluid materials.

Pasteur's most famous immunization was that developed against rabies (Fig. 1-3). The causative agent was not yet identified as a virus when Pasteur found he could perpetuate the disease in dogs or rabbits by injecting spinal cord extracts from rabid animals into normal animals. Extracts prepared from infected cords that had been dried for several days at room temperature were less infectious than those not dried, and infected cords that were dried for longer periods were not infectious at all. Pasteur correctly deduced, in parallel with his earlier studies with fowl cholera and anthrax, that injections of the inactive cord extract and then the weakened extracts with a progression toward more potent virus-containing extracts would protect his animals against otherwise fully active rabies virus.

The first human test occurred on July 6, 1885. A young boy named Joseph Meister had been bitten severely, some 14 times, just 2 days previously. After much persuasion from the boy's parents Pasteur initiated his treatment of 12 injections, gradually increasing the potency of the virus-cord extract over a 2-week period. Despite Pasteur's many fears, the boy survived the rabid dog bites and the active virus present in the final injections of the series.

A few weeks later Pasteur presented his report on rabies prevention to the Academy of Sciences. Within a year the Pasteur treatment was applied to 350 persons without one fatality. Pasteur's fame quickly spread around the world. Pasteur Institutes, first in Paris and then in other major European cities, were constructed with funds contributed for vaccine production and research. Many young physicians and scientists begged to come and study under Pasteur in Paris. The Pasteur Institutes quickly assumed a dominant role in the battle to control infectious diseases.

Pasteur died in 1895 after a lifetime of scientific accomplishment, first in chemistry and then in biochemistry, microbiology, immunology, and medicine. The impact of this one man on science can hardly be envisioned. He was born the son of a humble tanner in 1822; he first had an interest in art and later in chemistry. It is written that he was not an exceptional scholar even as a college student, but his keen observations, his willingness to test hypotheses experimentally, and his courage in the face of the unknown have rightfully earned him the title "father of immunology."

Pasteur's remains are housed at the Pasteur Institute in Paris. By a strange twist of fate, Joseph Meister became the gatekeeper there. In 1940, 55 years after being immunized with rabies vaccine, he took his own life. German military forces had requested his keys to Pasteur's crypt, and, rather

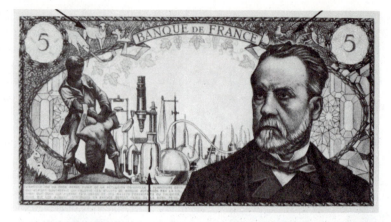

Fig. 1-3. French 5-franc notes illustrate many of Pasteur's scientific accomplishments in a true art form. Upper left and upper right arrows point to sheep and chickens that commemorate development of attenuated vaccines for anthrax and chicken cholera. Lower arrow indicates rabid rabbit spinal cord in a drying jar first used to treat Joseph Meister, the young boy shown battling a rabid dog. Rabbits in lower left corner possibly portray Pasteur's entry into bacterial warfare and his deliberate infection of rabbits who were burrowing into a friend's wine cellar and dislodging the masonry with disastrous results. Crystals at left and right center illustrate relationships of crystal structure to optic rotation. Grape clusters refer to Pasteur's study of diseases of wine and discovery of pasteurization, and swan-necked flask near Pasteur's portrait is a reminder of his disputation of the theory of spontaneous generation. Flagellated bacilli surrounding the number 5 in each upper corner of note refer to his discovery of anaerobic life. The reverse side of the bill is also beautiful and illustrates fungi, mulberry, and grapes with the portrait of Pasteur.

than surrender them to what he thought would be plunder and dishonor, he committed suicide.

At about the time of Pasteur's discoveries and shortly thereafter there emerged a strong conviction that immunity was totally dependent on certain body cells. These cells were described by the Russian zoologist Elie Metchnikoff (1845-1916) and were called phagocytic (cell-eating) cells (Fig. 1-4).

Metchnikoff was a brilliant student who studied zoology at the University of Kharkov. He studied in Germany before obtaining his doctorate at St. Petersburg and becoming a docent (assistent professor) at the University of Odessa. He married in 1868, and his wife died in 1873. In one of his periods of depression that followed the death of his wife, Metchnikoff made an unsuccessful attempt on his life by taking an overdose of morphine. After his recovery he returned to work but disliked certain changes in the university. A few years later (in 1881) he was again so despondent that he attempted suicide, this time by self-inoculation with the organisms that cause relapsing fever. Although he became seriously ill, it was not his fate to die. Within a year he resigned from the university and took his second wife and her orphaned brothers and sisters to Italy. While his family was away at a circus, he began to study the motile cells that he could see microscopically in transparent starfish larvae. He thought that these cells might be protective in a digestive way, much like the cells that gather at points of infection near splinters in human skin; he stuck some rose thorns into the larvae. The next day the thorns were surrounded by these ameboid cells. Shortly thereafter he returned to Russia, and while studying the water flea (Daphnia) he observed that phagocytic cells could ingest and destroy yeasts

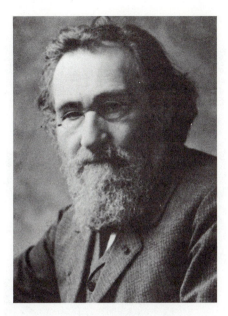

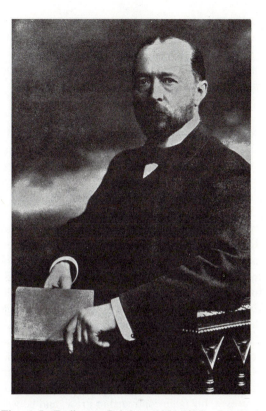

Fig. 1-4. Elie Metchnikoff (1845-1916). The electrifying and persistent personality of Metchnikoff allowed him to convert his discoveries of phagocytosis into a doctrine that gained many disciples from his coterie of students. His doctrine of cellular immunity eventually was united with the doctrine of humoral immunity approximately 10 years before his death. (From Dubos, R., and Hirsch, J.: Bacterial and mycotic infections of man, ed. 4, Philadelphia, 1965, J.B. Lippincott Co.)

Fig. 1-5. Emil von Behring (1854-1917). Behring's discoveries of antitoxin and the principles of antiserum therapy placed him strongly on the side of those favoring humoral substances as the cause of immunity. He established one of the first corporations to produce immunobiologic products. (From Parish, H.J.: A history of immunization, Edinburgh, 1965, E. & S. Livingstone, Ltd.)

(Monospora bicuspidata) that were pathogenic to the flea. A paper on these studies was published in 1884. Metchnikoff spent the rest of his life studying the phenomenon of phagocytosis in higher animals. In 1908 he shared a Nobel Prize with Ehrlich for his early contributions to immunity.

Those who supported the theory of phagocytosis as the prime source of immunity were not long without antagonists. Nuttall, an American bacteriologist working in Goettingen, Germany, found in 1888 that defibrinated blood was bactericidal in itself. Although phagocytosis also occurred, he suggested that the phagocytic white blood cells merely removed the bacteria killed by some heat-labile, serum substance. Others,

including Behring, began to study the bactericidal quality of blood for several different pathogenic microbes. Pfeiffer published a report of his studies of the cholera bacillus in 1894, which clearly showed that peritoneal fluids and immune serum would lyse the cholera vibrio (Pfeiffer's phenomenon).

Perhaps the greatest support for the humoral theory arose from the studies of Behring (1854-1917), who stated in 1890 that immunity to diphtheria and to tetanus was dependent on the capacity of blood to inactivate diphtheria or tetanus exo-toxin. It was easily proved that this antitoxic activity resided in the cell-free portion of the blood. In 1901 Behring became the first Nobel laureate in Physiology and Medicine for his work with anti-serum therapy (Fig. 1-5).

Behring led a life unlike that of Metchnikoff. Behring was born into a poor family. He nearly passed up medical school in favor of free university training in theology but was able to enter the army medical school in Berlin. As a military physician, he apparently had a rather unrestrained bachelorhood, but he was professionally able and worked diligently. He was transferred in 1889 to Robert Koch's laboratories in Berlin and moved later (in 1891) with Koch into the Institute for Infectious Diseases. After his successes with antitoxin therapy were proved in human beings, Behring achieved tremendous fame. After all, diphtheria and tetanus were the great killers of that day. Koch's jealousy of Behring and his discoveries forced a transfer of Behring's appointment from the Institute into the university system, but he was a poor teacher and soon resigned. However, his fame continued to grow, and he was honored first by being brought into the nobility and then by being awarded the Nobel Prize. Later he created the Behring Werke, which still exists today, for manufacturing biologic products.

By 1903 it had become apparent to Wright (1861-1947), an English physician and later teacher of Sir Alexander Fleming (the discoverer of penicillin), that neither the cellular theory nor the humoral theory was wrong and that both were correct. In 1903, with Douglass, he published convincing evidence that serum substances, which he termed *opsonins,* functioned by aiding phagocytosis of bacteria. By this simple discovery the differences between the humoralists and the cellularists were resolved.

Wright was an extremely interesting personality. He was a fine scholar, first in literature at Trinity College in Dublin and later in medical school. After completing his medical studies he continued postgraduate studies in Germany and

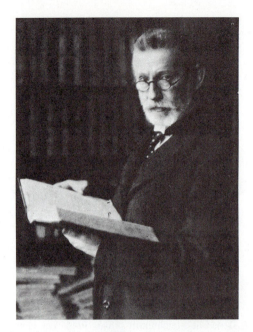

Fig. 1-6. Paul Ehrlich (1854-1915). An exact contemporary of Metchnikoff but of much different background and personality, Ehrlich has been described as the greatest scientific worker in medicine prior to World War II. He was a histologist, hematologist, chemotherapist, bacteriologist, physician, and immunologist. (From Burdon, K., and Williams, R.P.: Microbiology, ed. 6, New York, 1968, Macmillan, Inc.)

taught in Australia. He took an English Army Medical School appointment, where he conducted important studies of typhoid fever vaccines; later, at St. Mary's in London, he studied opsonins and leukocytes. It was at St. Mary's that he had Fleming as his student. Wright was a convincing speaker with a fantastic command of language; he was a solid conservative and an outspoken battler against women's suffrage.

During these same years a man named Ehrlich was making unique contributions to immunology, contributions that were both original and correlative in nature. Ehrlich (1854-1915) attended several schools, eventually earning his doctorate in 1878. As a student, he was noted for his intense love of histology and staining. One of his earliest

Table 1-2. Historical landmarks in immunity

1721	Lady Montagu	Smallpox immunization
1798	Edward Jenner	Smallpox immunization
1880	Louis Pasteur	Age attenuation of vaccines
1881	Louis Pasteur	Heat attenuation of vaccines
1884	Elie Metchnikoff	Discovery of phagocytosis
1885	Louis Pasteur	Rabies vaccination
1888	George Nuttall	Bactericidal property of blood
1890	Emil von Behring	Antitoxin therapy
1897	Paul Ehrlich	Studies in immunity
1903	Almroth Wright and Stewart Douglass	Role of serum in phagocytosis
1923	Gaston Ramon	Toxoid immunization
1957	Alick Isaacs	Interferon

scientific contributions was the discovery of mast cells. He was an addicted cigar smoker, note taker, and memo writer who had considerable disregard for his personal appearance and that of his laboratory. He was an original thinker and is honored as the founder of chemotherapy. Prior to his work with chemotherapeutics, especially during the years 1890 to 1896 after recovering from tuberculosis, he worked at the famous Institute for Infectious Diseases in Berlin, where he studied immunity. In studying immunology he discovered that there was a time lag after antigen injections before antibody was formed; he discovered the anamnestic or booster response and standardized antitoxins and toxins. He discovered that immunity could be transferred from mother to offspring. His theory of antibody formation, the side chain hypothesis, is still prominent. Ehrlich renamed complement (from Bordet's alexin), developed the concept of horror autotoxicus, and made many other contributions to immunology. For these he shared the Nobel Prize in 1908 with Metchnikoff (Fig. 1-6).

After Ehrlich it was approximately 25 years before another truly major contribution to immunity was made. Ramon, a Frenchman, observed in 1923 that toxins could be converted to toxoids with formaldehyde. The toxoids retained essentially all the antigenic activity of the toxin with-

out its noxious effects. Toxoids are much more stable than toxins and were quickly used to replace the toxin-antitoxin mixtures then used in immunization. Ramon also developed his own form of the precipitation test, which was based on antibody dilution. This is a truer measure of antitoxin than the animal protection tests developed by Ehrlich.

The final landmark to be considered in this resume of historically important contributions to immunity (Table 1-2) is the discovery of interferon. Interferons are substances excreted by cells harboring an intracellular parasite. The interferons then enter adjacent cells and protect them against the inducing and other antigenically unrelated intracellular parasites. The nonspecificity of interferons is an important difference between interferons and antibodies. The original interferon was discovered by Isaacs and Lindenmann in 1957; Isaacs continued his studies of interferons until his death in 1967.

SEROLOGY

Closely associated with the development of vaccines and immunizing preparations was the development of a dichotomy between those who believed immunity was dependent on cellular constituents of the body and those who believed in acellular serum components as the basis of immunity. Metchnikoff's contribution already has been described, as has Wright's resolution of the cellularist-humoralist polemic. Now it is essential to examine some of the earlier and later discoveries in serology (Table 1-3).

The first serologic reaction described was bacterial agglutination. The agglutination reaction, or the clumping of bacteria by specific antisera, was described by Grüber and Durham in 1896. In their paper they showed that the cholera vibrio was agglutinated by cholera antiserum, and the typhoid bacillus was agglutinated by antityphoid serum, but not vice versa. Immediately after this publication and in the same year Widal described the agglutination test as a diagnostic aid for typhoid fever. Bacterial agglutination became known as the Grüber-Widal test, but Grüber's name was dropped later. Certainly the agglutination test has had wide application in clinical bacteriology and microbial taxonomy. By the use of red blood cells as the antigen the test has been extended to hemagglutination, which is important in blood grouping and blood transfusion.

The second serologic test to be described, the precipitation test, like the agglutination test, was discovered in Austria; Kraus discovered that bacterial culture filtrates or glass ground extracts of bacteria were precipitable by bacterial antisera. He also determined the serologic specificity of the reaction between plague, typhoid, and cholera bacilli. The various modifications of the precipitin test have allowed its application in diagnostic microbiology and medicine, in bacterial taxonomy, and in the study of the serologic specificity of antigens and haptens.

The discovery that serologic precipitation tests could be performed in gels was announced during 1946 to 1948 by Ouchterlony, Elek, and Oudin in three separate laboratories in Sweden, the United States, and France, respectively. These immunodiffusion tests differed in their physical design but were based on the observation that antigens and antisera could diffuse from reservoirs placed in agar, through that agar until they met in concentrations adequate for precipitation. The fact that the Ouchterlony test is very simple to prepare and to interpret and that it has a somewhat more general application accounts for its greater popularity today. Gel immunodiffusion tests have been improved by several modifications.

The first of these modifications was immunoelectrophoresis, developed by Grabar and Williams in 1953. In this procedure an electrophoretic separation of antigens in a mixture of antigens precedes the immunodiffusion portion of the test, which is conducted essentially as in the Ouchterlony tests. The advantage of the method is that the antigens are displaced and segregate themselves according to their ionic properties, thus

Table 1-3. Historical landmarks in serology

1896	Max Grüber and Herbert Durham	Agglutination test
1896	G. Fernand Widal	Agglutination test for typhoid fever
1897	Rudolf Kraus	Precipitation test
1898	Jules Bordet	Complement
1901	Jules Bordet and Octave Gengou	Demonstrate complement fixation
1906	August von Wassermann	Complement-fixation test for syphilis
1942	Albert Coons	Fluorescent antibody
1945	R.R.A. Coombs	Antiglobulin tests
1946-1948	Örjan Ouchterlony, Jacques Oudin, and Stephen Elek	Gel diffusion tests
1953	Pierre Grabar and Curtis Williams	Immunoelectrophoresis
1959-1960	Solomon Berson and Rosalyn Yalow	Radioimmunoassay

facilitating the enumeration of the precipitates that form and easing their identification. Another useful modification of immunodiffusion referred to as radial or quantitative immunodiffusion was first described by Feinberg in 1957; however, the test is known as the Mancini test, since it was most extensively studied by Mancini. In this technique antigen diffuses radially from a well placed in an antibody-containing gel. The zone of precipitate that forms is an accurate measure of the quantity of antigen added. Other important variants of the immunodiffusion method such as crossed immunoelectrophoresis, counterimmunoelectrophoresis, and the Laurell, or rocket, technique are discussed in Chapter 15.

One of the major early contributions to the field of serology was made by Bordet (1870-1961), a Belgian who completed his medical studies by the age of 22 years and entered the Pasteur Institute under Metchnikoff in Paris. Within 3 years of his graduation he published his paper on alexin (later renamed complement by Ehrlich), a normal serum substance that was heat labile and that was strongly bactericidal when antibody was present. Bordet also found that complement did not increase in quantity during immunization. He made several contributions to medical bacteriology. He returned to Belgium as Director of the Pasteur Institute in Brussels. At the Free University he again returned to research in immunology. He studied the mechanism of in vitro serologic reactions and conglutination. Productive as he was, Bordet is most remembered for his discovery of complement, which allowed Wassermann to develop his famous test for syphilis. Of course the great advantage of the complement-fixation test is not in its single application to the serodiagnosis of syphilis but in its wide applicability to many diseases. The Nobel Committee recognized this and awarded the Prize to Bordet in 1919.

Anyone reading the current immunologic literature will be impressed by the repeated reference to the fluorescent antibody method developed by Coons in 1942. The covalent bonding of fluo-

rescein isocyanate or isothiocyanate with antibody molecules provided a remarkably useful histochemical reagent for locating antigen in tissue preparations. This technique required the use of ultraviolet microscopy but was immediately accepted as a superior technique to the use of azolabeled antigens for the same purpose. Later development of the indirect procedure, or immunologic sandwich technique, extended the method to one in which intracellular antibody was detectable as well. The fluorescent antibody procedure has been exploited extensively by those interested in the cellular events surrounding antigen metabolism and antibody synthesis.

In 1945 Coombs and his co-workers at Cambridge, England, published the first of their articles on the antiglobulin test that today bears Coombs' name. The Coombs test fulfilled an urgent need for a rapid and sensitive test to identify incomplete or monovalent antibodies, to prevent incompatible blood transfusions, to detect Rh incompatibilities, and to prevent and diagnose erythroblastosis fetalis. Modern blood banks use the Coombs test routinely for all crossmatch procedures.

The radioimmunoassay procedures in such widespread use today for detecting nanogram or even picogram quantities of antigens and haptens rely on the methods founded by Rosalyn Yalow and Solomon Berson in the years immediately after 1956. Their utilization of radioactive tracers for detecting insulin (the antigen) and antiinsulin greatly extended the sensitivity of serologic tests, which also are noted for their high specificity. The methods originally designed for insulin now have been applied to the detection and quantitation of a myriad of antigens and haptens, including human growth hormone, lactogenic hormone, corticosteroids, several different antibiotics, many enzymes, tumor antigens, and viruses. This remarkable advance also signaled the development of other labeled antigen (or antibody) tests, most notably enzyme immunoassays. For her contributions Yalow was awarded the Nobel Prize in Phys-

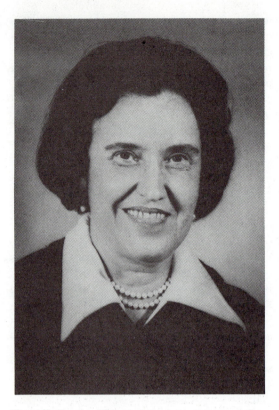

Fig. 1-7. Rosalyn Yalow, the first woman to receive a Nobel Prize in Physiology and Medicine (in 1977) for her research in immunology. With Solomon Berson she developed the first radioimmunoassays.

iology and Medicine in 1977, which she shared with two other persons who did research on a separate, although related, subject. Yalow is the first woman to receive this coveted award for studies in immunology (Fig. 1-7).

IMMUNOCHEMISTRY

Arrhenius was the first to use the term *immunochemistry,* in 1903; he published a monograph bearing that title in 1907. Other books emphasizing the chemistry of immunity and immunology were published by Wells in 1929, Landsteiner in 1936, Marrack in 1934, and Kabat and Mayer in 1948; immunochemistry has long been accepted as a subdivision of immunology. Currently it rep-

resents one of the most rapidly expanding subsections of the science as a whole (Table 1-4).

The first major contribution to immunology with a distinctive chemical imprint resulted from the study of haptens. The word *hapten* was originated by the famous Landsteiner (1868-1943) in 1921 to refer to small chemical groups that could be attached to already existing antigens and that would add an additional (the haptenic) specificity to the antigen. Earlier (in 1906) Obermayer and Pick had discovered that mild nitration or iodination of proteins would alter their serologic specificity; unlike Landsteiner, they did not learn that low molecular weight—nitrated or iodinated—compounds alone could react with antibodies to the chemically modified antigen. Landsteiner pursued the subject of chemically modified antigens and haptens for over 25 years, from his initial studies in 1917 until his death in 1943. Of his 167 publications in this interim, 95 can easily be cited as relating to haptens, conjugated antigens, and serologic specificity. Many of the remaining papers were devoted to blood grouping and blood group specificity (not included in the 95), and these, too, often were oriented toward antigen specificity. It was his work with blood groups that led to his Nobel Prize award in 1930 (Fig. 1-8).

During the 1920s and 1930s new insight into serologic reactions was developing from a chemical base. This is exemplified by the studies of Heidelberger with Avery and Goebel in their chemical descriptions of pneumococcal polysaccharide antigens. Later, with Kendall, Heidelberger devised the quantitative precipitin technique. The impact of this work was so great that immunochemists ever since have expressed the quantity of antibody in terms of milligrams of protein per milliliter in preference to the often meaningless quotation of antibody titer. The initial studies with quantitative precipitation were possible largely through the availability of the nitrogen-free pneumococcal polysaccharide antigen that Heidelberger had earlier helped to prepare.

Once Heidelberger and Kendall had established that analytical chemical techniques could be ap-

Table 1-4. Historical landmarks in immunochemistry

1906	F. Obermayer and E. Pick	Altered protein antigens
1907	S. Arrhenius	Monograph on immunochemistry
1917	Karl Landsteiner	Haptens
1929	Michael Heidelberger	Quantitative chemical serology
1934	J. Marrack	Antigen-antibody reaction
1938	Elvin Kabat and Arne Tiselius	Antibodies as globulins
1958	Rodney R. Porter	Structure of immunoglobulins
1959	Gerald M. Edelman	Structure of immunoglobulins
1966-1968	K. Ishizaka, H. Bennich, and S.G.O. Johansson	Studies with IgE

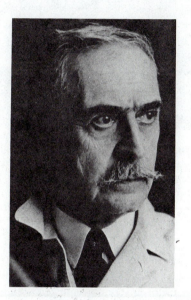

Fig. 1-8. Karl Landsteiner (1868-1943). This physician left the practice of medicine and yet made one of the most significant contributions to that science in the last 80 years: his discovery of the human ABO blood groups. (From Dubos, R., and Hirsch, J.: Bacterial and mycotic infections of man, ed. 4, Philadelphia, 1965, J.B. Lippincott Co.)

plied to the precipitation reaction, chemical procedures were applied to other serologic reactions. Kabat, one of Heidelberger's students, applied quantitative techniques to the agglutination reaction. While Kabat was doing postgraduate research in Sweden, he conclusively identified antibodies as being in the γ-globulin fraction of serum. This he determined by the use of the analytical ultracentrifuge that had just been developed in Sweden. Since that time (1939) Kabat has been especially concerned with the immunochemistry of the human blood group antigens.

Also in the 1930s Marrack, an Englishman, made an important contribution, of a more theoretic sort, to immunochemistry. In 1934 he proposed a new model for antigen-antibody reactions based on the multivalence (multiple combining sites) of each. With a combination of their specific reactive groups a latticework of alternating antigen and antibody molecules could be created. This concept of lattice formation is fundamentally an extension of some of Bordet's ideas on serologic reactions, but Marrack emphasized the genuine attractiveness of antigen and antibody for each other based on the special chemistry of each. Marrack's lattice hypothesis may be considered as proved today and has been very useful in explaining serologic reactions, not only with multivalent reactants but also with haptens and monovalent antibodies.

In 1972 two immunochemists, Rodney R. Porter and Gerald M. Edelman (Figs. 1-9 and 1-10) were recognized by the Nobel Committee for their outstanding contributions toward the solution of the structure of immunoglobulins. Both men worked on the same immunoglobulin, the one now known

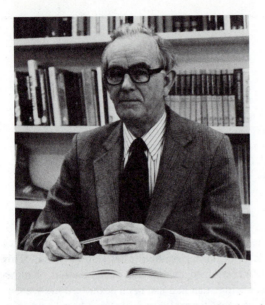

Fig. 1-9. Rodney R. Porter of Oxford University shared the Nobel Prize in Physiology and Medicine with Gerald M. Edelman. It is interesting that their fundamental studies in the chemistry of immunoglobulins should win an award in medicine, underscoring the dependence of advances in medicine on chemistry and immunology.

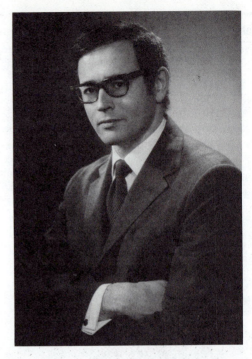

Fig. 1-10. Gerald M. Edelman of Rockefeller University was only 43 years of age when he shared the Nobel Prize with Rodney R. Porter in 1972. The discoveries for which the Nobel Prize was awarded were made by Edelman in the middle 1960s. (Photograph by Fabian Bachrach.)

as IgG, but each used slightly different methods. Porter utilized an enzyme method to cleave the antibody molecule into three parts, two that were identical and which contained the antibody activity and a third portion by which the antibody molecule attaches itself to cells. Edelman disrupted the normal structure of immunoglobulins by strong disulfide reagents in high-molarity urea. Under these conditions the molecule was fragmented into two types of polypeptide chains, one of which (L chain) was approximately half the size and weight of the other (H chain). Within 3 years of these discoveries it was possible to synthesize this information into a single structure for IgG. This is the four-peptide structure, which is similar for all five known immunoglobulins (Fig. 6-1).

It is quite probable that the discovery of IgE by Ishizaka and his co-workers and by Bennich and Johansson in the years 1966 to 1968 also

should be considered a landmark discovery in immunology. The fact that a unique immunoglobulin-like factor in serum was responsible or closely associated with various forms of allergic disease was known from the studies of Prausnitz and Küstner in 1921. A quarter of a century later these allergies were related to the activity of a new immunoglobulin, IgE, which is essentially destructive in behavior rather than protective, like the ordinary antibodies. Unraveling the mysteries of the in vivo activities of IgE undoubtedly will continue for several years, and it is hoped each year will open a new door to the prevention and treatment of allergic disease.

Progress in immunochemistry continues to be explosive and, like the study of human immunobiology, seems to be one of the most fashionable areas of immunologic research today. Proof that it is more than just fashion and that immunochemists have made genuinely giant contributions to immunology is seen in the special awards at the First International Congress of Immunology held in Washington, D.C., in 1971. Five men were selected for distinguished service awards: Burnet, Haurowitz, Grabar, Heidelberger, and Marrack. Of these, the first two were recognized for their contributions in immunobiology and the remaining three for their contributions in immunochemistry.

IMMUNOBIOLOGY

Since immunology is fundamentally a biologic science, every facet of immunology could be considered under an umbrella called immunobiology. Obviously the use of the word *immunobiology* here, as a subdivision of immunology, is intended for those segments of immunology which have not yet developed to the status (at least from a historical point of view) possessed by immunity, serology, and immunochemistry. When items such as allergy and hypersensitivity, theories of antibody formation, autoimmune disease, tissue transplantation, tumor immunology, immunologic tolerance, red blood cell grouping, and erythroblastosis fetalis are discussed under a single heading, the ramifications of immunology into the medical sciences become very apparent (Table 1-5).

The concept that disease could be caused by antibodies was a complete antithesis to the pioneer work of Behring, Ehrlich, Bordet, and the many others who had conclusively demonstrated that antibodies and serum substances were protective. Today there is no longer room for speculation; the whole subject of allergy and hypersensitivity is replete with documented examples of antibody-associated illnesses. Antibodies to foreign serum proteins, to plant pollens, to animal danders, and even to self-antigens are associated with and are in many cases the actual cause of a disease condition. Antibodies are not the only initiators of immune disease; there is a form of immune illness that is

cell dependent rather than humoral. This latter class, the delayed hypersensitivity, was the first to be described.

The discovery of delayed hypersensitivity was a direct outgrowth of Koch's studies of tuberculosis. Koch (1843-1910) noted that laboratory guinea pigs are highly susceptible to tuberculosis and that an inoculation of tubercle bacilli into these animals will kill them in 4 to 8 weeks. If such tuberculous guinea pigs are given a second subcutaneous injection of more tubercle bacilli, they are able to mobilize defenses that tend to wall off the new inoculum. The second injection site becomes reddened, tissue death follows, and the dead tissue and tuberculosis germs are sloughed off, leaving an ulcer that will heal. This is the Koch phenomenon. Although the record is somewhat incomplete and confused, Koch apparently thought that dead tubercle bacilli or growth products of these organisms, called tuberculin, could be injected into persons who already had tuberculosis and that a curative effect would be obtained. The idea was apparently that these injections would cause the tubercle bacilli, wherever they were located, to be sloughed, as in the Koch phenomenon in tuberculous guinea pigs. However, this did not occur.

Injections of tuberculin into the skin of tuberculous individuals caused a gradual reddening at the injection site, followed by induration. This process developed to its maximum at about 48 to 72 hours after the injection and did not occur in nontuberculous persons. This delayed hypersensitivity skin test is an example of an allergy of infection. Skin tests of this type are employed in epidemiologic studies of several infectious diseases, of which tuberculosis is a prime example. Similar delayed hypersensitivity tests are employed to determine drug hypersensitivity.

Koch made many contributions to medical bacteriology; it is unfortunate that his efforts to cure and to immunize against tuberculosis resulted in failure. He has many scientific credits, among which are proof of the life cycle of anthrax bacillus and its causative role in the disease, improvement

Table 1-5. Historical landmarks in immunobiology

1890	Robert Koch	Delayed hypersensitivity
1901	Karl Landsteiner	Human blood groups
1902	Charles Richet and Paul Portier	Anaphylaxis
1905	Clemens von Pirquet	Serum sickness
1908	Paul Ehrlich	Theories of antibody formation and other studies
1921	Carl Prausnitz and Heinz Küstner	Reagin discovery
1930	Felix Haurowitz and others	Template theories of antibody formation
1940	Karl Landsteiner and Alexander Wiener	Discovery of Rh antigens
1942	Karl Landsteiner and Merrill Chase	Cellular transfer of delayed hypersensitivity
1944-1960	Macfarlane Burnet and Peter Medawar	Immunologic tolerance
1956	Ernest Witebsky	Autoimmunity studies
1960	Baruj Benacerraf, Jean Dausset, and George Snell	Immunogenetics and histocompatibility

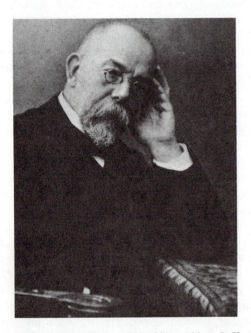

Fig. 1-11. Robert Koch (1843-1910). Although Koch is probably most famous as a bacteriologist, his discovery of delayed hypersensitivity always has been considered a hallmark in immunology. (From Burdon, K., and Williams, R.P.: Microbiology, ed. 6, New York, 1968, Macmillan, Inc.)

in staining procedures, identification of the tubercle bacillus, Koch's postulates, Koch's phenomenon, tuberculin, and discovery of the cholera bacillus.

As a youngster, Koch was active and keenly interested in nature. His family, although poor, mustered sufficient funds to send him through medical school. He practiced medicine in Berlin, Hamburg, and several small villages. Koch's extensive research was done in his own humble laboratories until 1880, when he received an appointment in the Imperial Health Office in recognition of his studies with anthrax. Later at the University Institute Pfeiffer, Behring, Ehrlich, and other noted immunologists were his students. In 1891 Koch became the first director of the research Institute for Infectious Diseases. In 1905 he was awarded the Nobel Prize in Physiology and Medicine for his research in tuberculosis (Fig. 1-11).

The next important mark in the history of immunobiology is the description of anaphylaxis by the French scientists Portier and Richet (1850-1935) in 1902. In 1913 Richet received the Nobel Prize for these studies. This work began on the French Mediterranean, where the sea anemone and the Portuguese man-of-war populations were dense. Both of these have fairly potent toxins. While trying to immunize dogs against the sea anemone toxin, Portier and Richet found that small sublethal quantities injected into a previously immunized dog could throw the dog into extensive convulsions and collapse, terminating in death. They suggested the term *anaphylaxis* (without or against protection). This was the first unequivocal demonstration that antibodies could be detrimental to one's health. This evidence had a tremendous impact on the practice of medicine; this was the era of antiserum therapy, and injections of antiserum were particularly likely to initiate anaphylaxis. The replacement of antiserum therapy with antibiotic therapy has not alleviated the dangers of anaphylaxis, which is all too often the result of antibiotic treatment.

At the beginning of the twentieth century several persons, including Ehrlich and Otto in Germany and Smith in the United States, were studying serum sickness, a kind of protracted anaphylaxis resulting from injections of large quantities of antitoxin. Serum sickness was a more gentle form of anaphylaxis than that described by Richet; although seldom fatal, it was quite common. Schick and von Pirquet subsequently summarized much of the available information on serum sickness, which they published in the form of a monograph in 1905. Because of this, they are generally, although erroneously, cited as the discoverers of serum sickness; the discovery probably should be credited to Smith. Even so, von Pirquet formulated many novel ideas about allergy, many of which are still valid today.

The Prausnitz-Küstner test is not widely used today, but few would dispute the importance of this test or the importance of the contributions that Prausnitz and Küstner made to the study of allergy. In 1921 they published their data on reagin, a serum antibody–like substance apparently associated with food allergies, hay fever, asthma, hives, and other allergic conditions. Until the 1960s nearly all the information we had about reagin came from the work of Prausnitz and Küstner and from experimentation with the Prausnitz-Küstner test. The chemical nature of reagin is now accepted as being identical to IgE.

Landsteiner was awarded the Nobel Prize in 1930 for his description in 1901 of the major human blood groups, the ABO system. Practically every student of biology is cognizant of the pivotal role this theory had in clarifying the problems in blood transfusion reactions and in solving them by the proper matching of blood. Eventually the solution to many tissue transplantation problems may be based on antigenic typing of cells. If this proves to be so, again we will be indebted to Landsteiner. After all, blood transfusions are a special form of transplantation.

Landsteiner teamed with Wiener in 1940 for another important contribution to immunohematology, the discovery of the Rh antigen system common to humans and to the rhesus monkey (for which the antigen was named). This discovery, amplified by Wiener, Levine, and others, provided the basis for a scientific understanding of certain transfusion reactions and erythroblastosis fetalis.

Beyond his contributions to blood group immunology and to the nature of antigenic determinants, Landsteiner also made with Merrill Chase in 1942 the discovery that a class of allergies known as the delayed hypersensitivities could be transferred from the allergic animal to a normal recipient with lymph node cells (lymphocytes). This was the initial step in unraveling the cellular and molecular basis of important phenomena such as contact dermatitis and certain other drug allergies, the tuberculin reaction and certain other allergies of infection, some aspects of transplantation immunology, and, of course, much of the cellular basis of other immunologic conditions.

Much of the original work on organ-specific antigens was initiated by Witebsky and his students, although the discovery of tissue-specific antigens dates back to Uhlenhuth's work in 1903. A fuller comprehension of these antigens is necessary before tissue transplantations can be successful on a routine basis. These histocompatibility antigens are under intensive study at the present time. Closely associated with this is the role of tissue antigens in autoimmune diseases. Witebsky established four criteria for proof of an autoimmune disease: (1) the autoimmune response must be regularly associated with the disease; (2) a replica of the disease must be inducible in laboratory animals; (3) pathologic changes in the human and experimental condition should parallel each other; and (4) transfer of the autoimmune illness should result from the transfer of serum or lymphoid cells from the diseased individual to a normal recipient. In 1956 examination of Hashimoto's thyroiditis in humans and rabbits by Witebsky confirmed that it was an autoimmune disease; this opened a new era of medicine.

The development of the modern theories of antibody formation is largely the result of the hypotheses and scientific investigations of Haurowitz and Burnet (Fig. 1-12). In 1930 Haurowitz formulated the template theory of antibody formation, which suggested that antigen was retained by the antibody-forming cells and served as a template or mold about which antibody was synthe-

sized. In this way antibody and antigen (the lock and key described by Ehrlich) have a physical compatibility that permits their later specific combination in serologic reactions. The template theory is an example of an instructive mechanism for antibody synthesis. Burnet's ideas about antibody formation evolved gradually, until in 1959 he conceived of the clonal selection theory, the essence of which is that cells are already endowed with the genetic ability to make a certain antibody, and the antigen, through combination with its specific cell, causes that cell to proliferate and hence result in observable antibody formation. The two theories have obvious irreconcilable differences, but this does not detract from their usefulness in stimulating immunologic opinion and experimentation.

An attractive portion of the clonal selection the-

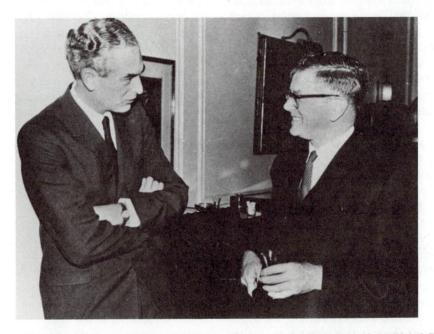

Fig. 1-12. Peter Medawar *(left)* and Macfarlane Burnet. This photograph of the Nobel Prize winners in Physiology and Medicine was taken about the time of their award in 1960 for developing the concept of immunologic tolerance. (From Burnet, F.M.: Changing patterns, St. Kilda, Australia, 1969, William Heinemann, Ltd.)

ory is its application to specific immunologic tolerance, the failure to make antibody to a normally antigenic material because of a previous exposure to the antigen. Burnet suggested that self-recognition occurs in neonatal life by contact of antibody-forming cells with new antigens as the fetus first forms them. The result in utero is a functional shutdown of such a cell, so that one does not make antibodies to his own antigens. Medawar tested this with neonatal exposure to non-self-antigens and measured the results the theory predicted, that is, that the animal, when grown to adulthood, will not respond to the antigen. For their contributions to immunology Burnet and Medawar shared the 1960 Nobel Prize (Fig. 1-12).

The 1980 Nobel Prize in Physiology and Medicine was shared by three scientists for their collective yet separate studies of immunogenetics and histocompatibility. George Snell, a geneticist, joined the staff at the Bar Harbor Laboratories in Maine in 1935 and devoted his life to the development of congenic mouse strains, that is, mice that differ at only a single gene locus (Fig. 1-13). From this effort, and in conjunction with Peter Gorer, he determined that genes controlled the synthesis of antigen II (later named H-2 for histocompatibility) and the success or failure of grafts between mice that were otherwise identical. Hence a genetic basis for the study of transplantation immunology and histocompatibility in experimental animal species was created.

Meanwhile Jean Dausset found that human patients who had received multiple blood transfusions usually produced antibodies to white blood cells of the donor. These antibodies reacted with antigens on the surface of the donor's leukocytes (human leukocyte antigens, or HLA) or with the same antigen on the leukocytes of other persons. The generation of an immune response to HLA soon was related to graft failure, parallel to the studies found with the H-2 system in mice.

Benacerraf began his progress toward the Nobel Prize by studying synthetic polypeptides as simplified models of more complex antigens. When he found that some guinea pigs made antibodies to a specific synthetic antigen but others failed to respond to the antigen, he theorized the presence of immune response genes in the responders that were not present in the nonresponders. Further studies localized the immune response gene on the same chromosome that controlled the synthesis of the histocompatibility antigens. McDevitt also had shown that this condition existed in mice. Thus the genes that regulate the synthesis of the transplantation antigens accompany the genes that regulate the immune response.

In the mid 1970s research conducted primarily at Cambridge University in England by Milstein and Köhler led to the description of immunoglobulin-synthesizing hybridomas. A myeloma cell—a neoplastic cell that normally secretes antibody and grows well in culture—is fused with a second cell to form the hybrid. In the experiment as it is now conducted, a nonsecreting myeloma cell is used as one parent. The second cell is a lymph node or spleen cell from an animal recently immunized with some antigen of special interest. The two cells are incubated together under conditions that allow their cell membranes to fuse, producing a binuclear hybrid. The hybrid usually discards some chromosomes after the fusion. The hybrid cells then are placed in a medium that contains compounds which prevent the growth of the parent myeloma cell. The cells that grow have retained the growth characteristics of the spleen cell. The growing cells are screened to determine if they have retained the spleen cell gene for antibody formation, that is, they are examined for their ability to synthesize antibody. Clones of active cells are then perpetuated in culture. Such cells will produce a monomolecular antibody that is specific for a single site of the antigen. Such monoclonal antibodies have application in studies of immunoglobulin chemistry and synthesis, antigen analysis, immunoassay, immunogenetics, and other areas. These antibody-producing hybridomas are one of the most exciting of the recent developments in immunology.

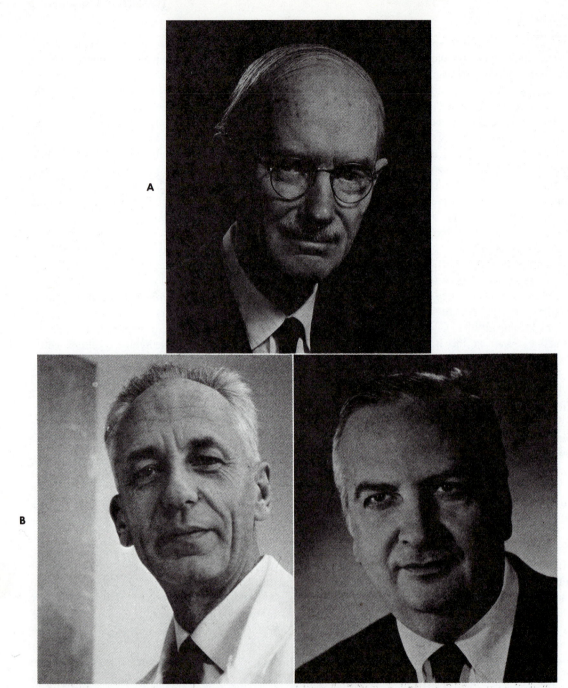

Fig. 1-13. The most recent immunologists to receive the Nobel Prize in Physiology and Medicine are George Snell (**A**), Jean Dausset (**B**), and Baruj Benacerraf (**C**). Separately these three conducted research on the transplantation antigens and the ability of an animal to develop an immune response. These characteristics were determined to be regulated by structural genes on the same chromosome.

BIBLIOGRAPHY

Baxby, D.: Jenner's smallpox vaccine, Exeter, N.H., 1981, Heinemann Educational Books, Inc.

Benacerraf, B.: Role of MHC gene products in immune regulation, Science **212:**1229, 1981.

Brock, T.: Milestones in microbiology, Englewood Cliffs, N.J., 1961, Prentice-Hall, Inc.

Bulloch, W.: The history of bacteriology, London, 1938, Oxford University Press.

Burnet, F.M.: Changing patterns, New York, 1969, American Elsevier Publishers, Inc.

Cope, Z.: Almroth Wright, founder of modern vaccine therapy, London, 1966, Thomas Nelson & Sons, Ltd.

Dausset, J.: The major histocompatibility complex in man, Science **213:**1469, 1981.

Dixon, C.W.: Smallpox, London, 1962, J. & A. Churchill, Ltd.

Dubos, R.J.: Louis Pasteur, free lance of science, Boston, 1950, Little, Brown & Co.

Edelman, G.M.: Antibody structure and molecular immunology, Science **180:**830, 1973.

Lechevalier, H.A., and Solotorovsky, M.: Three centuries of microbiology, New York, 1965, McGraw-Hill Book Co.

Marquardt, M.: Paul Ehrlich, London, 1949, William Heinemann, Ltd.

Parish, H.J.: A history of immunization, Edinburgh, 1965, E. & S. Livingstone, Ltd.

Parish, H.J.: Victory with vaccines, Edinburgh, 1968, E. & S. Livingstone, Ltd.

Porter, R.R.: Structural studies of immunoglobulins, Science **180:**713, 1973.

Rains, A.J.H.: Edward Jenner and vaccination, London, 1974, Priory Press, Ltd.

Snell, G.D.: Studies in histocompatibility, Science **213:**172, 1981.

Sourkes, T.L.: Nobel Prize winners in medicine and physiology 1901-1965, New York, 1966, Abelard Schuman, Ltd.

Wagner, R.: Clemens von Pirquet, his life and work, Baltimore, 1963, Johns Hopkins University Press.

Yalow, R.S.: Radioimmunoassay: a probe for the fine structure of biologic systems, Science **200:**1236, 1978.

2

A PREAMBLE TO IMMUNOLOGY

Any encounter with a new subject of study is aggravated by a need to acquire a totally new vocabulary and to become acquainted with the breadth of the subject. Because of this, students are uncertain and hesitant, not only about the range and intensity of their future course of study but also about their qualifications. Therefore this chapter is included to present a broad overview of immunology and to introduce the terminology needed for its study. In this way the new subject can be given a first-level evaluation as a topic worthy of scholarly pursuit for its own sake, and the contribution of the subject to neighboring disciplines can be estimated. This preamble is only a brief scan of the field of immunology; detailed information is presented in the other chapters.

IMMUNOCYTOLOGY

The primary focus of study in immunology is the adaptive response of cells of the *hematopoietic system* to macromolecules. Although there are many important variations to this, immunology is basically a study of cells and molecules. The macromolecules that activate the *lymphoid cells* of the body are known as antigens. *Antigens* may be either protein or polysaccharide in nature; they may exist as conjugates of each other (glycoproteins) or with other substances (lipopolysaccharides or lipoproteins). Any substance composed of these molecules, such as bacteria, viruses, erythrocytes, and tissue cells, also is described

as an antigen. Existing antigens may be chemically modified by the attachment to them of low molecular weight nonantigenic compounds to create *conjugated antigens or neoantigens*. If the lymphoid cells of the body that become exposed to the neoantigen react to its low molecular weight portion, that portion can be described as a *hapten*. By this mechanism the animal body is enabled to respond to foreign substances of both large and small size.

The adaptive response of the body to antigens or *hapten-antigen conjugates* is termed the *immune response* even though the antigen may have no relationship to immunity or disease. In the same sense exposure of an animal to an antigen is known as an immunization. Because of the historical use of these terms, antigens sometimes are described as *immunogens* (to generate an immune response). Relatively impotent antigens may invoke only a feeble immune response unless the animal is stimulated with *adjuvants* or is given booster doses of the antigen.

Three principal cell types respond to antigens: the *macrophages,* the *B lymphocytes,* and the *T lymphocytes*. The *tissue macrophages* are derived from the *monocytes* that are present in blood. Among the important functions of the macrophages is *phagocytosis*, the ability to engulf other cells. Macrophages also can imbibe soluble substances, and these, like the particulate substances, are degraded within the phagocyte by a battery of hydrolytic enzymes present in the *lysosomes*. By mechanisms that remain totally unknown, the macrophages spare critical portions of the antigens known as the *antigenic determinant sites*.

Other phagocytic cells, particularly the *polymorphonuclear neutrophil,* may engulf and degrade antigens, but the total contribution of these cells to the antigen-processing function is minimal. Other granulocytes such as the *eosinophil* and *basophil* are probably noncontributory to antigen processing, although both cells are important in other aspects of the immune response.

All the cells that are critical to the immune response are a part of the hematopoietic system, since they arise from stem cells of the bone marrow. The monocytes and macrophages comprise the *mononuclear phagocytic system,* which is but one line of development from this primitive cell. The neutrophils, basophils, and eosinophils represent a second line of development: the myeloid, or granulocytic, series. *Lymphocytes* represent the third, or lymphoid, series. The prelymphocytes leave the bone marrow and pass through the blood to the other parts of the *central lymphoid system*. In fowl this passage is to the *thymus* and the *bursa of Fabricius*. Mammals have no bursa but do have tissues that function the same as the bursa, which are referred to as the *bursal equivalent*. Understanding of the identity of these tissues is still incomplete. The thymus is a tissue in which one population of lymphocytes known as the *T lymphocytes* is imprinted with characteristics that distinguish them from the *B (bursal) lymphocytes*. Among the characteristics shared by T cells are the presence of unique surface proteins that are antigenic. In mice these are known as the Thy and Lyt markers. T cells also form rosettes spontaneously with sheep erythrocytes, respond to specific lectins such as concanavalin A with a cycle of growth and division, and have nonimmunoglobulin receptors on their surface for antigenic determinants. When antigens or lectins stimulate T cell growth, the T cells secrete low molecular weight proteins known as lymphokines. Among these *lymphokines* are *interferon, chemotaxin* for monocytes, a *macrophage migration inhibition factor,* a *blastogenic factor, lymphotoxins,* and others. All lymphokines are not produced by a single T cell; T cell subsets have separate functions. Lymphokines participate in *cell-mediated immunity,* expressed as resistance to viruses, fungi, tumor cells, and other foreign cells (graft rejection is mainly caused by T cells). T cells also contribute to *cell-mediated* or *delayed hypersensitivity* phenomena such as *contact dermatitis* (from cosmetics, poison ivy, etc.) and *allergies of infection*. The latter is exemplified by the tuberculin reaction.

Among the primary characteristics of B cells are the presence of Ia *(immune associated)* proteins on their cell surface and surface receptors for *immunoglobulins,* certain lectins (phytoagglutinins), and complement molecules. Antigen determinants that combine with their corresponding antibody on the B cell stimulate B cell proliferation and differentiation into *plasma cells* that actively secrete immunoglobulins (antibodies). Several B cell subsets are recognized, each forming a plasma cell specialized to synthesize only one molecular form (class, or *isotype*) of immunoglobulin (Ig). The five major immunoglobulin isotypes are designated as *IgG, IgM, IgA, IgD,* and *IgE*.

Interaction of macrophages, B cells, and *T cells* takes place in the *peripheral lymphoid organs* such as the lymph node, spleen, and tonsil. The first stage consists of antigen processing by macrophages and the transfer of antigen determinants to B and T cells. *Helper T cells* may assist B cells in producing antibodies to complex *(T cell–dependent)* antigens. *Suppressor T cells* regulate antibody formation so that it does not continue uncontrolled. B cells apparently make antibody to structurally simple *(T cell–independent)* antigens without the assistance of T cells.

Genes that influence helper, suppressor, and other T cell subsets are located on the chromosome that contains the structural genes for antigens found on all nucleated cells. Since these antigens stimulate the graft rejection response, they are known as the *transplantation* or *histocompat-*

ibility antigens, and their genes are named in the same way. Because helper, suppressor, and other genes are located near these histocompatibility genes, this area of the chromosome is referred to as the *major histocompatibility complex.*

Much of the *macrophage–B cell–T cell interaction* is assumed to occur in *germinal centers,* or growth centers of these cells, which develop in the peripheral lymphoid organs after antigenic stimulation. These clusters or clones of cells are the anatomic basis for the *clonal selection theory* of immune responsiveness, which suggests that lymphoid cells are prepatterned to respond to antigens, and this response causes their growth and division to form clones of cells that produce immunoglobulins or lymphokines. The alternative theory, the *instructive theory,* is that antigens instruct cells to make antibody only to the antigenic determinant that enters the cell.

IMMUNOLOGIC REAGENTS

The five immunoglobulin isotypes of the blood differ from each other in their physicochemical as well as their serologic activity. Special molecular varieties of two of these—IgA and IgM—are found in milk, saliva, nasal secretions, etc. and are known appropriately as *secretory IgA* and *secretory IgM.* Of these *γ-globulins,* the greatest attention is usually given to IgG, since it is present in a greater concentration in blood than the others and is known to have an important role in *immunity.* One of these roles is the *neutralization* of toxins, in which case the antibody is known as an antitoxin. IgG antibodies also can neutralize the infectivity of viruses and contribute to antibacterial immunity. IgM also is useful in improving phagocytosis, when its activity as an *opsonin* is important, or in consort with *complement* in *cytolytic functions.* The role of IgA in blood still is not totally defined. IgD seems to be an important antigen receptor on cells, and IgE is an important cause of allergic reactions.

The abundance of antibodies is increased beyond these basic five by the presence of *subclasses* or *allotypes* that vary from one another in their amino acid content or sequence in one of their peptide chains. This number is also enormously expanded by the realization that each antigenic determinant stimulates a separate cell of each isotype and allotype to produce a region in the molecule *(idiotype)* that will react only with that antigen.

These immunoglobulins may not be produced by persons with genetic defects in B cell or T cell development and who have *immunodeficiency diseases.* It is also possible to treat an animal with a chemical, biologic, or physical *immunosuppressant,* which will prevent or reduce the production of immunoglobulins. It is interesting that even small quantities of an antigen given at the proper time in the fetal development of an animal or in larger doses to adults may produce an *immune tolerance* (stimulate suppressor T cells). This is a condition in which the animal fails to respond to that antigen but responds typically to other antigens. Oncogenesis of plasma cells results in *immunoproliferative diseases* in which an excessive synthesis of one *(monoclonal)* or more *(polyclonal)* γ-globulins *(gammopathy)* occurs. These diseases are grouped as the *multiple myelomas.*

Several of these immunoglobulins may participate with antigen and several serum proteins that are part of the complement system to produce a variety of protective and inflammatory effects. This results from an activation of the complement molecules so that new activities are expressed. Among these are a *chemotactic* effect, *opsonic,* or phagocytosis-promoting, effect, *kinin* formation, an *inflammatory* or *anaphylatoxic* effect, and others, of which the best known is a cytolytic effect on certain cellular antigens. Complement activation may be initiated by the *classic pathway* (antibody method involving all nine components) or may progress through the *alternate,* or properdin, *pathway.* In this system a series of four proteins replaces the first three components of the classic complement system. The complement system normally is controlled by natural inactivators or inhibitors, but when these are genetically absent or inactive, immunodeficiencies of the complement system can be detected.

IMMUNOLOGIC REACTIONS

The union of an antigen with its antibody with or without the participation of complement or other accessory factors is the subject matter of serology. When the antigen is soluble, the reaction is described as a *precipitation* reaction. Serologic precipitates also can form when the reagents diffuse through gels and combine with each other. There are many variations to such *immunodiffusion* tests: *radial* (quantitative) *immunodiffusion,* double diffusion of the *Ouchterlony type, immunoelectrophoresis, crossed immunoelectrophoresis, counterimmunoelectrophoresis,* and others. When the antigen is cellular or particulate, the serologic reaction is an *agglutination* reaction or, as in the case of erythrocyte antigens, *hemagglutination.* Fluid antigens can be absorbed to cells to convert precipitation tests to *passive agglutination* tests. When complement is present, it is fixed in the serologic reaction *(complement fixation),* and this may be measured as a cytolytic reaction *(bacteriolysis* or *hemolysis).* When phagocytic cells are present, the serologic reaction may be seen to favor phagocytosis of the antigen. Occasionally no outward sign of an antigen- or hapten-antibody reaction is noted. This may demand the use of *fluorescent antibody* procedures, *radioimmunoassay, enzyme immunoassay,* or *antiglobulin* (double antibody) techniques.

The result of immunologic reactions in vivo that destroy or resist foreign cells or their products is usually classified as immunity. This explains the origin of the terms *transplantation immunity* and *tumor immunity,* that is, immunity to grafted cells and tumor cells. When the immune response is directed against self-antigens, an *autoimmune disease* is often the result. Self-proteins may become antigenic if they are modified to create antigenic determinant sites. When disease results from immune responses to external antigens, these diseases are usually labeled *allergies* or hypersensitivities. The *immediate* or *immunoglobulin-dependent allergies* rely on the attachment of *reagin (cytotropic IgE)* to the surface of *mast cells.* Combination of this IgE with antigen initiates *mast cell degranulation* with the liberation of *vasoactive amines* such as *histamine* and *serotonin.* The antigen-antibody reaction may trigger the *Hageman pathway* and the eventual release of *bradykinin* and other *kinins.* White blood cells also may release pharmacologically active substances. *Antihistamines* and *β-adrenergic drugs* such as epinephrine modify these toxic reactions. In their milder forms these reactions are associated with the *atopic illnesses,* hay fever or other *respiratory allergies,* and *food allergies.* In their more severe form these are seen as life-threatening *anaphylactic reactions.*

BIBLIOGRAPHY
Recent textbooks of immunology

Bach, J.F., editor: Immunology, ed. 2, New York, 1981, John Wiley & Sons, Inc.

Barrett, J.T.: Basic immunology and its medical application, ed. 2, St. Louis, 1980, The C.V. Mosby Co.

Bellanti, J.A.: Immunology II, Philadelphia, 1978, W.B. Saunders Co.

Bellanti, J.A.: Immunology, basic processes, Philadelphia, 1979, W.B. Saunders Co.

Benaceraff, B., and Unanue, E.R.: Textbook of immunology, Baltimore, 1979, Williams & Wilkins Co.

Bier, O.G., daSilva, W.D., Götze, D., and Mota, I.: Fundamentals of immunology, New York, 1981, Springer-Verlag New York, Inc.

Bigley, N.J.: Immunologic fundamentals, ed. 2, Chicago, 1981, Year Book Medical Publishers, Inc.

Carpenter, P.L.: Immunology and serology, ed. 3, Philadelphia, 1975, W.B. Saunders Co.

Clark, W.R.: The experimental foundations of modern immunology, New York, 1980, John Wiley & Sons, Inc.

Cunningham, A.J.: Understanding immunology, New York, 1978, Academic Press, Inc.

Fudenberg, H.H., Stites, D.P., Caldwell, H.L., and Wells, J.V.: Basic and clinical immunology, ed. 2, Los Altos, Calif., 1980, Lange Medical Publications.

Hood, L.E., Weissman, I.L., and Wood, W.B.: Immunology, Menlo Park, Calif., 1978, Benjamin/Cummings Publishing Co.

Kabat, E.A.: Structural concepts in immunology and immunochemistry, ed. 2, New York, 1976, Holt, Rinehart &
Winston, Inc.

McConnell, I., Munro, A., and Waldmann, H.: The immune
system: a course on the molecular and cellular basis of immunity, ed. 2, Oxford, 1981, Blackwell Scientific Publications, Ltd.

Nossal, G.: Antibodies and immunity, ed. 2, New York, 1978,
Basic Books, Inc., Publishers.

Roitt, I.M.: Essential immunology, ed. 4, Oxford, 1980,
Blackwell Scientific Publications, Ltd.

Rose, N.R., Milgrom, F., and van Oss, C.J., editors: Principles of immunology, ed. 2, New York, 1979, Macmillan,
Inc.

Schwartz, L.M.: Compendium of immunology, ed. 2, New
York, 1981, Van Nostrand Reinhold Co.

Sell, S.: Immunology, immunopathology and immunity, ed. 3,
New York, 1980, Harper & Row, Publishers, Inc.

Weissman, I.L., Hood, L.E., and Wood, W.B.: Essential
concepts in immunology, Menlo Park, Calif., 1978, Ben-
jamin/Cummings Publishing Co.

Journals in English devoted primarily to immunology

Acta Allergologica (Allergy)

Acta Pathologica et Microbiologica Scandinavica, Section C:
Immunology

Advances In Immunology

Annals of Allergy

Cancer Immunology and Immunotherapy

Cellular Immunology

Clinical and Experimental Immunology

Clinical Immunobiology

Clinical Immunology and Immunopathology

Contemporary Topics in Immunobiology

Contemporary Topics in Molecular Immunology

CRC Critical Reviews in Immunology

Current Topics in Microbiology and Immunology

Developments in Immunology

European Journal of Immunology

Human Immunology

Immunogenetics

Immunological Communications

Immunological Reviews

Immunology

Immunology Letters

Immunology Today

Immunopharmacology

Infection and Immunity

Inflammation

International Archives of Allergy and Applied Immunology

International Journal of Immunopharmacology

IRCS Medical Science: Immunology and Allergy

Journal of Allergy and Clinical Immunology

Journal of Clinical Immunology

Journal of Clinical and Laboratory Immunology

Journal of Immunogenetics

Journal of Immunological Methods

Journal of Immunology

Journal of Immunopharmacology

Journal of Reproductive Immunology

Journal of the Reticuloendothelial Society

Lymphokine Reports

Molecular Immunology

Monographs in Allergy

Progress in Allergy

Scandinavian Journal of Immunology

Springer Seminars in Immunopathology

Thymus

Tissue Antigens: Histocompatibility and Immunogenetics

Transplantation

Transplantation Proceedings

ANTIGENS, HAPTENS, AND THE MAJOR HISTOCOMPATIBILITY COMPLEX

GLOSSARY

active immunity Self-generated immunity

adoptive immunity Acquisition of immunity in the form of immunologically competent cells from an immune donor.

allele One of two genes at a common locus.

alloantibody An antibody that reacts with an antigen of the same species as the animal synthesizing it.

alloantigen An antigen present in another member of one's own species.

alloimmunization The immunization of an individual with antigens from within its own species.

antibody A globulin formed in response to exposure to an antigen; an immunoglobulin.

antigen A macromolecule that will induce the formation of immunoglobulins or sensitized cells that react specifically with the antigen.

antigen determinant sites Unique portions of the structure of the antigen that are responsible for its activity.

antiserum A serum containing antibodies.

autoantigen A molecule that behaves as a self-antigen.

autocoupling hapten One that can combine spontaneously with a carrier.

autoimmunization Immunization with self-antigens.

cross-reactive antigen An antigen so structurally similar to a second antigen that it will react with antibody to the second antigen.

epitope An antigenic determinant.

H-2 The major histocompatibility antigen system of mice.

hapten A nonantigenic material that, when combined with an antigen, conveys a new antigenic specificity on the antigen.

helper cell A subclass of T cells that assists B cells in antibody formation.

heteroimmunization Immunization of an individual with antigens from another species.

heterophil antigen One that is broadly distributed in nature.

HLA The major histocompatibility antigen system in humans (human leukocyte antigen).

Ia antigen An immune associated antigen.

immune associated antigen An antigen present on B lymphocytes and macrophages and inherited with Ir genes.

immune response gene A structural gene in the MHC that exerts a regulatory role on the immune response.

immunodominant region The most potent epitope in an antigen.

immunogen Antigen.

immunologic tolerance A failure or depression in the immune response on proper exposure to antigen, especially massive doses; probably synonymous with *immune paralysis*.

Ir gene An immune response gene.

isoantigen An antigen present in another member of one's own species.

isoimmunization Immunization of an individual with antigens of another individual of the same species.

LPS Lipopolysaccharide, the endotoxic portion of the cell wall of most gram-negative bacteria; mitogenic for B lymphocytes.

major histocompatibility complex A collection of structural genes associated with transplantation antigens and the immune response.

MHC Major histocompatibility complex.

passive immunization The acquisition of immunity through injection of antibodies or antiserum produced by another animal.

suppressor cell A subclass of T cells that suppresses the capacity of B cells to become immunoglobulin producers.

T cell–dependent antigen An antigen that requires T and B cell cooperation to induce specific antibody formation.

T cell–independent antigen An antigen which does not require that T cells assist B cells in the production of its specific antibody.

Th cell A helper T cell.

tolerance A failure to respond to an antigen.

tolerogen An immunogen used under circumstances that produce tolerance rather than immunity.

Ts cell A suppressor T cell.

xenoantigen An antigen present in another species.

xenoimmunization The immunization of an individual with antigens from another species; synonymous with heteroimmunization.

ANTIGEN-IMMUNOGEN

No one can define an antigen in exact terms. Rather, antigens are defined in terms of the antibodies they produce; unfortunately antibodies are defined in terms of the antigens that produce them. Still one can evolve a general understanding of what antigens are from an admittedly incomplete definition supplemented with descriptions of known antigens.

An antigen is traditionally defined as any substance that, when introduced parenterally into an animal, will cause the production of antibodies by that animal and will react specifically with those antibodies. Because it was feared that this definition emphasized the production of immunoglobulins (the B cell response), the term *immunogen* was introduced to include more definitely the response of T cells to antigens. This was probably unnecessary, since immunologists had long recognized that the response to antigens was divided into the humoral (immunoglobulin) and cell-mediated (T cell) response. In addition, the term *immunogen* seemed to signify that antigens were always related to immunity (immunogen meaning generating immunity in contrast to antigen, which means generating against). At present most authorities use *antigen* and *immunogen* as synonymous terms, but the latter is more common. This means that we now refer to the response to antigen as the immune response even though it only occasionally refers to immunity as such. Likewise, immunization refers to any productive exposure to an antigen, regardless of whether the antigen is related to disease.

As the term *immunogen* was being popularized, some immunologists began to refer to two classes of antigens: those which could stimulate the immune response (immunogens), and those which could react with immunoglobulins but not stimulate the immune response. The term *hapten* was created for the latter class of molecules nearly 60 years ago, and it seems unfortunate that its definition became confused by the introduction of immunogen. Haptens are discussed fully in a later section of this chapter.

The traditional definition of antigen or immunogen needs to be dissected so that we can see what is stated, what is implied, and what is omitted from the definition.

First, the word *parenteral* means "outside the digestive tract" and implies that materials given orally are not antigenic. This is not true. What is true is that digestive enzymes often hydrolyze and destroy the antigenic quality of many otherwise fully antigenic substances. When such an antigen is given parenterally, little can be destroyed before it is carried to the antigen-processing cells. Consequently more antibody results from the parenteral injection. The oral poliomyelitis vaccine is a notable exception. In this instance the virus, an active although attenuated strain, is taken orally, invades the cells lining the intestinal tract, and reproduces itself. Because of this reproduction, a larger antigenic dose is produced than in fact was administered. The natural result of this increased antigenic exposure is a heightened antibody response. These same conclusions would hold true for other antigenic materials that actually reproduce in the digestive tract. As a general rule, antigens are much more effective via parenteral routes such as intradermal, subcutaneous, intravenous, intramuscular, or intraperitoneal injection, but parenteral also may refer to inhalation.

Second, even when the immunogen is administered parenterally, it must be given in a correct dose to stimulate the immune response. Obviously too scant an amount will be insufficient, but, surprisingly, too large an amount also may be improper. Young animals in particular but also adult animals can have their immune response to an antigen temporarily suppressed by exposure to large quantities of antigen. This supression (tolerance) is antigen specific and does not encompass other antigens. When immune tolerance is the result of a large inoculum of antigen, the antigen may be referred to as a tolerogen.

Third, the definition of an antigen involves animals; plants do not make antibodies. Furthermore only certain types of animals produce true immunoglobulins. Although some invertebrates exhibit resistance to certain pathogens or their toxins, it is not at all certain that they do this through adaptive antibody formation. Consequently a vertebrate animal must be chosen for immunologic studies.

A last and extremely important part of the definition of an antigen is the specific reaction that occurs between the antigen and the antibodies it caused to be produced. Those antibodies do not react with other antigens except within very finite limits. This is a fact which is known to us from our everyday experience; after all, we are immunized with poliomyelitis vaccine to prevent polio, not to prevent diphtheria or tetanus. This specificity of serologic reactions is an overwhelmingly simple concept and is of underlying importance, if not the whole key, to serology. The actual extent of this specificity is discussed later in this chapter.

Several factors are omitted from the definition and should be mentioned. The initiation of antibody formation by antigens is not the only change produced in the animal by the introduction of an antigen. One usually can detect concomitant increases in immediate and delayed hypersensitivities. Aside from this, many antigens of an infectious or toxic kind provoke their special reaction to this additional biologic activity which they possess. If the antigen is administered with an adjuvant, which is often the case, side effects from the adjuvant often are detectable.

All vertebrates are not equally responsive to antigens. The mammals, birds, amphibia, and fishes all have a complex yet similar immune response involving both humoral and cell-mediated responses. The elasmobranchs (for example, sharks and sting rays) have a slightly more primitive response and do not produce as many molecular forms of the immunoglobulins as do the higher life forms. The cyclostomes are the lowest vertebrates that express an immune response. Animals phylogenetically lower than cyclostomes do not respond to antigens and lack B and T lymphocytes or their functional equivalents.

This leads to a second definition of an antigen as a substance that catalyzes B lymphocytes and T lymphocytes into specific adaptive responses. For B lymphocytes this is a transformation into plasma cells that synthesize and excrete immunoglobulins. For T lymphocytes this is the elaboration, also after cell growth and division, of lymphokines. Antigens also may alter the behavior of phagocytic cells directly during phagocytosis or indirectly in response to lymphokines.

HOST CONTROL OF IMMUNOGENICITY
Immune response genes

Even if the animal species chosen for active immunization is one that normally has a good antibody-forming capacity to the antigen used, it is possible that the individual selected will not respond or will respond poorly to the antigen. All the reasons that some animals are refractory to antigenic stimulation may yet be unknown, but the discovery of specific immune response (Ir) genes in inbred lines of laboratory animals indicates, as seen in the phylogenetic tree, that a specific inheritance is essential before an animal can respond to an antigen.

When injected with a complex antigen that contains many antigenic determinant sites, nearly all animals will respond with antibody formation. This occurs because some animals respond to one or more portions of the molecule, whereas other animals respond to the same or other portions. Thus both animals are labeled as responders, although potentially reacting to completely different portions of the antigen. A different situation exists if feeble antigens are given, a feeble antigen being defined as one with a limited number of antigenic sites. In this case the responding animals are more likely to respond to the same regions of the antigen. Since the capacity to respond to a given antigenic determinant is under genetic control, it can be claimed that the responders share a certain Ir gene. Any animal failing to respond lacks the necessary Ir gene.

The first antigens used in studies of Ir genes consisted of a linear polylysine chain to which side chains of polyalanine were attached. At the ends of the alanine side chains specific amino acids were added to fulfill the structure of the molecule. When histidine and glutamic acid were the terminal

amino acids, the abbreviation (H,G) A-L was used to distinguish the molecule from (T,G) A-L or (P,G) A-L when tyrosine and glutamic acid or when phenylalanine and glutamic acid were the terminal amino acids. The initial experiments revealed that CBA mice were good responders to (H,G) A-L but not to (T,G) A-L, whereas C57BL mice showed just the opposite response. This response gene was termed the *Ir-1 gene*. Other mouse Ir genes that have been studied include Ir-2, which regulates the response to Ea-1, an erythrocyte-borne antigen; Ir-3, which controls the response to (P,G) Pro-L (phenylalanine–glutamic acid–proline-lysine polymer); Ir-4, which affects the response to bacterial lipopolysaccharide (LPS), and Ir-5, which controls the response to Thy 1.1 antigen, an antigen on mouse thymocytes earlier known as the θ, or T, antigen.

The use of weak allogeneic antigens is a second approach that has uncovered Ir genes. A third approach to the identification of Ir genes is the use of standard antigens applied only in minimal doses so that only vigorous responders can be identified.

Currently Ir genes have been identified in mice, guinea pigs, rats, monkeys, and humans, and there is little reason to doubt that all immunocompetent species possess these genes. Most experimental studies have been conducted in mice, since they reproduce rapidly and because of the abundance of additional genetic information on this species. From these studies several interesting facts have been identified.

The first of these is that the Ir genes are transmitted as a single dominant gene. In guinea pigs this was demonstrated in the strain 2 high-responder matings with strain 13 low responders to a synthetic polymer of glutamic acid and alanine. All the first generation progeny (2×13 F_1) were high responders, but their mating with strain 13 yielded progeny that were equally divided between high and low responders. F_1 mating with strain 2 produced 100% high responders.

The identical genetic relationship has been recognized in mice. The CBA mouse is a low responder to a tripolymer of glutamic acid–lysine-alanine, which is highly immunogenic for the C57BL mouse strain. Breeding of these two strains produced mice which are all high responders. Back crosses of the F_1 generation mice with low-responder parents produced offspring of which half were high and half were low responders. This indicated that a single dominant gene was the basis of the response.

Mapping of the Ir gene location became possible in the mouse for which many inbred strains were available. These strains were the stock strains originally used by Snell and his associates to study tissue compatibility between strains. The survival of grafts between strains was attributed to their sharing of common transplantation antigens on their cells. The structural genes for these antigens were located on the mouse chromosome 17. Originally this was termed the H-2 gene for antigen II, the first gene associated with histocompatibility. Now it is known that mice have three major genes, the H-2K, H-2D, and H-2L genes, which regulate graft acceptance or rejection. Minor genes also contribute to transplantation success. The region around the H-2K, H-2D, and H-2L genes is known as the major histocompatibility complex (MHC). By virtue of the studies pioneered by Snell it was recognized that these genes were highly polymorphic, that is, that many alleles exist at each locus and thus these genes code for many different histocompatibility antigens. These are the Class I products of the MHC. Further details of this are described in the chapter on transplantation immunity, but the MHC is important here because the Ir genes were found to map within it. Within the Ir region subregions became identifiable when it was shown that the transmission of immunoresponsiveness to two separate antigens was controlled by separate loci. The exact nomenclature and spatial assignments of these loci may be altered as new information becomes available. At this writing, the regions A, E, and J are accepted. The A and E genes are the most important in controlling the immune response from

the positive, or helper, side and the J gene from the suppressor side. The K, D, and L genes contribute primarily to histocompatibility and graft rejection with a much weaker contribution to immune responsiveness.

T cells and macrophages

With this information at hand a question that can be asked is, "At what level of the immune response system do these genes function?" Of course their function ultimately is expressed as immunoglobulin formation, but do the Ir genes act directly on B cells? The answer to this is no. Only T cell–dependent antigens are under Ir cell control. T cell–independent antigens fall under Ir gene control only when they are conjugated to a T cell–dependent carrier antigen. Thymectomy of high-responder animals prior to immunization with a T cell–dependent antigen converts them to low responders. These experiments indicated the T cells helped the B cells. These T cells are known as helper, or Th, cells.

Further experiments indicated macrophages as an additional source of Ir gene control. For example, mice that respond to glutamic acid–alanine-tyrosine (GAT) polymers produce a typical primary antibody response when first immunized with this polymer. When B cells of these mice are properly reexposed to GAT, they will produce a secondary or booster response. They also will exhibit the secondary response when they are exposed to macrophages from high-responder mice if the macrophages previously were exposed to GAT. No secondary response resulted if macrophages from nonresponders were used even though these macrophages also had been previously exposed to GAT. Thus the macrophage is a second regulator of the immune response. In a somewhat similar experiment T lymphocytes from responder guinea pigs previously exposed to a synthetic antigen (glutamic acid–lysine-phenylalanine [GLP]) proliferated only if cocultivated with GLP-treated macrophages from high-responder guinea pigs. Macrophages from low responders were not stimulatory. These experiments conclusively demonstrate that Ir genes do not stimulate antibody formation by a direct action on B cells but do so indirectly through T lymphocytes and macrophages.

It was discovered later that T cells and macrophages interacted with B cells at the level of antigen presentation. If the Ir gene codes for a distinct surface protein in the same way that the H-2K, H-2D, and H-2L genes code for specific transplantation antigens, then this protein would be present on cells of high-responder animals but not on cells of low responders. Consequently alloimmunization could identify this protein if it existed as an antigenic macromolecule, that is, low responders should make antibody to the factor present on cells of the high responders because it would be foreign to them (the low nonresponders). These experiments led to the identification of immune associated (Ia) proteins or antigens. These are known as the Class II products of the MHC.

The Ia proteins

Animals that are high responders do have antigenic proteins—the Ia markers on their macrophages—and these are absent from cells of low responders. This same Ia antigen has been identified on the B cell, which the macrophage will help. The T cell does not possess the Ia marker but has receptors for it on its surface. Both the B cell and macrophage have immunoglobulin on their surfaces, which serves as a receptor for antigenic determinants. The macrophage ingests the antigen, processes it, and spares the antigenic determinants. These determinants are held by immunoglobulin receptors on the macrophage surface and passed to immunoglobulin receptors for the antigen on the B cell surface. Meanwhile the T cell is bridging the B cell and macrophage via its Ia receptors and their surface Ia proteins. From this cell interaction and by mechanisms not yet elucidated the immune response is stimulated.

The chemistry of the Ia proteins, which are products of the I-A and I-E genes, has been partial-

ly elucidated. Both genes clearly are associated with helper functions, since antisera to their gene products will react with the cells bearing them and suppress their helper activity. Products of the J gene have not yet been identified, but these are associated with down regulation of the immune response, or suppressor activity. This suppressor activity, like helper activity, is exerted through T cells (Ts). The I-A region codes for two polypeptides designated as Aα and Aβ, and the I-E region likewise codes for a pair of polypeptides, Eα and Eβ. The α-peptides have molecular weights of about 32,000 and the β-peptides near 28,000 (Fig. 3-1). The peptides of the I-A region coassociate through noncovalent bonding to form the protein product of that gene AαAβ, and the I-E region peptides coassociate in the same way to form EαEβ. There appear to be many allelic forms of the β-chains and fewer of the α-chains. This suggests that differences in the structure of the β-chains are associated with the antigen specificity of the immune response. When the macrophage and B cell have identical Ia proteins, the Th cell with receptors for that Ia protein helps the antibody response. It is assumed that the Ts cell will interact with I-J region products to downgrade the immune response. This is basis for the regulatory role of the MHC on the immune response.

The MHC and disease

Since the regulatory role of MHC genes on the immune response is so powerful, it was only natural to seek a relationship of the MHC with certain diseases. In the mouse such studies were quickly successful and identified an H-2 association with sensitivity to mouse leukemia. In humans the MHC genes regulating tissue transplantation success are the HLA genes, and these likewise are coinherited with an increased risk for certain diseases, particularly certain autoimmune diseases.

An interesting example of this is seen in the case of ankylosing spondylitis. This disease may be considered a variant of rheumatoid arthritis which is exceptionally difficult to diagnose. An-

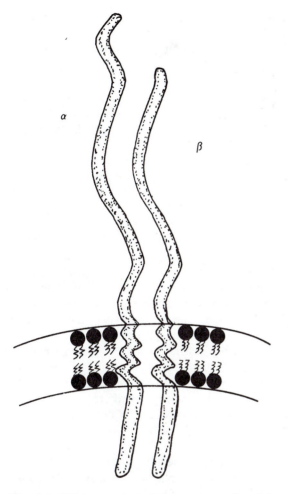

Fig. 3-1. This conception of the structure of an I-A protein could as easily represent the structure of an I-E or I-J protein. Notice that both the α-chain (32,000 mol wt) and β-chain (28,000 mol wt) are embedded in the lipid bilayer of the cell membrane by hydrophobic regions and are rooted in the cytoplasm. The two peptides are associated by noncovalent forces.

kylosing spondylitis is classified, like rheumatoid arthritis, as an autoimmune disease, a disease exhibiting several unusual immune phenomena. HLA-B27 antigen is so regularly associated with spondylitis that the identification of HLA-B27 antigen on cells of the individual is taken as a major criterion for the diagnosis of ankylosing spondylitis. Other details of the MHC-disease relationship are described in Chapters 11 and 21.

CHARACTERISTICS OF IMMUNOGENS

The definitions of immunogen previously presented explain what immunogens do but not what they are. In physicochemical terms immunogens are macromolecules that possess a high degree of internal chemical complexity. They are also soluble or easily solubilized by phagocytic cells of the immunized animal and are foreign to that animal.

Macromolecule

Macromolecule in terms of immunogenicity means the molecule should have a molecular weight of 10,000 or more. Proteins like insulin (5,700 mol wt), protamines and histones (6,000 mol wt), and low molecular weight fractions of gelatin (10,000 mol wt) are all poor antigens. Polysaccharides of this size are often nonantigenic; heparin (17,000 mol wt), for example, is not immunogenic. In general, polysaccharides are poorer antigens than proteins of the same size. This is because they usually are composed of only four or five monosaccharide units, whereas proteins normally contain 18 to 20 different amino acids.

Large proteins and polysaccharides of natural origin are excellent antigens. Ribonuclease (14,000 mol wt), tobacco mosaic virus protein (17,500 mol wt), egg albumin (40,000 mol wt), tetanus toxin or toxoid (66,000 mol wt), thyroglobulin (669,000 mol wt), and hemocyanin (6,000,000 mol wt) are examples of good protein antigens. Dextrans, ranging from 50,000 to 100,000 mol wt, are antigenic but not for all species. Mice and humans respond well to polysaccharide antigens, but guinea pigs are less responsive.

The greater the molecular weight of a substance, the more likely it is to function as an antigen. The reason for this is that the entire molecule does not function as an immunoglobulin- or lymphokine-inducing structure. Instead within each molecule there are specific regions of limited size that function as the antigenic determinant sites, also known as epitopes (see section on haptens and antigenic determinant sites). The larger a molecule is, the greater the number of these sites, and thus the greater the variety and quantity of antibody that will be formed.

Molecular complexity

Large molecular size alone is not enough to confer antigenicity on a substance. Organic chemists can produce synthetic polymers of virtually any size, such as polystyrene, nylon, Teflon, Saran, polyacrylamide, and homopolymers of amino acids, all of which are nonantigenic. Various reasons for this may be cited, but one explanation is that these polymers lack internal molecular complexity. The primary structure of these macromolecules is relatively simple: one or two different monomers are covalently linked into a repetitive structure, which ultimately reaches great size. Most naturally occurring macromolecules are often very complex because they are built from many different low molecular weight constituents; for example, proteins often are composed of 18 to 20 different amino acids. Variations in amino acid sequence allow a significant internal complexity to be developed in these molecules. Even polysaccharides, which are composed of fewer structurally similar units, are complex compared with the synthetic plastics.

From these descriptions of antigens it should be clear that proteins are usually antigenic, within the limits prescribed. Proteins are usually large, are often composed of 20 or more different amino acids, are soluble in body fluids or are easily degraded by proteolytic enzymes to that condition, and can be chosen to meet the restriction of foreignness. Oligosaccharides are frequently but not always antigenic; they ordinarily meet all the criteria except internal complexity. Polysaccharides, through their extensive side branching via glycosidic bonds, do exhibit a secondary and tertiary structural complexity equal to or even greater than that of proteins. Were it not for this,

polysaccharides might not be as good antigens as they are.

Despite much literature to the contrary, other biologic polymers in a pure chemical form are not antigenic. Ribonucleic and deoxyribonucleic acids (RNA and DNA) are haptenic, not antigenic. The same is true of lipids. Complexes of lipids or nucleic acids with proteins, or in some cases with polysaccharides, are excellent antigens. In these complexes the nucleic acids or lipids serve as haptens against which antibodies can be formed, provided the hapten is part of a complete antigen.

The composition and sequence of the building units is referred to as the primary (I^0) structure of the macromolecule. Secondary, tertiary, and quaternary structure also can influence antigenicity. In the case of proteins, II^0 structure refers to the α-helix formed by the coiled peptide chain; III^0 structure refers to the folding and bending of the α-helix to form spherical, ellipsoidal, or globular-shaped structures; and IV^0 structure refers to the contribution of multipeptide chains to the molecule. Examples of how these features modify or create antigenicity are described for several antigens in a later section of this chapter.

Solubility

Another argument used to explain the nonantigenicity of synthetic polymers is their insolubility in body fluids and their inability to be converted to soluble forms by tissue enzymes. Complex copolymers of the unnatural D-amino acids are poorly degraded, which may account for their low antigenicity. The relatively greater immunogenicity of pneumococcal polysaccharides for mice than for rabbits has been related to the greater hydrolytic activity of mouse liver enzymes for these polysaccharides. Practically all cellular antigens, bacteria, viruses, and red blood cells are quickly engulfed by phagocytic macrophages and digested to their soluble constituents. This participation of phagocytic cells is more than casual; if poor antigens are insolubilized or aggregated to ensure rapid engulfment, they become more potent antigens.

Foreignness

To be antigenic, the macromolecule must come from a foreign source, either an entirely different species or an animal of the same species antigenically different from the animal being immunized. The more distant or foreign the antigen source, the better it will be. Duck serum proteins are not good antigens for chickens, but antigens from plant sources are. Plant proteins are usually good antigens in any animal. This concept of foreignness was recognized by Ehrlich and was stated by him as the principle of horror autotoxicus (literally, a fear of self-poisoning); he used this theory to accommodate the observation that molecules which fulfill the characteristics of an antigen already listed but that are a normal part of an animal's circulation are not antigenic for that particular animal. Otherwise we would make antibodies against our own erythrocytes, serum proteins, etc. This would result in a condition incompatible with life, since the ensuing in vivo antigen-antibody reaction would destroy those erythrocytes or other antigens. The body has a built-in protective system that minimizes autoantibody development against normal circulatory antigens.

This is not to say that autoantibodies cannot be formed. They do exist, and their existence is not necessarily in conflict with the concept of horror autotoxicus. There are several mechanisms whereby an individual might produce autoantibodies. Antibodies of course could be formed against normally noncirculating antigens, for example, milk casein of the female, sperm of the male, or lens proteins of the eye. Second, antibodies might be developed against an altered circulating antigen, which would react with the normal form of the antigen. Such cross-reactive antibodies are well known and are purposely developed; antibodies to toxoids react with toxins, and these two are not chemically identical. Toxoids are used in immunization to prevent diseases such as diphtheria and tetanus because the toxins themselves are too dangerous to use in the immunization. In addition, an antibody could be formed against a foreign antigen with a chemical similarity to an autoantigen. These and other mechanisms for the formation of autoantibodies are discussed in more detail in Chapter 21.

ANTIGEN NOMENCLATURE

Some terms used by immunologists may be confusing. These include *autologous antigen, heterologous antigen, homologous antigen,* and *heterophil antigen.* An autologous antigen is one's own antigen, which under appropriate circumstances would induce autoantibody formation; autologous antigen is thus synonymous with autoantigen. A heterologous antigen is merely a different antigen from that which was used in the immunization; it may or may not react with the antiserum used, depending on its chemical similarity to the immunizing or homologous antigen. The homologous antigen is simply that antigen used in the production of antiserum. In serologic tests a heterologous antigen may be used as a negative control for any nonspecific reaction arising from errors in performing the serologic test or in the preparation of the serologic reactants.

Heterophil (heterogenetic) antigens are those antigens which exist in unrelated plants or animals but which are either identical or so closely related that antibodies to one will cross-react with antibodies to the other. In many instances heterophil antigens are polysaccharides, which by virtue of their limited chemical complexity are structurally similar even though derived from widely separated taxonomic sources. Two examples of heterophil antigens involve the human blood group antigens. Human blood group A antigen is cross-reactive with antibody to pneumococcal capsular polysaccharide type XIV, and human blood group B antigen reacts with antibodies to certain strains of *Escherichia coli,* the common colon bacillus. Ordinary cotton is related structurally to both type III and type VIII pneumococcal polysac-

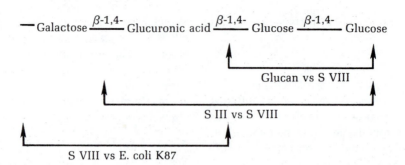

Fig. 3-2. This sequence of galactose, glucuronic acid, and two glucose residues is the basis of serologic cross-reactions, as noted by brackets.

Table 3-1. Serologic and sequence relationships of insulins

Species	Amino acid in A chain positions			Reaction with anti–beef insulin
	8	**9**	**10**	
Beef	Alanine	Serine	Valine	
Sheep	Alanine	Glycine	Valine	Yes
Pig	Threonine	Serine	Isoleucine	Yes
Whale	Threonine	Serine	Isoleucine	Yes
Horse	Threonine	Glycine	Isoleucine	Yes
Rabbit	Threonine	Serine	Isoleucine	Yes

Data from Moloney, P.J.: Antibodies to insulin. In Young, F.G., editor: The mechanism of action of insulin, Springfield, Ill., 1960, Charles C Thomas, Publisher; and from Pope, C.G.: The immunology of insulin, Adv. Immunol. **5:**209, 1966.

charides by virtue of their common cellobiuronic acid content (alternating D-glucose and D-glucuronic acid), and their antisera are mutually cross-reactive. Antisera to pneumococcal antigens III and VIII also cross-react with a polysaccharide from *E. coli* K87 and oat glucan (Fig. 3-2). Capsular cross-reactions have been observed between *Hemophilus influenzae* type a with pneumococcus type 6, *H. influenzae* type b and pneumococcus types VI, XV, XXVIII, and XXXV, and of type c with pneumococcus type XI.

Cross-reactions occur with protein antigens if the antigens are from closely related taxonomic sources. Antisera to hen egg albumin will react with duck egg albumin. Bovine and equine serum albumins, and bovine and human fibrinogens, are also cross-reactive. Cross-reactions of anti–beef

insulin with the insulins from pigs, sheep, whales, humans, and other species are known (Table 3-1). These insulins are very low molecular weight proteins with nearly identical structures differing from each other by only a few or by even a single amino acid residue. Sheep insulin, for example, differs from beef insulin only by the replacement of serine with glycine in position 9 of the A chain; pig insulin differs from beef insulin at positions 8 and 10; and horse insulin varies from beef insulin at positions 8, 9, and 10.

The best known of the heterophil antigens is the Forssman antigen, originally described as an antigen present in most guinea pig tissues (but not red blood cells), which would stimulate the production of sheep red blood cell agglutinins by rabbits. The Forssman antigen is truly heterogenetic, since it is found in human erythrocytes, *Streptococcus pneumoniae,* horses, dogs, tigers, whales, carp, toads, turtles, chickens, and other organisms. It is absent from the rabbit, and it is on this basis that the rabbit is able to make antibodies to the Forssman antigen. Another interesting observation is that it is a hapten, not an antigen, since injections of purified Forssman "antigen" alone will not induce antibody formation. Glucose, galactose, ceramide, and *N*-acetylgalactosamine have been identified in the Forssman haptens.

The generic or class names given to the antigens are supplemented by many additional variations. Among these are blood group antigen, transplantation antigen, tumor antigen, and blocking antigen. It seems that almost any adjective can be used to modify the description of an antigen.

The most important of the antigen-modifying terms are *T cell–dependent* and *T cell–independent* antigen. T cell–dependent antigens are those which are unable to stimulate B cells to synthesize antibody unless T lymphocytes are present. The nature of this T cell–B cell cooperation is discussed in a later chapter. T cell–dependent antigens are usually structurally more complex than the T cell–independent antigens. Bacterial LPS, pneumococcal capsular polysaccharides, polyvinylpyrrolidone, dextran, the bacterial flagellar protein flagellin, and other simple molecules are T cell–independent antigens. B cells destined to produce immunoglobulins of the IgM isotype are readily stimulated by the T cell–independent antigens. In fact there are two subclasses of T cell–independent antigens: the T1, or polyclonal, antigens, which stimulate all or nearly all B cells (LPS), and the weakly polyclonal or monoclonal T2 antigens (ficoll, polyvinylpyrrolidone), which primarily stimulate the B cell that will produce a specific corresponding antibody which will react with that antigen.

TYPES OF IMMUNIZATION

Now that the nature of antigens has been described, it is appropriate to turn to the responses of the body to these antigens. The response to antigens is known as the immune response; the process itself is immunization, and it can take several forms.

Autoimmunization

Autoimmunization is the response of one's T and/or B cells to proteins or polysaccharides that have begun to function as self-antigens, or autoantigens or which serve as targets for immunoglobulins and T cell–directed activities. This is usually expressed as some form of autoimmune disease or allergy.

Alloimmunization

Alloimmunization refers to immunization with antigens from an individual within one's own species. The genetic differences between individuals or races or strains within a species dictate the existence of unique antigenic specificities that are not shared by all members of the species. Exposure to these antigens is then an immunizing experience, and this is the basis for blood transfusion reactions and tissue graft rejection (when these are conducted within one species). The antigens responsible for this are known as alloantigens, and the antibodies are alloantibodies.

The prefix *allo-,* and its use in the terms introduced here, means "other." *Allo-* generally is used when the other is closely related to the term with which it is compared. Alloantigen, alloantibody, alloimmunization, etc. are rapidly replacing isoantigen, isoantibody, isoimmunization, etc., where the prefix *iso-* was used in the sense of equal or similar.

Xenoimmunization

Immunization of one species with antigens from a second species is xenoimmunization, or heteroimmunization. The antigens involved are xenoantigens, or heteroantigens, and the antibodies could be called xenoantibodies, or heteroantibodies. This is the usual kind of immunization conducted, with antigens used across the species barrier (*xeno-* means foreign). Since this is the standard form of immunization, the prefix *xeno-* or *hetero-* usually is dropped.

Active, passive, and adoptive immunization

These definitions and explanations of autoimmunization, alloimmunization, and xenoimmunization apply primarily to active immunization, in contrast to passive immunization. In the former situation the individual's own cells respond to the antigen by synthesizing antibodies or producing lymphokines. In the latter case antibodies or lymphokines produced by some donor individual are injected into a recipient who becomes passively immunized. On a practical basis passive immunization is limited to alloimmunization and heteroimmunization.

A third variety of immunization, more closely related to passive than to active immunization, is adoptive immunization. This term refers to the transplantation of immunocompetent tissue from one animal to an immunologically deficient animal. These tissues already may be in the process of immunoglobulin synthesis, or they merely may be ready for that activity when the recipient is later immunized. In either instance the result is actually a passive immunization, since it is not, strictly speaking, the cells of the immunized animal that synthesize the antibodies.

Adoptive immunization relies on the transplantation of tissue from one animal to another and consequently is subject to the immunologic principles governing transplantation (Chapter 11). Adoptively transferred tissue will survive only a few days in a graft recipient unless the donor and recipient are histocompatible or the recipient has been immunosuppressed to permit the survival of the adopted tissue.

HAPTENS AND ANTIGENIC DETERMINANT SITES

Heretofore the discussion has centered on what antigens do and what they are. Little or no attention has been devoted to the explanation of why one antigen is different from another. This can be indicated very cryptically by stating that antigens are different because they possess different antigenic determinant sites. The meaning of this is enlarged on in the following paragraphs.

There is considerable evidence that only a specific, limited part of an antigen molecule is the inducer of B cell and T cell responses. This portion, which is also the part of the antigen with which the antibody reacts, is known as the antigenic determinant site, or epitope. The number of antigenic determinants per molecule of antigen is referred to as the valence of the antigen. In this context valence has absolutely no relationship to the ionic condition of the antigen.

The antigenic valence of a molecule can be considered in two contexts: the total valence and the functional valence. The functional valence of all complete antigens is two or more and is roughly proportional to the molecular weight of the antigen, with one valence site existing for each 10,000 or so molecular weight. Functional valence sites are all on the outer surface of the antigenic molecule and can be measured by determining the number of antibody molecules that attach to the antigen. Total valence is the sum of the functional and nonfunctional (hidden) valence sites; this too is undoubtedly related to molecular size.

The whole antigen per se does not actually cause antibody formation; hydrolytic products of the antigen generated by phagocytes do this. This means that some antibodies can be formed against internal antigenic determinants that are not functional in the parent molecule. These hidden epitopes can be identified only when the antigen is structurally altered, which is possible by enzymatic hydrolysis, so that identifiable fragments can be examined for the number of their antigenic determinant sites. Serum albumins, which have molecular weights of about 70,000, contain six functional valence sites, but enzymatic digestion (of bovine serum albumin) produces nine peptides, each of which is capable of precipitating with an antibody. Since precipitation requires at least two valence sites, a total of 18 (minimum) determinant sites must be present in the original molecule. It is unknown how many additional determinant sites are destroyed by the hydrolysis, but the total valence of bovine serum albumin is at least three times the functional valence.

Monovalent fragments of a complete antigen can combine with an antibody (made against the complete antigen) but do not precipitate with it. Haptens behave like monovalent determinants but can be constructed to be divalent or even multivalent, in which case they will precipitate with antibody.

Efforts to increase the understanding of the nature of antigenic determinant sites have been based on three different approaches: the degradation of antigens, the synthesis of antigens, and the alteration, or haptenic modification, of antigens. Identification of the number, shape, size, and chemistry of antigenic determinant sites has been the goal.

Degradation of antigens

By a careful selection of proteases with restricted peptide-bond specificity, limited proteolysis of protein antigens will generate fragments that can be purified and then analyzed for their capacity to react with antisera prepared against the intact protein. Such studies are rather simply interpreted when linear proteins constitute the antigen; silk fibroin was one of the first to be examined in this manner. In this study ultimately one antigenic determinant site was identified to reside in an octapeptide consisting of Gly (Gly$_3$ Ala$_3$) Tyr. (The parentheses indicate that the sequence within them was not determined.) Removal of the carboxyterminal tyrosine halved the antibody-combining power of the peptide; thus this determinant consisted of a linear sequence of about seven or eight amino acids and was dominated by a terminal constituent (Table 3-2).

A similar hydrolysis of tobacco mosaic virus protein produced several peptides with antibody-binding activity, but one, peptide VIII, was far more potent than any of the others. Within this peptide a locus consisting of Leu-Asp-Ala-Thr-Arg seemed to be the immunodominant portion. Synthesis of this peptide readily confirmed this. Analogs which contained a single amino acid substitution revealed that such substitutions seriously affected the binding power. This reveals the highly discriminatory ability of certain antisera and again indicates the small size (five amino acids) of an antigen determinant.

In the globular protein ribonuclease the peptide bond between Ala and Ser at positions 20 to 21

Table 3-2. Characteristics of antigenic determinants

Antigen or hapten	Molecular weight	Determinant	Determinant size	Important observation
Natural antigens				
Silk fibroin	50,000 to 60,000	Octapeptide	748	Terminal amino acid
Tobacco mosaic virus protein	16,500	Pentapeptide	646	Hydrophobic group
Ribonuclease	14,000			Tertiary structure important
Dextran	50,000 to 100,000	Isomaltose	990	Little internal complexity
Synthetic antigens: polyamino acids				
$G_{52} A_{38} T_{10}$	4,100			Low molecular weight
$G_{60} A_{30} T_{10}$	13,300	Hexapeptide	792	Noncovalent bonding to form determinant site
Haptens	Generally less than 1,000	Variable	Less than 1,000	End and acid groups, tertiary structure important

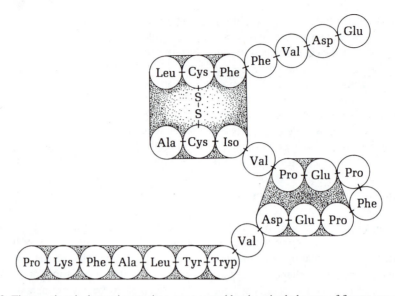

Fig. 3-3. Three antigenic determinants sites, represented by the stippled areas of five to seven amino acids in the peptide fragment shown, indicate that determinant sites may be either linear or nonlinear within a single peptide chain or across two peptide chains. Same features apply to polysaccharide antigens.

is hydrolyzed by subtilisin concomitant with inactivation or ribonuclease. A major epitope was identified in the eicosapeptide that represents the amino terminus of the enzyme, but this was not further delineated. Alteration of the secondary and tertiary structure of ribonuclease by disulfide bond reduction handicapped its performance with antiserum to the native protein, clearly identifying spatial configurations as critical to antigenic determinant sites. This observation has been made with protein and polysaccharide antigens where disturbance of the α-helix or cross-linking compromise antigen performance.

The importance of quaternary protein structure is exemplified in the hemoglobins, which each have two α–peptide and two β– or two γ–peptide chains, etc. Antisera against a complete human $\alpha_2\beta_2$ hemoglobin will not react with free α-chains but will with the hybrid human α_2-canine β_2. The antibody against $\alpha_2\gamma_2$ that will react with its α portion is different from the α-specific

antibody prepared against $\alpha_2\beta_2$. These experiments reveal how the association of one peptide chain with another alters the availability and reactivity of antigenic determinant sites and that antigenic determinants need not consist of amino acids in a linear sequence in a protein or of monosaccharides in an oligosaccharide (Fig. 3-3).

Synthesis of antigens

Studies similar to those discussed previously have been repeated with synthetic polymers of the L-α-amino acids. These are synthetic polyamino acids or polypeptides. The synthetic polyamino acids are much like native proteins but with some striking exceptions; for example, homopolymers containing but a single type of amino acid may be made, and the D isomers of the amino acids are as easily used as the L isomers. A third consideration is that the sequence of synthetic copolymers is exceptionally difficult to regulate and is nearly impossible to determine after synthesis.

Consequently copolymers are discussed in terms of their percentage composition: $Glu_{59} Lys_{41}$ refers to a copolymer of glutamic acid and lysine in which the former accounts for 59% and the latter accounts for 41% of the molecule.

The results of immunochemical studies indicate that neither D nor L homopolypeptides are antigenic, regardless of their molecular weight. This is not unexpected in view of the known nonantigenicity of other large molecules that lack internal complexity. A mixture of poly-L-glutamic acid and poly-L-lysine is antigenic for rabbits, although neither polymer alone causes antibody formation. In the case of the mixture it is possible that a noncovalent bonding of these oppositely charged polymers occurs. This could present a physical complexity to the antigen-processing cells that allows them to preserve chemical structures not seen in the individual polymers. A very similar mechanism is used to explain the ''antigenicity'' of nucleic acids that promote antibody formation when injected in complexes with acetylated bovine serum albumin but which are antigenically inert when injected alone. These studies support the conclusion that an antigenic determinant site need not be entirely a covalently linked structure.

Many copolymers of amino acids are antigenic. Larger molecular weight polypeptides are more antigenic than their lower molecular weight counterparts, even though both have the same qualitative composition. Polypeptides containing only two amino acids are usually poor antigens. The smallest pure polypeptide that is antigenic has a molecular weight of 4,100. Linear and multichain compounds are antigenic by virtue of this increased dimensional complexity. A polylysine, branched through the addition of polyalanine to the ϵ–amino group of some lysines, with the polyalanines in turn bearing a terminal Tyr-Glu, is antigenic. A polymer of the same composition in which the Tyr-Glu are attached to the polylysine core before the polyalanine is added is not antigenic. This clearly illustrates that strategic positioning of the amino acids is essential to confer antigenicity on a molecule. Synthetic polypeptides always have low valence, apparently because the same antigenic determinant site recurs periodically in the molecule.

Haptenic modification of antigens

Experiments conducted by Landsteiner completely rearranged immunologic thinking. From his studies emerged the concept of haptens as simple nonantigenic compounds, usually of low molecular weight, which could be covalently coupled to existing antigens to create new antigenic determinants. (In some instances it is possible to create antigens by adding many hapten groups to a nonantigen.) These hapten-antigen complexes, or conjugated or neoantigens, generated antibodies with specificity for the haptenic group.

A hypothetical hapten (H) combined with an antigen (Ag-1) forms the new complex H-Ag-1. Immunization of an animal with these substances will result in the formation of antisera (sera containing antibodies), as listed in Table 3-3. Injection of H alone is incapable of raising an antiserum, but the injections of Ag-1 and H-Ag-1 results in the formation of antisera in complete harmony with the fact that these substances are antigens. The reactivity of the antisera to Ag-1 (anti-Ag-1) and to the hapten antigen-1 conjugate (anti-H-Ag-1) is illustrated in Table 3-4. H will not react with anti-Ag-1 (line 1), but it will react with anti-H-Ag-1 (line 2). The portion of the antiserum reacting is that with a specificity for the hapten. As seen in lines 3 and 4, Ag-1 will react with anti-Ag-1 and anti-H-Ag-1, and in the latter case it is the portion of the antiserum directed against Ag-1 that participates. Occasionally this reaction, although logically expected, does not occur. This may be the situation when the haptenic modification of Ag-1 has been so extensive that every original antigenic determinant site is altered. In such an instance anti-H-Ag-1 actually has a totally new antigenic specificity, which is not similar to native Ag-1, and so no reaction occurs between these two. In line 5 we see, as expected, that H-Ag-1 reacts with anti-H-Ag-1. Line 6 again illustrates the specificity of anti-H-Ag-1 for H, since that is the common denominator between the antigen and the antiserum in this instance. Ag-2 can have no bearing on this reaction, as seen by the results of reaction 7.

The selection of haptens with known structures permitted Landsteiner to assess the specificity of the antibody response within very finite limits. Most of Landsteiner's studies involved the use of substituted azoproteins as antigens. Substituted aromatic amines were converted to diazonium salts, which then covalently combined with the tyrosyl residue in any antigenic protein to form the monosubstituted derivative. If the hapten was present in sufficient excess, the disubstituted product would be formed. Antisera formed to one azoantigen, possibly diazoarsanilic acid coupled to bovine γ-globulin, were made to react with diazoarsanilic acid coupled to another carrier such as ovalbumin so that only the hapten specificity would be measured. Then a series of closely re-

lated azohaptens coupled to ovalbumin would react with the antiserum. These reactions were graded on a simple plus-minus basis or estimated in terms of percentage to determine the specificity of the antisera.

A second method used to evaluate the specificity of these antisera was to preincubate them with the related hapten (in its nondiazotized form) prior to an incubation with the original hapten-antigen conjugate. The degree by which the second reaction was inhibited was used as a measure of the specificity of the antiserum for the second hapten.

From these studies several conclusions became evident. Historically it is only fair to state that they have probably been overemphasized. Certainly the following are not conclusions that can be fairly applied to all antigens, but in the framework within which they were developed—the diazohapten-antigen system—they are valid conclusions.

1. Strongly acid or basic groups are usually very decisive in regulating antibody specificity.

2. Nonionic groups of approximately equal size and shape are interchangeable without significant losses in serologic activity.

3. Spatial configurations of haptens (D-, L-, ortho-, meta-, para-, and other) are important.

4. Terminal components of an antigen often exert a controlling influence on the specificity of the antibodies formed.

Only two examples of these studies are described here. The dominance of acidic groups in

Table 3-3. Effects of hapten-antigen immunization

Material injected	Antibody formed
Hapten (H)	None
Antigen-1 (Ag-1)	Anti-Ag-1
Hapten-Antigen-1 (H-Ag-1)	Anti-H-Ag-1

Table 3-4. Reactions of hapten-antigen antisera

Hapten (H) or antigen (Ag)		Antiserum	Reaction	Portion of antiserum reacting
1 H	+	Anti-Ag-1	No	None
2 H	+	Anti-H-Ag-1	Yes	Anti-H
3 Ag-1	+	Anti-Ag-1	Yes	Anti-Ag-1
4 Ag-1	+	Anti-H-Ag-1	Yes	Anti-Ag-1
5 H-Ag-1	+	Anti-H-Ag-1	Yes	Anti-H-Ag-1
6 H-Ag-2	+	Anti-H-Ag-1	Yes	Anti-H
7 Ag-2	+	Anti-H-Ag-1	No	None

determining the specificity of the antibody formed is observable in Table 3-5. In this experiment antisera versus the para-positioned carboxylic, sulfonic, and arsonic acid residues on substituted anilines were prepared. These antisera were tested in mutual cross-reactions with these haptens conjugated to a different carrier protein. In every instance complete specificity for the type of acid was observed, and no cross-reactions occurred.

Positionings of haptenic substitutes have a critical effect on antibody specificity. Table 3-6 illustrates that ortho-, meta-, and para- placed carboxyl groups on the benzene ring of aniline pro-

duce monospecific azoproteins. The spatial configuration of the corresponding sulfonic acids yields similar results, although there is some cross-reactivity between ortho- and meta- positionings. Other meta-, ortho-, and para- isomers tend to be specific or exhibit very slight cross-reactivity.

It is always interesting to today's immunologists to note how well Landsteiner's studies have stood the test of more critical, modern serologic techniques. Nearly all the basic rules of hapten specificity were discovered by Landsteiner through the use of precipitation inhibition reactions, a crude serologic method by modern standards. Cer-

Table 3-5. Contribution of acidic radicals to serologic specificity

Antigen conjugated with	Antisera versus			
	Aniline (NH_2)	PABA (NH_2, $COOH$)	PASA (NH_2, SO_3H)	PAAA (NH_2, AsO_3H_2)
Aniline	+ + +	—	—	—
PABA	—	+ + + ±	—	—
PASA	—	—	+ + + ±	—
PAAA	—	—	—	+ + + ±

From Landsteiner, K.: The specificity of serologic reactions, revised ed., New York, 1962, Dover Press, Inc.

Table 3-6. Contribution of spatial arrangement to serologic specificity

Antigen conjugated with	Antisera versus			
	Aniline (NH_2)	OABA (NH_2, $COOH$)	MABA (NH_2, $COOH$)	PABA (NH_2, $COOH$)
Aniline	+ + +	—	—	—
OABA	—	+ + +	—	—
MABA	—	—	+ + + +	—
PABA	—	—	—	+ + + ±

From Landsteiner, K.: The specificity of serologic reactions, revised ed., New York, 1962, Dover Press, Inc.

tain further additions, of course, have been made to hapten immunology by recent experimentation, but these have had little influence on the tenets established by Landsteiner.

An example of more modern contributions is that insulin, which contains only one lysine, can be conjugated with dinitrofluorobenzene. The antiserum produced by immunization with the conjugate displays specificity for the haptenic ligand. Therefore a single haptenic group may suffice to alter the specificity of an antigen. More than one hapten moiety per antigen molecule is required for precipitation. Analysis of serologic reactions of divalent haptens with their antibodies suggests that a complex of three divalent haptens with three antibody molecules to form an equilateral triangle is the most common complex formed.

The immunochemical study of haptens and low molecular weight compounds remains a fertile and active area of reasearch. Biologic and medical scientists currently are applying the principles of hapten immunology to the solution of many problems in which the detection or quantitative determination of low molecular weight compounds is the key determination. Nearly all these compounds, which are classified among the peptide or nonpeptide hormones, coenzymes, vitamins, and therapeutic drugs, by virtue of their low molecular weight are either nonantigenic or very poor antigens. By handling them as haptens, one can produce antisera suitable for their detection and quantitation.

Autocoupling haptens

A number of highly reactive low molecular weight compounds, which on the basis of size

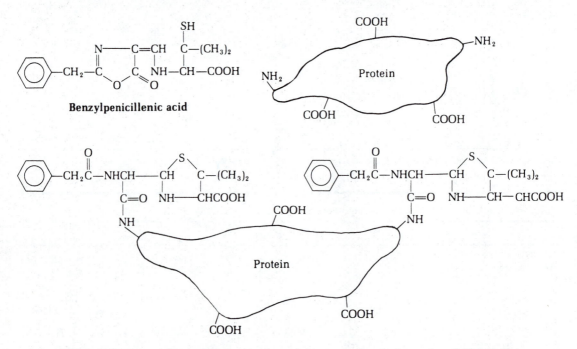

Fig. 3-4. Benzylpenicillenic acid is one of many decomposition products of penicillin G. This acid can form peptide bonds with the amino groups of tissue proteins, creating neoantigens in which the penicillin derivative is most closely related to penicillenic acid. Conjugates of penicillin derivatives can also form easily by — S — S — exchange with the sulfur atom in the thiazolidine portion of the antibiotic structure, but these are less important as allergens.

alone must be considered as haptens, will produce antibodies if injected alone into an animal. Representative of such compounds are free diazonium salts, fluoro- and chloro-substituted dinitrophenyl compounds, acid anhydrides, and others. Decomposition products of penicillin have this property, and this is one way antibodies to penicillin are formed (Fig. 3-4). These compounds all have one property in common: the ability to form spontaneous covalent bonds with tissue proteins or polysaccharides to create neoantigens in vivo. These conjugates represent novel antigens to the animal, and the animal responds with antibody. In any discussion of haptens, autocoupling haptens must be considered as a unique class of haptens that, because of their special chemical reactivity, do not conform to the general description of haptens.

Unlike the response to the usual hapten-antigen complexes, which are no more offensive to an animal's health than the injection of other antigens, the response to autocoupling haptens can have serious consequences. One of these is the anaphylactic reaction based on IgE antibodies formed as a result of the autocoupling hapten's ability to conjugate with tissue macromolecules. Subsequent reinjection of the autocoupling hapten results in an in vivo serologic reaction between the IgE and the hapten that can be fatal or near fatal within minutes after the injection. This is the subject of Chapter 18. The application of autocoupling haptens to the skin can induce contact dermatitis, a form of drug allergy. This is related to the sensitization of T cells and the products they release. This subject is dealt with in Chapter 20.

BIBLIOGRAPHY

Ahlstedt, S., and others: New aspects of antigens in penicillin allergy, CRC Crit. Rev. Toxicol. **7:**219, 1980.

Atassi, M.Z., editor: Immunochemistry of proteins, vols. 1 and 2, New York, 1977, Plenum Publishing Corp.

Atassi, M.Z.: Precise determination of protein antigenic structure has unravelled the molecular immune recognition of proteins and provided a prototype for synthetic mimicking of other protein binding sites, Mol. Cell. Biochem. **32:**21, 1980.

Atassi, M.Z., and Stavitsky, A.B., editors: Immunobiology of proteins and peptides, New York, 1978, Plenum Publishing Corp.

Benacerraf, B., and Germain, R.: The immune response genes of the major histocompatibility complex, Immunol. Rev. **38:**70, 1978.

Clement, L.T., and Shevach, E.M.: The chemistry of Ia antigens, Contemp. Top. Mol. Immunol. **8:**149, 1981.

Dorf, M.E., editor: The role of the major histocompatibility complex in immunobiology, New York, 1981, Garland Publishing, Inc.

Feldman, M., and Kontiainen, S.: Antigen specific T cell factors, Mol. Cell. Biochem. **30:**117, 1980.

Hemmings, W.A., editor: Antigen absorption by the gut, Baltimore, 1978, University Park Press.

Hildemann, W.H., and Benedict, A.A., editors: Immunologic phylogeny, New York, 1975, Plenum Publishing Corp.

Hildemann, W.H., Clark, E.A., and Raison, R.L.: Comprehensive immunogenetics, New York, 1981, Elsevier/North Holland Biomedical Press.

Kano, K., and Milgrom, F.: Heterophile antigens and antibodies in medicine, Curr. Top. Microbiol. Immunol. **77:**43, 1977.

Katz, D.H., and Benacerraf, B., editors: The role of products of the histocompatibility gene complex in immune responses, New York, 1976, Academic Press, Inc.

Klein, J.: H-2 mutations: their genetics and effect on immune functions, Adv. Immunol. **26:**56, 1978.

Klein, J., and others: The traditional and a new version of the mouse H-2 complex, Nature **291:**455, 1981.

Landsteiner, K.: The specificity of serologic reactions, revised ed., New York, 1962, Dover Press, Inc.

McDevitt, H.O., editor: Ir genes and Ia antigens, New York, 1978, Academic Press, Inc.

McDevitt, H.O.: The role of H-2 I region genes in regulation of the immune response, J. Immunogenet. **8:**287, 1981.

Möller, G., editor: Ir genes and T lymphocytes, Immunol. Rev. **38:**1, 1978.

Nairn, R., and others: Biochemistry of the gene products from murine MHC mutants, Annu. Rev. Genet. **14:**241, 1980.

Reichlin, M.: Amino acid substitution and the antigenicity of globular proteins, Adv. Immunol. **20:**71, 1975.

Rosenthal, A.S.: Regulation of the immune response—role of the macrophage, N. Engl. J. Med. **303:**1153, 1980.

Rudbach, J.A., and Baker, P.J., editors: Immunology of bacterial polysaccharides, New York, 1979, Elsevier/North Holland Biomedical Press.

Schwartz, B.D., and Cullen, S.E.: Chemical characteristics of Ia antigens, Springer Semin. Immunopathol. **1:**85, 1978.

Sela, M., editor: The antigens, vols. 1-5, New York, 1973, Academic Press, Inc.

Tada, T., and Okumura, K.: The role of antigen-specific T

cell factors in the immune response, Adv. Immunol. **28**:1, 1979.

Taussig, M.J.: Antigen-specific T-cell factors, Immunology **41**:759, 1980.

Unanue, E.R., and Rosenthal, A.S., editors: Macrophage regulation of immunity, New York, 1980, Academic Press, Inc.

Vitetta, E.S., and Capra, J.D.: The protein products of the murine seventeenth chromosome: genetics and structure, Adv. Immunol. **26**:148, 1978.

Winchester, R.J., and Kunkel, H.G.: The human Ia system, Adv. Immunol. **28**:222, 1979.

SITUATION: THE GRANT REQUEST

You attended the first meeting of Microbiology 450—"Host-Parasite Relationships: Pathogenic Mechanisms." The instructor distributed his lecture schedule and course outline, examination schedule, and a page titled "Research Grant Topics." His explanation of these items was routine except for his discussion of the last item. He stated that within 2 weeks each student would be required to select one of the topics and develop a research grant proposal on that subject. To assist in this, he distributed copies of some of his own research grant proposals and guidelines for the preparation of these proposals.

After some discussion with a couple of predental students at the dormitory and a cursory library search you learned that enzymes of certain streptococci were related to their ability to cause dental caries. For your research grant proposal you selected the subject "Cross-reactive Antibodies to Enzymes and Dental Caries." In this proposal you intend to develop the hypothesis that enzymes in noncariogenic streptococci might be useful in vaccines against dental caries.

Questions

1. Are enzymes as fully antigenic as other proteins?
2. Do antibodies to enzymes neutralize the catalytic activity of the enzymes?
3. Are enzymes with identical substrate specificities but from different species serologically cross-reactive?
4. What kind of immunization routes would favor the appearance of neutralizing antibodies in oral secretions?

Solution

As long as enzymes meet the general criteria of antigens, they are able to elicit an immune response. This was discussed in this chapter in terms of ribonuclease and lysozyme. Lysozyme is especially important because it has a molecular weight of only 14,000. Many enzymes exceed this in size and are globulins with a complicated amino acid sequence and varied composition so that they easily fulfill the requirements of antigenicity. Antisera have been prepared against trypsin, chymotrypsin, pepsin, carboxypeptidase A, carboxypeptidase B, ficin, chymopapain, papain, bromelin, clostridiopeptidase, collagenase, elastase, cathepsins of several types, kallikrein (kininogenase), plasmin, thrombin, streptococcal proteinase, staphylococcal coagulase, and subtilisin, just to list a few antigenic proteases.

Antibodies to enzymes will neutralize the catalytic activity of the enzyme under the proper conditions. Clearly factors such as high salt concentration, acid pH, high temperature, and other physical forces will dissociate antigen-antibody complexes, and enzymes would provide no exception to these. On the other hand, even under ideal conditions the serologic complex is in a state of constant dissociation and reassociation, with the result that a few molecules of enzyme would be free from its neutralizing antibody at any chosen instant. Thus the recovery of a modicum of enzyme activity in any enzyme-antienzyme mixture is not unexpected. Even within the limits of expectation from these observations, antienzymes are often potent inhibitors of their respective enzymes so that 90% inhibition or more can be achieved. Antienzymes are usually more successful as inhibitors when they combine with an antigenic determinant that is a part of or a neighbor to the catalytic site. In the latter instance steric effects prevent or reduce the opportunity for the substrate to approach the catalytic site. Because of this, antienzymes are better enzyme inhibitors when the substrate is of great rather than low molecular weight.

Serologic cross-reactions among enzymes follow the same ground rules as with other antigens. Proteins serving similar functions in closely related species are often highly cross-reactive. This has been demonstrated for many serum proteins and hormones and also for enzymes, including trypsins, chymotrypsins, lactic dehydrogenases, galactosidases, and others. Contrariwise, multiple serotypes of enzymes serving similar functions occasionally are identified within a single species.

In the example considered here it has been recognized that the glucosyltransferase of *Streptococcus mutans* is a contributing enzyme to tooth decay. The enzyme synthesizes extracellular glucose polymers (glucans), which contribute to formation of dental plaques. Within these plaques, and under them, dentin-eroding activities lead to the appearance of caries. Serologic types of *S. mutans* are seven in number (a through g), and the glycosyltransferases of types a, d, and g are serologically related, as are the enzymes of types b, c, and e. However, there is little serologic cross-reactivity between the two subgroups. It is poten-tially possible to use these enzymes, or serologically cross-reactive enzymes from nonpathogenic species, in prophylactic immunization against tooth decay. Since the principal antibody found in saliva is secretory IgA in company with secretory IgM (Chapter 6), immunization routes which favor production of these immunoglobulins should be used. Instillation of killed *S. mutans* into sites near the major salivary glands and into the parotid gland ducts of monkeys already has been demonstrated as a successful prophylactic for caries in monkeys.

The concept to use cross-reactive glucosyltransferases from nonpathogenic bacteria for this purpose has merit and should result in a high-quality research proposal for the requirement in this course on pathogenic mechanisms.

References

Arnon, R.: Antibodies to enzymes—a tool in the study of antigenic specificity determinants, Curr. Top. Microbiol. Immunol. **54**:47, 1971.

Evans, R.T., Emmings, F.G., and Genco, R.J.: Prevention of *Streptococcus mutans* infection of tooth surfaces by salivary antibody in Irus monkeys *(Macaca fascicularis),* Infect. Immun. **12**:293, 1975.

Salton, M.R.J., editor: Immunochemistry of enzymes and their antibodies, New York, 1977, John Wiley & Sons, Inc.

Smith, D.J., and Taubman, M.A.: Antigenic relatedness of glucosyltransferase enzymes from *Streptococcus mutans,* Infect. Immun. **15**:91, 1977.

CHAPTER

4

MACROPHAGES AND ANTIGEN-PROCESSING CELLS

GLOSSARY

activated macrophage Macrophage from antigen-sensitized or otherwise stimulated animals.

alveolar macrophage An aerobic macrophage of the lung.

bacteriotropin An immune opsonin that stimulates phagocytosis of a bacterium, other cell type, or particle.

basophil A blood granulocyte whose granules release histamine during anaphylactic reactions.

chemotaxis Attraction of leukocytes or other cells by chemicals; synonymous with *leukotaxin* in reference to white blood cells.

ECF-A Eosinophilic chemotactic factor of anaphylaxis.

eosinophil A white blood cell that contains cytoplasmic granules with an affinity for acid dyes; synonymous with *acidophil*.

eosinophilic chemotactic factor of anaphylaxis A mast cell peptide that is chemotactic for eosinophils.

granulocyte A collective term for leukocytes with pronounced cytoplasmic granulation.

HETE Hydroxyeicosatetraenoic acid, a chemotaxin derived from arachidonic acid.

HHT Hydroxyheptatrienoic acid, a chemotaxin derived from arachidonic acid.

hydroxyl radical A toxic form of oxygen produced by phagocytes; · OH.

IL-1 Interleukin 1.

IL-2 Interleukin 2.

IFN Interferon.

interferon Protein(s) released from a cell that is infected by an intracellular parasite, which protects neighboring cells from invasion by the same or other intracellular parasites.

interleukin A monokine that acts on other leukocytes.

interleukin 1 A monokine that activates T cells and possibly B cells.

interleukin 2 A monokine that serves as a growth factor for T cells.

Kupffer's cell A macrophage of the liver.

Langerhans' cells Macrophages found in the skin.

LC Langerhans' cells.

macrophage Tissue or blood phagocytes, 20 to 80 μm in diameter, containing lysosomes, vacuoles, and partially digested debris in their cytoplasm.

monocyte White blood cells, 12 to 30 μm in diameter, with rounded nucleus, precursor to macrophages.

monokine A protein elaborated by a monocyte or macrophage that acts on other host cells.

myeloperoxidase An enzyme in lysosomes that aids intraphagocyte killing.

neutrophil A leukocyte with granules that are not predominant in their affinity for acid or basic dyes.

opsonin An antibody that attaches to a cellular or particulate antigen and which "prepares" it for phagocytosis.

phagocytic index (in vivo) $\dfrac{\text{Log concentration of particles at } T_1 - \text{Log concentration of particles } T_2}{T_2 - T_1}$

where T = time.

phagocytosis The engulfment of cells or particulate matter by leukocytes, macrophages, or other cells.

PMN polymorphonuclear neutrophilic leukocyte.

polymorphonuclear neutrophilic leukocyte A white blood cell with a granular cytoplasm and multilobed nucleus that is very active in phagocytosis.

RES Reticuloendothelial system.

reticuloendothelial blockade Malfunction of phagocytic cells by prior exposure to phagocytosable particles.

reticuloendothelial system A collective term for cells of varying morphology and tissue residence with the common feature of being actively phagocytic.

singlet oxygen A toxic form of oxygen produced by phagocytes; $^1O_2$.

superoxide radical A toxic form of oxygen produced by phagocytes: $\cdot\, O_2$.

TBX$_2$ Thromboxane 2, a chemotaxin derived from arachidonic acid.

T cell growth factor Interleukin 2.

TCGF T cell growth factor.

tuftsin A chemotactic tetrapeptide derived from a γ-globulin.

The cells of the body that respond to antigens are variously categorized as belonging to the hematopoietic, the reticuloendothelial, the phagocytic, or the lymphoid system. The organs and tissues that make up these systems are not as well defined as those of the nervous, skeletal, endocrine, or other systems, which exist as distinct structural organs and have a clear, often singular, physiologic role. The organ systems of interest to immunologists are often dispersed and may have multiple functions. This is certainly true for cells of the mononuclear and granulocyte phagocytic system described in this chapter.

THE HEMATOPOIETIC SYSTEM

For most purposes the hematopoietic system is an appropriate beginning study for the immunocytologist. Cells of the immune response system are formed and mature and are dispersed from the bone marrow. They are then reclassified as cells of the phagocytic, lymphoid, or other system according to the new functions they acquire or express outside the bone marrow (Fig. 4-1).

In mammals the bone marrow, if considered as a single tissue, is the largest tissue of the body.

In the average human adult the total weight of the bone marrow is about 3 kg. Marrow fills the central core of all long bones, but other bones, especially in the cranium, contribute significantly to its total mass. Marrow is divisible into two parts: the vascular and adipose portion and the portion directed to hematopoiesis, or blood cell formation. The vascular tissue is simply the circulatory system that supplies the nutrients and removes the wastes from these actively growing cells. This tissue plus the fat represent about half the weight of bone marrow.

The remaining half of the bone marrow is the source of erythrocytes, platelets, granulocytes, monocytes, and lymphocytes. These arise from a primitive, undifferentiated stem cell, the reticulum cell, which differentiates into a separate precursor for each cell line. Within each of these cell lines, or systems, a further developmental series of cells, intermediate between the precursor and the end cell, has been recognized. Of these cell series, only those of the granulocytic, monocytic, and lymphocytic series are effector cells of the immune response. Cells of the erythroid and megakaryocytic (platelet) series often are affected by the

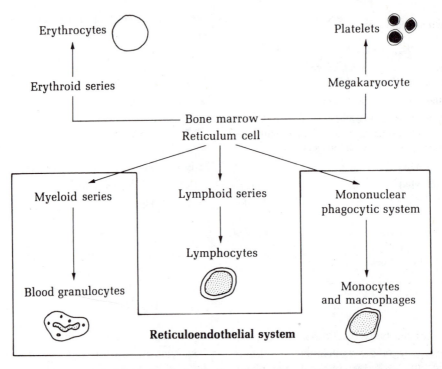

Fig. 4-1. Origin of immunologically vital cells from bone marrow. Granulocytes and monocytes traditionally have been considered as the two halves of the reticuloendothelial system (RES), but the latter are now being treated as a separate unit. The lymphoid system represents the third important cell line. Cells of the erythroid series and megakaryocytes are important as antigens.

immune response and may serve as targets for it. In bone marrow the white blood cells surpass the number of red blood cells by a ratio of 3:1.

THE RETICULOENDOTHELIAL SYSTEM

The term *reticuloendothelial system (RES)* is nearly archaic and lacked a satisfactory definition even when it was a more useful and timely term. At the present the RES can be considered as a collection of cells of different origin and morphology that are united by their common property of phagocytosis. Two major subdivisions exist within the RES: the mononuclear phagocytic system and the granulocytic phagocytes. The mononuclear cells are the more active of the two phagocytic systems.

Mononuclear phagocytic system

The mononuclear phagocytic cell system consists of the blood monocytes and the free (motile) and fixed (nonmotile) macrophages of the tissues. Monocytes arise from precursor promonocytes of the bone marrow, from which they are released into the blood, although monocytes also can be found in the marrow. Most, if not all, of the tissue macrophages arise from the blood monocytes.

Monocytes. The monocytes represent 1% to 3% of the circulating leukocytes in the adult human, or about 300 cells per cubic milliliter of blood. Monocytes have a circulating half-life of only 8 to 10 hours. They must be synthesized at a rate of about 1.7×10^8 cells per kg of body weight per day to maintain their normal circulating population. These cells vary between 10 and 20 μm

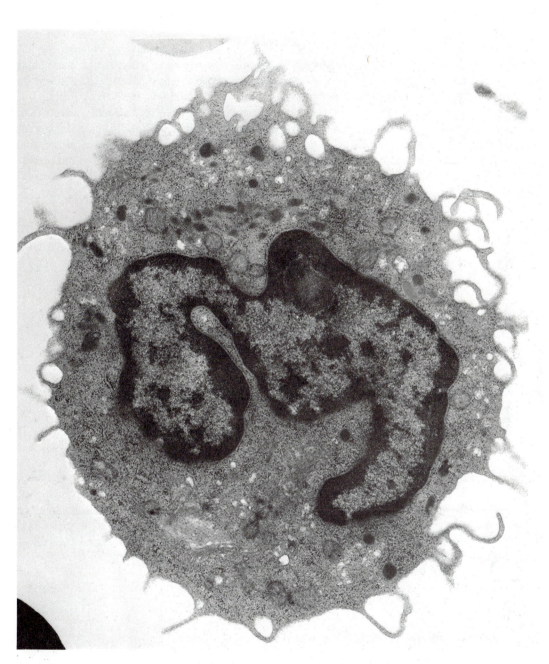

Fig. 4-2. This electron microscopic view of a blood monocyte was cut at a plane which reveals a large cleft in the dark nucleus. Notice the many different types of cytoplasmic inclusions. (Courtesy Dr. E. Adelstein.)

in diameter; their nucleus is large and usually occupies about half the space within the cell. The nucleus may be oval, indented, crude horseshoe, or kidney shaped. The cytoplasm is abundant and has a fine granular texture as a result of its generous content of lysosomal granules (Fig. 4-2).

Macrophages. Monocytes that disappear from the blood are not removed from the body as dead or damaged cells. Instead these cells enter the tissues and become macrophages. There are more macrophages per gram of tissue in the spleen than in any other organ, but there are more total macrophages in the liver because of its larger size. Tissue macrophages have a life span of many months or years. Macrophages have specific tissue names that vary according to their tissue location (for example, histiocytes in connective tissue, Kupffer's cells in liver, alveolar macrophages or dust cells in lung, and microglial cells in the neural system). The tissue macrophages will not have an identical morphology, even though they all arise

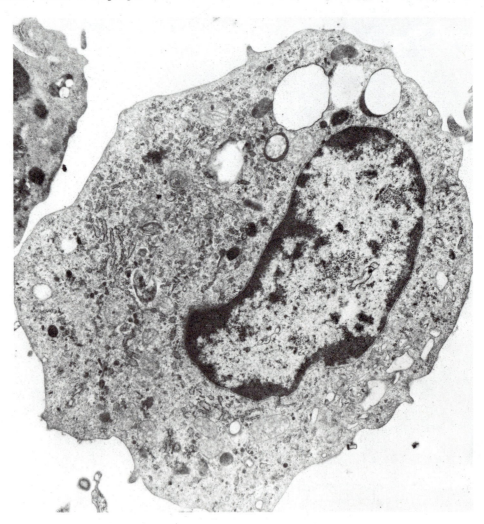

Fig. 4-3. Electron micrograph of a macrophage. Note the large cytoplasmic space and the numerous types of granules. (Courtesy Dr. E. Adelstein.)

from a common precursor, the peripheral blood monocyte. When the monocyte enters tissues, it undergoes a metamorphosis, during which there is a rapid increase in size, in protein synthesis, and in lysosome content. The extent of these changes is modified by the tissue in which the alteration takes place, thus leading to individual characteristics and separate names for the macrophages that arise in the different tissues. In addition, their appearance is regulated by their ameboid motility and the exact moment that fixed preparations are made in relationship to this motility (Fig. 4-3).

Unlike the blood monocytes, which have a half-life of only a few hours, tissue macrophages have a life span of many months or years. This may not be true in inflammatory lesions, in which many cells undoubtedly die or fuse with other macrophages to form multinucleate giant cells or epithelioid cells. In areas of chronic inflammation, where granulomas typically arise, giant and epithelioid cells are almost invariably present, surrounding a central necrotic core that is devoid of true cellular structure because of the death of cells originally present there.

Macrophages serve many roles. They are the most active of the body's phagocytic cells and are important in antigen processing (Fig. 4-4). Macrophages and Th cells cooperate with B cells in a process that has been called antigen-focusing, which regulates the immune response to T cell–dependent antigens. Macrophages are important secretory cells, producing and secreting components of the complement system, hydrolytic enzymes, toxic forms of oxygen, and the monokines described later. The macrophage surface bears unique proteins that serve as identifying markers. Among these are receptors for IgM and two subclasses (1 and 3) of IgG. Antibody present on the macrophage surface obviously would serve as receptors for antigen, aiding both phagocytosis and antigen processing. Binding of complement components C3b and C3d to the macrophage surface is done by specific receptors for these proteins. Perhaps the most important proteins on the macrophage surface are Ia proteins. These proteins and their role in the helper response (I-A and I-E proteins) or suppressor response (I-J proteins) are described in Chapter 3.

Within germinal centers where clones of T cells or B cells develop after exposure to antigen, macrophages and dendritic reticular cells are also present. The former can receive, ingest, and process free antigens. The latter can receive antigen in the form of antigen-antibody complexes but does not seem to ingest or process antigens. Dendritic cells are not ameboid either and thus are not macrophages. Their exact function is uncertain, but their presence seems essential to the perpetuation, if not the initiation, of the germinal center.

Peritoneal macrophages. Macrophages (resident macrophages) washed from the untreated peritoneal space, along with other cells normally present there, approach twice the diameter of the monocyte and have an oval or indented nucleus and a lightly granular cytoplasm. Rough endoplasmic reticulum also can be seen in electron micrographs of these cells. These cells adhere readily to surfaces over which they move by ameboid motion. Unstimulated, or resident, peritoneal macrophages are active phagocytes and cytodestructive to cells that they ingest.

Irritation of the peritoneal cavity with suspensions of agar, starch, mineral oil, etc. stimulates the immigration of macrophages into the peritoneal cavity. The "stimulated" macrophages are basically the same as the resident macrophages; however, they are present with a different proportion of neutrophils, monocytes, mast cells, and lymphocytes. These proportions are influenced by the factors such as choice of irritant, the time it is present in the peritoneal space, and animal species. For this reason comparisons of cellular activities in unfractionated, stimulated peritoneal washings with those of the resident cell population are tenuous.

This is not intended to deny the existence of the well-recognized activated macrophage. This type of macrophage represents the most motile, most actively phagocytic, most enzyme laden,

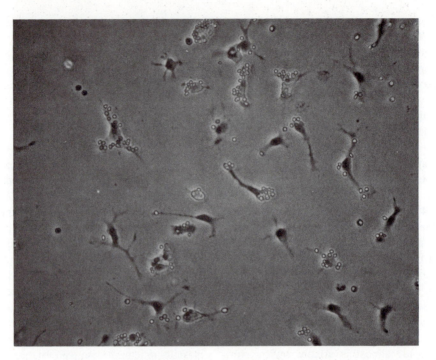

Fig. 4-4. Macrophages in culture. Note their elongated form, indicative of their motility. The clear refractile bodies are erythrocytes that the macrophages are phagocytosing. (Courtesy Dr. E. Leonard.)

and most cytocidal of the macrophages. It is known variously as the activated, armed, angry, or professional macrophage. It is a third-level cell, exceeding the monocytes and ordinary macrophages in activities associated with phagocytosis. Generation of activated macrophages relies on a message from antigen- or mitogen-exposed T cells.

Kupffer's cells. Macrophages of the liver are represented by Kupffer's cells. These cells attach to or embed themselves within the endothelial lining of the small blood vessels. Here they are ideally situated for clearance of foreign particles that enter the blood. Their cytoplasm, already granular because of its lysosome content, becomes even more uneven in appearance as engulfed particles in various states of decomposition reflect their phagocytic activity. These characteristics enable an easy identification of Kupffer's cells despite variations in their shape and size, which

is usually in the range of 40 to 50 μm in diameter.

Alveolar macrophages. Alveolar or pulmonary macrophages are unique among their kind because they roam freely on the outer surface of the lung in a fully aerobic atmosphere where they are exposed to constant supply of phagocytosable particles that are inhaled. Somewhere between 3 and 15 million of these cells are present in each gram of lung, depending on the animal species studied. The alveolar macrophage is 15 to 50 μm in diameter and contains many types of intracytoplasmic inclusions, some of which are lysosomes. These cells move over the alveolar surface scavenging dust particles, microorganisms, and other debris. Their aerobic metabolism and enzyme content indicate that these bone marrow–derived cells, like macrophages in other tissues, contribute significantly to body defenses and immunity.

Langerhans' cells. Langerhans, who first de-

scribed the pancreatic islet cells that secrete insulin, also discovered cells in the epidermis, since
named for him. These Langerhans cells represent
3% to 8% of the cells in the epidermis, or approximately 500 to 1,000 per square millimeter. In
tissues Langerhans' cells are irregular, even
branching in profile, are about twice the diameter
of monocytes, and have a deeply indented nucleus.
Rod-shaped granules are present in the cytoplasm
and on electron microscopy are seen as a laminated
structure swollen at one end like a tennis racket.
This granule is a reliable marker for Langerhans'
cells. Langerhans' cells arise from the bone marrow and are distributed largely to the skin but
are found at other sites: lymph nodes, tonsil, and
mucous membrane, for example.

Langerhans' cells sequester antigen after its
intradermal injection and are a prime source of
haptens (dinitrochlorobenzene) that have been
deposited on the skin. Exposure of the skin to ultraviolet light depletes it of Langerhans' cells,
after which the provocation of contact dermatitis
with haptens is virtually impossible. The evidence
indicates that Langerhans' cells behave as antigen-
presenting substitutes in the skin like the more
classic macrophages.

Giant and epithelioid cells. Variants of giant
cells may be seen in granulomas provoked by
different irritants, but the typical giant cell is a
polykaryon containing multiple nuclei. These
nuclei are typically 2 to 10 in number, but cells
with 30 or more nuclei have been observed. These
nuclei are arranged as a peripheral ring enclosing
lysosomal granules, mitochondria, and other cellular substructures. Giant cells may be 100 μm
or more in diameter and have numerous fine cytoplasmic processes extending from their surface
with which they interdigitate with other cells.

Giant cells arise from cell fusion of macrophages, the number of nuclei present identifying
the number of parent cells. The giant cells retain
several of the properties of macrophages: phagocytosis, motility, and antigen degradation, for
example.

Within human granulomas a secretory form of
macrophage known as the epithelioid cell is often

seen. Only phagocytosing macrophages become
epithelioid cells; the inactive macrophages do not.
The role of these cells in immunology needs much
clarification.

THE GRANULOCYTIC PHAGOCYTES
Neutrophils

The polymorphonuclear neutrophilic leukocytes
(PMN) represent about 60% to 65% of the 5,000 to
10,000 circulating white blood cells in each cubic
milliliter of blood. This amounts to about 3 to 6 $\times$
10^3 PMNs per milliliter of blood. PMNs are easily
recognized in stained blood smears by their multilobed nucleus composed most often of three lobes
connected by thin strands of nuclear material
(Fig. 4-5). These cells are about 11 to 14 μm in
diameter, or about twice the size of erythrocytes.
The abundant cytoplasm is filled with small granules that do not stain intensely with either acidic
or basic dyes (Fig. 4-6). The granules are seen as
neutral staining violet-hued structures.

PMNs originate from the bone marrow through
a series of mitotic divisions that begin with the
myeloblasts, which transform first to promyelocytes and then to myelocytes. This requires about
1 week and is followed by another week of post-
mitotic maturation. During this phase nuclear
changes permit the recognition of the metamyelocyte, the band cell, and the mature neutrophil.
These nucleated cells represent approximately two
thirds of all nucleated cells in the bone marrow.
More than 10^{11} neutrophils leave the bone marrow
and enter the blood of a 70-kg individual each
day. In the blood the neutrophils have a half-life
of only 4 to 10 hours. Many cells are lost from
the blood into urine, oral and pulmonary secretions, the gastrointestinal tract, and tissues that
they enter in response to inflammatory stimuli. By
virtue of their ameboid motion, PMNs penetrate
between the endothelial cells of the venules and
collect in the inflammatory exudate, where they
may live for an additional 1 or 2 days.

The granules in PMNs are of two different
types. The primary granules are so named because
they are the first recognized, at the promyelocyte
stage. These are also known as the azurophilic

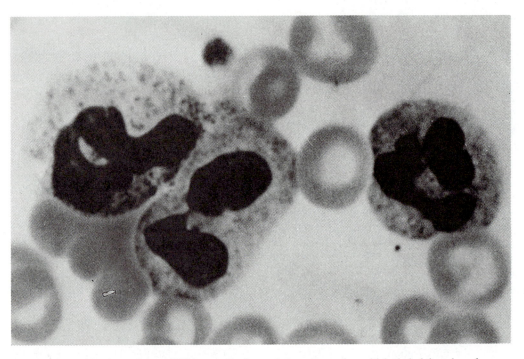

Fig. 4-5. This view of three PMNs reveals the varied conformation which their lobated nucleus can assume. (Courtesy Dr. E. Adelstein.)

granules because they stain light blue with Wright's blood stain. These represent about one third of the granules in the mature neutrophil. Myeloperoxidase, neutral proteinases, lysozyme, acid hydrolases, β-glucuronidase, and several other classes of enzymes characteristic of lysosomes are found in these granules, in addition to the cationic protein. The secondary or specific granules become numerous during the promyelocyte-myelocyte stage and are characterized by their inclusion of lysozyme, neutral proteinases, and lactoferrin and by their lack of myeloperoxidase. During phagocytosis the granules of the neutrophil disappear (degranulation), and the enzymes stored within them are discharged.

Eosinophils

Acidophilic leukocytes also are called eosinophils because eosin, an acid dye used in staining blood smears, stains their granules intensely. Eosinophils represent about 3% of the circulating white blood cells, or 70 to 450/ml. These cells are about 10 to 15 μm in diameter. Their nucleus is eccentrically located within the cytoplasm and is usually bilobed or ellipsoid (Fig. 4-7).

Bone marrow serves as the source of the eosinophil. Eosinophils are first recognized in the form of promyelocytes that contain acidophilic granules. Maturation to the eosinophilic myelocyte and eosinophilic metamyelocyte requires about 40 to 60 hours. After this the cells, now indistinguishable from blood eosinophils, remain in the marrow from 1 to 3 days before they emerge. The half-life of the eosinophil in blood is 8 to 12 hours. Eosinophils may leave the bloodstream and enter tissues, where their half-life is about 24 hours.

The granules of eosinophils are unlike those of neutrophils. By light microscopy one notices the difference in their staining properties. By electron microscopy the larger granules can be seen to

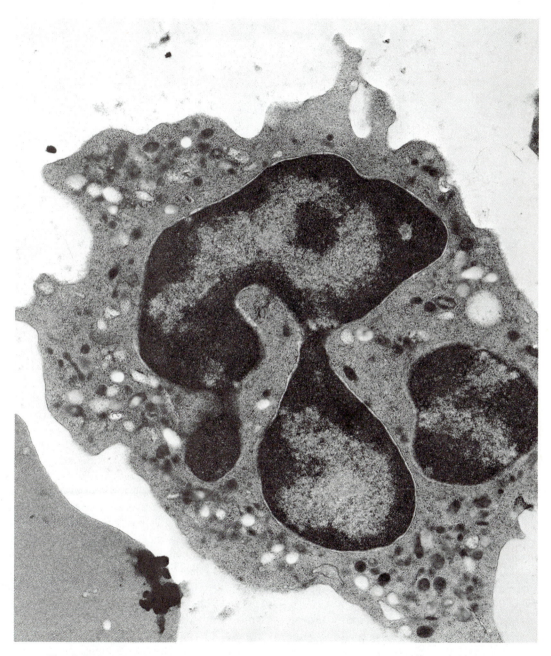

Fig. 4-6. Cytoplasmic granulation and a multilobulated nucleus are visible in this electron micrograph of a neutrophil. (Courtesy Dr. E. Adelstein.)

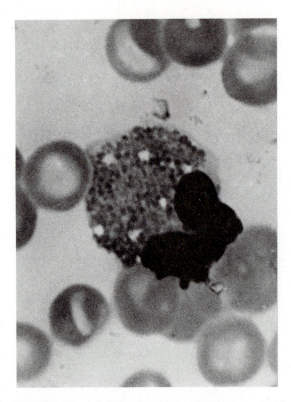

Fig. 4-7. The dark, bilobed nucleus of the eosinophil is often an important key to its identification. (Courtesy Dr. E. Adelstein.)

have a distinct crystalloid core composed largely of the major basic protein. This protein (about 6,000 mol wt) is found as a cross-reactive antigen common to eosinophils of different animal species. Smaller granules lacking the crystalloid bar also are seen in eosinophils (Fig. 4-8).

Eosinophil granules contain many enzymes, including acid phosphatase, peroxidases, histaminase, aminopeptidase, ribonuclease, deoxyribonuclease, and proteinases.

Eosinophils possess ameboid motility and are phagocytic, but less so than neutrophils. Degranulation and oxidative metabolism are associated with phagocytosis, but these are less cytocidal than those of neutrophils.

Basophils

The basophils of human blood are 14 to 18 μm in diameter and are so named because their cytoplasm contains granules that are receptive to the basic dyes. Basophils constitute 1% or less of the white blood cells; there are perhaps 40 to 50 per cubic millimeter of human blood. The nucleus of basophils is not always well segmented and may be obscured by its numerous cytoplasmic granules (Figs. 4-9 and 4-10). The granules are 0.3 to 0.8 μm in diameter and round or oval in profile. On electron microscopy an indentation of the limiting membrane of the granules is noticeable. The inner structure of the granule is fine grained and consists of minute particles about 100 Å in diameter.

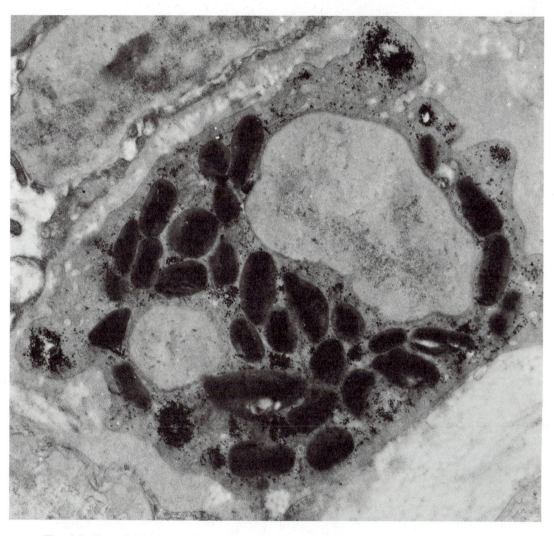

Fig. 4-8. Crystalloid bars can be seen by electron microscopy in many of the granules of this eosinophil. (Courtesy Dr. E. Adelstein.)

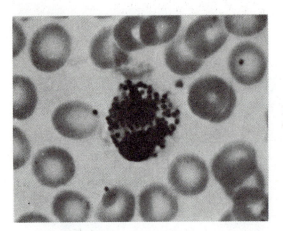

Fig. 4-9. Dense granules can be seen within basophils. (Courtesy Dr. E. Adelstein.)

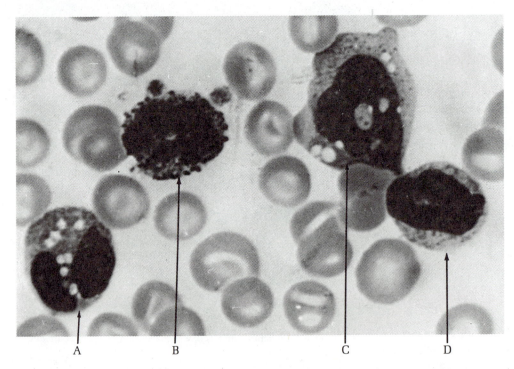

Fig. 4-10. The nucleated cells in this stained blood film illustrate their relative size and structure. *A*, Eosinophil; *B*, basophil; *C*, monocyte; *D*, lymphocyte. (Courtesy Dr. E. Adelstein.)

These granules are very important because they are delicate structures whose outer membrane is easily disrupted. When granulolysis occurs, the contents of the granule are released into the surrounding tissue and bloodstream. Among the important contents of the granule are heparin and histamine. Heparin is a powerful anticoagulant, and histamine is a vasoactive amine that contracts smooth muscle. These products also are found in tissue mast cells. Blood basophils contain 1 pg of histamine per cell, about one twentieth the histamine content of tissue mast cells but more than 20,000 times that of platelets. The histamine of blood basophils and mast cells contributes to the severity of the IgE-dependent allergies. Basophils are also important in basophilic cutaneous hypersensitivity reactions but have little or no phagocytic capacity.

PHAGOCYTOSIS
History

The Russian-born immunologist Metchnikoff is credited with the clarification of the relationship of phagocytosis to natural immunity. Metchnikoff's theories evolved from his observation in 1882 that starfish larvae possessed a group of highly mobile ameboid cells which congregated at points of inflammation, which he induced by inserting thorns into the animals. He also observed that these cells would engulf carmine particles and immediately suspected that they might devour other types of particles such as microbes and digest them. This supposition was supported by his observations of an infectious disease in the transparent water flea of the genus *Daphnia,* caused by the yeast *Monospora biscuspidata.* The outcome of this disease was directly related to whether phagocytic cells of the flea could destroy the yeasts, which was the case when the yeast inoculum was kept small. Overpopulation by yeasts after large inoculations resulted in the death of the fleas. Metchnikoff quickly expanded his research to higher animals and found phagocytosis to be an effective natural defense mechanism; he was awarded the Nobel Prize in 1908 for these studies.

The phagocytic process

Quantitating phagocytosis. To study phagocytosis, one must first decide what particles will be used as the subject particles. A wide choice of materials is available, including living or dead bacteria, living or dead yeasts, foreign erythrocytes, lipid emulsions, colloidal silver, colloidal carbon, iron oxide particles, spheres of polystyrene, polyacrylamide or methyl methacrylate, thorotrast, and others. These cells or particles may be radiolabeled to aid in tracing their in vivo behavior or to ease quantitation. Nonantigenic materials are preferred, since they preclude any possible contribution by the immune system. The particles should have a known and reasonable uniform size distribution, since larger particles are more easily ingested by phagocytic cells. The most widely chosen material is colloidal carbon in the form of washed india ink.

Since two classes of cells, the circulating cells and the fixed cells, are involved in phagocytosis, two separate procedures have been developed to measure their activity. Phagocytosis of circulating cells is most commonly studied in vitro. In this method whole blood or peritoneal washings treated with an anticoagulant are incubated with a suspension of bacterial cells or other particles in a 37° C water bath for a measured interval, usually 30 minutes. At the end of this time blood films are prepared and stained with Wright's or another appropriate stain and are examined microscopically. The average number of bacteria (or particles) per phagocytic cell is determined and reported as the phagocytic or opsonic index.

An in vivo phagocytic index, which measures primarily phagocytosis in the liver and spleen, also may be calculated. This usually is done by intravenous injection of an inert particle such as carbon or metal. Periodically thereafter blood samples are removed, and the concentration of the residual, free particle is determined. The phagocytic index is expressed as K where

$$K = \frac{\text{Log concentration at } T_1 - \text{Log concentration at } T_2}{T_2 - T_1}$$

and where T_1 and T_2 are the times at which the concentrations were determined. Corrections may be inserted for the body weights of different animals if comparative studies are desired. When this is done, most species of laboratory animals have phagocytic indexes within fivefold to tenfold of each other. In one experiment in which 8 mg of colloidal carbon was given to mice and rabbits for each 100 g of body weight, K mouse = 0.047 and K rabbit = 0.008. The explanation for the greater K value for mice is that they have a relatively larger liver: it is the liver Kupffer cells that take up 90% of injected materials. A correction for differences in liver size by the formula

$$\alpha = \frac{\text{Total body weight}}{\text{Weight of liver and spleen}} \cdot \sqrt[3]{K}$$

has been developed by Benacerraf from his experiments with phagocytosis. Application of this formula for corrected phagocytic index yields α mouse = 5.4 and α rabbit = 5.4; it is equally applicable to other species or situations.

Factors that influence phagocytosis

In vitro system. A number of physical parameters govern the rate or extent of phagocytosis. Clearly, before comparative studies between experimental and control groups or between species of animals are possible, the ratio and actual concentration of phagocytic and ingestible cells must be held constant. Stated more directly, physical contact between phagocytes and cells is necessary before this function can occur; simple dilution will decrease both the rate and extent of phagocytosis. Phagocytosis is a surface phenomenon. Slight changes in acidity or alkalinity, alterations in surface tension or ionic strength, and temperature displacement from 38° to 40° C all will decrease phagocytosis by interfering with the glycolytic system of the phagocytic cell and depriving it of the energy necessary to conduct this process, as was indicated earlier.

In general, physical forces detrimental to phagocyte vitality diminish phagocytosis. Those forces ensuring frequent or extended contact between the two cells will promote phagocytosis. The duration of contact between the phagocytic partners is increased by a number of normal serum factors. Chemotactic fractions of complement may operate to promote phagocytosis in this way. Antibody to the surface antigens of the cell to be engulfed is the single most stimulatory factor for phagocytic function.

In vivo system. Although many of the factors that alter the phagocytic index in vitro do the same in vivo, some of these effects have been more fully studied and thus are reserved for discussion under this latter category.

Reticuloendothelial blockade is most often studied in the in vivo system. It is possible to engorge the RES with inert colloidal particles, for example, carbon or thorotrast, prior to injection of bacteria. When this is done, the first response is one of marked depression in the phagocytic removal of bacteria from the bloodstream. This is followed in a few hours by total recovery or even hyperphagocytic activity. It has been suggested that this is the result of cell proliferation, but only circumstantial proof is available.

The injection of purified LPSs, which are the chemical equivalents of bacterial endotoxins, stimulates phagocytosis. Administration of cortisone and estrogens is also stimulatory. Certain fatty acid esters promote RES uptake of particles, but others have no effect or may depress the phagocytic index.

Chemotaxis. When one considers the phagocytic process from beginning to end, the first item is how the phagocytic cell and the victim cell or particle make contact. This requires little explanation if the victim cell is injected into the bloodstream, since immediate contact with the circulating granulocytes is possible. Moreover, as the blood passes through the internal organs, the fixed macrophages will have an opportunity to contact and engulf their prey. Because motile phagocytes do migrate toward bacteria and will accumulate at inflammatory loci in tissues even if microorganisms are not present, it is thought that bacteria and injured tissue cells excrete chemoattractants for phagocytes. Such substances are called chemotaxins or leukotaxins.

Methods for studying chemotaxis. Although it is often difficult to identify or characterize chemotaxins in vivo, the phenomenon of chemotaxis can be observed without undue difficulty. In experimental animals the ear window, which involves a small abrasion on the ear surface covered by a sterile microscopic coverglass, can be used. Cells that accumulate on the inflamed surface attach to the coverglass. The rate and type of phagocyte infiltration can be determined by periodic microscopic examinations. Presumed chemotaxins can be applied to the abraded skin to determine their influence on the rate, type, and numbers of phagocytic cells recovered on the coverglass.

Several techniques have evolved to facilitate the study of chemotaxis in vitro. The first and thus one of the most important of these was the development by Boyden of the chemotaxis chamber, of which there are now several physical modifications (Fig. 4-11). All consist of a chamber or tube that possesses two compartments. The upper compartment contains the cells to be analyzed for their chemotactic response, and the lower compartment contains the substance with presumed chemotactic activity. The two compartments are separated by a semipermeable filter with pores of a selected diameter, perhaps 5 or 8 μm, as chosen by the investigator. These pores are so small that phagocytic cells which exceed 10 μm in diameter can penetrate the filter only by active motility. After a brief incubation the filter is removed and stained to determine how many cells are present on its underside or, in the case of thick filters, how far through the filter the cells have migrated. These data are compared with those of control

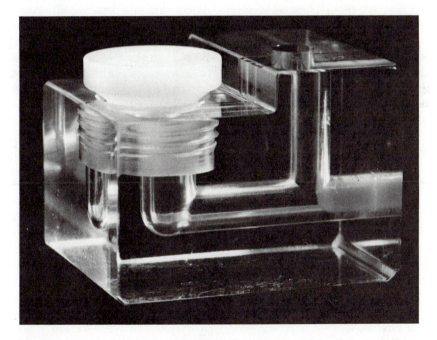

Fig. 4-11. Boyden's chemotaxis chamber. The cell preparation is placed in the hollow core of the white screw-type plug, which is holding a filter in place at its base. The putative chemotactic solution is in the tubular structure of the chamber below the plug and is held in the chamber by another plug at the right, invisible in photograph.

chambers to determine the chemotactic activity of the test substance (Fig. 4-12).

In another assay system plugs are cut and removed from an agarose gel formed in a petri dish. The phagocytic cell suspension is added to one reservoir and control solutions or presumed chemotaxins to neighboring reservoirs. During an ensuing incubation the phagocytes move through pores in the gel. Later this gel film can be stained and observed for the distance the cells have migrated from the reservoir toward the various solutions. By comparing the attractiveness of control and test solutions it is possible to calculate a chemotactic index.

Whichever method is chosen to measure chemotaxis, care must be taken to distinguish it from simple chemokinesis. Chemotaxis refers to directional motility and chemokinesis to an increase in random motility.

Chemotaxins. Chemical agents that promote the directional motility of cells are chemotaxins or leukotaxins. A partial list of chemotaxins active on selected leukocytes is as follows:

I. Monocytes/macrophages
  A. Soluble bacterial factors
  B. C5a
  C. C(5,6,7)
  D. T cell chemotaxin
  E. Tuftsin
  F. Cationic peptides from neutrophils

II. Neutrophils
  A. Soluble bacterial factors
  B. C5a
  C. C(5,6,7)
  D. Tuftsin
  E. Formyl peptides
  F. Thromboxane B_2
  G. 5-HETE
  H. 12-HETE

III. Eosinophils
  A. Soluble bacterial factors
  B. C5a
  C. C(5,6,7)
  D. ECF-A
  E. ECF-L

  F. Thromboxane B_2
  G. 12-HETE
  H. HHT
  I. Histamine
  J. Fibrin peptides

Chemotaxins do not always exist in an active form but may be derived from inert precursor molecules, the chemotaxinogens. The change is often the result of an enzyme hydrolysis of the chemotaxinogen to release the chemotaxin.

Although several chemotaxins stimulate several different types of phagocytic cells, others act on only one or a few of such cells. This may be caused by the absence of receptors for the chemotaxin on the cell surface, failure of the chemotaxin to penetrate the cell surface, or other factors.

Two chemotaxins are generated from the complement system. This results from the combination of antigens with certain isotypes of IgG or with IgM, which then activates the complement system. A cleavage product of the fifth component of complement is chemotactic for macrophages, neutrophils, eosinophils, and basophils. This molecule, C5a, is an example of a chemotaxin derived from a chemotaxinogen, C5. C5a is a protein with a molecular weight of approximately 11,000 and consists of 77 amino acids in a linear sequence. Its amino terminal arginine is critical to the anaphylatoxic role of C5a but not to its chemotactic role.

The characteristics of a second chemotaxin originating in the complement system somewhere in the C5, C6, C7 complex are still vague. It is active on macrophages, neutrophils, and eosinophils. It is not C5a, but its chemistry has not been defined yet.

Although there is a substantial amount of scientific literature ascribing a chemotactic function to C3a, a peptide derived from the third component of complement, this is now believed to be in error. The similarities of C3a and C5a did not allow purification of C3a without trace contamination by C5a, which is now considered the cause of chemotactic activity in C3a preparations.

Tuftsin is the name assigned in 1974 to a tetra-

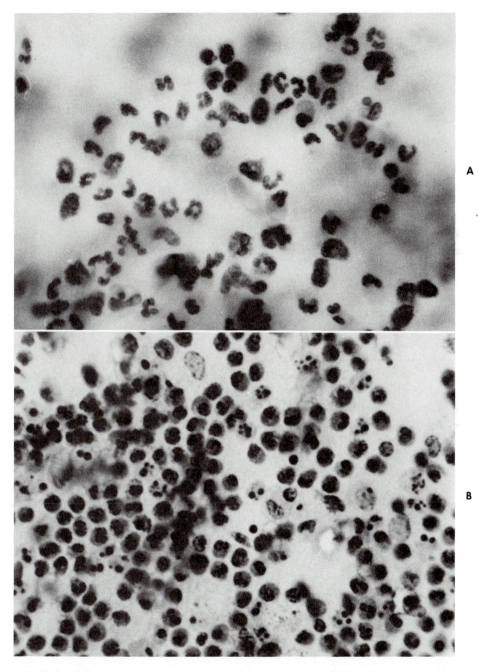

Fig. 4-12. A, Cells that have migrated through a chemotaxis control filter. **B,** Cells collected in the same manner in a positive experiment. The cell nuclei are stained well in both preparations, which eases the identification of the cells even though the cytoplasm is not well defined in **A.**

peptide discovered by researchers at Tufts University that was chemotactic for both granulocytes and macrophages. Tuftsin is a tetrapeptide consisting of Thr-Lys-Pro-Arg derived from a unique globulin described as leukokinin. The amino acid sequence of tuftsin is found at or near residues 289 through 292 in the crystallizable fragment (Fc) region of most γ-globulins. Tuftsin is released from globulins first by a cleavage at the carboxyl terminal side of the arginine followed by hydrolysis of a lysine-threonine bond by the enzyme leukokininase present on the outer membrane of macrophages and neutrophils.

Receptors for tuftsin present on neutrophils and macrophages bind the chemotaxin prior to its internalization. It has been suggested this is the same as the receptor for LPS. Tuftsin not only stimulates phagocyte motility but also improves antigen processing and aids oxidative metabolism of the cells, thus making them more cytocidal.

Peptides of low molecular weight in which the amino group on an amino terminal methionine is formylated are also chemotactic for human, rabbit, and guinea pig granulocytes. Formyl Met-Leu-Phe and formyl Met-Met-Phe are examples of these substituted tripeptides. The presence of the formyl group is critical, since the unsubstituted peptides are not chemotactic. These molecules stimulate the secretion of lysosomal enzymes and oxidative metabolism within granulocytes, in addition to being chemotactic.

Mast cells that undergo degranulation during allergic reactions release the eosinophil-specific ECF-A (eosinophilic chemotactic factor of anaphylaxis). Two tetrapeptides, Val-Gly-Ser-Glu and Ala-Gly-Ser-Glu from mast cells, demonstrate ECF-A activity. These peptides exist preformed in mast cell granules and are not synthesized just at the time of the allergic reaction. Because of their low molecular weight and amino acid structure, the ECF-A peptides are resistant to several proteases.

Fatty acids contained within the phospholipids of mammalian cell membranes are released by various stimuli. One of these fatty acids is a 20-carbon acid with four unsaturated bonds, that is, an eicosatetraenoic acid, better known by its common name arachidonic acid. Arachidonic acid is further metabolized by two separate pathways (Fig. 4-13). In the lipoxygenase pathway hydroxyl groups are added to form the hydroxyeicosatetraenoic (HETE) acids. Of these, the 12 hydroxy and 5 hydroxy (12-HETE and 5-HETE) are powerful chemotaxins for granulocytes. The leukotrienes in the B series are also chemotactic. (Leukotrienes [LT] C, D, and E are anaphylatoxic. See Chapter 18.) In the cyclooxygenase pathway both oxidative and cyclization reactions occur to produce the prostaglandins (PG), thromboxanes, and related compounds. Thromboxane B_2 and hydroxyheptatrienoic acid (HHT) both are derived from platelets, and both are chemotactic for neutrophils and eosinophils.

Antigen or mitogen stimulation of T lymphocytes causes them to release a chemotaxin that is active on macrophages. This chemotaxin has the electrophoretic mobility of an albumin and a molecular weight between 35,000 and 55,000. These characteristics separate this chemotaxin from lymphocyte-derived chemotactic factor (LDCF), which may be produced by either B or T lymphocytes and has a molecular weight of only 12,500. Another T cell–derived chemotaxin is also a low molecular weight protein (about 25,000 to 50,000 mol wt) and is referred to as ECF-L, since it is an eosinophilic chemotactic factor from lymphocytes.

Many bacteria produce chemotaxins during growth in culture or during infection. Several different capsular serotypes of *Streptococcus pneumoniae* produce a chemotaxin with a molecular weight of about 3,600. Unrelated bacteria such as those in the genus *Proteus* apparently produce the same leukotaxin. This substance obviously is not related to the capsular antigens of the diplococcus, which have long been accorded a negative or antichemotactic activity. *Staphylococcus aureus* produces a molecule whose molecular weight is less than 10,000, which is chemotactic.

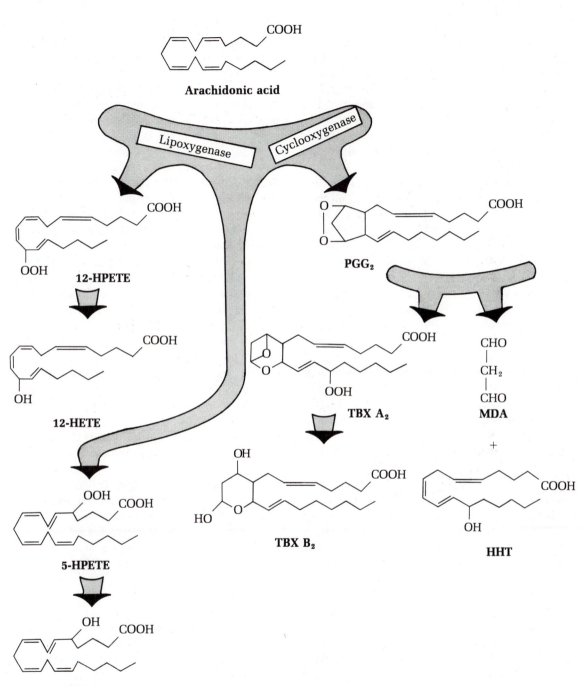

Fig. 4-13. In the metabolism of arachidonic acid by the lipoxygenase pathway two chemotaxins (*5-* and *12-HETE*) are produced. By the cyclooxygenase pathway, thromboxane B_2 *(TBX B_2)* and HHT are the chemotaxins produced.

A wide array of other compounds are also chemotactic. These include fibrin, collagen, lysosomal enzymes, kallikreins (proteases), bacterial endotoxin (LPS), and plasminogen activator.

Negative chemotaxis. Some substances are negatively chemotaxic; that is, they prevent the attraction of leukocytes to known active chemotactic agents. Some of these are outright cell poisons that interfere drastically with cellular functions involving energy metabolism. Examples are fluoride salts, arsenite ions, and iodoacetate, all three of which are inhibitors of the glycolytic system of the phagocytic cell. Phagocytic cells depend on anaerobic glycolysis for their main energy source; when this pathway is interrupted, chemotaxis fails. As a consequence, these chemicals prevent the migration of leukocytes toward the usual positively chemotactic compounds.

The virulence of several different bacteria can be equated with their resistance to phagocytosis. The most fully studied of these situations has been experimental infections of laboratory mice with *Streptococcus pneumoniae.* A single, encapsulated pneumococcus is sufficient to initiate a lethal infection for mice, which can resist infection by several thousand nonencapsulated bacteria. The most obvious difference in the behavior of these two bacterial cell types in vivo is the ease by which the unencapsulated organisms are phagocytosed and destroyed, whereas the encapsulated organisms are very resistant to phagocytosis. The capsule of these bacteria is totally polysaccharide, differing in chemistry from one antigenic type to another but usually consisting of D-glucose, D-glucuronic acid, and/or other simple monosaccharides.

The mechanism of chemotaxis. In the ameboid motility of phagocytes, actin filaments form just under the cell membrane. These serve as a microskeleton which becomes concentrated in the broad anterior lamellipodium of the cell and over which the cell draws its cytoplasm. Cytochalasin B is a drug that blocks the actin rearrangement and thus halts chemotaxis. Calcium ions are needed for the shortening of actin from its precursor, and any

action that halts a Ca^{2+} flux into the cell will depress chemotaxis. This is the structural basis for chemotaxis.

The chemical mechanism of chemotaxis is under continual study. The initial reports of the expression of new esterase activities in cells responding to chemotactic stimuli suggested that changes in the lipids of the cytoplasmic membrane could be correlated with the response. Agents that influence the intracellular cyclic nucleotides modulate chemotaxis. Decreasing cyclic adenosine monophosphate (cAMP) levels decreases chemotaxis, whereas increasing cyclic guanosine monophosphate (cGMP) levels increases chemotaxis. Methylation reactions are associated with chemotaxis, and the conversion of *S*-adenosyl-L-methionine to *S*-adenosyl-L-homocysteine is one reaction that has been identified. Exactly how this influences chemotaxis is unknown.

Cells gain their chemical energy for chemotaxis from anaerobic glycolysis by a shift to the aerobic oxidation of carbohydrates. This shift is also important in providing the cytotoxic forms of oxygen that are essential to intraphagocytic killing.

Attachment and opsonization. Contact between the phagocytic cell and its victim is not always sufficient to cause phagocytic engulfment. Some intended victims escape. This is reduced if phagocytosis takes place in a fibrin clot, on a blood vessel wall, or on another surface where the ameboid motion of the phagocyte favors recontact of the two cells. Phagocytosis is a surface phenomenon and is much less efficient in a fluid medium.

Molecular factors that promote attachment of phagocytes and the object they will engulf are called opsonins (from the Greek word that means to prepare for eating). The earlier term *bacteriotropin,* once almost synonymous with opsonin, is outdated.

The most potent opsonins are immunoglobulins, and these can be considered from two viewpoints. The immunoglobulins that bind to the surface of neutrophils, macrophages, and eosinophils are predominantly IgG1 and IgG3. These cytophilic antibodies, when possessed with specificity for an engulfable antigen (such as bacteria, yeast, virus, and erythrocyte), bind its exposed antigenic determinants and hold the antigen only one molecule in length from the phagocyte surface. This binding is possible because the Fc portions of IgG1 and IgG3 are the parts held to the phagocyte, leaving its antigen-binding fragments (Fab) free to attach to antigen.

Humoral antibodies that attach to bacteria encourage phagocytosis by neutralizing ionic charges on the bacterial cell surface, making them more approachable by the phagocyte. The negative chemotactic force of encapsulated bacteria such as the pneumococcus, *Klebsiella pneumoniae,* and *Hemophilus influenzae* clearly is related to their capsule; nonencapsulated variants are easy prey for phagocytic cells. But when the capsules of the pathogenic form of these bacteria are coated with antibodies, they are no longer able to repel phagocytes and are as easily engulfed as the nonencapsulated forms.

The opsonic activity of circulating antibodies is largely caused by IgG and IgM, with the latter being about 500- to 1,000-fold more potent than the former in stimulating phagocytosis of bacteria. This may reflect only the tendency of polysaccharide capsular and somatic antigens to favor IgM formation, since gram-negative bacteria and encapsulated pneumococci often were used as the phagocytic subjects in these studies.

When complement component C3 is split to release the anaphylatoxin C3a during serologic reactions, the residue C3b remains attached to the antigen-antibody complex. Both cytophilic and circulating immunoglobulins can initiate reactions leading to C3b formation. In addition, C3b can be formed from the alternate pathway of complement activation that is initiated by complex oligosaccharides such as those found on the surface of bacteria in the form of teichoic acids, LPS, or bacterial capsules. Receptors for C3b that adheres to antigen surfaces also are found on phagocytic cells. In this way C3b links the phagocytic cell

with its victim and serves as an important opsonin.

A number of other substances have been described as opsonins. Fibronectin, one of the most recent of these, is a serum glycoprotein with a molecular weight of about 200,000 to 250,000. Fibronectin can exist also in a dimeric form. Macrophages synthesize fibronectin, and this is believed to aid their phagocytosis. When serum levels of fibronectin fall, after surgery or burns, phagocytic activity falls. Many other proteins, when added to simple buffers used to study phagocytosis in vitro, will stimulate phagocytosis and could be described as opsonins, although their activity is far below that of the molecules previously described.

Engulfment. Exactly how the phagocytosed particle is taken into the cell without rupturing the cytoplasmic membrane of the phagocyte continues to be a mystery. The phagocyte cell cytoplasm apparently flows completely around the engulfed cell and fuses with itself. The victim cell is held inside this phagocytic vesicle, or phagosome, which is surrounded by an everted cell membrane cover. This phagosome is displaced centrally, and contact with cytoplasmic lysosomal granules occurs. Fusion of the lysosome and phagosome follows, and the lysosome disintegrates, releasing a multitude of hydrolytic enzymes into what is now referred to as the phagolysosome.

Intracellular killing

The original concept that hydrolytic enzymes released from lysosomes were responsible for the cytocidal events within phagocytes now has been largely abandoned. Instead attention has been directed at oxygen-dependent and oxygen-independent avenues for cell death, with the former being the most fully explored.

Oxygen-dependent reactions. The resting phagocytes, with the exception of the alveolar macrophage, use anaerobic glycolysis as their major energy source. In this pathway of carbohydrate metabolism sugars are converted to lactic acid, and no oxygen is consumed. During and after the phagocytic act the phagocytes begin to consume oxygen as they shift their pathway of carbohydrate metabolism to the greater energy-yielding hexose monophosphate (HMP) shunt (Fig. 4-14). Associated with this pathway is the enzyme nicotinamide-adenine dinucleotide phosphate (NADPH) oxidase, which removes a hydrogen from NADPH to form $NADP^+$ while simultaneously converting ordinary oxygen (O_2) to the superoxide radical ($\cdot O_2^-$), which is an anion. The superoxide anion is a one electron–reduction product of oxygen; it has an unpaired electron and is very reactive, which is typical of free radicals. The enzyme superoxide dismutase scavenges these radicals and converts them to hydrogen peroxide (H_2O_2) and singlet oxygen ($^1O_2$). The superoxide dismutase reaction is:

$$\cdot O_2^- + \cdot O_2^- + 2H^+ \rightarrow H_2O_2 + {}^1O_2$$

An indication that $\cdot O_2^-$ acts as a microbicide within phagocytes is found in experiments in which phagocytes fed superoxide dismutase bound to engulfable particles were less cytocidal.

The H_2O_2 produced by superoxide dismutase is degraded by another enzyme, myeloperoxidase, in the presence of Cl^- or I^- to produce hypochlorite (OCl^-) or hypoiodite (OI^-).

$$H_2O_2 + Cl^- \rightarrow H_2O + OCl^-$$

When radioactive I_2 was added to mixtures of phagocytes and bacteria, the bacteria became iodinated as they were being killed. Hypochlorite is a known bactericide; it is the agent produced by chlorine used to purify drinking water.

Hypochlorite ions and hydrogen peroxide interact spontaneously to produce water, the chloride ion, and singlet oxygen.

$$OCl^- + H_2O_2 \rightarrow H_2O + Cl^- + {}^1O_2$$

Ordinary oxygen has two unpaired electrons that rotate in the same direction. A shift of the elec-

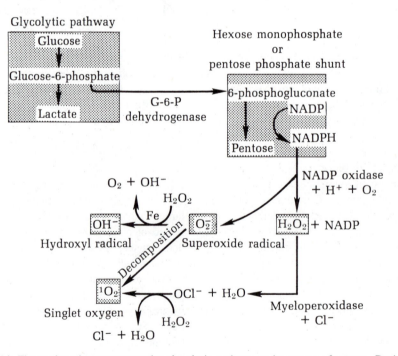

Fig. 4-14. The resting phagocyte uses the glycolytic pathway as its source of energy. During and after phagocytosis it shifts to the hexose monophosphate (HMP) shunt. This enables the cell to accumulate several potent oxidizing agents, which can contribute to cell killing.

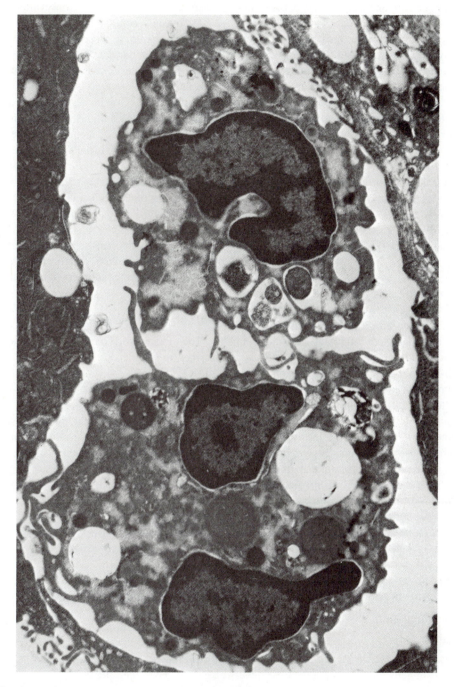

Fig. 4-15. These two neutrophils seen in an electron microscopic photograph have depleted their cytoplasmic granules during phagocytosis. The upper cell contains bacteria at different levels of destruction in the phagolysosomes just below its nucleus.

trons to a higher orbit and an inversion of the directional spin of one electron creates singlet oxygen. When singlet oxygen returns to its ground state of ordinary oxygen, light is emitted. This chemoluminescence is observed during phagocytosis. Certain dyes and carotenoid pigments that react with $^1O_2$ absorb its energy and quench this luminescence. Bacteria that contain a high concentration of carotenoid pigments are more resistant to intraphagocytic death than are cells that lack carotenoids.

One other toxic form of oxygen is produced within phagocytes when hydrogen peroxide reacts with the superoxide radical in the presence of iron. The products are oxygen, hydroxyl ions, and the hydroxyl radical ($\cdot OH$).

$$\cdot O_2^- + H_2O_2 \rightarrow O_2 + OH^- + \cdot OH$$

The hydroxyl radical is a one electron–reduction product of hydrogen peroxide and is the most potent oxidizing agent produced in biologic systems. Thus it is considered an important contributor to intraphagocytic killing.

Oxygen-independent reactions. The intracellular accumulation of lactic acid and the lowering of the pH to about 4.5 within the phagosome create a definite bacteriostatic if not bactericidal pH. The enzyme lysozyme that can hydrolyze the cell wall of gram-positive bacteria is present within phagocytic cells. Cationic proteins within these cells may bind to the surface of microorganisms, most of which are negatively charged, and interfere with cell transport functions. Phagocytin, although still poorly described, is a unique cytocidal agent. Transferrin that is contained within phagocytes and lactoferrin bind iron and remove it from the nutrient supply of microbes, thus preventing their growth.

Intracellular digestion

Nonviable antigens within phagocytes are quickly digested within the phagolysosome. Viable, cellular antigens are digested after their death from exposure to toxic forms of oxygen and the oxygen-independent pathways. Many living microbes are resistant to lysosomal enzymes and become sensitive to them only after cell death.

Lysosomes contain a vast array of hydrolytic enzymes, including those which are active on proteins, polysaccharides, nucleic acids, lipids, and other biopolymers. Among these enzymes and substances are β-acetylglucosamine hydrolase, acid phosphatase, acid ribonuclease, acid deoxyribonuclease, arylsulfatase, cathepsin, collagenase, cytochrome c reductase, elastase, esterases, β-galactosidase, α-glucosidase, β-glucuronidase, hyaluronidase, lipase, lysozyme, α-mannosidase, neuraminidase, and phagocytin.

These enzymes ultimately digest the phagolysosomal contents until they are unrecognizable debris (Fig. 4-15). These residual bodies at different stages of digestion are seen within active phagocytes. Meanwhile the phagocyte regenerates its lysosomes in preparation for the next phagocytic event.

Phagocytic deficiency disease

The phagocytic deficiency diseases are described in Chapter 22.

Secretory function of macrophages: monokines

Low molecular weight proteins secreted by monocytes and lymphocytes that act on other host cells are referred to as monokines and lymphokines, respectively. These secretory products of macrophages are the following:

  I. Enzymes
    A. Arginase
    B. Lysozyme
    C. Collagenase
    D. Elastase
    E. Cathepsins
    F. Plasminogen activator
    G. Esterases
    H. Acid hydrolases
    I. Angiotensin-converting enzyme
 II. Products of oxygen
    A. Hydrogen peroxide
    B. Hydroxyl radical
    C. Singlet oxygen
III. Complement components

A. C1q

B. C2

C. C3

D. C4

E. C5

F. A·C3bINAC

G. C3bINAC

H. Factor B

I. Properdin

IV. Miscellaneous

A. Arachidonic acid derivatives

B. IFN

C. IL-1 and IL-2

D. Pyrogenic factor

Most of these molecules are incompletely described in chemical terms, but this is being improved, and it will be possible to add this information to what is now largely a description of biologic activities. In addition, certain of these molecules are produced both by monocytes and lymphocytes and can justly be described as both or either monokines or lymphokines. Some resolution of this problem has come from the suggestion that those kines which are derived from and act on other white blood cells be called interleukins.

IL-1. A macrophage-derived peptide previously known as lymphocyte-activating factor, B cell–activating factor, macrophage-derived T cell–replacing factor, and a host of other descriptive terms is now designated as *interleukin 1* (IL-1). Biochemical studies of mouse and human IL-1 indicate it is a protein with a molecular weight in the range of 12,000 to 16,000. The mouse protein has a more acidic isoelectric point (near 5) than the human product, whose isoelectric point is approximately 7. Isoelectric heterogeneity of highly purified murine IL-1 has identified three biologically active forms, IL-1α, β, and γ, all of which have isoelectric point values near 5. The amino acid composition of the α molecule has been determined, and its relatively high content of aspartic and glutamic acids is consistent with its isoelectric point.

IL-1 from macrophages has several biologic activities, as indicated by its several synonyms: the activation of B lymphocytes, stimulation of Th cells, and the replacement of or stimulation of cytotoxic T cells (CTC cells). These activities are neither antigen nor histocompatibility restricted; that is, the B cell or T cell response to any antigen is sensitive to IL-1, which functions across animal strain and species barriers. Monocytes and macrophages produce IL-1 when stimulated by antigens or mitogens.

IL-2. IL-2 is also an antigen-unrestricted, genetically unrestricted, antigen- or mitogen-induced product of macrophages but is also produced by T cells. Among the earlier synonyms of IL-2 were killer cell helper factor, T cell mitogenic factor, and T cell growth factor (TCGF), and the latter has remained as popular as IL-2. Mouse IL-2 has a molecular weight near 30,000 and an isoelectric point between pH 4 and 5. IL-2 from other species may be quite different; gibbon IL-2 has a reported molecular weight of 21,500. IL-2 is of considerable interest because it will prolong the growth period of T cells in culture.

Interferons. Low molecular, nonantibody lymphocyte-derived peptides that interfere with viral replication are termed interferons (IFN). Monocytes also produce IFN, but these are described in a later chapter with the lymphokines.

Other macrophage products. An extensive list of products released by macrophages can be cited, but these are not active on other leukocytes, lack a specific activity on such cells, and thus are not classified as lymphokines. This list would include virtually all the lysosomal enzymes, complement factors C1q, C2, C3, C4, C5, and C7, factor B, or C3 proactivator, properdin, C3bINAC (C3b inactivator), plasminogen activator, arachidonic acid derivatives (PGs and prostacyclins), fatty acids, leukocyte pyrogens, and others.

BIBLIOGRAPHY

Beeson, P.B., and Bass, D.A.: The eosinophil, Philadelphia, 1977, W.B. Saunders Co.

Butterworth, A.E., and David, J.R.: Eosinophil function, N. Engl. J. Med. **304:**154, 1981.

Carr, I.: The macrophage: a review of ultrastructure and function, New York, 1973, Academic Press, Inc.

Carr, I.: The biology of macrophages, Clin. Invest. Med. **1**:59, 1978.

Carr, I., and Daems, W.T.: The reticuloendothelial system: a comprehensive treatise, vol. 1, Morphology, New York, 1980, Plenum Publishing Corp.

Cline, M.J.: The white cell, Cambridge, Mass., 1975, Harvard University Press.

Cohen, S., Pick, E., and Oppenheim, J.J., editors: Biology of the lymphokines, New York, 1979, Academic Press, Inc.

de Weck, A.L., Kristensen, F., and Landy, M., editors: Biochemical characterization of lymphokines, New York, 1980, Academic Press, Inc.

Escobar, M.R., and Friedman, H., editors: Macrophages and lymphocytes: nature, functions, and interaction, New York, 1980, Plenum Publishing Corp.

Friedman, P.S.: The immunobiology of Langerhans cells, Immunol. Today **2**:124, 1981.

Gabig, T.G., and Babior, B.M.: The killing of pathogens by phagocytes, Annu. Rev. Med. **32**:313, 1981.

Gadebusch, H.H., editor: Phagocytes and cellular immunity, Boca Raton, Fla., 1979, CRC Press, Inc.

Gallin, J.I., and Quie, P.G., editors: Leukocyte chemotaxis: methods, physiology, and clinical implications, New York, 1978, Raven Press.

Greenwalt, T.J., and Jamieson, G.A., editors: The granulocyte: function and clinical utilization, New York, 1977, Alan R. Liss, Inc.

Güttler, F., Seakins, J.W.T., and Harkness, R.A., editors: Inborn errors of immunity and phagocytosis, Baltimore, 1979, University Park Press.

Havemann, K., and Janoff, A., editors: Neutral proteases of human polymorphonuclear leukocytes, Baltimore, 1978, Urban & Schwarzenberg, Inc.

Herscowitz, H.B., and others, editors: Manual of macrophage methodology: collection, characterization, and function, New York, 1981, Marcel Dekker, Inc.

Hocking, W.G., and Golde, D.W.: The pulmonary-alveolar macrophage, N. Engl. J. Med. **301**:580, 639, 1979.

Klebanoff, S.J.: Oxygen metabolism and the toxic properties of phagocytes, Ann. Intern. Med. **93**:480, 1980.

Klebanoff, S.J., and Clark, R.A.: The neutrophil: function and clinical disorders, Amsterdam, 1978, Elsevier/North Holland Biomedical Press.

Lisiewicz, J.: Human neutrophils, Bowie, Md., 1980, Charles Press Publishers, Inc.

Mahmoud, A.A.F., and Austen, K.F., editors: The eosinophil in health and disease, New York, 1980, Grune & Stratton, Inc.

Möller, G., editor: Accessory cells in the immune response, Immunol. Rev. **53**:3, 1980.

Murphy, P.: The neutrophil, New York, 1976, Plenum Publishing Corp.

Najjar, V.A., and Schmidt, J.J.: The chemistry and biology of tuftsin, Lymphokine Rep. **1**:157, 1980.

Natelson, S., Pesce, A.J., and Dietz, A.A., editors: Clinical immunochemistry, Washington, D.C., 1978, American Association of Clinical Chemists, Inc.

Neidel, J.E., and Cuatrecasas, P.: Formyl peptide chemotactic receptors of leukocytes and macrophages, Curr. Top. Cell. Regul. **17**:138, 1980.

Nelson, D.S., editor: Immunobiology of the macrophage, New York, 1976, Academic Press, Inc.

O'Flaherty, J.T., and Ward, P.A.: Chemotactic factors and the neutrophil, Semin. Hematol. **16**:163, 1979.

Quastel, M.R., editor: Cell biology and immunology of leukocyte function, New York, 1979, Academic Press, Inc.

Quie, P.G., Mills, E.L., and Holmes, B.: Molecular events during phagocytosis by human neutrophils, Prog. Hematol. **10**:193, 1977.

Rocklin, R.E., Bendtzen, K., and Greineder, D.: Mediators of immunity: lymphokines and monokines, Adv. Immunol. **29**:56, 1980.

Rosenthal, A.S.: Regulation of the immune response—role of the macrophage, N. Engl. J. Med. **303**:1153, 1980.

Sbarra, A.J., and Strauss, R.R., editors: The reticuloendothelial system, vols. 1 and 2, New York, 1980, Plenum Publishing Corp.

Schadelin, J., Schadelin, R., and Mandell, G.L.: Chemiluminescence of phagocytic cells, CRC Crit. Rev. Clin. Lab. Sci. **13**:1, 1981.

Schiffman, E., and Gallin, J.L.: Biochemistry of phagocyte chemotaxis, Curr. Top. Cell. Regul. **15**:203, 1979.

Siskind, G.W., Litwin, S.D., and Weksler, M.E., editors: Developmental immunobiology, New York, 1979, Grune & Stratton, Inc.

Synderman, R., and Goetzl, E.J.: Molecular and cellular mechanisms of leukocyte chemotaxis, Science **213**:830, 1981.

Unanue, E.R.: Secretory function of mononuclear phagocytes: a review, Am. J. Pathol. **83**:396, 1976.

Unanue, E.R., and Rosenthal, A.S., editors: Macrophage regulation of immunity, New York, 1980, Academic Press, Inc.

VanOss, C.J., Gillman, C.F., and Neuman, A.W.: Phagocytic engulfment and cell adhesiveness as cellular surface phenomena, New York, 1975, Marcel Dekker, Inc.

Vernon-Roberts, B.: The macrophage, Cambridge, England, 1972, Cambridge University Press.

Waksman, B.H.: Atlas of experimental immunobiology and immunopathology, New Haven, Conn., 1970, Yale University Press.

Waldman, R.H., editor: Clinical concepts of immunology, Baltimore, 1979, Williams & Wilkins Co.

Weller, P.F., and Goetzl, E.J.: The regulatory and effector roles of eosinophils, Adv. Immunol. **27**:339, 1979.

Weller, P.F., and Goetzl, E.J.: The human eosinophil: roles in defense and tissue injury, Am. J. Pathol. **100**:791, 1980.

Wilkinson, P.C.: Chemotaxis and inflammation, Edinburgh, 1974, Churchill Livingstone.

THE B AND T LYMPHOCYTES

GLOSSARY

B cell A lymphocyte from the bursa of Fabricius or that is of the immunoglobulin-forming type.

bursa of Fabricius A cloacal organ in fowl from which the immunoglobulin-synthesizing B lymphocytes originate.

capping phenomenon The movement of antigens on the surface of B lymphocytes to a single locus.

central lymphoid tissue Bone marrow, thymus, and bursa of Fabricius.

Con A Concanavalin A.

concanavalin A A mitogen highly specific for T lymphocytes.

CTC A cytotoxic T cell.

FTS Facteur thymique serique (serum thymic factor).

GALT Gut-associated lymphoid tissue.

helper cell A subclass of T cells that assist B cells in antibody formation.

immunoblast A cell intermediate between the lymphocyte and plasma cell.

lectin An agglutinin of plant origin.

lymphocyte The agranular leukocyte with sparse cytoplasm and round nucleus derived from the thymus (T type) or bone marrow or bursa (B type) found in lymph, lymph nodes, blood, spleen, etc.

lymphocyte transformation The active nucleic acid metabolism and nuclear enlargement of a lymphocyte on contact with antigen.

Lyt marker An antigen marker on T lymphocytes.

memory cell A cell that responds more quickly to the second exposure to antigen than to the primary exposure and is responsible for the anamnestic response.

mitogen A substance that stimulates mitosis.

peripheral lymphoid tissue Lymphoid tissues other than bone marrow, thymus, and bursa.

PHA Phytohemagglutinin.

phytohemagglutinin An extract of plant, usually legumes, that will agglutinate erythrocytes.

plasma cell A cell 10 to 20 μm in diameter that can actively synthesize immunoglobulins and can be distinguished morphologically from similar cells.

rosette technique 1. A test involving antibody-producing or antibody binding cells and a cellular antigen. 2. Adsorption of normal T cells to sheep erythrocytes.

runt disease A graft-versus-host (GVH) reaction in a newborn animal exposed to immunocompetent graft tissue.

suppressor cell A subclass of T cells that suppresses the capacity of B cells to become immunoglobulin producers.

T lymphocyte A thymus-derived lymphocyte that is responsible for cell-mediated hypersensitivity.

Tc A cytotoxic T cell.

Tdh A T cell that participates in delayed hypersensitivity (DH) reactions.

Th A helper-inducer cell.

Thy 1 antigen An antigen found on T cells.

thymopoietin A thymic hormone.

thymosin A hormonelike substance from thymus believed to be the active component of T lymphocytes.

thymus A gland located near the parathyroid and thyroid whose lymphocytes (T type) regulate cell-mediated hypersensitivity and interact with B cells for immunoglobulin formation.

Ts A suppressor cell.

wasting disease A failure to grow or thrive in neonatally thymectomized animals.

terms of the central and peripheral lymphoid tissues. The two central lymphoid tissues of mammals are bone marrow and thymus. Lymph nodes, spleen, tonsil, intestinal lymphoid tissue (Peyer's patches), and other collections of lymphocytes constitute the peripheral lymphoid tissues. In addition to marrow and thymus, fowl have a third central lymphoid organ, the bursa of Fabricius, which is critical to the development of immunoglobulin-producing cells.

The central lymphoid organs

Bone marrow. The structure of bone marrow is described in the section on hematopoietic tissue in Chapter 4.

THE LYMPHOID SYSTEM

The lymphocyte is the dominant cell of the lymphoid system, which is generally discussed in

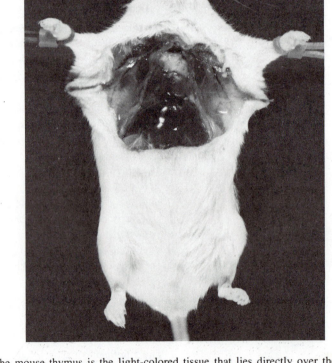

Fig. 5-1. The mouse thymus is the light-colored tissue that lies directly over the heart. The bilobed nature of the mouse thymus is not easily seen here, since the left lobe is lying over the right lobe. (Courtesy T. Ellis.)

Thymus. The human thymus is a flat, bilobed organ situated below the thyroid gland along the neck and extending into the thoracic cage. In the mouse it is also bilobate and lies over the heart (Fig. 5-1). In some species the thymus tissue is distributed along the neck and thorax in several small lobules. In the chicken and other fowl the thymus is a multilobed structure rarely extending into the thoracic cavity and usually lying along the neck (Fig. 5-2). Likewise the guinea pig thymus is basically extrathoracic, but it exists as a single major lobe. The thymus emerges from the third and fourth branchial pouches during embryonic development and is a fully developed organ at birth. At this time the human thymus will weigh 15 to 20 g. By puberty it will reach 40 g, after which it will atrophy, becoming less significant structurally and functionally. Atrophy of the thymus with age is a characteristic of all species.

Anatomically the thymus may be considered as a pouch of epithelial cells filled with lymphocytes (the thymic, or T, lymphocytes, in contrast to the bursal, or B, lymphocytes), nourished and drained by the vascular and lymphatic systems. The epithelial cells and other structural cells divide the thymus into a complex assembly of continuous lobes, each of which is heavily laden with lymphocytes. The lymphocyte population is greatest in the cortex, or outer portion, of each lobule, whereas the inner section, the medulla, is relatively free of these important cells. The medullary portion is continuous from one lobe to another, and, in addition to its content of vascular structures, reticulum cells, and lymphocytes, it is the most common site for the thymic corpuscles known as Hassall's corpuscles. These are concentric, cellular structures that stain lightly and have as yet no functional identity; however, they are a histologic hallmark of thymus tissue.

The thymic cortex, between the septa, is rich in lymphocytes of all sizes. These thymocytes are not morphologically distinguishable from lymphocytes in other tissues, but they are antigenically identifiable by the presence of the Thy 1 antigen,

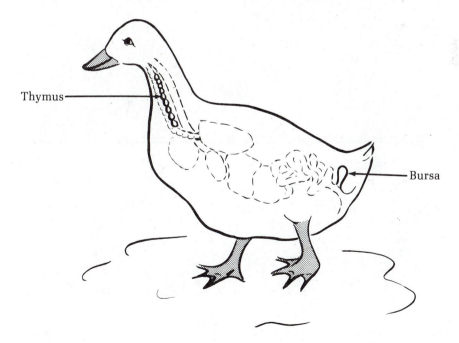

Fig. 5-2. The bursa of Fabricius is present in the cloacal region. The avian thymus is a multilobed structure laying along the esophagus.

a distinctive surface marker antigen that separates them from B lymphocytes. Not all lymphocytes in the thymus are T cells; some are B cells, but B cells represent only a minor portion of the whole. The thymus relies on the bone marrow as the source of the T cell precursors, which differentiate and become T cells in the thymus.

The nude mouse. The nude mouse is a hairless mouse with the combined genetic fault of an inability to grow hair or to develop a thymus (Fig. 5-3). In 1968 this strain of mouse was observed to produce paired thymus sacs in the normal anatomic position, but the glands were devoid of lymphocytes. The thymic-dependent areas of the lymph nodes also are lacking in T cells. Nude mice are not absolutely lacking in T cells; usually a few can be detected in peripheral blood, but this is rarely as much as 5% of the total lympho-

cyte population. It generally is not possible to note a mitogenic effect of concanavalin A (Con A) or phytohemagglutinin (PHA) in nude mice, although LPS, a B cell stimulant, is as active in nude as in normal mice. Thymus grafts into nude mice will restore the normal T cell population, and it has been determined that these are of nude mouse, not donor mouse, origin. Bone marrow grafts from nude mice to normal mice that have had their thymus irradiated will repopulate the recipient with T cells. These experiments indicate there is no stem cell defect in the nude mouse, only a defect in the maturation of these stem cells.

Nude mice, although customarily cited as being immunodeficient only in the T cell–related activities, also have lowered immunoglobulin levels compared with their normal littermates. The IgA and IgG1 concentration in nude mouse sera is less

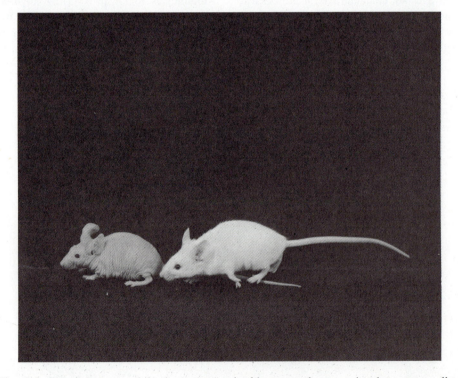

Fig. 5-3. The nude mouse *(left),* here compared with a normal mouse, has been an excellent source of information about the role of the thymus in immunology, since it lacks this organ. (Courtesy Dr. H. Mullen.)

than 10% of that of controls. IgG2a and IgG2b are reduced to about 20% of the level of normal littermates. The IgM levels are not influenced by the T cell loss. As might be expected, nude mice respond typically to T cell–independent antigens, including LPS, pneumococcal type 3 capsule, and dinitrophenyl flagellin.

Since nude mice are more severely penalized in the T arm of their immune response than in the B arm, they often are discounted as mixed immunodeficients and considered only as T cell deficient.

Bursa of Fabricius. The bursa of Fabricus is a lymphoid organ situated near the terminal end of the gut in fowl; higher animals do not possess a bursa (Reading 2; Fig. 5-2). It is a saclike structure about 3 cm in diameter at the time of its maximal development, when the chicken is about 4 months of age. After that time the bursa begins to atrophy. A cross section of a young bursa reveals that it, like the thymus, is subdivided into follicles. Within each follicle there are cells of many types, among the most prominent being macrophages, lymphocytes, and plasma cells. The lymphocytes are morphologically similar to the lymphocytes seen in the thymus but differ significantly from them in function. These are the B (bursal) cells, which have their own unique antigen, the β, or B, antigen, which they acquire in the bursa. B cells lack the Thy 1 antigen. The bursa relies on the bone marrow as the source of the precursor cells that will eventually become B cells.

Mammals do not have a bursa, yet they have lymphocytes that perform the same functions as B lymphocytes and which are given the same name. As one might imagine, there has been a considerable research effort toward identifying the bursal equivalent in mammals. One line of inquiry assumed that the bursal equivalent, like the bursa, might reside along the gastrointestinal tract. Removal of gut-associated lymphoid tissue (GALT) early in the life of experimental animals will impair their immunoglobulin response. Because of this severe effect on the physiologic homoestasis of the animal, it remains somewhat uncertain if GALT is the bursal equivalent. Bone marrow is used as a source of B cells in most experimental studies.

The peripheral lymphoid organs

The central lymphoid organs are not a repository of lymphocytes. These cells leave the thymus and bursa, pass through the bloodstream, and enter the tissues, including a reentry into the thymus and bursa. Some of these tissues are dominated by a lymphoid structure and are collectively termed the *peripheral lymphoid organs*. The most prominent organs of this type are the spleen and lymph nodes, but others, including the tonsils and appendix, have a pronounced lymphocytic character.

Lymph nodes. Lymph nodes are complex, cellular stations situated along the lymphatic ducts, which lead from the tissue to the thoracic duct and empty into the circulatory system just as the vessels enter the heart. Each node serves as a central collecting point for the lymph from a discrete, adjacent anatomic region. Lymph nodes are numerous near the joints and where the arms and legs join the body. Some animals, notably fowl, are almost totally lacking in lymph nodes. All lymph nodes are irregular spheres surrounded by a tough capsule and often embedded in adipose tissue (Fig. 5-4). Afferent lymph ducts carry lymph into the gland that serves partially as a filtering or settling basin. The macrophages, granulocytes, and lymphocytes flow slowly through the gland because of the reduction in flow created by the vast spongelike meshwork arrangement of the gland. This reticular meshwork provides the surface on which macrophages may impinge and phagocytose antigens arriving from the tissue. The lymphocytes are gathered into follicles or nodules in the cortex. Lymphocytes are also present in the medullary portion of the gland, but here the septa between the follicles are inapparent. This anatomic similarity of thymus, bursa, and lymph nodes is very striking. The T lymphocyte is more apt to reside in the medullary region and the B lymphocytes in the cortical region of lymph nodes. The T lym-

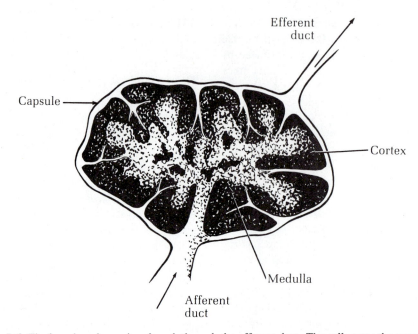

Fig. 5-4. The lymph node receives lymph through the afferent duct. The cells enter the spongelike lobules and concentrate according to their specificity for the cortex (B cell region) or medulla (T cell region) and then leave by way of the efferent duct.

phocytes proliferate on antigenic stimulation and create germinal centers after antigenic stimulation, but these are situated nearer the center of the node than are B cell germinal centers, which are cortical or far cortical in location. T cell germinal centers contain macrophages, growing T lymphocytes, and smaller adult lymphocytes, but no plasma cells.

The function of the lymph node as a filtering basin for infectious organisms collected from the surrounding tissue is demonstrated by the observation that areas of local inflammation caused by infectious bacteria or fungi often progress up the lymph channels and produce reddened and swollen cords extending up the arms or legs. This is customarily followed by an enlargement of the lymph nodes as they concentrate the infectious organisms. In instances in which the infection is not successfully combated, the lymph nodes may even suppurate and drain to form open lesions; but the more frequent situation is that these swollen and

tender nodes gradually subside as healing takes place, in large part resulting from local phagocytosis and antibody production. Basically this same scene is repeated when antigens of any type are deposited in the tissue. The lymph node enlarges, and phagocytosis and antibody formation—the prime functions of lymph nodes—are a part of this continuum.

Spleen. The spleen, situated in the abdominal cavity, may be ovoid or rather fingerlike in shape, depending on the species. It is a vital organ early in the life of an animal, but the spleen may be removed from adults without much influence on normal health. Nevertheless the spleen does contribute to several important body functions, particularly the removal of aged cells of most classes but especially erythrocytes, the phagocytosis of blood-borne particles and antigens, and the synthesis of immunoglobulins. Except for the splenic removal of erythrocytes, these same functions are carried out by the lymph nodes. What the

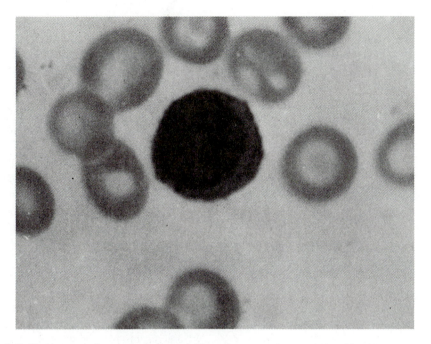

Fig. 5-5. The large nucleus and small rim of cytoplasm are characteristic of lymphocytes as they appear in blood films. (Courtesy Dr. E. Adelstein.)

lymph node is to the lymphatic system, the spleen is to the circulatory system.

The spleen has a fibrous outer capsule enclosing the body of the organ. Traditionally the spleen is considered to be composed of two parts: the red pulp and the white pulp. The red pulp is well supplied with arteries and is that portion of the organ in which injured erythrocytes are engulfed by phagocytic cells and destroyed. The red pulp usually constitutes about 50% of the organ, but this and the size of the spleen can change dramatically in disease states. The white pulp contains nodules or follicles of lymphocytes surrounding the lymphatic sheaths. On repeated antigenic stimulation germinal centers develop in the white pulp, where lymphocytes, plasma cells, and their important cell products are fabricated. Although T lymphocytes may be found in the spleen, its function as a B cell–containing organ is more evident.

Other lymphoid organs. The tonsils are lymphoid tissues that, like the thymus, are rather large

in childhood and tend to diminish in size with age. The internal structure of tonsils is very reminiscent of the thymus, bursa, and lymph nodes, being divided into follicles that are more lymphoid in nature near their outer, cortical perimeter. Tonsillar lymphocytes are largely B cells. Other potentially important collections of lymphoid tissue exist in the appendix, lamina propria, and Peyer's patches of the intestine. The lymphocyte population of Peyer's patches is a mixture of B and T lymphocytes. The lamina propria contains T cells and a large population of plasma cells.

Lymphocytes

The important cell common to all lymphoid tissue is the lymphocyte. Lymphocytes are derived from lymphoblasts in bone marrow and are dispersed into the blood where they represent 20% to 30% of the circulating leukocytes. Lymphocytes carried by the blood course through many organs, but critical events take place in the thymus and bursa of Fabricius (or its mammalian equivalent) that appear to imprint the lymphocytes with special functions and regulate the response of the lymphocytes, as either T or B lymphocytes, to antigens.

Lymphocytes are traditionally classified according to their size. The smaller variety usually ranges from 6 to 10 μm in diameter and the large class from 10 to 20 μm in diameter (Fig. 5-5). An intermediate class also is sometimes designated. All lymphocytes have a rounded nucleus or a nucleus that has a single identation. The nucleus is large in comparison to the cytoplasm, which may appear as a mere fringe about the nucleus. In the large lymphocytes the cytoplasm is a more significant portion of the total cell volume. The nucleus of lymphocytes is characterized by an irregular clumping of chromatin into darkly staining linear arrangements, which may give the nucleus a vague cartwheel appearance. The cytoplasm is slightly basophilic because of its content of ribosomes, but the arrangement of ribosomes into polysomes or into the rough endoplasmic reticulum typical of cells endowed with active protein-synthesizing capabilities is not prominent. A few cytoplasmic mitochondria and lysosomes are visible in electron micrographs of lymphocytes (Fig. 5-6).

Lymphocytes are feebly motile. A pseudopod-like structure, the uropod, is the means by which lymphocytes are motile and is used to establish contact with macrophages, tumor cells, or other cell types. The uropod sometimes is seen as a long, narrow projection and at other times as a more blunt, footlike structure.

Life-span studies of lymphocytes of most mammalian species divide them into two fractions: those with a short span (mostly large lymphocytes) of 5 to 7 days and the small lymphocytes with a life span measured in months or even years. The former are B cells, and the latter are T cells. This is only one of the many differences between B and T cells.

T lymphocytes

Ontogeny and surface markers. T lymphocyte precursors are present in the bone marrow and are recognized by the presence of an enzyme terminal deoxynucleotidyl transferase (Tdt). This enzyme adds a terminal nucleotide to existing nucleotides. This enzyme is lost as the cell matures in the thymus or under the stimulus of thymic hormones. The immature T cell leaves the bone marrow via the blood and eventually passes into the thymus. Within the thymus these thymocytes reduce in size to about 7 μm in diameter. This change is accompanied by the loss of the TL and Qa2 antigens, the markers of immature T cells. The TL marker is the product of the T1a gene, which is situated on the mouse MHC chromosome 17 near the Qa gene set. After leaving the thymus the peripheral lymphocytes express the Qa3 and Thy 1 antigen specificities. The Thy 1 antigen, formerly known as the θ or T antigen, is divisible into Thy 1.1 and Thy 1.2, of which the latter is most widely distributed among the various mouse strains. Small glycoproteins of about 20,000 mol wt are responsible for these specificities, whose structural gene is on chromosome 9.

The Lyt alloantigens exist in a series of which the most important seem to be Lyt 1, Lyt 2, and Lyt 3. The structural gene for Lyt 1 is on mouse chromosome 19, and that for Lyt 2 and 3 is on chromosome 6. Lyt 2 and 3 are closely linked and are usually inherited as a pair. Consequently T lymphocytes are Lyt 1,2,3 positive, Lyt 1 positive, or Lyt 2,3 positive. The Lyt 1 antigen density is approximately the same on thymocytes and peripheral T cells, but the Lyt 2,3 density is lower on the latter. These antigens are found on leukemic (young) T cells and cannot be considered as maturation antigens. The Lyt 1,2,3–positive cells represent about 50% of the peripheral blood T cells and are considered the precursors of the Lyt 1 cells and Lyt 2,3 cells, which represent approximately 30% and 10%, respectively. The Lyt antigens thus are useful in segregating the mouse T cells into subsets that are now known to have different functions.

Thymic hormones. The differentiation and maturation of cells from the bone marrow that terminate in the recognition of a mature T cell are

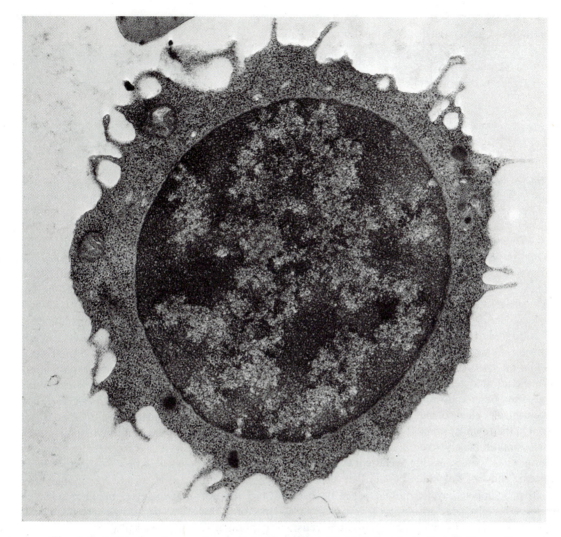

Fig. 5-6. A lymphocyte seen by electron microscopy. The lymphocyte tends to lack a well-developed endoplasmic reticulum; biochemically this must be interpreted as a handicap to protein (antibody) synthesis by this cell. Note the cytoplasmic extensions. (Courtesy Dr. E. Adelstein.)

regulated by a number of peptides, which have been described as thymic hormones.

Many different preparations from thymus glands, from purified T cells, and even from serum have been identified to contain a thymic hormone. Only a few of these hormonelike molecules have been purified sufficiently to permit the assignment

of a specific biologic activity to a specific compound (Table 5-1).

Thymic humoral factor is prepared from calf thymus where it is present as a heat-labile protein consisting of 31 amino acids. Its isoelectric point is between that of thymic serum factor (facteur thymique serique, or FTS) and thymosin α_1 at

Table 5-1. Characteristics of thymic hormones

	Source	Molecular weight	Isoelectric point	Major activities
Thymosin α_1	Calf thymus	3,108	4.2	Increases Con A response, red blood cell rosettes, Thy 1−positive cells
Thymic humoral factor	Calf thymus	About 3,300	5.6	Enhances Th numbers and response to Con A
FTS	Serum	859	7.3	Enhances red blood cell rosettes, Thy 1−positive cells
Thymopoietin II	Calf thymus	5,562	—	Induces Thy 1− and Lyt-positive cells
Serum factor	Serum	<500	—	Several T cell−enhancing activities

5.6. Thymic humoral factor has been demonstrated to repair T-cell deficits in thymectomized mice, to augment Th cell activity, to stimulate the mixed leukocyte culture (MLC) response, and to stimulate responsiveness to T cell lectins.

Thymosin is a mixture of 15 or more proteins, of which one, thymosin α_1, has been fully described. Thymosin α_1 is a peptide with a molecular weight of 3,108 and an isoelectric point of 4.2. The amino acid sequence of thymosin is unlike that of any other known protein. Immunologic and biochemical evidence indicates that it is synthesized in the thymus, possibly in the form of a precursor approximately fivefold its own size. Thymosin is heat stable possibly because it contains no cysteine and lacks disulfide bonds. It is also free of aromatic or heterocyclic amino acids. Thymosin restores T cell characteristics to T cell−deficient mice, as measured by an increase in rosetting cells, increase in the response to T cell lectins, increased number of Th cells, enhanced MLC activity, induction of Thy 1−positive and Lyt-positive cells, and the induction of Tdt activity. Additional active molecules present in the original thymosin preparations, such as thymosin α_7, have been less well characterized, but thymosin β_4 has been sequenced. It is unlike thymosin α_1 in structure.

FTS is the smallest of the chemically characterized thymic hormones. It has a molecular weight of only 859 and is composed of only 9 amino acids. Its isoelectric point is 7.3. This small pep-tide is apparently synthesized in Hassall's corpuscles, the round refractile structures regularly seen in the thymus. When injected into T cell−deficient animals, FTS induces the appearance of the Thy 1 antigen, increases sheep cell rosetting by lymphocytes, and diminishes the Ts cell population.

Thymopoietin II, the largest of the well-characterized thymic hormones, has a molecular weight of 5,562; it is a heat-stable protein composed of 49 amino acids. Among its activities is the ability to induce Thy 1 and Lyt antigen expression on immature lymphocytes. These cells are positive for Tdt activity until thymopoietin binds; then the cells mature and lose this enzyme while expressing the typical antigens of mature T cells. Thymopoietin is a product of the thymus epithelium and not of thymocytes or other cells. Thymectomy removes this hormone from the blood within hours.

Other factors have been described that have thymic replacing activity. These include serum factor, a small peptide of less than 500 mol wt from human blood, and lymphocyte-stimulating hormones from calf thymus. Macrophage and T cell factors IL-1 and IL-2, although chemically distinct from the thymic hormones, share some of their functions.

The several antigens on T cell surfaces mentioned previously have become useful markers for recognizing, identifying, and purifying T cells and their antigenic subsets, but as yet none of them

Table 5-2. Differences between T and B lymphocytes

Characteristic	T lymphocyte	B lymphocyte
Tissue where modified	Thymus	Bursa of Fabricius or bursal equivalent
Unique surface antigen	Thy 1, Lyt, and OKT antigens	Lyb antigen
Surface immunoglobulin	V_H	Readily detectable IgM and/or IgD
Phytoagglutinin receptors	Yes, especially Con A	Yes, especially LPS
Complement receptors	No	Yes: C1q, C3b, C3d, C4b
Antigen receptors	Yes, V_H domains	Yes, through surface immunoglobulin
Functional subsets	Th, Ts, Tc, Tdh, Ta	Bμ, Bγ, Bα, Bδ, Bϵ
Tissue distribution	High, in thoracic duct lymph, blood	High in spleen, low in blood
Life span	Long	Short
Lymphocyte transformation	Yes, to small lymphocytes	Yes, to plasma cells
Mixed lymphocyte reaction (MLR)	Responder cell	Stimulator cell
Cell product	Lymphokines	Immunoglobulins
Germinal center location	Paracortical and medullary regions of lymph nodes	Far cortical regions of lymph nodes
Sensitivity to immunosuppression	Less than that of B cells	Greater than that of T cells
Response to conjugated antigens	Mostly to carrier	Good hapten response
Immune tolerance	Early, persistent, and to low antigen doses	Less sensitive than T cells

has been associated with antigen recognition. Efforts to identify an antigen receptor on T cells have presented conflicting evidence. Most studies with antisera against immunoglobulins have failed to identify such immunoglobulins on the T cell surface, and stripping of the T cell surface with enzymes has not significantly changed these results. Antibodies that are specific for just the antigen-combining portions of immunoglobulins will bind to T (and B) cells. (See Chapters 6 and 8.) These regions in an immunoglobulin are known as the V domains, and it is now widely accepted that one of these V domain fragments, V_H, is the antigen receptor that permits the T cell response to antigens (Table 5-2).

The situation regarding the presence of immunoglobulin on the surface of human T cells is much different than just described for mouse T cells. IgM is present on one set of T cells (Tμ) and IgG on another (Tγ). The Tμ cells function as Th cells and represent 10% to 20% of peripheral blood

T cells. The Tγ population accounts for 5% to 15% of the circulating T cells and serve as Ts cells.

The response of T cells to antigens is reflected in a cycle of growth and division known as lymphocyte transformation until a clone of T cells responsive to the antigen is created (Fig. 5-7). These cells appear morphologically like the unstimulated cell but are physiologically different. This is reflected in their ability to synthesize transfer factor and to secrete lymphokines. (See Chapter 7.) These clones of T cells often can be identified as cell clusters or germinal centers in the paracortical or medullary regions of lymph nodes.

Other important markers are present on the surface of peripheral T cells. One of these is a receptor for sheep red blood cells. Incubation of such erythrocytes with T cells results in the spontaneous formation of E-rosettes consisting of a T cell surrounded by a cluster of erythrocytes (Fig. 5-8). Enumeration of T cells by this method in-

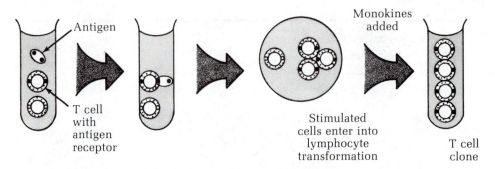

Antigen

T cell
with
antigen
receptor

Monokines
added

Stimulated
cells enter into
lymphocyte
transformation

T cell
clone

Fig. 5-7. A clone of T cells can be generated only with difficulty, unlike that of macrophages and B cells. Antigen-stimulated T cells will reproduce for several generations if supplied with monokines or lymphokines. Unstimulated cells slowly die.

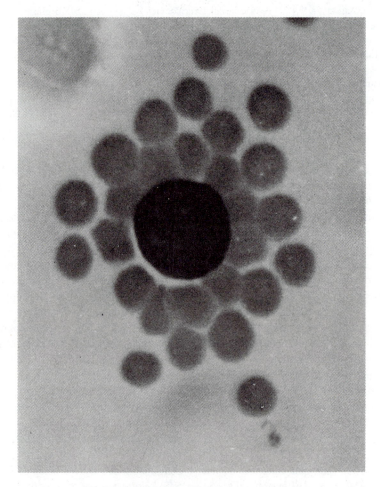

Fig. 5-8. This rosette reveals how large the number of sheep erythrocytes that attach to lymphocytes can be. (Courtesy Dr. E. Adelstein.)

dicates that 70% to 80% of the circulating lymphocytes in a normal mature animal are T cells. The basis for spontaneous rosette formation between these cells is not known, but T cells from the mouse, human, and a few other species share this property. On the basis of the rosetting criterion nearly 90% of the lymphocytes in thoracic duct fluid are T cells. Peyer's patches contain approximately 50% T and 50% B cells. The T cell population is high in the lymph node medulla but lower in its cortical region. T cells are also low in the tonsil.

A second important characteristic of certain T cells is a surface receptor for Ia proteins. The chemical nature of this receptor is not known. It is important, since it permits cell-to-cell cooperation, when the cooperating cell has the Ia protein on its surface. T lymphocyte transformation is associated with the T cell response to Ia proteins on B cells when they are coincubated in culture; this is the MLR (mixed lymphocyte reaction) or MLC.

T lymphocyte transformation is also the result of T cell surface contact with certain mitogens.

T cell mitogens. Mitogens are substances that induce mitosis and several plant proteins, known as phytoagglutinins, because they also agglutinate mammalian cells, or PHA, if they agglutinate erythrocytes also stimulate mitosis in either or both B and T cells, depending on their specificity. Con A and PHA are lectins (another synonym) that activate T cells. Con A is the most specific T cell mitogen in current use. PHA activates T cells but also will activate B cells in some species if the lectin concentration is high. Pokeweed mitogen (PWM) is stimulatory to both T and B cells. The B cell–specific mitogens are described under the section on B cells.

Con A. Con A was first extracted from jack bean *(Canavalia ensiformis)* in 1919 and was identified as a lectin for erythrocytes in 1935. It was not until 1970 that it was found that it would bind to lymphocytes. Con A is a protein existing predominately as a tetramer above a pH of 7 and as a dimer below a pH of 6 (Table 5-3). The peptide subunits have a molecular weight of 25,500, and each one binds one Mn^{2+} and one Ca^{2+} ion. The presence of the metals is required for Con A binding to saccharides; again, each monomer can bind to one saccharide unit. The amino acid sequence of the monomer units has been determined but is not especially revealing. Salt bridges between 114 and 116 on one dimer and glutamic acid 192 on the other hold the tetramer together. Succinylation of free amino groups in Con A converts it to the stable dimer.

Both Con A and succinyl Con A are potent mitogens for T lymphocytes, and a dose of 3 $\mu g/$

Table 5-3. Characteristics of selected mitogens

	Abbreviation	Source	Molecular weight	Lymphocyte receptor	Susceptible cell
Concanavalin A	Con A	*Canavalia ensiformis* (jack bean)	102,000	Mannosides and glucosides	T cells
Phytohemagglutinin	PHA or PHA-L	*Phaseolus vulgaris* (red or yellow beans)	115,000 to 140,000	*N*-acetyl-D-galactosamine	B and T cells; some species predominantly T cells
Pokeweed mitogen	PWM	*Phytolacca americana* (pokeweed)	32,000	Unidentified	T and B cells
Lipopolysaccharide	LPS	Gram-negative bacteria	About 4,000	Unidentified	B cells

ml is optimal. Both B and T lymphocytes bind Con A, and each lymphocyte has about 10×10^6 receptors per cell, but only the T cell is sensitive to Con A–induced lymphocyte transformation. The T cell receptors for Con A are α-D-manno-pyranosides and α-D-glucopyranosides. This statement is based on the pronounced ability of methyl-α-D-mannoside and methyl-α-D-glucosides to inhibit Con A binding and mitogenicity.

PHA. PHA is a protein extracted from the red kidney bean, *Phaseolus vulgaris.* It has a powerful hemagglutinating property and in 1960 was discovered to induce lymphocyte activation. The optimal concentration of the reagent needed to demonstrate the maximum amount of mitogenic activity is only 1 to 5 μg/ml.

Most preparations of PHA used as mitogens have been crude extracts of kidney beans. Fractionation of these extracts by ion-exchange chromatography and molecular sieving has separated the lymphocyte-stimulating component, PHA-L, from the hemagglutinin, PHA-H. Both molecules are proteins with molecular weights between 115,000 and 140,000. The PHA-L fraction is a glycoprotein and attaches to other glycoproteins, which are its receptors on sensitive cells.

PHA binds to and activates both B and T cells, with some degree of specificity being exhibited in certain species. The ability of PHA to stimulate only 70% of mouse lymphocytes is indicative of a specificity for T cells in this species. Both B and T lymphocytes of the human are PHA sensitive.

PWM. Extracts from the roots, leaves, stems, and berries of the pokeweed, *Phytolacca americana,* have a feeble erythrocyte-clumping property. These extracts have a potent mitogenic activity for lymphocytes. The active ingredient in these extracts is a protein composed of a single peptide chain with a molecular weight of 32,000. The receptor site on lymphocytes for PWM is not known. PWM activates both B and T lymphocytes of mice.

Other mitogens. Lectins extractable from the peanut *(Arachis hypogaea),* soybean *(Glycine max),* pea *(Pisum sativum),* and red and yellow was bean *(Phaseolus vulgaris)* are all protein-aceous. The peanut agglutinin, soybean agglutinin, and wax bean agglutinin are of tetrameric peptide structure and have molecular weights varying between 110,000 and 130,000. All are specific for polysaccharides on the surface of cells to which they bind. These mitogens vary in their specificity for T and B cells.

T cell functions. Neonatal thymectomy of experimental animals causes a number of immunodeficiency symptoms. Such animals fail to make antibodies to the T cell–dependent antigen. They also may fail to reject tumors or tissue transplants or may do so more slowly. Certain of the allergic responses, notably the delayed hypersensitivity response, may not develop, but all these functions are regained by adoptive immunization with T cells.

Studies of fractionated T cells have revealed that there are several functional subsets, each of which is restricted to one or only a few of the activities exhibited by the total T cell population.

The helper T cell (Th). The helper cell function of T lymphocytes has been demonstrated in several animal models. For example, the nude mouse is congenitally deficient in a thymus and must receive thymic grafts or mature T cells to display full immunocompetence. Likewise neonatally thymectomized animals and animals lethally irradiated and then reconstituted only with B cells require help from the T cell compartment of a normal animal to regain immune normalcy.

In the late 1960s it was shown that thymectomized mice given certain antigens failed to respond with the expected amount of immunoglobulin. The T cell–dependent antigens are generally more complex molecules than the T cell–independent antigens, which stimulate B cells without the participation of T cells. This experiment revealed that, to respond to T cell–dependent antigens, the B cell must receive two signals, one from the antigen and a second from the T cell. It also was found that lethally irradiated mice, in which both T and B cells have been destroyed, make no antibody to sheep red blood cells (which are T cell dependent) even when reconstituted with T cells. If both T cells and bone marrow cells were provided, a near normal antibody response followed. Bone marrow cells alone were feebly stimulatory because of their supply of pre–T cells that could mature in the irradiated mouse's thymus gland. These experiments conclusively demonstrated a role for a B cell–assisting, or helper, T cell. By the use of cytotoxic immunoglobulins specific for antigenic subsets of T cells, the human $T\mu$ and the mouse Lyt 1 cells have been identified as the helper cells. The Lyt 1 helper cell population has been divided into two compartments, the Lyt 1–positive, Qa1-negative helper and the Lyt 1–positive Qa1-positive inducer. The latter induces pre–Tc cells to mature, induces Lyt 1,2,3 cells to differentiate into suppressor Lyt 2,3 cells, induces monocytes to engage in delayed hypersensitivity reactions, and helps B cells. The Lyt 1–positive, Qa1-negative cell seems only to be a pure helper. Since the T inducer cell stimulates the generation of Ts cells, it is obvious that it plays a central role in modulating the response to T cell–dependent antigens. It is not yet known if the human helper cell—the $T\mu$ and OKT4 antigen–positive cell—represent a single or a dual set of helper cells. The human helper cell represents 40% to 60% of the peripheral blood T lymphocytes and the mouse helper cells about 30%. These figures are much greater than for suppressor cells, which are about 5% to 15% of the circulating T lymphocytes in each species.

The suppressor T cell (Ts). The identification of the Ts cell emerged from several different types of experiments. In one experiment it was discovered that thymectomy enhanced the B cell response to a T cell–independent antigen. In this instance the B cell needed no assistance from the Th cell but was affected by the Ts cell. In another study large doses of antigen were used to thwart the antibody response in a phenomenon known as immunologic tolerance. T cells taken from these "tolerized" animals and injected into normal animals along with antigen penalized the antibody

response. The dependence of tolerance in part on Ts cells can be demonstrated by another experiment in which a lethally irradiated thymectomized mouse is reconstituted with B cells and given a dose of a T cell–independent antigen that produces tolerance in a normal mouse. In the treated mouse, antibody is produced unless T cells are supplied, and then tolerance is observed.

Fractionation of the T cell population used to supplement these mice revealed that the Lyt 2,3 lymphocyte was the critical suppressor cell. The Ts cells are regulated by products of the I-J gene and this distinguishes them from the Tc Lyt 2,3 cells which are not I-J restricted. These Ts cells are derived from Lyt 1,2,3, cells possibly by the action of the inducer Th cell. There may be as many as three subsets of Ts cells separable by their surface markers and drug sensitivity. A contra-suppressor cell has been theorized to control the mouse Ts cell. The human Ts cell is the $T\gamma$ cell. The $T\gamma$ cell is probably a subpopulation of the OKT8 antigen–positive cells, since the former represents about 30% to 40% of the circulating T cells and the $T\gamma$ less than half that.

Kinetic studies have shown that the Th function is demonstrable soon after antigen exposure in normal doses, followed by a Ts function when the antibody peak is reached. The Th cells persist for only a few days after antigen exposure, but the Ts cells, when once generated, remain functional for approximately 2 months in mice. Ts cells will respond to low doses of antigen, much lower than required to stun B cells. The Ts cells exert their action on B cells, on Th cells, on Tdh cells, and also on macrophages. The means they use for this are described in the later section on cellular interactions.

The cytotoxic T cell (Tc or CTC). The ability of antigen-primed T cells to attack and destroy the target cell is a phenomenon described as cell-mediated cytotoxicity (CMC) or cell-mediated lympholysis (CML). A subset of T cells, termed the CTC (or *Tc*) or *Tk* (cytotoxic or killer) cells, is responsible for this phenomenon. These mouse cytotoxic T cells (CTC) bear the Lyt 2,3 antigen set on their surface. Tc cells can be distinguished from Ts cells, which are also Lyt 2,3 positive, by the additional presence of I-J region products on Ts cells. Human CTCs are Tγ, OKT4-positive cells. Target cell destruction by CTCs can be distinguished from similar activities of other cells by several features: (1) it is antigen restricted and develops only after antigen stimulation, (2) it is MHC restricted, meaning the Lyt 2,3 cell kills only cells with the same histocompatibility antigen on their surface as the CTCs possess, and (3) killing is often slower, usually requiring 2 or 3 days in culture to develop significant killing. Foreign tissue in the form of transplants, tumor cells, virus-infected host cells, or cells infected by other infectious agents are the best targets. The CTC contacts the primary antigen and the histocompatibility antigen as the dual recognition signal to initiate cell killing.

The delayed hypersensitivity T cell (Tdh). The mouse T cells that contribute to the delayed hypersensitivity (DH) reactions share with the Th cells the Lyt 1 antigen but lack the Lyt 2,3 set. Human Tdh cells are the Tμ, OKT4-positive cells. These cells are poorly described in terms of other characteristics. Their response is antigen specific, and they are the source of several lymphokines, such as migration inhibition factor (MIF) and macrophage chemotaxin, which participate in the hypersensitivity reaction. (See Chapter 7.)

The amplifier T cell (Ta). The amplifier T cell (Ta) is a recently described cell that causes Th, Ts, and B cells to exaggerate their normal activities. These cells have Ia determinants on their surface unlike all but the Ts subset of thymus-derived lymphocytes. The Ta cell is reported to carry the complete Lyt 1,2,3 antigen set on its surface.

B lymphocytes

Ontogeny and surface markers. B line stem cells are present in the bone marrow and are the source of the pre–B cell. The pre–B cells, even in the animal not yet stimulated by an antigen, synthesize IgM. This globulin is confined to the cytoplasm of the cell and is not secreted. This feature distinguishes the pre–B cell from the immature B cell, which does secrete IgM and has it on its surface. The pre–B cell loses some of its cytoplasm and becomes a smaller cell when it transforms into an immature B cell. Many of these cells also express surface IgD. At this stage the B cell can be identified by surface receptors for molecules of the complement system, especially C1q, C3b, C3d, and C4b, and receptors for the Fc region of IgG. The I-A and/or I-E proteins are also present in these cells.

After antigen exposure the B cell differentiates into a mature B cell that secretes a single class of immunoglobulin molecule. This also will be specific for a single determinant on the antigen. Accompanying this physiologic shift there will be a morphologic differentiation into the plasma cell, the animal's most proficient antibody-forming cell.

The pre–B cells are first found in the fetal liver and later in the bone marrow. This may occur as early as the ninth gestational week in the human being and at the end of the second week in mice. The immature B cell also may be found in the bone marrow and also is detectable in the peripheral lymphoid organs and blood. Mature B cells are located in the blood and peripheral lymphoid tissues presumably after a differentiating pass through the bursa or its equivalent. In the latter site they will be accompanied by plasma cells, but these cells are not found in blood or normal bone marrow.

In the blood approximately 20% to 30% of the circulating lymphocytes can be identified as B cells on the basis of their surface immunoglobulin marker. Nearer to 50% of tonsillar and splenic lymphocytes are B cells.

B lymphocytes contain other surface markers in addition to immunoglobulins. They contain the I-A or I-E gene products, the histocompatibility antigens (H-2 in the mouse, HLA in humans), antigens of the β or B series, now known as the Lyb antigens, and others. All these can be used to aid in the identification of B cells. The I-A proteins of the mouse or their counterpart in humans, the D/DR proteins, are the stimulator molecules for T cells that cause transformation of foreign T cells in the MLR or MLC.

It should be emphasized that, whereas these B cells may have many common features, they can be subdivided into major subsets on the basis of the class of immunoglobulin that they are patterned to synthesize. Thus from the pre–B cell separate B cell lineages are derived that synthesize only IgM as adult cells (Bμ lineage), IgG (Bγ lineage), etc., to create Bα, Bδ, and Bϵ lineages. Within each major B cell line, subdivisions depend on two features: the type of light chain that is present in the immunoglobulin, either κ or λ, and the subclass of the heavy chain. (See Chapter 6.) In this way B$\mu\kappa$ and B$\mu\lambda$, and B$\gamma\kappa$ and B$\gamma\lambda$, can be distinguished from each other. Since there are four separate γ-chains known, the B$\gamma\kappa$ actually exists as B$\gamma1\kappa$, B$\gamma2\kappa$, B$\gamma3\kappa$, and B$\gamma4\kappa$. Beyond this a B cell recognizes only one determinant on an antigen, so the B cell lineage expands to a vast number of such cells.

All B cells are not necessarily fixed into synthesis of just one class of immunoglobulin, since class switch from IgM to IgG has been recognized. The stimulus for this may be a reexposure to antigen and an assistance from a Th or Ta cell.

Immunoglobulin on the B cell surface behaves as the specific receptor for antigen. Histochemical techniques reveal that this immunoglobulin is randomly distributed over the B cell surface. When antigen is added, the immunoglobulin begins to accumulate in distinct foci that further blend into one agglomerate. This is referred to as lymphocyte capping, which precedes a gradual disappearance of the antigen and the immunoglobulin as the complex is internalized.

Lymphocyte capping is a B cell phenomenon not demonstrated by T cells. It signals a phase of cell differentiation into actively secreting plasma cells and memory cells. Memory cells cannot be described in cytologic terms, but they are functionally responsible for the recognition of antigen on reexposure and the rapid antibody response which follows this second as compared with the first exposure. Plasma cells are easily recognized both morphologically and functionally.

B cell mitogens. Certain mitogens also stimulate B cell transformation into plasma cells. Whereas antigen is categorized as a monoclonal stimulant, since it stimulates only cells in the functional B subsets that have the specific immunoglobulin receptor for that antigen on their surface, other mitogens are described as polyclonal. Polyclonal mitogens stimulate all B cells regardless of their antigen specificity. This reflects a shared ability of these mitogens to affect the plasticity of the B cell cytoplasmic membrane in the same manner accomplished by antigen.

LPS. The most specific of the commonly used B cell mitogens is the LPS that is extracted from the cell wall of many gram-negative bacteria where it functions as the somatic or O antigen and as an endotoxin. The lipid portion of LPS is the site of its mitogenic activity. This lipid, lipid A, contains a 14-carbon saturated fatty acid, β-hydroxymyristic acid, and other long-chain fatty acids joined to a phosphorylated dissacharide composed of glucosamine. Its mitogenic potency may reside in its ability to fuse with lipids in the membrane of B cells.

Other mitogens for B cells include protein A, a protein that is found on the surface of the bacterium *Staphylococcus aureus*. This protein combines with immunoglobulin on the B cell by a different mechanism than antigen, but nevertheless this sparks lymphocyte transformation.

Before considering plasma cells as the end cell of the B cell lineage, it is important to contrast several properties of B and T cells not yet considered. In general, B cells are more sensitive to irradiation than are T cells. Cytotoxic drugs as a rule are not noted for their B or T cell specificity, but cyclophosphamide is an exception that is recognized as more effective on B than on T cells. In contrast, antigen-induced unresponsiveness (immunotolerance) is much easier accomplished in T cells and lasts for a long time even when induced by minute quantities of antigen (low-dose tolerance). It is also possible to demonstrate that

B cells focus on the hapten portion of hapten-antigen conjugates, whereas the opposite is true of T cells.

The plasma cell. The plasma cell is about the same size as the small lymphocyte (6 to 10 μm) and can be confused with it in simple stains of tissue preparations. This is less likely in blood stains, since plasma cells are quite scarce in blood. All plasma cells are not the same size; some may approach 20 μm in diameter. Plasma cells have their nucleus centrally placed, and the cytoplasm, which is usually sparse in relation to that of other cells, is often gathered at one side. The nucleus stains intensely, and the lumpy strands of chromatin give the nucleus a cartwheel appearance. This is much more prominent in the plasma cell than in the lymphocyte, where the chromatin also may be unevenly distributed within the nuclear membrane. The cytoplasm of the plasma cell has a strong affinity for basic (cationic) dyes such as pyronin. When used in combination with methyl green, pyronin is an excellent stain for plasma cells. The plasma cell nucleus takes on a blue-green color and its cytoplasm an intense red because of the binding of methyl green and pyronin to these cell structures. This pyroninophilic character of the plasma cell cytoplasm results from its highly acidic nature, which in turn results almost entirely from its content of RNA. This statement is amply supported by electron microscopy, which reveals that the cytosol of plasma cells is literally filled with rough endoplasmic reticulum (Fig. 5-9). This complex intracellular system consists of two serpentine, parallel membranes heavily laden with ribosomes. The ribosomes contain considerable RNA of their own and serve as the site of messenger RNA attachment during protein synthesis. It is here that immunoglobulin synthesis proceeds.

Relatives of the lymphocytes

Natural killer (NK) or null cells. In mouse, rat, guinea pig, human, and other animal species a cell has been recognized to display a cytotoxic activity on tumor cells in vivo and in vitro without prior exposure to antigens of the target cell. This behavior separates it from the CTC, which becomes cytotoxic only after antigen exposure. This natural killer (NK) activity is potentially the first line of immune surveillance against neoplastic cells and virally infected cells.

The exact identification of NK cells has been difficult, in part because several different cell types have NK activity, and possibly because NK cells lack fidelity in terms of their markers. Morphologically NK cells are about the size of lymphocytes (12 to 15 μm in diameter) but have a larger cytoplasm-to-nucleus ratio. Their nucleus is indented rather than round, as in lymphocytes. Some NK cells will rosette with sheep red blood cells, but their affinity for the erythrocytes is weak, and these rosettes are easily dispersed (Fig. 5-8). Mouse NK cells vary in their reaction with anti–Thy 1 or anti–Lyt 1, whereas all mouse T cells bind these antibodies. NK cells generally lack surface receptors for complement, and some reports indicate they have no immunoglobulin receptors, although reports are conflicting on this point. These features plus the lack of I-A proteins indicate that NK cells are not B cells. Since NK cells are not phagocytic, they cannot be macrophages. NK cells are thus cytotoxic non-B, non-T, and nonmacrophages and sometimes are referred to as null cells. About 0.5% to 2.5% of all mononuclear cells behave as NK cells, but these numbers are increased if the lymphoid cells are activated by IFN, lectins, or IL-2. A mutant mouse—the beige strain—is deficient in NK cells, and its sensitivity to transplantable tumors indicates the protective role of NK cells. The nude mouse has NK cells but few, if any, T cells.

NK cells have a spontaneous cytotoxicity for tumor cells almost regardless of the target cell source. Membrane-labeled target cells release their label within a few hours after exposure to NK cells, much faster in fact than when exposed to CTCs.

The attack of NK cells on their targets is blocked by gangliosides, which may represent their natural receptor.

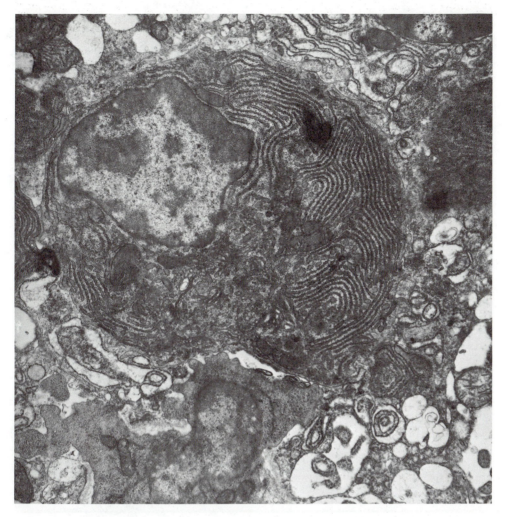

Fig. 5-9. Electron microscopic view of a plasma cell. The cytoplasm is literally filled with endoplasmic reticulum, which is seen as parallel curving lines. This is the site of immunoglobulin synthesis. (Courtesy Dr. E. Adelstein.)

K cells. Several morphologically distinct cells have been assigned a key role in antibody-dependent cell cytotoxicity, or ADCC. Macrophages and neutrophils participate in ADCC, but they are easily distinguished from a population of lymphocyte-like cells that also cooperate with antibody to destroy cellular targets. These killer, or K, cells are not T cells, since they are present in neonatally thymectomized and nude mice. Anti–Thy 1 sera do not deplete their numbers in vivo. K cells have been described as null cells (non-T and non-B) despite their acknowledged role as receptors for immunoglobulin. K cells have receptors for IgG that, when this is specific for cell surface antigens, serve as a focal point for a cytolytic destruction of the target cell. K cells are unable to kill target cells except in the presence of specific antibody and are not MHC restricted in target cell killing as the CTCs are.

PURIFICATION OF IMMUNOLOGICALLY ACTIVE CELLS

Numerous methods have been employed to harvest and separate macrophages, B cells, and T cells. Reconstitution of these cells into artificial mixtures, as described in the next section of this chapter, allows investigators to identify the cellular requirements for the basic immunologic functions, to examine behavioral alterations

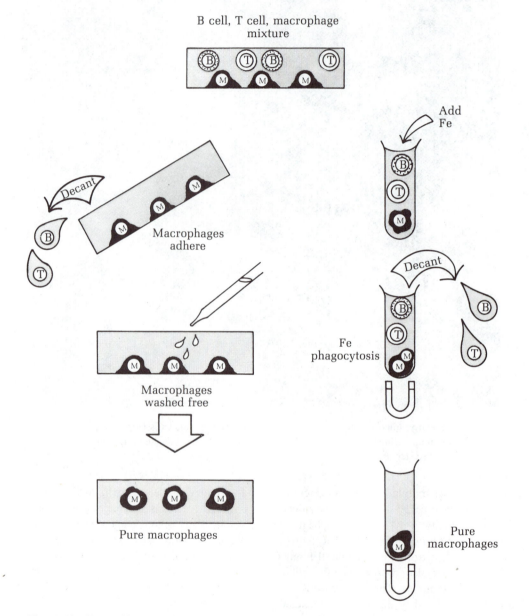

Fig. 5-10. The purification of macrophages is relatively simple, since they adhere to surfaces and engulf particles that aid in their recovery.

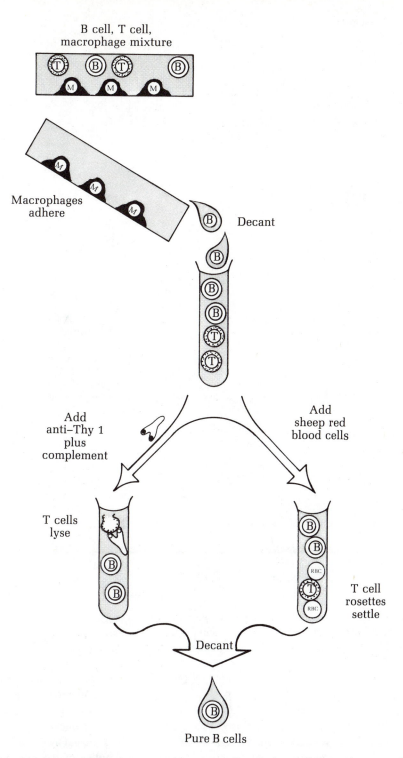

Fig. 5-11. One avenue toward the preparation of pure B cells is to eliminate the macrophages by adherence and then lyse the T cells with anti–Thy 1 sera and complement. A second approach is to sediment the T cells in rosettes, which leaves the B cells in suspension.

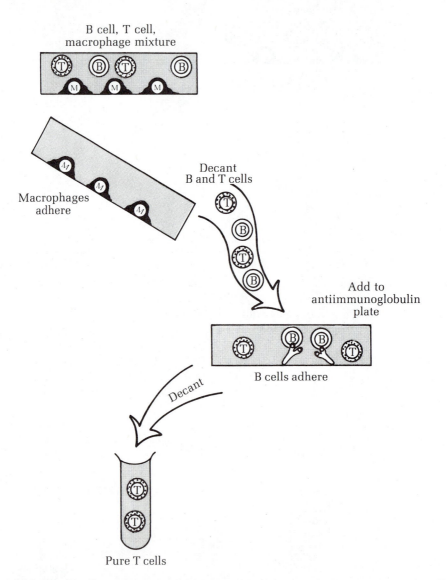

Fig. 5-12. Pure T cells can be prepared from macrophage-free preparations by panning B cells. In panning the immunoglobulin on the B cell surface is held to an antiimmunoglobulin on the pan. This holds the B cells firmly to the pan, facilitating recovery of the T cells.

of these cells when subjected to various stimuli, to evaluate the separate cell subsets, and to perform other important experiments.

Since macrophages have several properties not shared by lymphocytes, they can be prepared relatively free from these cells as contaminants. The

chemotactic response of macrophages in vivo enables their accumulation in the peritoneal cavity when it has been inoculated with irritants such as glycogen, starch, or mineral oil. Use of the last of these has been abandoned, since macrophages will engulf droplets of the oil, and oils may interfere with subsequent assays. Macrophages collected under these conditions are activated and display the heightened responses of such cells. Resident macrophages can be collected by peritoneal lavage without prior stimulation, but the cell harvest is smaller. Bronchopulmonary lavage can be used to collect alveolar macrophages.

Depending on the procedure, the macrophage population will be contaminated with neutrophils, mast cells, and a few other cell types, including lymphocytes. The ability of macrophages to adhere to surfaces, which they use so efficiently in phagocytosis, leaves most contaminating cells free in the suspending fluid, with which they can be decanted (Fig. 5-10). The phagocytic activity for bacteria, yeasts, or other particles is useful in the enumeration of macrophage but also can be used to purify them from a mixed population. Macrophages that have ingested iron filings can be held in place by a magnetic force while other cells are washed away. Unfortunately iron-ladened phagocytes are not useful in all studies.

Because of the similarity of B and T cells, they are more difficult to separate physically from each other than from macrophages. Purified B cell preparations can be achieved by adding cytotoxic anti–Thy 1 sera and complement to B and T cell mixtures. The T cells will be lysed, and the B cells will remain free. Advantage also can be taken of the sheep cell rosetting by T cells, which will produce aggregates that can be separated physically from B cells (Fig. 5-11). The simplest procedure for securing pure T cells is by "panning" (Fig. 5-12). Antibody molecules will adhere spontaneously to glass or plastic surfaces, and B cells have immunoglobulins on their surface. If a dish is coated with an antibody to globulins, it will bind B cells to the dish so that pure T cells can be collected by decantation.

CELLULAR INTERACTIONS IN THE IMMUNE RESPONSE

The interactions between macrophages, T cells, and B cells are exceedingly complex and incompletely known. New data are adding rapidly to our knowledge of this area, and in the future significant additions to the following paragraphs undoubtedly will be required.

Macrophage requirement

It was demonstrated nearly 25 years ago that macrophages were necessary for the expression of B cell activities, and a few years later they were found to cooperate with T cells in immunologic functions. The primary role of the macrophage is in antigen processing. Antigenic determinants prepared by macrophages are passed as such or in a complex with RNA to the effector B and T cells. Macrophage–B cell contact is not necessary for a response to antigens. Cell-free filtrates of macrophage-antigen cultures contain RNA complexed with an antigen fragment that is so stimulatory for B cells that it has been labeled as superantigen.

Is a soluble factor sufficient for macrophage–T cell interaction? The answer seems to be that it depends. Antigen-primed macrophages do release into their culture fluids molecule(s) that are essential for the T cell subsets to exhibit their unique functions. Purification of these molecules indicates that these are the I-A, I-E, or other gene products. These I-A products, the Ia antigens, are known to be present on the macrophage surface from which they are shed in culture. It is quite possible that this shedding could occur in vivo, but it may not be required.

In vivo experiments with transferred cells also have shown that the macrophage–T cell interaction is MHC restricted by genes in the Ir region.

T cell requirement

The requirement of T cells for the B cell response to certain antigens was the mechanism by which antigen came to be identified as T cell dependent or T cell independent, the latter requiring B cell assistance only from the macrophage. Some antigens may stimulate B cells directly, particularly if they are also mitogenic. Certain immunopotentiators may function by altering B cell permeability to intact antigen.

When a T cell requirement exists, it need not be by means of direct B cell–T cell contact. Soluble factors are liberated by T cells that stimulate or suppress B cells, and this can be demonstrated by separating B and T cells from each other by cell-impermeable membranes. This was demonstrated by an increased response of hapten-antigen-primed B cells to the hapten when T cells on the opposite side of the membrane had been exposed only to the carrier. In this experiment macrophages also were present, and it is known that macrophages can act across membranes to stimulate T cells.

In a contrasting experiment in which T cells and B cells were diluted in a series of wells in a microculture plate, antibody was produced only when B and T cells were simultaneously present. This was expected, but the number of B cell subsets that were stimulated was directly related to the number of T cells contained in that culture. This experiment negates the presence of a cell-free activator, since a single T cell could seemingly stimulate many B cells by this method.

An MHC restriction to T–B cell cooperation in the antibody response was revealed when it was discovered that T cells and B cells from histoincompatible strains did not cooperate to produce antibody. This restriction has since been defined to reside in the Ir gene segment of the MHC and not in the genes most dominant in graft-rejection phenomena. Our current concept is that T cells modified by originating in a mouse of one I-A (or I-E) gene develop receptors for the corresponding Ia antigen. When this antigen is present on the B cell and macrophage, B cell stimulation results, possibly by T cell receptors for the I-A protein binding to this protein on the other two participants (Fig. 5-13).

Macrophage-macrophage interactions are difficult to study and have been ignored, as have B cell–B cell interactions. However, the opposite is the case in regard to T cell–T cell interactions, which are numerous and complex. The complex interactions of T cell subsets centers on the interplay of Ts and Th cells previously discussed.

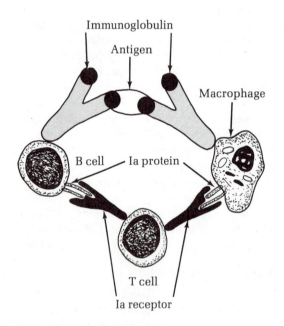

Fig. 5-13. One concept of macrophage, T cell, and B cell cooperation in the immune response envisions T cell receptors for I-A proteins binding to these proteins on the macrophage and the B cell. Surface immunoglobulins on the macrophage and B cell hold the antigen. In this way the dual signal of antigen and T cell help is transmitted to the B cell.

BIBLIOGRAPHY

Aiuti, F., and Wigzell, H., editors: Thymus, thymic hormones and T lymphocytes, London, 1980, Academic Press. (London), Ltd.

Bach, F.H., and others, editors: T and B lymphocytes: recognition and function, New York, 1979, Academic Press, Inc.

Bach, J.F., and Carnaud, C.: Thymic factors, Prog. Allergy **21:**342, 1976.

Battisto, J.R., and Knight, K.L., editors: Immunoglobulin genes and B cell differentiation, Dev. Immunol. **12:**1, 1980.

Bona, C., and Cazenave, P.A., editors: Lymphocytic regulation by antibodies, New York, 1981, John Wiley & Sons, Inc.

Cantor, H., and Boyse, E.A.: Regulation of the immune response by T-cell subclasses, Contemp. Top. Immunobiol. **7:**47, 1977.

Chess, L., and Schlossman, S.F.: Human lymphocyte subpopulations, Adv. Immunol. **25:**213, 1978.

Cohen, E.P., and Köhler, H., editors: Membranes, receptors, and the immune response, New York, 1980, Alan R. Liss, Inc.

Cone, R.E.: Molecular basis for T lymphocyte recognition of antigens, Prog. Allergy **29**:182, 1981.

Dickler, H.B.: Lymphocyte receptors for immunoglobulin, Adv. Immunol. **24**:167, 1976.

Dorf, M.E., editor: The role of the major histocompatibility complex in immunobiology, New York, 1981, Garland Publishing, Inc.

Dwyer, J.M.: Identifying and enumerating human T and B lymphocytes, Prog. Allergy **21**:178, 1976.

Eichmann, K.: Expression and function of idiotypes on lymphocytes, Adv. Immunol. **26**:195, 1978.

Friedman, H., editor: Subcellular factors in immunity, Ann. N.Y. Acad. Sci. **332**:1, 1979.

Goodwin, J.S., editor: Suppressor cells in human disease, New York, 1981, Marcel Dekker, Inc.

Greaves, M.F., Owen, J.J.T., and Raff, M.C.: T and B lymphocytes; origin, properties and roles in immune responses, Amsterdam, 1973, Excerpta Medica.

Herberman, R.B.: Natural killer (NK) cells, Prog. Clin. Biol. Res. **58**:33, 1981.

Herberman, R.B., and Ortaldo, J.R.: Natural killer cells: their role in defenses against disease, Science **214**:24, 1981.

Hume, D.A., and Weidemann, M.J.: Mitogenic lymphocyte transformation, Amsterdam, 1980, Elsevier/North Holland Biomedical Press.

Janeway, C.A., Jr.: Idiotypes, T-cell receptors and T-B cooperation, Contemp. Top. Immunobiol. **9**:171, 1980.

Katz, D.H.: Lymphocyte differentiation, recognition and regulation, New York, 1977, Academic Press, Inc.

Katz, D.H.: Adaptive differentiation of lymphocytes: theoretical implications for mechanisms of cell-cell recognition and regulation of immune responses, Adv. Immunol. **29**:138, 1980.

Kindred, B.: Nude mice in immunology, Prog. Allergy **26**:137, 1979.

Krakauer, R.S., and Clough, J.D., editors: Suppressor cells and their factors, Boca Raton, Fla., 1981, CRC Press, Inc.

Kung, P.C., and others: Monoclonal antibodies defining distinctive human T cell antigens, Science **206**:347, 1979.

Loor, F.: Plasma membrane and cell cortex interactions in lymphocyte functions, Adv. Immunol. **30**:1, 1980.

MacKenzie, I.F., and Potter, T.: Murine lymphocyte surface antigens, Adv. Immunol. **27**:151, 1979.

Marchalonis, J.J.: The lymphocytes, structure and function, New York, 1977, Marcel Dekker, Inc.

Mishell, B.B., and Shiigi, S.M., editors: Selected methods in cellular immunology, San Francisco, 1980, W.H. Freeman & Co., Publishers.

Moretta, L., Mingari, M.C., and Moretta, A.: Human T subpopulations in normal and pathologic conditions, Immunol. Rev. **45**:163, 1979.

Oppenheim, J.J., and Rosenstreich, D.L.: Signals regulating in vitro activation of lymphocytes, Prog. Allgery **20**:65, 1976.

Owen, J.J.T., and Jenkinson, E.J.: Embryology of the lymphoid system, Prog. Allergy **29**:1, 1981.

Ralph, P.: Functional subsets of murine and human B lymphocyte cell lines, Immunol. Rev. **48**:107, 1979.

Reinherz, E.L., and Schlossman, S.F.: Regulation of the immune response—inducer and suppressor T-lymphocyte subsets in human beings, N. Engl. J. Med. **303**:370, 1980.

Roder, J.C., Karre, K., and Kiessling, R.: Natural killer cells, Prog. Allergy **28**:66, 1981.

Ruddle, N.H.: T cell tumors, clones, and hybrids, Prog. Allergy **29**:222, 1981.

Sigal, N.H., and Klinman, N.R.: The B-cell clonotype repertoire, Adv. Immunol. **26**:255, 1978.

Warr, G.W.: Membrane immunoglobulins of vertebrate lymphocytes, Contemp. Top. Immunobiol. **9**:141, 1980.

Wedner, H.J., and Parker, C.W.: Lymphocyte activation, Prog. Allergy **20**:195, 1976.

SITUATION: A VISIT TO THE ANIMAL QUARTERS

You are on your way through the animal quarters to check your rabbits when the animal caretaker stops you in the hall and asks for your advice. A litter of mice has recently been born in which each animal had a malformed hind leg. One of the young was born dead and was given to a professor of comparative anatomy for examina-tion. In his report he described the anatomy of the limb malformation and the results of his examination of other organs and tissues. The striking result of his study was the detection of a total absence of splenic tissue in the afflicted mice. The animal caretaker was aware that the spleen had something to do with immunity and asked you if the loss of a spleen meant that the rest of the litter would die from infectious disease. He was curious, if the animals could be kept alive and bred with a perpetuation of the spleenless condition, whether the animals would be valuable in immunologic experimentation.

Questions

1. What is the role of the spleen in the immune defense system, and what would be the life expectancy of a spleenless animal?
2. What experiments come to mind as potential immunologic adventures with these unique mice?

Solution

The spleen is a lymphoid organ that is often divided for purposes of discussion into the white pulp and the red pulp. The latter is important in the clearance of defective or aged erythrocytes from the bloodstream and has no significant role in immunity. The white pulp is the lymphoid portion of the organ, and it is divided into sectors or lobules of lymphocytes surrounded by connective tissue. The lymphocyte population of the spleen is dominated by cells of the B type. In the human about 55% of splenic lymphocytes are of the B type and 15% of the T type, with the remainder unidentified. A slightly higher percentage of T cells is found in rat and mouse spleen.

As with other peripheral lymphoid tissues, the spleen is seeded with B and T lymphocytes before the birth of an animal. Since numerous other peripheral lymphoid tissues are present in mammals, including lymph nodes, tonsil, appendix, Peyer's patches, and other more diffuse tissues, the loss of the spleen generally has little influence on the resistance of adult animals to infectious disease. The removal of a ruptured spleen from human beings is not really a rare medical event and is not associated with an increased incidence of infectious disease. This may be caused by the seeding of other tissues with cells escaping through the rupture, since "clean" surgical splenectomy of children does carry some risk for an increased incidence of infectious disease. This may be related to the containment of splenocytes during clean surgery. Congenitally spleenless mice should be examined regularly for disease but are not under extreme risk for disease.

This discussion does not imply that immunologic experiments with spleenless animals would be fruitless. These unusual animals would be useful in evaluating the spleen as a source of immunologically active hormones; for example, extracts of splenic lymphocytes could be injected into spleenless animals to determine if the spleen influenced their immune response. Purified B and T lymphocytes from the spleens of congenic donors could be injected into spleenless animals for the same purpose. Purified B and T lymphocytes from the spleens of congenic donors could be injected into spleenless mice to determine the tissue homing pattern of these cells. The capacity of spleenless mice to perform phagocytic functions could be evaluated, since an important role of the spleen is phagocytosis. The immunoglobulin class or subclass distribution IgG1 versus IgG2 versus IgM might differ between normal and spleenless mice. Other experiments are without doubt of value to those with special areas of interest.

References

Battisto, J.R., Borek, F., and Bucsi, R.A.: Splenic determination of immunocompetence; influence on other lymphoid organs, Cell. Immunol. 2:627, 1971.

Battisto, J.R., and others: Immunoglobulin synthesis in hereditarily spleenless mice, Nature 222:1196, 1969.

Bucsi, R.A., Borek, F., and Battisto, J.R.: Splenic replenishment of synergistic ability to bone marrow and thymic cells of neonatally splenectomized CBA mice, J. Exp. Med. 136:761, 1972.

Lozzio, B.B., and Wargon, L.B.: Immune competence of hereditarily asplenic mice, Immunology 27:167, 1974.

CHAPTER 6

THE IMMUNOGLOBULINS

GLOSSARY

α-chain The H peptide chain of IgA.

Am marker An allotypic determinant in α-chains.

antibody fragment A portion of an antibody molecule as created by enzymatic hydrolysis or chemical dissociation.

Bence Jones protein An immunoglobulin L chain, that is, κ- or λ-chain, as found in urine or blood of patients with a myeloma.

C_H1, C_H2, C_H3, and C_H4 The portions of the H chains of immunoglobulins with constant amino acid sequences.

C_L The portions of κ- and λ-chains with constant amino acid sequences.

constant domain A region in an immunoglobulin whose amino acid sequence is identical to the sequence in another region.

δ-chain The H chain of IgD.

domain A section or region in the peptide chain of an immunoglobulin.

ε-chain The H chain of IgE.

Fab fragment A fragment of an immunoglobulin consisting of one L chain and half of the H chain.

F(ab′)₂ fragment Two Fab fragments plus an additional portion of the H chain of the immunoglobulin joined by disulfide bonds between the H chain portions of the fragment.

Fc fragment A polypeptide fragment of an immunoglobulin representing the carboxyl half of both H chains joined by disulfide bonds, as after papain treatment of IgG.

Fc′ fragment The carboxyl half of both H chains after pepsin treatment of IgG.

Fd fragment That portion of the H chain in an Fab fragment.

Fd′ fragment The portion of the H chain in the F(ab′)₂ fragment.

FR Framework region.

framework region The section in the V_L and V_H domains between the HV regions.

γ-chain The H chain of IgG.

γ-globulin A portion of the serum proteins in which the immunoglobulins are found; characterized by low electrophoretic mobility at pH 8.3.

gammopathy An imbalance in immunoglobulin concentration.

Gm group An allotypic group based on antigenic changes in H chain antigens of IgG.

H chain The heavy chain of an immunoglobulin.

heavy chain The large polypeptide chain, of which two exist, in the basic four-peptide structure of an immunoglobulin.

hinge region The region in the H chain of an immunoglobulin near where the L chain joins it and near the sites of papain and pepsin cleavage.

HV Hypervariable region.

hypervariable region A section of intense variability in the V_L or V_H domain.

immunoglobulin A (IgA) One of five serum immunoglobulins, possessing α H chains.

immunoglobulin D (IgD) The immunoglobulin in lowest concentration in serum, possessing δ H chains.

immunoglobulin E (IgE) The serum immunoglobulin with a potent homocytotropic tendency for mast cells, possessing ϵ H chains; synonymous with *allergic reagin*.

immunoglobulin G (IgG) The serum globulin in greatest concentration (75% to 95% of the total) and possessing γ H chains.

immunoglobulin M (IgM) The serum immunoglobulin of greatest molecular weight (about 900,000) formed earliest after antigen exposure and possessing μ H chains.

isotype Synonym of class when referring to immunoglobulins.

J chain A polypeptide chain found attached to secretory IgA and IgM that may function as a joining chain.

κ-chain One of two types of L chain found in an immunoglobulin.

Km A κ-chain allotypic marker: Km1, Km2, and Km3.

L chain Light chain of an immunoglobulin.

λ-chain An antigenic form of L chain of the immunoglobulins.

light chain The smallest of the two types of polypeptide chains (light and heavy) of immunoglobulins; two exist in the four-peptide unit.

M component The serum protein produced in excessive concentration in cases of myeloma or macroglobulinemia.

μ-chain The H chain of IgM.

multiple myeloma *see* Myeloma.

myeloma A plasma cell neoplasm resulting in excessive production of one or more immunoglobulins.

paraproteinemia The presence of protein molecules in plasma that are antigenically similar to but which lack the biologic activity of normal molecules, especially regarding immunoglobulins.

SC Secretory component.

secretory component A portion of secretory IgA and secretory IgM not present in serum IgA or IgM and not produced in plasma cells.

secretory immunoglobulin An immunoglobulin found in colostrum, saliva, mucous secretions, etc. as secretory IgA or secretory IgM.

variable domain A region in an immunoglobulin whose amino acid sequence is inconstant from one molecular species to another.

Waldenström's macroglobulinemia A myeloma involving IgM or IgM-like molecules.

In the human there are five molecular classes of the immunoglobulins. These are designated as IgG, IgA, IgM, IgD, and IgE; in each, Ig refers to immunoglobulin and the third letter to some distinctive property of that immunoglobulin. IgE is not dealt with here but is described in Chapter 18. The immunoglobulin classes also are called isotypes on the basis that within each isotype or class the molecules share antigenic determinants. Thus an antisera prepared in a rabbit by immunizing it with human IgG would react with all samples of human IgG because they share isotypic determinants.

STRUCTURE AND CHEMISTRY OF IgG

Immunoglobulin G, abbreviated IgG, is the best known and most fully studied of the immunoglobulins. It is the immunoglobulin referred to when reference is made simply to γ-globulin without further specification (Table 6-1). It is also known as γ_2-globulin and 7Sγ-globulin. The γ indicates its position in the serum electrophoretic profile, which is actually a rather broad region compared with the albumins. The 7S refers to its $S_{20,w}$ sedimentation coefficient (Svedberg coefficient), a number that indicates its sedimentation rate in the analytic ultracentrifuge. The true $S_{20,w}$ value of

IgG is closer to 6.6 than to 7. In the human IgG represents about 80% of the total antibody in an antiserum. Expressed in concentration this amounts to 1275 ± 500 mg/dl of serum. This high serum level is a reflection of both the rate of synthesis and the rate of elimination of IgG. It is produced at the rate of about 28 mg/kg body weight/day and has a half-life of approximately a month. IgG has a molecular weight of approximately 150,000, 2.5% of which is in the form of carbohydrate.

Fragments and chains

The history of the chemical structure of the IgG molecule is quite fascinating and is the model after which the study of other immunoglobulins has been patterned. The two studies that contributed most decisively to unraveling the structure of the immunoglobulins were those by Edelman in the United States at Rockefeller University and by

Table 6-1. Chemical and physical properties of immunoglobulin G

Current designation	IgG
Older names	γ-Globulin, 7Sγ-globulin
Molecular weight	150,000
$S_{20,w}$ value	6.6
Electrophoretic mobility	γ
Carbohydrate content	2.5% to 4%
Resistance to —SH reagents	High
Concentration (mg/dl serum)	$1,275 \pm 500$
Amount of serum immunoglobulins	75% to 85%
Half-life (days)	25 to 35
Rate of synthesis (mg/kg body weight/day)	28
Light chain types	κ or λ
Heavy chain class	γ
General formula	$\gamma_2\kappa_2$ or $\gamma_2\lambda_2$
Light chain allotypes	Km
Heavy chain subclasses	$\gamma_1, \gamma_2, \gamma_3, \gamma_4$
Heavy chain allotypes	Gm
Stable at 56° to 60° C	Yes

Porter at Oxford University in England. In 1972 the Nobel Prize Committee in Physiology and Medicine recognized the contributions of these two scientists by awarding them a joint Nobel Prize. The main observation of Edelman was that purified preparations of IgG were resistant to reductive cleavage by sulfhydryl reagents unless the molecule was unfolded by high concentrations of urea or guanidine. These two compounds at 7M or 8M are known to interrupt hydrogen bonds, which hold globular proteins in their unique shapes. When unfolded by 7M urea, proteins become more linear and expose groupings that were previously situated inside the molecule. This permits compounds such as mercaptoethanol (CH_2OHCH_2SH) to engage in oxidation-reduction reactions with disulfide groups that were previously masked. The —S—S— bonds of IgG are converted to two free —SH moieties while mercaptoethanol is oxidized and dimerized to a disulfide ($CH_2OHCH_2S)_2$. When IgG is examined in an analytic ultracentrifuge after such a treatment, the original 7S protein is absent, and two new peaks are seen. The heavier of these is a 3.5S molecule, and the other is about 2.2S. Calculation of the molecular weights of the heavy (H) and light (L) components indicates that they are about 50,000 and 20,000, respectively. Comparison of these values with the calculated molecular weight of IgG at 150,000 reveals that two H and two L components would make up essentially all the original molecule. Each IgG thus has two H chains and two L chains held together by disulfide bonds, and its structure is represented by the simple formula H_2L_2.

The Nobel Prize–winning discovery of Porter was based on his use of the proteolytic enzyme papain and a mild reducing environment to cleave the IgG molecule into three portions, two of which were identical. Papain digestion of IgG reduces it to polypeptides that behave as 3.5S molecules in the analytic ultracentrifuge. No 2.2S peak is observed. This 3.5S product of papain cleavage differs sharply in its immunochemical characteristics from the 3.5S product arising from disulfide reduction in urea. Carboxymethyl cellulose ion exchange chromatography will separate the papain cleavage products in two types of fragments, one of which, the *Fc fragment,* crystallizes spontaneously at 4° C. This fragment is deficient in antigen-binding ability and is now known to represent the carboxyl half of two H chains still held together by one or more interchain — S — S — bonds. The Fc fragment has a molecular weight of approximately 50,000. The sedimentation coefficient of the remaining portion, also 3.5S, indicates that it also should have a similar molecular weight. Since this remaining fragment is antigen-binding, it is called the *Fab fragment.* In the intact IgG molecule it is known that there are two loci capable of binding antigen, and, with the molecular weight borne in mind, it is clear that IgG = 1 Fc + 2 Fab. Each Fab fragment consists of the amino terminal half of the H chain (Fd) plus an L chain. It is thus possible to design a structure which represents these findings (Fig. 6-1).

Pepsin cleavage of IgG yields a fragment that is nearly identical to the Fc fragment, called the Fc' fragment. The difference between Fc and Fc' is that the former is slightly larger, retaining somewhat more of the H chain than does the latter. Those amino acids in the region between the Fc and Fc' cleavage points are termed the *hinge peptides.* This term is more meaningful than it would appear at first. Morphologic evidence indicates that the H chains actually are bent at this position when the antibody combines with antigen.

The remainder of the IgG molecule, after removal of the Fc piece, is basically two Fab pieces held together by an — S — S — bond plus the hinge peptide. It is designated as F(ab')$_2$, since it contains a small additional part of the H chain that the Fab fragments lack. That portion of the H chain found in the F(ab')$_2$ fragment is Fd', differing from Fd in that it contains a portion of the hinge region. F(ab')$_2$ fragments have an S$_{20,w}$ of approximately 5.

Since the L chains are fairly small, it was thought reasonable to begin amino acid sequence studies with this portion of IgG. Besides providing an exciting biochemical challenge, it was thought that the result also might unravel some of the mystery of how an antibody combines with an antigen. It had been demonstrated that the total amino acid composition of different antibodies was not identical, and sequence studies probably would add more understanding to where and how these differences existed.

The possibility of amino acid sequence studies of immunoglobulin L and H chains was greatly increased by the discovery of two unique conditions. The first of these was the availability of human myeloma proteins; the second, the recognition of homogeneous antibodies. More recently hybridomas have been used as a source of pure immunoglobulins.

Multiple myelomas

Multiple myeloma is a neoplasm of proliferating immunocytes or plasma cells. These plasma cell tumors proliferate in the bone marrow and erode away the surrounding hard bone. On radiographic examination discrete holes are apparent in the osseous tissue. This can become so extensive that the long bones of the body fracture when moderate weight or stress is applied. Meanwhile plasma cell infiltration of the soft tissues also develops.

Diagnosis of multiple myeloma relies on radiographic examination of the skeletal bones, tissue examination, especially of bone marrow, and analysis of serum proteins. In bone marrow or other lymphoid tissue heavy sheets of plasma cells can be detected, accounting for as much as 10% of all cells in the marrow in advanced cases. In the normal individual, plasma cells are relatively uncommon in bone marrow. The plasma cells may be either of two types; the first is the typical plasma cell with sparse cytoplasm and the classic pyroninophilic staining behavior, and the other exhibits a swollen cytoplasm containing globules of protein known as Russell bodies. These Russell bodies are inclusions of immunoglobulin, and this is a reflection of the ambitious protein-synthesizing activity of these plasma cells. This re-

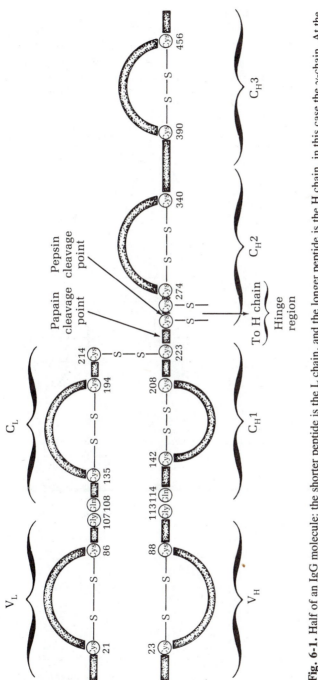

Fig. 6-1. Half of an IgG molecule: the shorter peptide is the L chain, and the longer peptide is the H chain, in this case the γ-chain. At the left, or amino terminal, end a variable domain is present on both the L and H chains. These are the V_L and V_H domains, which consist of approximately 107 amino acids. The next 107 amino acids of the L chain form the constant domain (C_L). The H chain has three constant domains, C_H1, C_H2, and C_H3, with the hinge region situated between C_H1 and C_H2. Each domain contains approximately 107 amino acids. The two H chains are joined where indicated to form the four-chain structure. The points of papain and pepsin cleavage also are indicated.

sults in an unusually high serum concentration of γ-globulin, which can be detected by ordinary serum electrophoretic analysis. This analysis may reveal that practically all the excess γ-globulin has migrated to a specific point in the γ-β portion of the serum electrophoretic profile (Fig. 6-2). A quantitative tracing of the serum proteins will in-

dicate this point by a pronounced absorption spike. This nearly monophoretic protein is known as an M (myeloma) component or M protein. When a single spike is seen, it is indicative that the gammopathy (disease of γ-globulin) is related to the excessive replication of a single type of plasma cell to produce a clone of such cells, all of which are

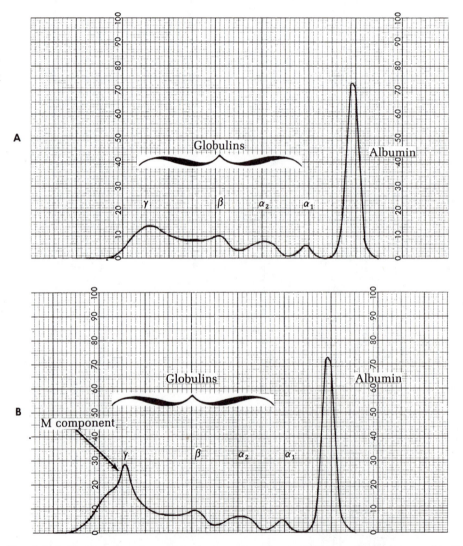

Fig. 6-2. A, Tracing of an electrophoretic separation of a normal serum. **B,** Same type of tracing of a serum from a patient with multiple myeloma. Notice the monoclonal nature of the disease.

excreting the same kind of γ-globulin. This is appropriately described as a monoclonal gammopathy or monoclonal immunoproliferative disease, which indicates the homogeneity of the cells involved and their serum product. In contrast to this situation, when several peaks are seen in the serum profile, or when the entire region is elevated, several different clones of plasma cells are simultaneously engaged in overproduction of immunoglobulin. Accordingly several kinds of γ-globulin are being produced, resulting in electrophoretic heterogeneity. This type of myeloma is referred to as a polyclonal gammopathy.

In certain instances the position of the M component in the electrophoretic profile of the serum will suggest that the M component is of the IgG, IgA, IgM, or other class. If the M component were situated at the far end of the IgG range, it would suggest that it is an IgG myeloma and not an IgA or IgM type, since these latter immunoglobulins typically migrate more toward the β side of the γ-β gulf. However, the electrophoretic positioning of the M components(s) is unreliable in determining the class of immunoproliferative disorder. This can be done only by using antisera that are specific for the different classes of γ-globulin. Only then can one refer to the γG, γA, γM, etc. myeloma. Of these myelomas, 60% are of the IgG class, 16% are IgA, and 14% are IgM. IgD myelomas represent less than 1% of the total.

Waldenström's macroglobulinemia. In the case of the γM myeloma the term *Waldenström's macroglobulinemia* is preferred. This is not because of any gross immunologic difference in this disorder but because of the higher viscosity of IgM compared with other immunoglobulins. Consequently the clinical features of γM myeloma differ from those of the others, and the early descriptions of the disease by Waldenström are honored by continuance of his name.

Bence Jones protein and L chains. Thus in the multiple myelomas and in Waldenström's macroglobulinemia there exist the conditions of hyperimmunoglobulinemia, in some instances from a single plasma cell type. Consequently a source of

a single molecular form of immunoglobulin is available from these unfortunate persons. Many of these patients will have in their blood and excrete in their urine a protein termed the *Bence Jones protein*. In fact in about 10% of all myelomas only the Bence Jones protein is produced, with no complete IgG, IgA, or IgM. Bence Jones proteins are unusual in their response to heat. They are soluble at room temperature, become insoluble near 60° or 70° C, and then resolubilize at 80° C. This pattern reverses when the temperature is lowered, so that one can recover Bence Jones protein again. This unique reversible denaturation permits a speedy identification of Bence Jones protein in urine from persons with multiple myeloma. Structurally the Bence Jones proteins are single-peptide chains with a molecular weight of 20,000 or 22,000, but dimerization to a 40,000 or 44,000 mol wt form occurs spontaneously. Serologically the Bence Jones proteins will react with antisera to the L chains of IgG, and L chains will react with antisera to Bence Jones proteins. This stringent serologic test conclusively identifies L chains as Bence Jones proteins. Subsequent serologic tests revealed that all Bence Jones proteins (L chains) are not identical and that there are two types, designated as κ and λ. After the purification of these proteins from urine, amino acid sequence studies were begun with the hope of uncoding the unique antibody behavior of the immunoglobulins.

Early in the studies of the myeloma proteins and the Bence Jones proteins the criticism was offered that the sequence studies were of little value, since false immunoglobulins were being studied. In fact these proteins were termed *paraproteins*, to indicate that, although they were antigenically and structurally related to immunoglobulins, they lacked the antibody function typical of true immunoglobulins.

This problem has been resolved with the discovery that many of the myeloma proteins do react with known antigens. The original problem was simply to identify the antigen, a search that has now been completed for many human myeloma proteins. IgG myeloma proteins have been recognized to neutralize streptolysin O; others have been identified that react with staphylolysin, transferrin, dinitrophenyl hapten, and *Leptospira* and *Brucella* organisms. Serum albumin, human blood group antigens A_1, and I, cardiolipin, *Klebsiella* organisms, and dinitrophenyl groups are among the antigens known to react with different IgM myeloma proteins. Fewer antigens have been identified to correspond with IgA myelomas because the IgA myelomas are rarer, but these include human blood group I and dinitrophenyl groups. In many instances the Fab fragment of the myeloma protein has been demonstrated to combine with the antigen. The knowledge that myeloma proteins have serologic activity strengthens the clonal selection concept of antibody formation. The binding affinity of these paraproteins for the antigen often was lower than that of normal antibodies (one was only 2.3×10^{-4} M), but this was not true for all of them. One paraprotein of the IgM class has been identified to have a specificity for IgG. It has a valence of 10 and a dissociation constant of 7×10^{-4} M, more in the range of ordinary antibody molecules.

Homogeneous antibody

Among the first antibodies with molecular uniformity to be studied were homogeneous antibodies specific for polysaccharides of the streptococcal cell surface. These immunoglobulins had a uniform electrophoretic mobility that gave them the general appearance of M components on serum electrophoresis. Cleavage of the antibodies to release the H and L chains followed by gel electrophoresis confirmed the high level of homogeneity, since only two to four protein bands were detected when 10 to 12 formerly were noted. It has now been learned that many polysaccharides situated on the outer surface of bacterial cells, including meningococci, staphylococci, and pneumococci in addition to the streptococci, will encourage formation of homogeneous antibodies. Polysaccharide antigens tend to favor antibodies with restricted heterogeneity because of their limited number of antigenic sites, a factor that forces the response toward molecular constancy. To secure the homogeneous antibody, rabbits of proper genetic background must be selected, and whole bacterial cells should be administered by the intravenous route. Purified polysaccharides usually are not suitable, and other immunization methods are less efficient.

Hybridoma

One of the best sources for pure immunoglobulins is the cultured myeloma cell, but even this procedure has been improved by the hybridoma technique. The hybridoma technique is described fully in Chapter 8, but in its simplest form spleen cells, which cannot grow continuously in culture, are taken from a mouse immunized with a chosen antigen. These cells are incubated with a mouse myeloma cell, which can grow continuously in culture provided the proper nutrients are present. Mutants of the myeloma cell are selected that no longer secrete immunoglobulin. These cells are incubated in the presence of a chemical, polyethylene glycol (PEG), which causes cell membranes to become destabilized. This permits some cells to fuse. If the cell mixture is transferred to a tissue culture medium, the spleen cells fail to grow, and the myeloma cells fail to grow because the medium has been adjusted to prevent their growth. The cells that do grow are hybrids or hybridomas. They grow because they have some of the nutrient properties of the parental spleen cell, which overcome the medium composition, and the property of continuous growth in culture from the myeloma cell. These hybridomas will secrete into the growth medium an antibody with a specificity for the antigen used to immunize the mouse. Moreover this antibody will be specific for a single determinant of that antigen. About 100 μg of this immunoglobulin can be recovered from each milliliter of culture fluid. If the hybridoma is inoculated into the peritoneal cavity of a mouse, it will grow and produce an ascites fluid containing as much as 10 mg of immunoglobulin per milliliter. Such hybridomas have been an important source of a single molecular species of immunoglobulin produced by a single cell. These immunoglobulins are now the starting material for many chemical and genetic studies.

Constant and variable domains in L chains

One of the most interesting aspects emerging from the L chain sequence studies was the discovery that the carboxyl terminal half of all the λ-type L chains is nearly identical. The κ-chains also have a constant amino acid sequence in their carboxyl half. The constant half of the κ-chain is very similar but not identical to the constant half of the λ-chains. These regions are designated C_κ and C_λ, or more generally as C_L (constant light). The amino halves of the λ-chains vary in structure from one to another; the same is true for the κ-chains. These regions are designated V_κ and V_λ, or as V_L (variable light). Thus the 214 amino acids of all L chains are arranged in a unique way, with a constant amino acid sequence in the carboxyl half and variable sequence in the amino half. These regions are now customarily referred to as domains, that is, the constant domain and the variable domain. Constant and variable domains of the H chains also are known and are discussed later in the chapter.

Within the first 107 amino acids of L chains the variability of the amino acid sequence fluctuates from residue to residue. Although the sequence of the V_L domain is variable, it is not equally variable at all positions, and the regions of greatest inconstancy are referred to as the hypervariable (HV) regions. Three such HV regions exist in each V_L domain, and these normally encompass amino acids 30 to 35, 50 to 55, and 95 to 100 with slight variations (Fig. 6-3). It is exactly these sequences which protrude from the end of the peptide chain and serve as part of the antigen-binding site. These regions differ in amino acid sequence according to the specificity of the immunoglobulin. These are the idiotypic regions of immunoglobulins.

These idiotypic regions are separated by the framework (FR) sequences, of which there are four in each V_L domain. These embody the first 29 amino acids from the amino terminal end, the last seven amino acids of the V_L, and the intervening sequences between the three HV regions.

The λ-type L chain has 213 to 216 amino acids, depending on whether certain additions or deletions of amino acids exist. The penultimate amino acid of the carboxyl terminus is cysteine, one of only five cysteines in this polypeptide (Fig. 6-4). This cysteine is the site of dimerization in Bence

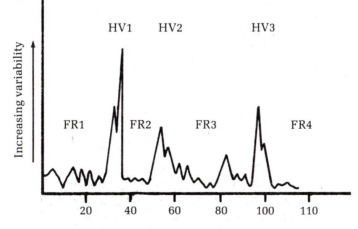

Fig. 6-3. A variability tracing of an L chain. The three major HV regions are identified, with the framework *(FR)* regions on each side.

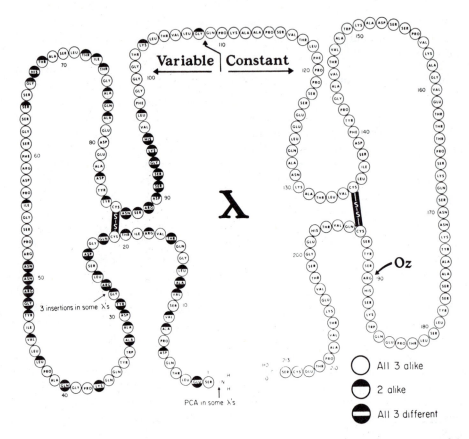

Fig. 6-4. Entire amino acid sequence of three human λ-type L chains. Notice the symmetry of the molecule, in terms of zones of constant and variable sequence, and the placement of disulfide bonds. The location of the Oz determinant at position 190 is noted. (See Fig. 6-5.) (From Putnam, F.W.: Structural evolution of kappa and lambda chains. In Killander, J., editor: Gamma globulins, New York, 1967, Interscience Press.)

Jones proteins and the point at which L chains are covalently linked to H chains in normal IgG. Two of the other four cysteines engage in intrachain disulfide bonding, between residues 135 and 194 in the constant region and between residues 21 and 86 in the variable region. The exact location of the internal disulfide bonds may vary by a few amino residues in different κ- or λ-chains. This double cystine formation creates two nearly symmetric loops of 60 amino acids each in the L chain. The amino terminal acid is serine, but this may be blocked by pyrrolidone carboxylic acid, a cyclized form of glutamic acid.

κ L chains are in many ways similar to λ-chains (Figs. 6-5 and 6-6). They have cysteine as the terminal amino acid on the carboxyl end, and this serves for attachment to the H chain or for dimer Bence Jones protein formation. Two intrachain disulfide bonds occur, between 134 and 194 and between 23 and 88, again creating symmetric loops of approximately 60 amino acids each. These — S — S — bonds and loops are at almost

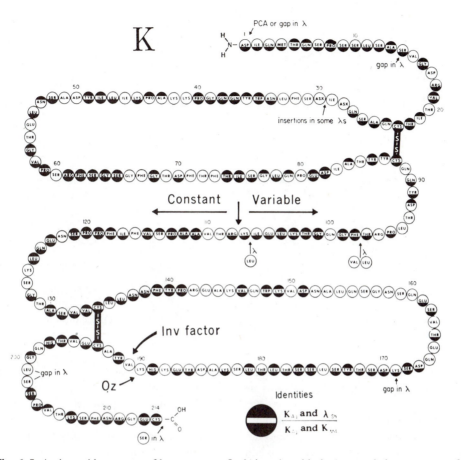

Fig. 6-5. Amino acid sequence of human κ-type L chains. As with the λ-type chain, symmetry of the constant and variable sequence portions and disulfide linkages are apparent. Key at bottom of illustration indicates the homology with human and murine κ-chains and a human λ-chain. (From Putnam, F.W.: Immunoglobulin structure variability and homology, Science **163**:633, 1969.)

exactly the same position as those found in λ-chains. This suggests a common genetic origin of the two L chains from which the λ and κ varieties have evolved with the retention of many common structural characteristics. The amino terminal acid is not blocked with pyrrolidone carboxylic acid and is usually aspartic acid.

In a given individual both κ- and λ-chains are produced and found in antibody molecules; however, they are not found simultaneously in a single antibody molecule. Two structural formulas now can be written for IgG: $H_2\kappa_2$ and $H_2\lambda_2$. These two types exist in a ratio of about 2:1 in any one individual.

L chain allotypes

Human κ-chain allotypes have been identified that permit a finer identification of these L chains. Allotypic proteins are structurally and functionally similar molecules that differ from each other antigenically. The allotypic determinants of κ-chains reside in the C_L domain. The Km1 (κ-marker) L

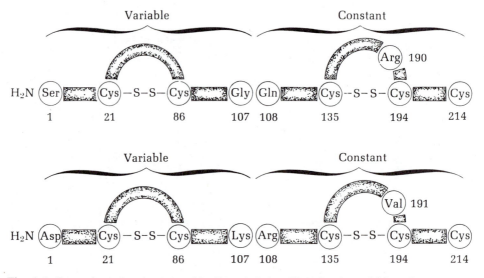

Fig. 6-6. Comparison of κ- *(upper)* and λ- *(lower)* chains. Note that the variable and constant regions are the same size, that the intrachain disulfide loops are comparably positioned, and that the Km factor in the κ-chain is placed at essentially the same location as the Oz factor in the λ-chain, at positions 190 and 191.

chain has valine at position 153 and leucine at position 191. These are replaced by alanine and valine, respectively, in the Km3 molecule. Km2 has alanine and leucine in positions 153 and 191.

Antigenic variants in human λ-chains have been identified and were once described as allotypes (Oz, Kern, and Mcg determinants) but are no longer accepted as such. These molecules contained antigenic differences which can be described as private markers rather than the more general allotypic markers.

γ-CHAINS

The H chains of IgG are designated as γ-chains to distinguish them from the H chains of the other immunoglobulins. The carbohydrate portion of IgG (2.5% of the total weight of the molecule) is equally divided between the two γ-chains and is situated on the Fc portion of the H chain. Monosaccharide units found in the carbohydrate portions include mannose, galactose, *N*-acetyl-D-glucosamine, *N*-acetyl-D-galactosamine, and sialic acid. None of the polysaccharide side chains seems to

contain more than five or ten constituent units, although this may be the result of destructive hydrolysis in the preparation of these structures for assay. Attachment of the polysaccharide to the peptide backbone is primarily through asparagine, although one serine-borne unit has been identified.

Constant and variable domains of γ-chains

The complete amino acid sequence for γ-chains has been determined, and some fascinating parallels to L chain structure have been revealed. The amino terminal portion of the γ-chain, consisting of about 121 amino acid residues and residing in the Fab fragment, is of variable amino acid sequence from one γ-chain to another. This variable domain (V_H or V_γ) is essentially the same length as V_L of κ- and λ-chains. In the first 107 amino acids of the V_H domain are three HV regions at essentially the same positions that hypervariability is located in the V_L domains, that is, near residues 30 to 35, 50 to 55, and 95 to 100. The HV V_L and V_H sequences create a wedge within which determinants of the antigen contact the binding sites of the antibody molecule. The amino acid sequences of the V_H and V_L HV regions are not identical. As with the V_L HV regions, those in the V_H domain are separated by FR sequences. The carboxyl terminal region of γ-chains, consisting of about 375 amino acid residues, can be divided into three subregions that have amino acid sequences very similar to each other. These are designated C_H1, C_H2, and C_H3, or $C_\gamma1$, etc. C_H1 is immediately adjacent to V_H, and numbering proceeds toward the carboxyl terminus. The regions 114 to 223, 246 to 361, and 362 to 496 represent the C_H1, C_H2, and C_H3 domains, respectively. Within each is a 60–amino acid disulfide bridge—at 142 to 208 in C_H1, 274 to 340 in C_H2, and 390 to 456 in C_H3. These C_H zones have approximately a 30% to 40% homology with C_L regions of κ- and λ-chains. This has interesting genetic implications, suggesting that genes derived from a common precursor gene have evolved for the C_L and C_H regions and for the separate C_H regions.

Amino acid sequence and enzyme digestion studies indicate that the cleavage point of papain is between threonine 225 and cysteine 226. Cysteines at positions 226 and 229 in IgG1 bridge to the same amino acids in the companion γ-chain to hold them together as the Fc subunit. Cysteines at position 220 serve as the links to the L chains. Pepsin hydrolyzes the γ-chains between two leucine moieties at positions 234 and 235. The disulfide bonds remaining at 226 and 229 enable the Fab units to be preserved as $F(ab')_2$.

The hinge region

This general region of the γ-chains—roughly between cysteine 220 and argenine 241—is known as the hinge region. It is characterized by one interchain disulfide bridge between an L and the H chain and two interchain disulfide bridges between the two H chains. It also contains the unusual sequence Pro-Pro-Pro-Cys-Pro, and the incorporation of proline into an amino acid chain is known to interrupt the normal α-helix configuration and restrict folding of the chain. It is perhaps this which makes the hinge region so sensitive to proteolysis.

γ-Chain subclasses

Four major subclasses of the human γ-chain are detectable by specific antisera. These are designated IgG1, IgG2, IgG3, and IgG4 and occur in the proportions of approximately 15:8:1.5:1, respectively. The chemical basis for the subclasses is differences in the number and position of disulfide bridges between the two γ-chains. For example, IgG1 has two, IgG2 has four, IgG3 has eleven, and IgG4 has two inter-γ-chain disulfide bridges. IgG3 has an extended hinge region that gives it a higher molecular weight than the other IgG subclasses. These separate subclasses are recognizable by specific antisera; an antiserum prepared against one human γ-chain will react with all other human γ-chains, but the extent of this reaction will not be the same for all chains. There actually will be four levels of reactivity, and on this basis the four subclasses were designated.

γ-Chain allotypes

The discovery of human IgG H chain allotypes arose from the identification of subgroups in the sera of patients with rheumatoid arthritis. These individuals commonly have an IgM antibody that reacts with their own IgG. This IgM, also known as rheumatoid factor (RF), also will react with pooled human IgG, and indeed this is the serologic device used to identify RF and assist in the diagnosis of rheumatoid arthritis. However, it was found that the IgG of different individuals functioned unequally as the antigen for RF, and subgroups of IgG known as Gm (γ) subgroups or allotypes were created. These Gm allotypes, earlier designated by letters Gma, Gmb, etc., are now numbered, Gm1, Gm2, etc. These Gm allotypes are unequally distributed among the four IgG subclasses (Table 6-2). IgG1 includes four Gm subgroups, IgG2 has but two, and IgG3 includes twelve. IgG4 does have Gm allotypes, but these have not been fully correlated with the other

Table 6-2. Subclasses of human IgG

	Percent	Gm antigens
IgG1	60.9	Gm1, 2, 3, 17
IgG2	29.6	Gm8, 23
IgG3	5.3	Gm5, 6, 10, 11, 13, 14, 15, 16, 21, 24, 26, 27
IgG4	4.2	Present but not yet correlated with existing Gm system

known allotypes. The chemical basis for the differences in antigenicity of the Gm allotypes is known in several instances. In IgG3 the Gm5 allotype has phenylalanine at amino acid residues 296 and 436. When tyrosine replaces phenylalanine at both positions, then a different antigenic specificity, Gm21, is created. In IgG1, when the arginine at position 214 is replaced by a lysine, the Gm determinant is lost. Similar exchanges regulate the other Gm determinants as well, and these amino acid substitutions can occur in C_H1, C_H2, or C_H3 domains.

These Gm phenogroups are of interest to population geneticists and demographers who study migration and "gene dilution." Nearly 100% of all Finnish and about 60% to 65% of all Swedes, Norwegians, and English contain the Gm1 antigen on their γ-globulins. Central Europeans have this antigen at a level of about 50%; southern Europeans, less than this.

The complications added to the original structure of IgG written as H_2L_2 now can be expanded to include the known variations in H and L chain allotypes. The two major L chain forms of IgG are $\gamma_2\kappa_2$ and $\gamma_2\lambda_2$. These formulas indicate that L chains of either the κ or λ type may be present in IgG. We know that further variations in the κ-chain are possible by variations in the Km marker. Thus one could write formulas such as $\gamma_2(\kappa, Km1)_2$ or $\gamma_2(\kappa, Km2)_2$. But these structures do not distinguish between γ-chain variations. For example, $(\gamma Gm1)_2$ $(\kappa Km1)_2$ and $(\gamma Gm 18)_2$ $(\kappa Km1)_2$ would be distinguishable by specific Gm antisera. The limit of these variations in one individual is not known, but it is apparent that in the human population many different types of IgG can be produced. If we accept four possible types of L chains and four IgG subclasses and only 18 Gm allotypes, then $4 \times 4 \times 18$, or 288, different forms of IgG could hypothetically be present in one individual. Each differs from every other in antigenic reactivity and amino acid composition. Further variations, perhaps several thousand in number, would result from amino acid differences in the antigen-combining sites of these antibodies (idiotypic differences) that are not detectable by ordinary H or L chain antisera. It is little wonder that IgG is so electrophoretically heterogeneous. This heterogeneity indicates a vast heterogeneity of the plasma cell population, since only one kind of antibody molecule is produced by a single plasma cell. Plasma cell heterogeneity is expanded even further, since the other immunoglobulins yet to be discussed also arise from plasma cells.

STRUCTURE AND CHEMISTRY OF IgA
Serum IgA

IgA of serum is known as γA and β_2A because of its tendency to position between the true γ and β regions on electrophoresis (Table 6-3). It ranges between 7S and 11S in the analytic centrifuge. The predominant portion is 7S, and the cause of the polydispersed behavior is at least partially clarified by the known structures of IgA. IgA represents only 5% to 15% of all serum γ-globulins. This is equivalent to 225 ± 55 mg/dl of serum. IgA has a half-life of about 5 days and is synthesized at a rate of about 22 mg/kg body weight/day.

Structural studies have revealed that IgG and IgA possess several common features. Both are composed of four peptide chains, two L chains and two H chains. The L chains in both molecules are identical, that is, κ- and λ-chains, and their known subtypes occur in both molecules. The H chains of IgA, the α-chains, differ from the γ-chains of IgG by having a greater carbohydrate

Table 6-3. Chemical and physical properties of immunoglobulin A

Current designation	IgA
Older names	γA, β_2A
Molecular weight	160,000*
$S_{20,w}$ value	7*
Electrophoretic mobility	Fast γ, slow β
Carbohydrate content	10%
Resistance to — SH reagents	Low
Concentration (mg/dl serum)	225 ± 55
Amount of serum immunoglobulins	5% to 15%
Half-life (days)	5
Rate of synthesis (mg/kg body weight/day)	22
Light chain types	κ or λ
Heavy chain class	α
General formula	$\alpha_2\kappa_2$ or $\alpha_2\lambda_2$
Light chain allotypes	Km
Heavy chain subclasses	α1 and α2
Heavy chain allotypes	A2m(1) and A2m(2)
Heavy chain constant domains	3
Stable at 56° to 60° C	Yes
Secretory type exists	Yes

*Polymeric forms of greater molecular weight and S values are known.

content, approximately 10% of the total molecule, and a different amino acid sequence. α-Chains lack the Gm determinants, but two subclasses of α-chains, IgA1 and IgA2, do exist. IgA1 accounts for 90% of the total serum IgA. IgA1 has intrachain and interchain disulfide linkages of the standard type. These are refractory to reductive cleavage except when in high-molarity urea solutions. IgA2 is unique in that it is completely devoid of H-L interchain — S — S — bonding. The two chains are held together by strictly noncovalent linkages. Allotypic variation in the α-chain of IgA2 depends on the presence or absence of two antigens: A2m(1) and A2m(2). α-Chains in IgA1 do not express allotypic variation.

The α-chain of IgA1 contains 472 amino acid residues. This is sufficient to include a V_H and

three C_H domains. α-Chains have 34 cysteines, compared with 22 in IgG1. The H chains are joined by cystine formation through the cysteines at 242 and 301. Cysteine 471 is the probable source of the linkage of polymeric IgA to J chain. Oligosaccharide subunits are attached to five serines and three asparagines, and most of this occurs in the hinge region—specifically at serine residues 224, 230, 232, 238, and 239. IgA1 has a duplicated hinge region.

Papain and pepsin digestion of serum IgA yields the expected Fab or F(ab')$_2$ units, but the Fc and Fc' units are difficult to isolate because of their sensitivity to further digestion by papain or pepsin. Certain bacterial proteases cleave only IgA1. Reductive cleavage to release H and L chains is also possible.

Secretory IgA

The ratio of IgG to IgA in serum is 6:1; this is true for synovial fluid, cerebrospinal fluid, aqueous humor, and other internal secretions. In the external secretions—that is, in colostrum and early milk, nasal and respiratory mucus, intestinal mucus, saliva, etc.—IgA is usually present in a much higher concentration than either IgG or IgM. Secretory IgA is a nearly equal mixture of IgA1 and IgA2 in contrast to the IgA composition of serum.

Table 6-4 presents the distinguishing characteristics of human serum IgA, human secretory IgA, and two proteins associated with the latter, termed *secretory component* (SC) and *J chain*. As can be seen, human secretory IgA is a much larger molecule than its serum counterpart, having twice its molecular weight plus about 80,000. The major difference is the addition of SC and J chain and a second IgA unit to secretory IgA. Serum IgA and secretory IgA are not in simple equilibrium. Supporting data for this argument are that radiolabeled serum IgA does not appear in the secretions and that IgA administered to agammaglobulinemic patients does not always elevate the secretory IgA. From this it has been deduced that there is a separate cellular origin of serum and

Table 6-4. Comparison of serum IgA, secretory IgA, SC, and J chain

	Serum IgA	Secretory IgA	Secretory component	J chain
Current designation	IgA	SIgA	SC	J
Molecular weight	160,000	405,000	70,000 to 75,000	$15,000 \pm 500$
$S_{20,w}$ value	7	11	5	About 2
Carbohydrate content (percent)	10	10	9.5	7.5
Comment	Polymeric forms common	Formulas $(\alpha_2\kappa_2)_2SC \cdot J$ or $(\alpha_2\lambda_2)_2SC \cdot J$	High glycine content	Prealbumin

secretory IgA. When fluorescent antibody against serum IgA is used as a histochemical reagent, it is found that the plasma cells closely situated beneath the epithelium of excretory glands are stained. If fluorescent antibody against SC is used, the neighboring epithelial cells stain. The fluorescent antibody experiments indicate that plasma cells strategically situated near the body cavities are IgA synthesizers, and epithelial cells produce SC. J chain is produced in the plasma cells.

SC. The identification of an antigenic difference between serum IgA and IgA in milk is credited to Hanson in 1961, and later studies by Tomasi and others eventually identified this as being caused by the SC present in IgA found in secretions. SC is found as a part of the secretory IgA in all species examined, including dog, cow, sheep, goat, rabbit, mouse, and chicken, as well as the human. More recently SC has been identified as a part of human IgM in external secretions. SC bound to secretory IgA or to secretory IgM can be liberated by disulfide reducing compounds (such as 2-mercaptoethanol at a concentration of 0.2M). Free SC exists in secretions of those persons who are hypogammaglobulinemic in regard to IgA, and SC from this source is considered the most suitable for chemical characterization.

The molecular weight of SC is 70,000 to 75,000 (Table 6-4). It exists as a single peptide chain with an $S_{20,w}$ of 5. Electrophoretically the molecule moves to the position occupied by the fast β-globulins. Human SC (and presumably that of other

species) is lacking in methionine but has a high glycine content. About 11% of the weight of SC is in the form of carbohydrate.

IgA that is destined to become secretory IgA is released from submucosal plasma cells which neighbor the external mucosal tissue and diffuses toward the epithelial surface (Fig. 6-7). SC on the epithelial cells serves as a receptor for IgA. On attachment of this IgA to the cell a concentration gradient from the IgA-synthesizing cells is established. This encourages further migration of IgA toward the mucosal surface and its conversion to secretory IgA. The dimeric IgA may enter the epithelial cells (enterocytes, for example) and be transported across the cell in endocytic vesicles. Bile is a rich source of IgA that arises from the blood. Some of this is converted to secretory IgA in the liver before being discharged in the bile, where it has been referred to as biliglobulin.

Although 70% to 85% of secretory IgA has SC attached via disulfide linkages, some 15% to 30% of the SC is noncovalently bonded with SC. SC appears to contact the hinge region of both IgA four-peptide units involved in the complex and probably elsewhere in the Fc region. Since SC has a high content of glycine, it could easily possess the snakelike flexibility required for this union.

The functional role of SC remains enigmatic. It has not yet been proved to have a secretory role, and it is not required for J chain bonding, since this precedes SC attachment.

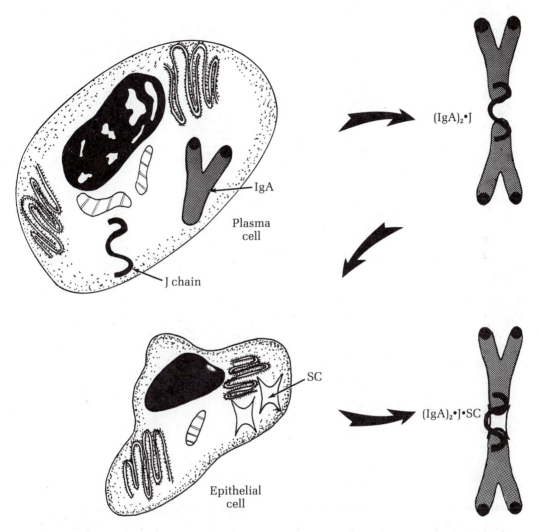

Fig. 6-7. The synthesis of secretory IgA begins in the plasma cell that secretes the J chain combined with two molecules of IgA. This contacts an epithelial cell where it acquires SC to become the complete secretory IgA.

SC is antigenic and possesses determinant sites known as I determinants, which are inaccessible when SC is combined into IgA, and A determinants that are accessible. The A determinants are subdivided into those which are resistant and those which are susceptible to reduction by 0.15M 2-mercaptoethanol.

J chain. In 1970 it was definitely concluded that a protein originally believed to be a degradation product of SC from secretory IgA was in fact a new, previously undescribed protein. Since this protein is found only in immunoglobulins composed of more than one four-peptide unit, it was named J chain (joining chain).

J chain has a molecular weight of 15,000 ± 500 (Table 6-4) and consists of 129 amino acid residues, of which 20 are aspartic acid (Fig. 6-8). This confers a high net negative electrical charge

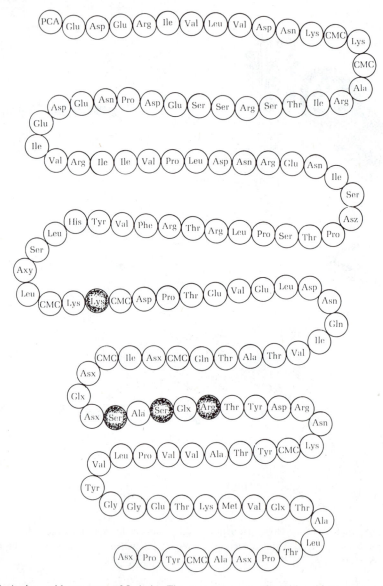

Fig. 6-8. Amino acid sequence of J chain. The numerous aspartic acid residues are apparent, and the shaded amino acids are points of carbohydrate linkage.

on the molecule, which migrates as a prealbumin. The amino acid composition of J chains of human, rabbit, pig, and dog origin is very similar, and all have about 7.5% carbohydrate. Rabbit and human J chains appear to be immunologically identical and partially related serologically to J chains of lower animals. J chain is attached to the α-chains of secretory IgA by virtue of S—S bonding to the penultimate cysteine at the carboxyl terminus, which is present in these H chains. There is one J chain per two IgA units. J chain is also found in serum and secretory IgM at one J chain per five IgM 75 units. This stoichiometry suggests that J chain does not merely join the four-peptide units of the immunoglobulins together; if this were the case, IgM should have five J chain units. Plasma cells that synthesize L and α-chains also synthesize the J chain, yet free J chain is scarce in these cells and is almost entirely bound into the immunoglobulin polymer. This is the basis for suggesting that the biologic role of J chain is to initiate polymerization of secretory IgA (and of the IgM globulins as well). Exactly how this polymerization begins and why it ends at different stages for IgA and IgM is not known; but since it is not accomplished randomly, it may be via specific disulfide interchange enzymes. Synthesis of J chain is apparently the rate-limiting step in the synthesis of polymeric IgA and IgM, and this is the reason it is rarely found as a free protein.

The molecular formula for exocrine IgA is $(\alpha_2\kappa_2)_2SC \cdot J$ or $(\alpha_2\lambda_2)_2SC \cdot J$.

STRUCTURE AND CHEMISTRY OF IgM

The only immunoglobulin with an $S_{20,w}$ value of 19 is the macroglobulin IgM (Table 6-5). This molecule has a molecular weight of approximately 950,000. The electrophoretic positioning of IgM is in the zone between the clear-cut γ- and β-globulins; IgM has been denoted both as a γ_1M and β_2M molecule. This molecule constitutes about 5% to 10% of the total immunoglobulins in the adult human, or about 125 ± 45 mg/dl of serum. This low serum content of IgM is the combined result of its short half-life (10 days) and low synthetic rate (5 to 8 mg/kg body weight/day). The carbohydrate content of IgM is about 10% to 11%. Because its molecular weight, protein content, and sedimentation value are all five times those of IgG, a structure of IgM consisting of 10 L and 10 H chains was quickly postulated. These peptide chains are held together by disulfide bonds and the J chain, which are easily separated by reducing agents. IgM is very sensitive to dissocia-

Table 6-5. Chemical and physical properties of immunoglobulin M

Current designation	IgM
Older names	$19S\gamma$, γ_1M, β_2M
Molecular weight	950,000
$S_{20,w}$ value	19
Electrophoretic mobility	Fast γ, slow β
Carbohydrate content	10%
Resistance to — SH reagents	Low
Concentration (mg/dl serum)	125 ± 45
Amount of serum immunoglobulins	5% to 10%
Half-life (days)	9 to 11
Rate of synthesis (mg/kg body weight/day)	5 to 8
Light chain types	κ or λ
Heavy chain class	μ
General formula	$(\mu_2\kappa_2)_5 \cdot J$ or $(\mu_2\lambda_2)_5 \cdot J$
Light chain allotypes	Km
Heavy chain subclasses	$\mu1$, $\mu2$ (M1, M2)
Heavy chain constant domains	4
Stable at 56° to 60° C	Yes
Secretory type exists	Yes

tion by dilute solutions of — SH reagents such as 2-mercaptoethanol.

When the 19S IgM molecule is treated with reducing agents and the newly formed — SH groups are blocked to prevent recombination, molecules of 6.5S to 7S are formed. This dissociation does not require unfolding of the molecule with urea, since IgM is so sensitive to reducing agents. The 7S fragments (γM_S) have a molecular weight of 190,000 and are similar in structure to IgG in the sense that each is composed of two H and two L chains. The H chains have been isolated and their molecular weight determined as 65,000 to 70,000. The H chains consist of 576 amino acid residues. Cysteine 140 is the link of the H chain to L chains, and cysteines 337 and 575 link the H chains to each other. Five oligosaccharide units have been identified, each being attached to an asparagine. Because of its size and sequence studies, it is agreed that the H chain contains four C domains, rather than three, plus the V domain. Consequently H chains of IgM differ from the H chains of IgG and are referred to as μ-chains. Two IgM subclasses, IgM1 and IgM2, are based on differences in the μ-chain.

The L chains prepared from IgM are identical to the L chains of the other immunoglobulins, that is, κ- or λ-chains. Since the L chains are identical to those of other immunoglobulins, it is assumed that they are linked to the H chain by the COOH terminal (or penultimate) cysteines.

By enzymatic digestion of the γM_S units, structures corresponding to the Fab and F(ab')$_2$ fragments of IgG are formed. These are designated as the Fab-μ and F(ab')$_2\mu$ fragments. Their molecular weights have been estimated as 47,000 and 114,000, respectively.

The molecular formula of serum IgM is written $(\mu_2 k_2)_5 \cdot J$ or $(\mu_2 \lambda_2)_5 \cdot J$ (Fig. 6-9). A secretory form of IgM has recently been described. Its distribution in body fluids parallels that of secretory IgA. Its molecular formula is that of serum IgM plus SC.

STRUCTURE AND CHEMISTRY OF IgD

IgD was first identified as a unique immunoglobulin in human serum in 1965 as the result of the discovery of a myeloma protein that was antigenically dissimilar from other immunoglobulins. Since that time several dozen examples of γD myeloma have been reported, and 135 cases were described in one article, although γD myelomas appear at an incidence of less than 3% of all myelomas. The failure to describe IgD earlier can be related to its paucity in normal human serum, where its normal mean level is 0.03 mg/ml. As a further consequence of this, most of the chemical data available on IgD have been derived from the γD myeloma proteins.

IgD is a typical immunoglobulin constructed from two H and two L chains. Both κ- and λ-type L chains are known, but the λ-type myelomas predominate (80%, compared with 20% κ-type). The H chain of IgD is structurally and antigenically different from the H chains of other immunoglobulins and has been designated the δ-chain. The κ- and λ-chains do not differ from their kind found in other antibodies, but the δ-chain has a molecular weight of 70,000 or some 12,000 greater than γ-chains. This led to the suggestion that the δ-chain possessed a fourth C_H unit. The additional size of the δ-chain may be associated with an extended hinge region in the molecule. Because of its large δ-chain, the entire IgD molecule has a molecular weight of 180,000 rather than 160,000. Its average $S_{20,w}$ is 6.55 (Table 6-6).

The H and L chains are easily recovered from the parent molecule after its exposure to 0.1M mercaptoethanol or 0.02M dithiothreitol for 1 or 2 hours at room temperature to reduce the —S—S bonds if the newly formed —SH units are blocked by iodoacetamide. Papain releases the expected two Fab and one Fc fragments, but the latter is rapidly degraded further and is difficult to isolate intact.

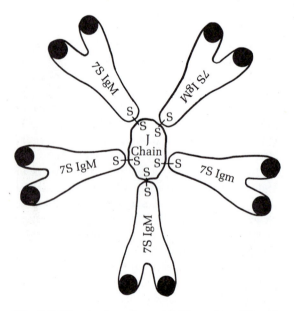

Fig. 6-9. The structure of serum IgM consists of five of the four-peptide or 7S IgM units linked to J chain.

IgD contains about 12% of its weight in the form of polysaccharide, all of which is attached to the δ-chain. This seems to be divided into three discrete sectors, one located at the Fc-Fd interface, or hinge region, and the other two in the Fc region.

IgD at a level of 30 μg/ml of serum is synthesized at the rate of 0.4 mg/kg body weight/day. This is about 100-fold less than the synthetic rate of IgG. The half-life of IgD is only 2 to 3 days.

Two features that have restricted our understanding of IgD in addition to its scarcity in serum are its heat and acid lability. Holding sera at 56° C for 1 hour reduces its IgD content by 50%, and after 4 hours only 10% is recoverable. This behavior is very remindful of IgE, which is also heat labile. A pH of 3 denatures IgD, and this feature means that it cannot be eluted from immunoadsorbent columns by the usual means of acid dissociation without simultaneously destroying the molecule. A third feature that must be held in

Table 6-6. Chemical and physical properties of immunoglobulin D

Current designation	IgD
Older names	None
Molecular weight	180,000
$S_{20,w}$ value	6.5
Electrophoretic mobility	Fast γ
Carbohydrate content	12%
Resistance to —SH reagents	Low
Concentration (mg/dl serum)	3
Amount of serum immunoglobulins	<1%
Half-life (days)	2 to 3
Rate of synthesis (mg/kg body weight/ day)	0.4
Light chain types	κ or λ
Heavy chain class	δ
General formula	$\delta_2\kappa_2$ or $\delta_2\lambda_2$
Light chain allotypes	Km
Heavy chain subclasses	None
Heavy chain constant domains	4
Stable at 56° to 60° C	No
Stable in dilute acid	No

mind is that IgD aggregates very readily, which can alter its biologic activity as well as its structure.

STRUCTURE AND CHEMISTRY OF IgE

A discussion of the structure and chemistry of IgE is presented in Chapter 18.

BIOLOGIC FUNCTION RELATIVE TO IMMUNOGLOBULIN STRUCTURE

The behavior of immunoglobulins follows the general tenets of protein behavior, being closely related to their amino acid sequence and structure. This has become especially clear with the immunoglobulins, since fragments and domains are easily prepared that simultaneously preserve certain structural elements and biologic activities.

The early separations by Porter and Edelman clearly demonstrated that the antigen-binding property of an immunoglobulin resided in its amino terminal end. Since neither free H nor free L chains possessed significant binding activity, this was clearly a joint venture. Later identification of the V_L and V_H domains indicated that antigen specificity must reside within them, since C domains were present in the nonbinding Fc fragment. Eventually the HV regions in the V_L and V_H domains were identified as the exact loci.

The constant domains were recognized as the loci for allotypic variations in both L and H chains that could not reside in the variable regions because the allotypic markers were regularly expressed.

Although the Fc fragment initially was described in terms of its ease of crystallization, it is emphasized now as the site of receptors for molecules of the complement system and cell surfaces. Only certain subclasses of IgG and IgM have receptors for the complement system, and the exact sequences essential to this function are not entirely agreed on but are probably in or near the hinge reigon and C_H2. Likewise the C_H2 domain is associated with the binding of IgG and IgM to the cell surfaces of phagocytic cells, of IgM and IgD to lymphocytes, and of IgE to mast cells and basophils.

The hinge region has a unique amino acid composition containing several prolines, which renders this section uncoiled and exposes it to enzymatic attack. This region actually flexes when antigen combines with the antibody molecule and is the hinge for joining the L and H chains.

In those polymeric IgM and IgA molecules the linking protein is the J chain. No further activity of the J chain has been described yet.

The function of SC is enigmatic, since there is no evidence that it enhances secretion. Instead it may improve the cohesiveness of the secreted immunoglobulin for the mucosal surface that it bathes.

IMMUNOGLOBULINS OF
LOWER MAMMALS

In general, the higher mammals reflect closely the immunoglobulin variations of humans. As one progresses to the lower vertebrates, IgA and IgE are lost, then IgG is lost, and finally IgM is preserved. All vertebrates synthesize secretory IgA.

The mouse, which is said to be the experimental animal in 70% of all occasions when a mammal is used, has eight distinct serum immunoglobulins. In addition to IgA, IgM, IgD, and IgE, four varieties of IgG exist: IgG1, IgG2a, IgG2b, and IgG3. The numbering of the mouse IgG subclasses is not intended to reflect a homology with human IgG. Except for the lack of IgG3 the rat immunoglobulin profile is the same as that of the mouse. Canines have IgA, IgM, and IgE but no IgD. Four IgGs also exist in dogs but are numbered IgG1, IgG2a, IgG2b, and IgG2c. Horses have four IgG-like globulins, labeled IgGa, IgGb, IgGc, and IgGT.

PURIFICATION OF
IMMUNOGLOBULINS

There are basically two different methods by which immunoglobulins can be purified. The general, or nonspecific, methods simply treat the immunoglobulins as γ-globulins and separate them from other serum proteins on the basis of their unique biophysical properties. In the specific methods the separation of the antibody globulins is accomplished through procedures that take advantage of the special antigen- or hapten-combining powers of immunoglobulins.

Nonspecific methods

The general methods for the purification of immunoglobulins are based on the discovery of Kabat over 30 years ago that antibodies are found in the γ-globulin fraction of the serum proteins. Although some of the antibodies are more properly called β-globulins, their chemical behavior is sufficiently like that of the γ-globulins to permit their isolation by many procedures designed for the latter class of proteins.

The γ-globulins are insoluble in half-saturated ammonium sulfate solutions; thus mixing of antiserum in equal proportions with saturated ammonium sulfate produces a globulin precipitate. Sodium sulfate may be used as the precipitant instead of ammonium sulfate. This precipitate is soluble in distilled water and can be reprecipitated for additional purification. Dialysis or gel filtration to remove sulfate ions yields a purified antibody preparation. Fractionation of serum by cold ethanol (Cohn's procedure) has been widely used to prepare human and animal serum proteins commercially. Because of the strict temperature and ionic strength requirements, however, it is not convenient for occasional use. γ-Globulins also may be precipitated from serum by lower concentrations of heavy metal ions than needed to precipitate other proteins. Rivanol at 0.4% concentration will precipitate most serum proteins other than the γ-globulins, which remain in the supernatant.

In addition to the solubility differences displayed by γ-globulins and other serum proteins, differences in ionic behavior also permit purification of antibodies. Preparative zone electrophoresis with polyvinyl resins as the solid phase allows greater recovery and less contamination of the antibody fraction with other proteins than the use of agar or starch as the solid phase. Beds of sponge rubber or chemical sponges such as polyurethane also are usable as the carrier phase.

Ion exchange chromatography, particularly with diethylaminoethyl (DEAE) cellulose and carboxymethyl (CM) cellulose, is a very useful purification procedure for antibodies. A simple batch procedure is based on the observation that, at pH 7.5, γ-globulins do not attach to DEAE cellulose, whereas all other proteins do. Filtration or centrifugation of an antiserum–DEAE cellulose mixture will leave the immunoglobulins in the fluid phase. The release order of serum proteins from DEAE, when they have been bound at pH 8.5, is in the order of their decreasing isoelectric points; so the γ-globulins are among the first to elute when the pH is lowered. Later fractions also will contain appreciable antibody, especially the β-globulins fraction.

Separation of the 19S immunoglobulins from the 7S immunoglobulins is possible by several simple techniques. Two of these are mentioned. The first is the molecular sieving or gel filtration technique, which divides serum proteins into three major peaks. Macroglobulins are excluded from Sephadex G-200 columns and are in the void volume peak eluted first from the column. In the second peak the 7S immunoglobulins are present. The other technique, sucrose density gradient centrifugation, is based on the greater density of the 19S antibodies compared with the 7S antibodies. If a 40% sucrose solution is carefully overlayered with a 10% sucrose solution and diffusion is allowed, a continuous 10% to 40% sucrose gradient will be established. If an antiserum is layered on top of the gradient and subjected to ultracentrifugation, the 19S globulins will sediment to the bottom of the tube (specific gravity 1.175). The 7S globulins, specific gravity 1.10, will equilibrate very near the middle of the tube. Careful removal of the fluid by use of a fraction collector will achieve separation of the two size-density classes of antibody.

Specific methods

All the specific methods for the purification of antibodies depend on a specific serologic reaction of the antibody with its antigen or hapten, after which the antibody is separated from the complex. This is easiest when the antigen in question is a polysaccharide, since polysaccharides have grossly different chemical properties from those of globulins. Certain haptens also present unique opportunities for the purification of antihaptens.

Antisera to polysaccharides may be purified by first preparing the antigen-antibody precipitate, harvesting it by centrifugation, and washing it free of contaminating serum proteins. If a specific enzyme such as dextranase or lysozyme is available to digest the antigen substrate, the antibody is left in a relatively pure state. Restrictions to the technique are quite obvious and very limiting. If no such enzyme is available, the polysaccharide antigen-antibody aggregate may be dissociated by increasing the salt concentration, raising the temperature, or altering the pH. Either acid or alkaline pH may result in dissociation, depending on the system. Dissociation is followed by a chemical procedure adapted to the precipitation of the polysaccharide or the immunoglobulin, or it may take place in a medium designed to hold one of the reactants in an insoluble condition. For example, dissociation in acid followed by salt precipitation of the globulin with $(NH_4)_2SO_4$ has been used. The polysaccharide, which remains in the supernatant, is washed from the antibody. The dissociated antigen-antibody complex can be subjected to electrophoresis, gradient centrifugation, gel filtration, or ion exchange chromatography to separate the two reactants, provided that they differ appreciably in size or ionic charge.

The most recent innovation in the purification of antibodies is the use of immunoadsorbents in affinity columns, which may be of several types: gels in which the antigen is entrapped but that have pores large enough for some physical contact between the antigen and antibody; inert polymers to which the antigen is bound covalently; or

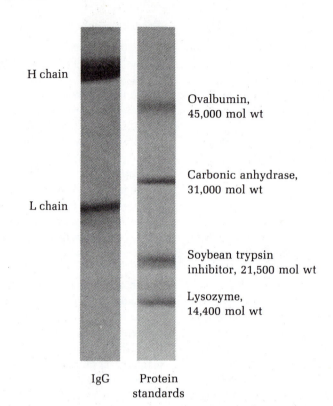

H chain

Ovalbumin,
45,000 mol wt

Carbonic anhydrase,
31,000 mol wt

L chain

Soybean trypsin
inhibitor, 21,500 mol wt

Lysozyme,
14,400 mol wt

IgG   Protein
standards

Fig. 6-10. An IgG purified from a protein A immunosorbent column was reduced to separate the H and L chains. These then were electrophoresed in a polyacrylamide gel under conditions that prevented reassociation. The positions of the H and L chains can be identified relative to the position of proteins of known molecular weight. (Courtesy Dr. C. Parker.)

cellulose derivatives or other chemicals to which the antigen is bound covalently. One of the first cellulose immunoadsorbents used was *p*-amino-benzylcellulose. If diazotized, this substituted cellulose will bond to any protein containing tyrosyl residues. If such a cellulose-protein is mixed with an immune serum to the protein, the antibody will attach to it. The cellulose derivative is then removed and washed, and the antibody is eluted, usually by lowering the pH. In this way *p*-amino-benzylcellulose diazotized to bovine serum albumin was used to prepare rabbit anti–bovine serum albumin that was 89% pure. A similar procedure using *p*-aminobenzyloxymethylcellulose will produce antibodies between 90% and 100%

pure to protein antigens such as rabbit globulin, human serum albumin, and hen egg albumin. Protein A columns will bind IgG regardless of its antigen specificity, and the immunoglobulins can be eluted later. This is a useful method for purifying IgG from a hyperimmune serum (Fig. 6-10).

BIBLIOGRAPHY

Allen, P.C., Hill, E.A., and Stokes, A.M.: Plasma proteins, Oxford, 1977, Blackwell Scientific Publications, Ltd.

Amzel, L.M., and Poljak, R.J.: Three-dimensional structure of immunoglobulins, Annu. Rev. Biochem. **48:**961, 1979.

Dorrington, K.J., and Bennich, H.H.: Structure-function relationships in human immunoglobulin E, Immunol. Rev. **41:** 3, 1978.

Edmunsdon, A.B., Ely, K.R., and Abola, E.E.: Conformational flexibility in immunoglobulins, Contemp. Top. Mol. Immunol. **7**:95, 1978.

Fudenberg, H.H., and others: Basic immunogenetics, ed. 2, New York, 1978, Oxford University Press, Inc.

Goding, J.W.: Allotypes of IgM and IgD receptors in the mouse: a probe of lymphocyte differentiation, Contemp. Top. Immunobiol. **8**:203, 1978.

Jefferis, R., and Matthews, J.B.: Structural studies of human IgD paraproteins, Immunol. Rev. **37**:25, 1977.

Kabat, E.A.: The structural basis of antibody complementarity, Adv. Protein Chem. **32**:1, 1978.

Kabat, E.A., Wu, T.T., and Bilofsky, H.: Sequences of immunoglobulin chains, NIH pub. no. 80-2008, 1979, Washington, D.C., U.S. Department of Health, Education, and Welfare.

Leslie, G.A., and Martin, L.N.: Structure and function of serum and membrane immunoglobulin D (IgD), Contemp. Top. Mol. Immunol. **7**:1, 1978.

Litman, G.W., and Good, R.A., editors: Immunoglobulins, New York, 1978, Plenum Publishing Corp.

Solomon, A.: Bence Jones proteins and the light chains of immunoglobulins, N. Engl. J. Med. **294**:17, 1976.

Steinberg, A.G., and Cook, C.E.: The distribution of the human immunoglobulin allotypes, Oxford, England, 1981, Oxford University Press.

Winkelhake, J.L.: Immunoglobulin structure and effector functions, Immunochemistry **15**:695, 1978.

SITUATION: MULTIPLE MYELOMA

Brian, a 60-year-old white man, was admitted to the hospital with pains in his back and legs. Enlarged lymph nodes were noted in the cervical, axillary, and groin areas. His hemoglubulin level was 12.4 g/dl, the white blood cell count was 9,200/mm^3, and the serum bilirubin level was increased. Urinalysis was 1+ for protein. Serum protein electrophoresis indicated a possible polyclonal gammopathy of the A and G classes. Total serum protein levels were normal. Skeletal x-ray films, bone marrow aspiration, and quantitative immunoglobulin determinations were ordered.

Questions

1. What is the probable nature of the proteinuria?
2. How does the total serum level remain normal with a concurrent polyclonal gammopathy?
3. How can a polyclonal gammopathy be suggested only from serum electrophoresis?
4. What is the preferred procedure for immunoglobulin quantitation?

Solution

The proteinuria undoubtedly is caused by Bence Jones protein. To test for Bence Jones protein, it may be necessary to acidify the urine to pH 4.5 with dilute acetic acid. The exact temperatures at which precipitation and dissolution will occur vary from patient to patient; some Bence Jones proteins do not dissolve at 100° C. The frequency of Bence Jones protein in urine has varied from as low as 30% to as high as 88% of myeloma cases. This wide range undoubtedly is caused by differences in technique (acidity of urine), protein concentration, and temperature criteria. The electrophoresis of fivefold to tenfold concentrated urine has done much to improve the urinary identification of Bence Jones protein. Systematic investigation indicates an incidence in urine in excess of 50%. The Bence Jones protein is frequently the only protein in the urine, where it is situated in the electrophoretic position occupied by the γ-globulins. It is the L chain of the immunoglobulins or dimeric or polymeric forms of the molecule.

As an aside, it it interesting that the name of Sir Henry Bence Jones has been perpetuated by this protein. Bence Jones was a clinical pathologist who recognized the protein in a urine sample supplied by Dr. Dalrymple, and another physician, Dr. Watson, later cared for the patient. The names of the patient and the two attending physicians have fallen into obscurity.

Polyclonal and monoclonal M components do not necessarily disturb the total γ-globulin concentration of the serum; in fact hypogammaglobulinemia is seen in 12% of all patients with myeloma. This has been interpreted as an elimination of normal plasma cells by cells of the plasmacytoma. Serum electrophoresis may identify the class of the hypogammaglobulinemic as well as the hypergammaglobulinemic protein. Simple serum electrophoresis often will distinguish an IgG myeloma from the others. Mixed IgA and IgM proteins will appear in nearly the same electrophoretic position and obscure the identification of the condition as a polyclonal disease. IgG with either IgA or IgM is more easily identified, although whether the second protein is A or M is often difficult to decide. In the recent past this distinction has been made via immunoelectrophoretic determinations of a crude quantitative nature with specific antisera against IgG, IgA, and IgM with normal strength and diluted serum. If the serum IgG and IgA are no longer detectable with specific antisera tested against diluted serum but the IgM is, then the indication is that the myeloma is of the IgM class. Radial immunodiffusion tests are now preferred because they are more sensitive and quantitative. In the patient described the Mancini test recovered 3.2 g/dl of IgG and 0.6 g/dl of IgA. Normal values should approximate 1.3 g/dl for IgG and 0.3 g/dl for IgA; thus the patient had a combined IgG and IgA myeloma.

References

Engle, R.L., and Wallis, L.A.: Immunoglobulinopathies, Springfield, Ill., 1969, Charles C Thomas, Publisher.

Osserman, E.F.: Plasma-cell myeloma. II. Clinical aspects, N. Engl. J. Med. **261**:1006, 1959.

Waldenström, J.: Diagnosis and treatment of multiple myeloma, New York, 1970, Grune & Stratton, Inc.

LYMPHOKINES

GLOSSARY

blastogenic factor A lymphokine that stimulates T cell growth.

CT Chemotaxin.

IFN Interferon.

interferon A family of lymphokines that protects neighboring cells from invasion by intracellular parasites.

leukocyte-inhibitory factor A lymphokine that arrests neutrophils.

LIF Leukocyte-inhibitory factor.

LT Lymphotoxin.

lymphotoxins A family of lymphokines that are cytolytic for target cells.

macrophage-activating factor A lymphokine that stimulates more aggressive properties in macrophages.

macrophage chemotaxin A leukoattractant lymphokine.

MAF Macrophage-activating factor.

MIF Migration inhibiting factor.

migration inhibiting factor A macrophage-arresting lymphokine.

mitogenic factor Synonym of blastogenic factor.

OAF Osteoclast-activating factor.

SIRS Soluble immune response suppressor.

soluble immune response suppressor A lymphokine that suppresses B cells.

TF Transfer factor.

In the preceding chapter the chemical nature of the major protein products of cells from the B cell line is presented with a brief note about their biologic functions. In this chapter the products of the T cell line are described, but chemical descriptions are limited and less definite than with the B cell products. The reason for this is simply that T cell products are active at very low concentrations, and the cells do not produce or excrete large quantities of these molecules. Procedures for massive, long-term cultures of T cells are just now achieving success, and of course the possibility of cloning T cell DNA into microorganisms expands the probability that the T cell products will be in greater supply and more easily characterized in the near future.

T cell products of a protein nature that affect or regulate the activities of other cells are classified as lymphokines. Since some lymphokines are stimulatory and others inhibitory, it is suspected that several of the T cell subsets (Th, Ts, Tc, etc.) are involved. It is generally not known if one T cell subset can produce all or multiple lymphokines characteristic of that subset or whether individual lineages within each subset are specialized to produce only one or a few lymphokines. Several studies also have identified B cells as a source of lymphokines.

Another uncertainty is whether lymphokine molecules are restricted to act on a single cell type. Many, probably several dozen, biologic ac-

129

tivities have been ascribed to lymphokines, yet to some it seems unlikely that so many different molecules would be produced even by the several specificities of T cells now recognized. Either some lymphokines act on diverse cell types, or T cells are more versatile in their production of excretory products than heretofore recognized, perhaps producing different lymphokines at different phases of their growth cycle.

TRANSFER FACTOR

After a T cell responds to an antigen, it has within it a substance that is extractable by cell lysis and which will convert naive T cells to the same antigen responsiveness as the extract donor. This substance is known as transfer factor, or TF. The chemical nature of transfer factor remains enigmatic. It behaves like both a polypeptide and nucleic acid; thus it is not chemically the same as lymphokines, which are protein. (See Chapter 20.) Neither is transfer factor a precursor of lymphokines in the sense of chemical structure, although it may be so in a semigenetic and functional sense. Exactly how transfer factor functions is unknown, but Tdh lymphocytes cannot produce lymphokines without being endowed with this factor. Whether the other major T cell subsets produce transfer factor is currently under investigation. Whether transfer factor converts only other Tdh cells to antigen responsiveness is also uncertain. There is an association of transfer factor competence and the production of some lymphokines, but this relationship is unclear.

MACROPHAGE CHEMOTAXIN

T cells apparently produce chemotaxins that are active on several cell types. The first of these to be identified acted on monocytes and macrophages (Fig. 7-1). Stimulation of antigen-sensitized T cells in culture with the specific antigen or a T cell mitogen initiates synthesis of chemotaxin within 24 hours. The physical character of chemotaxin is related to its species origin: guinea pig chemotaxin purified from Sephadex gel columns elutes in the molecular weight range of 25,000

to 55,000, but human chemotaxin is near 12,500 mol wt. The chemotaxin of both species is heat stable at 56° C for 30 minutes and is antigenically distinct from complement component C5, which is chemotactic for neutrophils (Table 7-1).

Guinea pig chemotaxin activity sometimes has been assigned to a fraction of culture fluid that has a migration inhibitory activity (MIF) on macrophages. The question was whether these activities were caused by one or two molecules. One supposition was that macrophages might be highly sensitive to chemotaxin, migrate toward its source, enter a higher concentration of the chemotaxin, and be specifically desensitized and arrested in their migration. It is now certain that these activities rely on separate molecules. Guinea pig chemotaxin acts on both guinea pig and rabbit macrophages, but its MIF is species specific. Moreover the chemotaxin is electrophoretically separable from the migration inhibitor.

MIF

One of the earliest described examples of the in vitro response of T cells to antigen was the inhibition of cell migration. This phenomenon was rediscovered and perfected in the 1960s. In its present form animals previously exposed to antigen are injected intraperitoneally with sterile paraffin oil or some other mild irritant such as an agar, starch, glycogen, or casein solution. After 2 to 4 days the peritoneal exudate is collected, washed, and drawn into capillary tubes that contain tissue culture media. Alternative sources of cells include peripheral white blood cells and spleen cells. Circulating white blood cells taken from the buffy coat frequently are not as suitable as peritoneal exudate cells, and spleen must be minced carefully and tediously until a sufficient supply of single cells is prepared. Regardless of the source, after the cells are drawn into the capillary tubes, the tubes are centrifuged and then cut precisely at the cell-fluid interface. The portion bearing the cells is placed in a special chamber filled with a suitable tissue culture medium that contains the sensitizing antigen in a concentration

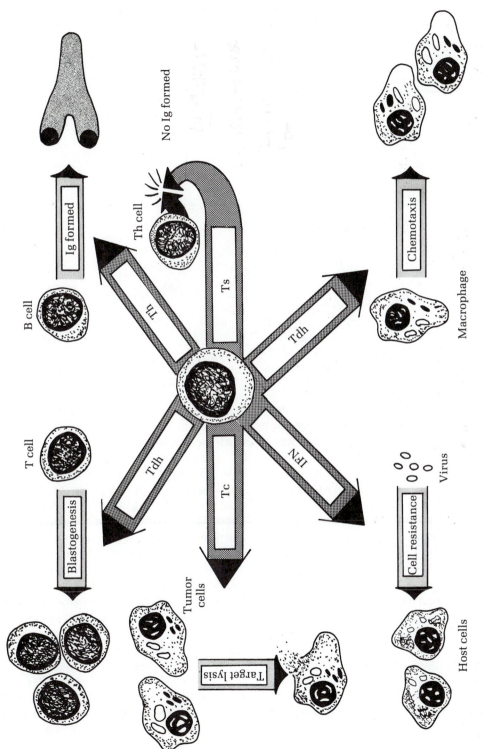

Fig. 7-1. Various T cell subsets are involved in the production of lymphokines that influence other T cells, B cells, macrophages, and other host or foreign cells. The best described of these activities are illustrated.

Table 7-1. Biochemical characteristics of the lymphokines

	Macrophage chemotaxin	MIF	LIF	Lymphotoxins	Blastogenic factor
Function	Attracts monocytes and macrophages	Inhibits macrophage motility	Inhibits PMN motility	Lyses target cells	Stimulates cell growth
Molecular weight	Human: 12,500 Guinea pig: 25,000 to 55,000	Human: 23,000 to 55,000 Guinea pig: MIF I, 65,000 MIF II, 25,000 to 40,000 Mouse: 48,000 to 67,000	68,000	α H: 110,000 to 140,000 α L: 60,000 to 90,000 β: 40,000 to 50,000 γ: 10,000 to 20,000	Human: 20,000 to 50,000 Guinea pig: 15,000 to 30,000
Heat resistance		Stable at 56° C for 30 minutes	Stable at 56° C for 30 minutes Labile at 80° C	Stable at 56° C for 30 minutes Labile at 80° C	Stable at 56° C for 30 minutes
Comment	Albumin	1. Has MAF activity 2. Guinea pig and human are albumins; mouse is a β-globulin	Albumin	Arise from a common precursor	

of 1 to 50 μg/ml. The chambers holding the tubes are incubated for 1 to 2 days, after which they are examined microscopically. The area of cell migration is calculated and compared with a control consisting of sensitized cells incubated in the absence of antigen. Typically the latter will exhibit a mushroom like button of cells at the opening of the tube, whereas the experimental tubes will not (Fig. 7-2). Based on areas of migration, migration inhibition of 50% to 75% or higher may be expected. Total (100%) inhibition is never achieved.

Antigen specificity of the test has been demonstrated with diphtheria toxoid, egg albumin, tuberculin or a purified protein derivative (PPD), histoplasmin, bovine γ-globulin, β-lactoglobulin, keyhole-limpet hemocyanin, and many other antigens, but the most important tests are probably those which involved hapten-protein conjugates. Cells from guinea pigs sensitized to dinitrophenyl guinea pig albumin were inhibited from migrating by that complex but not by the hapten attached to

bovine γ-globulin. The reverse was true in animals sensitized to dinitrophenyl bovine γ-globulin, which was the only migration inhibitor, whereas the hapten conjugated to other proteins was ineffective. These studies confirm that the T cell response is directed to the carrier, not toward the hapten portion (on which B cells focus).

It has been conclusively demonstrated that two cell types are necessary in the migration assay: sensitized lymphocytes and macrophages. Direct observations reveal that it is primarily cells of the macrophage type which emigrate from the capillary tubes. Moreover peritoneal exudates are composed predominantly of macrophages, which represent 80% to 90% of the total exudate population. Peritoneal exudate cells poured into plastic or glass dishes divide themselves into two categories: those which adhere (macrophages) and those which remain free (lymphocytes). In this manner populations of each exceeding 90% purity can be obtained. When purified lymphocytes from

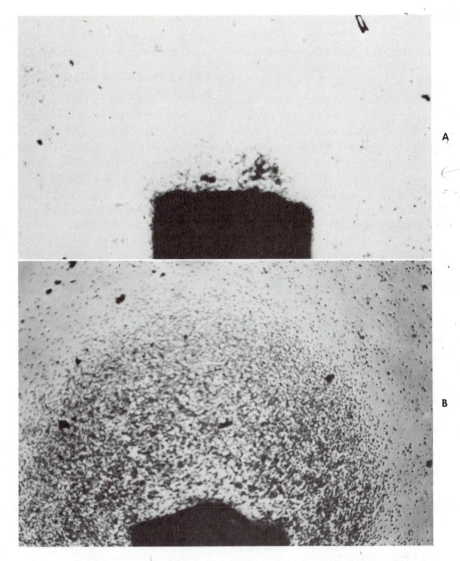

Fig. 7-2. A macrophage migration inhibition test. Peritoneal exudate cells from a guinea pig possessing a delayed hypersensitivity to histoplasmin were used. **A,** Little or no migration is seen in the presence of histoplasmin. **B,** Abundant migration in the presence of tuberculin. (Courtesy Dr. W. Irvin.)

a normal donor are mixed with antigen and macrophages from either a normal or sensitized donor, migration proceeds normally. In the reverse experiment, in which lymphocytes are taken from a sensitized donor, macrophage migration inhibition is the result, whether the macrophages are harvested from normal or sensitized donors. In fact the extent of inhibition can be correlated with the percent of sensitized lymphocytes in the final mixture. It has been estimated that one active lymphocyte can affect the migration of about 1,000 macrophages.

MIF is not present in lymphocytes prior to their exposure to antigen but is synthesized after exposure. Puromycin, actinomycin, and other inhibitors of protein synthesis provided the first clues that MIF was a protein. Guinea pig, human, and mouse MIFs all have been partially purified from Con A or antigen-treated cultures (Table 7-1).

Two guinea pig MIFs are known and can be distinguished by several features. MIF I has a molecular weight near 65,000, has an isoelectric point of 3 to 4, and is trypsin sensitive. MIF II is smaller, 25,000 to 40,000 mol wt, has an isoelectric point between 5 and 5.5, and is trypsin resistant. The resistance of MIF II to proteases is related to a protective role of its sialic acid. Both guinea pig MIFs are stable at 56° C.

Human MIF activity is restricted to a single protein with the electrophoretic mobility of an albumin (isoelectric point 4 to 6) in the molecular weight range of 23,000 to 55,000. Mouse MIF has an apparent molecular weight of 48,000 to 67,000 and is a heat-stable β-globulin.

MIF is adsorbed to the surface of macrophages but not to granulocytes. This adsorption is inhibited by the monosaccharide fucose, indicating a potential role for this sugar in the natural receptor.

MACROPHAGE-ACTIVATING FACTOR (MAF)

When macrophages come under the influence of T cell products, they become more actively phagocytic and more cytodestructive to engulfed bacteria or tumor cells, develop an increased number of lysosomal granules, adhere more firmly to surfaces, increase their oxygen consumption, and in general display more aggressive properties. These activated macrophages, also known as armed or "professional" macrophages, have been stimulated by a molecule that is indistinguishable from MIF. The macrophage-activating factor (MAF) response appears in these cells later than the MIF response, but this does not necessarily indicate a

separate molecular basis; it could be a concentration effect or simply the expression of two different responses to a single stimulus.

LEUKOCYTE-INHIBITORY FACTOR (LIF)

A second white blood cell migration inhibitor from T cells acts on the PMN. Leukocyte-inhibitory factor (LIF) is a distinct molecule separable from MIF on the basis of molecular weight, since LIF has a molecular weight of 68,000. Otherwise the molecules are much alike: both are stable at 56° C but not at 80° C, both are destroyed by proteases, and both behave electrophoretically as albumins (Table 7-1). Human LIF activity is destroyed by diisopropylfluorophosphate and other inhibitors that bind to serine. This has indicated that LIF belongs with the serine-containing esterase and protease enzymes, all of which contain a sensitive serine residue in their active site. How this putative enzyme activates the target neutrophils is open to conjecture. Monosaccharides found on the neutrophil surface (fucose and acetylglucosamine) serve as part of the LIF receptor.

LYMPHOTOXINS

The ability of antigen-trained or lectin-stimulated T cells, probably CTC cells, to destroy target cells has been identified both with cell-free substances defined as lymphotoxins, or LTs, and direct cell to cell contact (Figs. 7-1, 12-2, and 12-4). Conflicting evidence about the ability of antisera to lymphotoxin to neutralize its activity may be attributed to differences in specificity and potency of the antisera.

Mouse lymphotoxins have been the best characterized and have been subdivided into the α-, β-, and γ-lymphotoxins. All these arise from a complex precursor molecule (C_X) with a molecular weight in excess of 200,000. The α-lymphotoxin derivatives now have been further subdivided into the heavy (α H-LT) and light (α L-LT) forms, which have molecular weights between 110,000 and 140,000 and 60,000 and 90,000, respectively. Although these have not been evaluated individually, collectively as α-lymphotoxins they are resistant to 56° C but sensitive to 80° C and destroyed by certain proteases. The β-lymphotoxins are the next smaller (40,000 to 50,000 mol wt), and the γ-lymphotoxins are the smallest (10,000 to 20,000 mol wt). The α- and β-lymphotoxins are unstable in the cold, and this has handicapped further characterization. The lymphotoxin systems of the guinea pig and rabbit parallel that of the mouse.

The human lymphotoxin system is also very similar to that of the mouse. The human C_X molecule has a reported molecular weight of 200,000 from which the active lymphotoxins are derived. The first cytolytic molecule has been termed a precursor of the α heavy lymphotoxin, or $P_{\alpha H}$. It has a molecular weight of approximately 150,000. Loss of a peptide of 10,000 to 20,000 mol wt yields the α heavy lymphotoxin. From it the β-lymphotoxin and γ-lymphotoxin (molecular weights near 65,000 and 17,500, respectively) are derived (Fig. 7-3).

That lymphotoxins attach to the cell surface of target cells has been conclusively demonstrated by the use of radiolabeled molecules. The biochemical basis of this attachment either in the

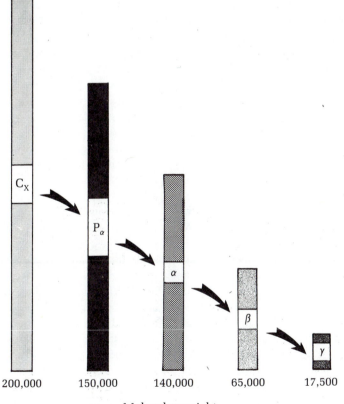

Molecular weight

Fig. 7-3. The stepwise formation of the lymphotoxins begins with the C_X molecule (200,000 mol wt) and proceeds through the precursor to the α-, β-, and γ-lymphotoxin molecules. Only one of the two forms of the α-lymphotoxin molecule is shown.

lymphotoxin molecule or its receptor is unknown. Within a few hours after lymphotoxin binding to the target cells, they become spherical, increase in size as they lose their osmotic balance, show evidence of nuclear and cytoplasmic degeneration by "vacuolization," detach from the vessel surface, and lyse.

BLASTOGENIC FACTOR

The formation of large, pyronin-staining immunoblasts from small lymphocytes is termed *lymphocyte transformation* and is a property of a lymphokine known both as blastogenic factor and mitogenic factor (Fig. 7-1). These lymphoblasts are morphologically similar to cells seen in vivo after antigen stimulation; they develop a larger and lighter staining nucleus, they are double the size of the small lymphocyte, or about 15 to 20 μm in diameter, and their cytoplasm acquires a more basophilic staining property, including a greater affinity for pyronin dyes, although they have very little fully developed, or rough, serpentine endoplasmic reticulum. Lymphoblasts are easily confused morphologically with mononuclear phagocytes in tissues or mixed cell cultures but can be differentiated form them by adding inert particles to viable cell populations. The particles are engulfed by and identify the monocytes.

Transforming lymphocytes are in a condition of hyperactive metabolism, synthesizing DNA, RNA, and protein at a rapid rate. DNA synthesis in transforming cells proceeds at approximately three times the rate of that in nonactivated lymphocytes. Therefore the uptake of tritiated thymidine, which is incorporated into the DNA of the cell nucleus, is used as an index of transformation. RNA synthesis also is accelerated and can be assayed by isotopic techniques with radiolabeled purine and pyrimidine bases. Both these changes are surprisingly slow in tissue cultures of lymphocytes, which may require 3 to 5 days of cultivation before statistically significant changes from control cultures become apparent. A change in the rate of protein formation can be detected within 4 hours and may replace nucleic acid–de-

pendent systems, which is a measure of transformation.

Biochemical characterization of blastogenic factors of guinea pig and human origin has indicated slight differences in size. The guinea pig factor has a 15,000 to 30,000 mol wt, and the human molecule has a molecular weight of 20,000 to 50,000. Both are stable at 56° C, and both are proteins and thus sensitive to proteases but resistant to ribonucleases and deoxyribonucleases.

IFN

The discovery of IFN in 1957 by Isaacs and Lindenmann revealed for the first time that animals had a second form of acquired immunity, other than immunoglobulins, which was based on excreted cell products. The first IFN described was excreted by T cells that had been exposed to an inactivated virus; its antiviral activity was detected by the ability of the cell culture fluids to protect animals or tissue cultures against virus infection. The idea that IFNs were unique antiviral substances stimulated solely by virus has long since been abandoned. Viruses are potent IFN inducers, and among them the myxoviruses and arboviruses are the most potent. Many other microbes, particularly those with an intracellular phase to their growth cycle, are IFN inducers: *Brucella abortus, Listeria monocytogenes,* and *Francisella tularensis* among the bacteria, but also rickettsia, malarial parasites, and other intracellular animal parasites. In addition to these natural inducers, many pure chemical substances will induce IFN: bacterial endotoxins, complex polysaccharides, PHA, anionic polymers of maleic anhydride, acrylic acid and pyrans, and, among the most studied, double-stranded RNA (dsRNA). Several cell poisons, including bacterial endotoxins and exotoxins, and actinomycin D will stimulate IFN production. Note that many of these inducers are not antigenic. What does this myriad of substances have that permits them to share a common activity? In the middle of the 1960s it was concluded that the natural inducers functioned because of their common content of dsRNA. Many synthetic

RNA pairs and modified pairs were tested; among them the polymers of polyinosinic acid and polycytidylic acid (poly I · C) were the most potent. Other polyanionic inducers are structural mimics of poly I · C or dsRNA. Cell poisons act because they cause cell death and the release of cellular dsRNA, which then stimulates the surviving cells to produce IFN.

The early chemical studies of IFN identified it as an acid-stable molecule with an isoelectric point near 5.5 in the broad molecular weight range of 18,000 to 100,000 that possessed antiviral activity. Eventually this molecular weight heterogeneity was related to the ease by which monomeric IFN can aggregate to form truly giant forms. Although the problem of size heterogeneity of IFN was resolved, new studies indicated heterogeneity of other types. All IFNs were not resistant to a pH of 2 overnight in the cold. Serologic studies identified an antigenic heterogeneity, and it was possible to demonstrate IFN production by T cells, macrophages, fibroblasts, and other cell types. Eventually it became necessary to define IFNs as proteins that were antigen nonspecific with a wide range of activities against viruses and intracellular parasites, that acted intracellularly and not by masking host cell receptors for virus, that were synthesized only after the proper stimulus and were not endogenously produced, and that displayed several biologic activities in addition to the inhibition of viral replication.

Many of the problems and uncertainties about IFN heterogeneity have been resolved by the recognition of three major forms of IFN and the identification of subspecies within these groups. The α-IFN is of leukocyte (T cell) origin and was formerly classified as a type I IFN along with β-IFN because both were acid stable. Fibroblasts are the source of β-IFN. Acid-labile IFN, or γ-IFN, is produced by T cells exposed to antigen or mitogens and is synonymous with type II, or immune, IFN. Immunoregulation may be a primary function of γ-IFN. All forms of IFN so far identified are proteins of about 17,000 mol wt. Differences in their size can be attributed to modest differences in their amino acid composition and the extent of glycosylation. The α-IFNs are not glycosylated, but the β molecules are. Both the α- and β-IFNs consist of approximately 165 amino acids and γ-IFN of 146 amino acids (Table 7-2).

The extremely low concentration of IFN in culture fluids, mentioned earlier as a handicap to the purification and characterization of most lymphokines, may no longer prove to be a limitation. Gene splicing and the implantation of mammalian DNA or mRNA coding for IFN into microbial cells have been successful, and IFN of microbial origin is now available. Already interesting genetic information has arisen from these studies with the finding of eight different genes code for eight different α-IFN molecules. Thus the heterogeneity of IFN is much broader than previously supposed.

Although the IFNs have the common ability to arrest viral infections or infections promoted by other intracellular parasites, even more excitement has been generated by the cell growth–regulating action of IFN. The ability of IFN to slow the growth of oncogenic tissues is a significant therapeutic finding, since it allows other host defense factors to rid the body of the cancerous growth.

Table 7-2. Distinctive characteristics of the IFNs

Current designation	Type	Cell source	Inducer	Molecular weight	Acid stability (pH 2)	Number of variants
α-IFN	I	T cells	Viruses, dsRNA	17,000	Yes	8
β-IFN	I	Fibroblasts	Viruses, dsRNA	17,000	Yes	5
γ-IFN	II	T cells	Antigens, mitogens	15,000	No	Unknown

Preliminary trials with bacterial IFN have indicated it is as suitable for this purpose as natural IFN.

IFN produced by host cells diffuses from these cells and binds to receptors on neighboring cells. This triggers the synthesis of viral inhibitors, which remain inactive until a virus enters the cell. Until that time the IFN-treated host cell can continue its normal metabolic processes.

When it was found that IFN or dsRNA was inhibitory to protein synthesis, several potential enzymes were screened as possible targets for IFN. One of these which has been identified is a protein kinase that adds phosphate groups taken from adenosine triphosphate (ATP) to proteins. When IFN is present, the kinase "erroneously" phosphorylates a protein-initiating factor. Phosphorylation of the initiating factor interrupts synthesis of the proteins needed for viral replication.

A second target molecule proved to be a nuclease that is activated by a molecule derived from ATP. The current hypothesis is that dsRNA or IFN activates a 2'5'-adenosine polymerase which degrades ATP to form short chains of adenosine linked by 2'5'-phosphodiester bonds (Fig. 7-4). The polymerase is active only after viral derived dsRNA is present. The product, 2'5'-adenosine, or 2'5'A, reacts with an endonuclease that cleaves RNA, and the newly synthesized messenger that arises after viral infection and which is needed for viral replication is destroyed. The failure of the protein kinase, the 2'5'-adenosine polymerase, and endonuclease to halt host cell growth is attributed to the operation of these three enzymes in a microenvironment near the viral invader.

Now that the mode of action of IFN is being unraveled and the ability to produce "bacterial" IFN has been realized, it may become possible

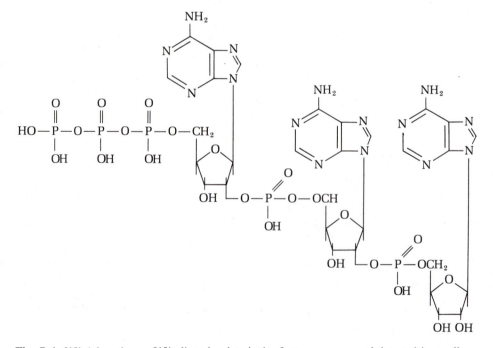

Fig. 7-4. 2'5'-Adenosine or 2'5'-oligoadenylate is the first new compound detected in a cell exposed to IFN, and it catalyzes a sequence of reactions that prevent viral replication.

to use IFNs to treat cancer, stimulate phagocytosis, halt viral infections, and treat other medical problems ecomonically and safely.

OSTEOCLAST-ACTIVATING FACTOR (OAF)

Although perhaps not of as much interest to immunologists as other lymphokines, a low molecular weight factor produced by T cells causes the loss of Ca^{2+} from bone in culture. This bone resorption is attributed to an osteoclast-activating factor (OAF). Biophysical measurements of OAF indicate it may have a molecular weight as low as 140, which can self-associate to produce molecultes between 1,300 and 3,500 mol wt. These may complex to form large molecules or bind nonspecifically to protein carriers and appear in a vast array of sizes. Although OAF is not yet well described, it can be distinguished from other bone-resorbing agents on the basis of differing heat lability, lipid solubility, and antigen specificity.

SOLUBLE IMMUNE RESPONSE SUPPRESSOR (SIRS)

The secretory product of Ts cells that provides an antigen-nonspecific suppression of B cells has been partially characterized. Soluble immune response suppressor (SIRS) may not act directly on B cells. Instead it may be altered by macrophages, probably by oxidation, to become the active molecule. This SIRS is a protein of 35,000 to 67,000 mol wt, which is readily destroyed by trypsin and chymotrypsin but resistant to ribonucleases and deoxyribonucleases. It is labile at pH 2 and about 70° C but is stable at 56° C for 1 hour. SIRS from Con A–stimulated mouse spleen cultures also displays MIF activity.

SIRS is definitely different from a soluble immune suppressor supernatant (SISS) found in cell-free filtrates of T cell cultures. SISS has a molecular weight of 60,000 to 80,000. This molecule is heat labile at 56° C and stable at pH 2.5.

The antigen-specific immune response supres-

sors that are shed or extracted from T cells are products of the I-J gene and are found on macrophages and B cells. The molecular weight of these products is about 70,000, which is entirely compatible with I-A and I-E protein structure. The structure of the I-J gene product is like that of the I-A and I-E products: a bimolecular protein consisting of an α- and β-chain.

MISCELLANEOUS LYMPHOKINES

Several other lymphokines have been described in biologic terms and to various degrees in biophysical terms. These include the interleukins, a chemotaxin for PMNs, a chemotaxin for eosinophils, a colony-stimulating or growth-stimulating factor, a monocyte growth factor, and others that are too incompletely described to be included here.

BIBLIOGRAPHY

Bendtzen, K.: Biological properties of lymphokines, Allergy **33:**105, 1978.

Cohen, S., Pick, E., and Oppenheim, J., editors: Biology of the lymphokines, New York, 1979, Academic Press, Inc.

deWeck, A.L., Kristensen, F., and Landy, M., editors: Biochemical characterization of lymphokines, New York, 1980, Academic Press, Inc.

Gately, M.K., and Mayer, M.M.: Purification and characterization of lymphokines: an approach to the study of molecular mechanisms of cell-mediated immunity, Prog. Allergy **25:**106, 1978.

Gillis, S.: Interleukin 2 dependent culture of cytolytic T cell lines, Immunol. Rev. **54:**81, 1981.

Goldstein, A.L., and Chirigos, M.A., editors: Lymphokines and thymic hormones: their potential utilization in cancer therapeutics, New York, 1981, Raven Press.

Pierce, C.W.: Activities of nonspecific and specific suppressor T cell factors in immune responses, Agents Actions (Suppl.) **7:**126, 1980.

Rocklin, R.E., Bendtzen, K., and Greineder, D.: Mediators of immunity: lymphokines and monokines, Adv. Immunol. **29:** 55, 1980.

Smith, K.A.: T-cell growth factor, Immunol. Rev. **51:**337, 1980.

Sorg, C.: The biochemistry and in vitro activity of soluble factors of activated lymphocytes, Mol. Cell. Biochem. **28:** 149, 1979.

Stewart, W.E., II: The interferon system, Vienna, 1979, Springer-Verlag.

Stringfellow, D.A., editor: Interferon and interferon inducers: clinical applications, New York, 1980, Marcel Dekker, Inc.

Watson, J.D.: Lymphokines and the induction of immune responses, Transplantation **31:**313, 1981.

Watson, J., and Mochizuki, D.: Interleukin 2: a class of T cell growth factors, Immunol. Rev. **51:**257, 1980.

Yabrov, A.A.: Interferon and nonspecific resistance, New York, 1980, Human Sciences Press, Inc.

CHAPTER 8

BIOLOGIC ASPECTS
OF THE IMMUNE RESPONSE

GLOSSARY

adjuvant A substance, usually injected with an antigen, that improves the immune response, either humoral or cellular, to the antigen.

alkylating agent An agent that reacts with electronegative centers in another compound and forms covalent bonds with it during the reaction; such compounds are often immunosuppressants.

ALS Antilymphocyte serum.

anamnestic response The rapid rise in immunoglobulin following a second or subsequent exposure to antigen; synonymous with *booster* or *secondary response*.

antigen competition Failure of a mixture of antigens to produce as high a titered antiserum to one or more of the antigens, as when the antigens are administered singly.

antilymphocyte serum An antiserum prepared against lymphocytes of either the B or T type or (usually) a mixture of them.

ATS Antithymocyte serum.

booster response *see* Anamnestic response.

clonal selection theory A theory of immunoglobulin formation which suggests that an antigen causes the replication of a cell to form a clone of cells producing antibody to that antigen.

corticosteroids Natural (or synthetic) compounds from the adrenal cortex that are antiinflammatory and immunosuppressive.

folic acid antagonist Structural analogs of folic acid that function as immunosuppressants, such as aminopterin and methotrexate.

Freund's adjuvant An adjuvant consisting of an oil and emulsifying agent (incomplete Freund's adjuvant) with which antigen solutions are emulsified; for the complete adjuvant, mycobacteria also are incorporated into the mixture.

germinal center A discrete cellular structure in lymphoid organs of antigenically stimulated animals containing macrophages, T or B lymphocytes, and/or plasma cells.

immunologic tolerance A failure or depression in the immune response on proper exposure to antigen, especially massive doses; probably synonymous with *immune paralysis*.

immune suppression Suppression of an immunologic response by chemical, physical, or biologic means.

memory cell A cell that responds more quickly to the second exposure to antigen than to the primary exposure and is responsible for the anamnestic response.

PEG Polyethylene glycol.

purine and pyrimidine analog Structural analogs of the bases of DNA and RNA that function as immunosuppressants.

As in Chapter 6, the primary focus in this chapter is on antibodies and how they are synthesized by the body in response to an antigenic stimulus.

IMMUNOGLOBULIN RESPONSE

The injection of an antigen into an animal may initiate several important changes. The immunoglobulin response is to some extent preceded by a period of antigen elimination. These two topics introduce us to other biologic aspects of the immunoglobulins.

Antigen elimination curve

For intravenously injected antigen three phases of antigen removal are easily detected (Fig. 8-1). The first phase occupies only 10 to 20 minutes if particulate antigens are used and represents the time required for equilibration of the antigen with tissues and fluids. Because of extensive phagocytosis in the liver, lung, and spleen, nearly 90% of the antigen is removed from the circulation in its first passage through these organs. Examination of sections from these tissues shortly after antigen administration will reveal that the macrophages have engorged themselves with antigen. Soluble antigens are not removed from the blood quite so quickly because of their slower pinocytic uptake by cells. If the antigen is aggregated, it is removed faster, indicating that size is important in phagocytosis and pinocytosis.

The second phase of antigen elimination is a phase of gradual catabolic degradation and removal of the antigen. This continues over a period of 4 to 7 days and represents the gradual enzymatic hydrolysis and digestion of the antigen. Consequently the limits of this period are regulated by the enzymatic capability of the host for the particular type of substrate that the antigen represents. Polysaccharide antigens survive for fairly long periods in rabbits. The extended half-life of poly-D amino acids is explained on the basis that most animals are deficient in enzymes which can degrade unnatural stereoisomers of amino acids. In animals that fail to produce antibody (become tolerant to the antigen), this second phase is extended for several weeks and represents the last phase of the antigen elimination curve.

The third portion of the curve, in which there is again an accelerated removal of antigen, is the immune elimination segment. This phase is the result

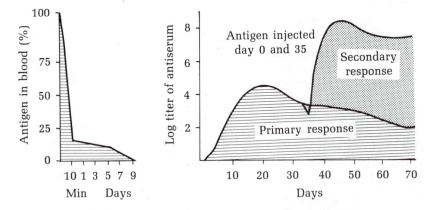

Fig. 8-1. Antigen decay (elimination) and primary and secondary immunoglobulin formation curves. The antigen elimination curve shows the three phases of equilibration, metabolic elimination, and immune elimination, the last beginning at about the fifth day. Circulating immunoglobulins are not detectable until about the fifth day. Notice how the secondary immunoglobulin response following the readministration of antigen at the thirty-fifth day reaches a very high titer compared with the primary response.

of the newly formed antibody molecules combining with the antigen, enhancing phagocytic engulfment, digestion, and removal of the antigen. Although the antigen decay shown in Fig. 8-1 progresses to zero between the fifth and fourteenth days, this is meant to reflect only the quantity of detectable antigen in blood. The absolute removal of all antigen from an immunized animal may take many months or years. Certainly, as serologic and chemical tests of greater and greater sensitivity have been applied to the detection of antigen in vivo, antigen has been recovered for longer periods of time after injection.

Immunoglobulin formation

Primary response. By restricting this discussion to the appearance of antibodies in the blood and to the total quantity of antibodies in the blood and by not considering the individual immunoglobulins, it can be seen that the antibody response plotted against time will approximate the curve seen in Fig. 8-1. After the first injection of antigen there is a lag of several days before antibody is detectable. This latent period, or induction period, varies from several hours to several days, depending on the kind and amount of antigen given, the route of administration, the species of animal and its health, and the sensitivity of the test used to measure the antibody. Antibody should appear sometime from the fifth to tenth day.

The latent period is not a reflection of the time it takes to begin antibody production at the cellular level. When antibody-forming cells are removed from the immunized animal, antibody synthesis can be detected within 20 minutes after the exposure to antigen. Since only a few cells are producing antibody at this time, it may take several days before antibody is measurable in the blood. Another important consideration is that those first antibody molecules to appear in the blood may find residual antigen still in the circulation. If these antigen and antibody molecules combine, the antibody will be difficult to measure by the usual serologic tests. Excretion of these antigen-antibody complexes will be rapid, so the first evidence of free antibody is not until a few days after the first antibody molecules were elaborated into the bloodstream. In this way overly large injections of antigens may tend to extend the latent period.

As the latent period ends, the primary antibody response becomes visible. The titer of antibody gradually increases over a period of a few days to a few weeks, plateaus, and begins to drop. The general shape of the primary response curve is the typical sigmoid curve, with an extended decay phase. The exact shape of the response curve is dictated by many variables, some of which are stated earlier.

Secondary response. If an additional exposure of antigen subsequently is given to the same animal, the antibody response differs dramatically from the primary antibody response. This secondary response is at first one of a sharp drop in circulating antibody because of its complexing with the newly injected antigen. Immediately thereafter, certainly within 2 or 3 days under ordinary circumstances, a marked increase in the antibody content of the blood becomes evident. This increase continues for several days, and ultimately the titer far surpasses that of the primary response. The secondary response is often called the memory, anamnestic (without forgetting), or booster response. It is as though the previously immunized animal became primed for that antigen and was prepared to respond to it in an accelerated way. All the variables that regulate the primary response also influence to some degree the booster response, but the booster response has an abbreviated latent period, a heightened titer, and an extended duration of detectable antibody when compared with the primary response curve (Fig. 8-1).

Several additional interesting facts about the anamnestic response should be cited.

1. It is not the result of a sudden release of preformed antibody that has been stored; it is the result of the bulk synthesis of new antibody. Proof of this is found in experiments in which a radiolabeled amino acid is injected at the same time as the antigen. When the antibody is studied after a few days, it is found to be heavily labeled with

isotope, indicating that it was produced recently.

2. The anamnestic response may be induced at almost any time after the primary response. Even many years after the primary response, when the primary titer has dropped to zero, the anamnestic response is still inducible. It may not be quite as striking as a booster nearer in time to the initial response, but the true secondary response will develop.

3. The secondary response is repeatable many times until the physiologic limit of that particular animal to that particular antigen is reached. This may not occur until three to five booster injections of antigen have been given.

4. Cross-reactive antigens will induce the response. In this case the degree of anamnesis will be correlated with the sameness of the two antigens; the more they are alike, the better the response.

5. Nonspecific anamnesis may occur. The origin of antibody is in lymphoid tissue. Any treatment of the immunized animal that will cause lysis or hyperplasia of the antibody-forming cells will cause a (minimal) anamnestic response.

6. The decrease in antibody titer after the secondary response seems to be more gradual than after the primary response. This is probably the result of two factors; one is that more cells are involved in antibody production in the secondary antibody response. If some of these cells are relatively long lived and continue functioning, then antibody will be formed over a longer period after the secondary than the primary response. The second factor involved is that the antiserum in the secondary response is qualitatively different from that after the initial response. It contains relatively more IgG, which has a half-life of 25 to 35 days. The primary antiserum is relatively rich in IgM, which has a half-life of only 8 to 10 days. The relative contribution of IgG and IgM to the primary and secondary response is illustrated in Fig. 8-2. The IgM secondary response in only one tenth that of IgG; for this reason hyperimmune sera are predominantly IgG in nature. IgG has been referred to as the memory component, implying that IgM anamnesis does not occur. This is true in a relative sense only, since secondary IgM levels are in fact somewhat greater than primary levels.

7. Reactivation of the immunoglobulin response is not entirely without danger, especially when soluble antigens or autocoupling haptens are employed. A certain proportion of the antibody produced after the primary antigenic exposure has the capacity to fix to tissue cells. These cell-bound

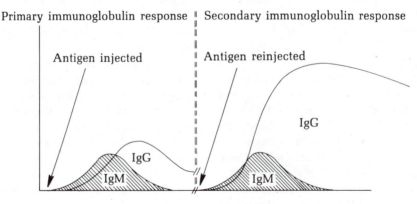

Primary immunoglobulin response | Secondary immunoglobulin response

Antigen injected | Antigen reinjected

IgG

IgG

IgM | IgM

Time scale

Fig. 8-2. Difference in the IgG response to primary and secondary exposure to antigen indicates why it is termed the memory antibody. IgM, illustrated to exhibit no "memory" usually shows a slight anamnestic response.

antibodies, for which there are several terms—for example, anaphylactic antibody, mast cell degranulating antibody, cytotoxic antibody, and homocytotropic antibody—can attach to the injected antigen while still attached to the tissue cells. In some instances this in vivo cell-bound antigen-antibody reaction can trigger a set of reactions that may be lethal to the animal. This syndrome is known as anaphylactic shock and under certain conditions is a hazard to reimmunization.

Adjuvants

Aside from the intrinsic variations in the immune response governed by the immunized animal and the antigen, the antibody response also can be modified by specific treatments of the animal. Some of these treatments may enhance the antibody response, whereas others may have the exact opposite effect.

Adjuvants (Latin *adjuvare,* to help) are agents used to potentiate the immune response. Although this often is thought of merely in terms of the immunoglobulin response, it is clear that many adjuvants also stimulate the activities of T lymphocytes (cell-mediated immunity [CMI]) and activate macrophages. Stimulation of the immune response generally is measured in terms of a greater antibody response than that produced without adjuvants or in the conservation of the quantity of antigen needed to achieve an optimal immune response. Adjuvants customarily are administered with the antigen; although this is not an absolute necessity, it generally avoids the need for a second injection of the adjuvant alone. Adjuvants may or may not be antigens in their own right.

Among the repository adjuvants, the aluminum and calcium salts, including aluminum phosphate, aluminum hydroxide, aluminum potassium tartrate (alum), and calcium phosphate, are the best known. When these materials are incorporated with antigen, they form an insoluble complex with the antigen. This slows the escape of antigen from a subcutaneous or intramuscular depot (which can be as great as 99% complete in 24 hours without adjuvant); by increasing the physical

size of the antigens, they also enhance phagocytosis. The original antigenic stimulus is prolonged over a period of 3 to 4 weeks because of the gradual dissolution and release of antigen from its insolubilized form. This creates the effect of multiple, microbooster exposures.

Water-in-oil emulsifying adjuvants have had a restricted use in humans, but the prospects for developing new and superior adjuvants of this type are great. The emulsified adjuvants allow only a slow release of the antigen from the oil-covered droplets into the true physiologic milieu of the animal, since the droplets, being of a broad size range, disintegrate at different rates. The second role of water-in-oil adjuvants is to provide microdroplets of antigen in oil to phagocytic cells. Again phagocytes can imbibe these antigen droplets more easily than antigen in solution.

A classic example of the water-in-oil emulsion adjuvant is Freund's adjuvant. The incomplete form of this adjuvant consists of a mixture of a light mineral oil and an emulsifier such as mannide monooleate. To this, the antigen in aqueous solution is added, and the emulsion is produced in a pharmaceutical blender or by passing the mixture repeatedly through a small-bore needle and syringe assembly. Freund's complete adjuvant contains 0.5 mg/ml of killed mycobacteria as a supplement to the incomplete adjuvant. The bacteria available in commercial preparations are either *Mycobacterium butyricum* or *M. tuberculosis.* Experimental formulations often substitute *Corynebacterium parvum (Propionibacterium acnes)* or BCG vaccine for the usual mycobacteria. Freund's complete adjuvant produces such serious granulomas that it is not recommended for human use. The adjuvant property of tubercle bacilli has been identified to reside in an unusual peptide, *N*-acetylmuramyl-L-alanyl-D-isoglutamine, or muramyl dipeptide (MDP) (Fig. 8-3). MDP does not produce granulomas. It and several of its chemical modifications are being compared for their adjuvant effect.

Newer water-in-oil emulsions prepared from highly purified and metabolizable ingredients

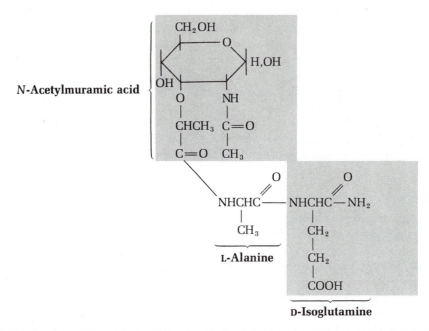

Fig. 8-3. The structure of *N*-acetylmuramyl-L-alanyl-D-isoglutamine, the adjuvant peptide isolated from the tubercle bacillus.

soon may be sanctioned for human use. Since the ingredients are fully metabolizable, disfiguring granuloma formation is not a complication as it is with other emulsifying adjuvants. Microscopic, uniformly sized water-in-oil droplets are referred to as liposomes. When phospholipids that are normally present in the host's cells are used as the oil base, the liposomes are completely biodegradable.

LPSs, or endotoxins, from nearly all gram-negative bacilli are stimulants of IgM production. The polysaccharide portion is relatively noncontributory to adjuvanticity, with the dominant biologic activity residing in the lipid A fraction, which appears to be common to all LPS molecules. Pure lipid A is pyrogenic and is probably a central cause of the fever observed during infections with gram-negative bacteria. This is also a handicap to the use of LPS in human medicine as an adjuvant. The primary role of LPS is as a polyclonal stimulant of the IgM class of B lymphocytes.

A bacterium used successfully as an adjuvant is *Bordetella pertussis*. The smooth, or phase I, *B. pertussis* cells contain a lymphocytosis-promoting factor that seems to mobilize both T and B cells, possibly favoring the number of Th cells released into the circulation. These gram-negative bacteria also contain an LPS that stimulates IgM synthesis.

An additional class of molecules with adjuvant action consists of those which labilize lysosomes. Substances such as vitamin A, beryllium salts, toxic forms of silica, and certain quaternary ammonium salts are all potent activators of macrophages and stimulate lysosomal enzyme release by these cells. Presumably this improves antigen processing.

Theoretically adjuvants may act by one or more of the following mechanisms: (1) directly increasing the number of cells involved in antibody formation, (2) ensuring a more efficient processing of the antigen, (3) prolonging the duration of the antigen in the immunized animal, and (4) increasing the synthesis and release of antibody from the antibody-forming cells. There is good evidence that adjuvants may function by the first three methods, but there is no known method of stimulating antibody-synthesizing cells to a greater rate of synthesis. Agents that lyse antibody-containing cells will cause the release of antibody into the serum and temporarily increase the antibody titer, but the long-term effect, resulting from destruction of the cells directly concerned with antibody synthesis, is depression of antibody titers.

The ultimate effect of adjuvants on the immune response curve is to blend the primary and booster responses together. Antibody will appear after about the same latent period and will rise at about the same rate but will continue to rise over an extended period compared with the usual primary response. Enhancing the immune response by incorporation of the antigen into an adjuvant-antigen mixture is a very practical way to spare expensive antigens, since small quantities of the mixture will ensure high-titer antisera. The application of adjuvant-antigen mixtures in immunization against infectious diseases creates a better and longer lasting immunity.

REGULATING IMMUNOGLOBULIN SYNTHESIS

How does the body control the synthesis of immunoglobulins? Certainly there is a physiologic limit to antibody synthesis that an animal will not exceed, and further booster doses of antigen will prove nonproductive. Several explanations have been forwarded to account for the slowdown in antibody synthesis.

One possibility is that the high concentration of circulating antibody itself functions as a feedback inhibitor to cause a halt in antibody synthesis. This is described more fully later in this chapter. A more recent explanation is based on a shift in the T cell population during the immune response.

Th versus Ts cells

Soon after antigen exposure Th cells dominate the T cell population. This can be proved by transfer experiments to the nude mouse, which responds feebly to T cell–dependent antigens because of its T cell deficiency. If the nude mouse is given a T cell–dependent antigen and T cells from a normal animal recently immunized, a substantial immune response will follow. If instead the T cells are collected late in the anamnestic phase of the donor's response, these cells plus antigen engender little or no antibody response in the nude recipient. This experiment not only establishes the presence of Th and Ts lymphocytes but also reveals that their equilibrium favors the helper cells near the time that antigen is first given and the suppressor cells after the immune response is well under way.

The idiotypic network theory

When an antibody is produced in response to an antigen, the antibody contains HV regions with unique amino acid sequences, which create the combining site for that antigen. These idiotypic HV regions are unique antigenic determinants which the animal has not previously confronted; therefore the animal responds with an antiidiotypic antibody. But even the antiidiotypic antibody contains unique idiotypic regions, and these stimulate a second generation antiidiotypic antibody. In this process a sequence of antiidiotypic globulins are formed, each capable of reacting with the previous one in the sequence. This sequence of serologic reactions may serve to slow or halt antibody synthesis, as first suggested by Jerne.

Several experiments have supported the idiotypic network theory as a mechanism for the control of antibody synthesis. For example, it is possible to passively immunize an inbred animal with antibodies to an idiotypic antibody normally produced by that animal in response to an antigen. If the animal is immunized with the antigen after this passive immunization, it will form antibodies that react with it, but these antibodies will be idiotypically different from those normally produced and against which the animal was passively immunized.

ANTIBODY PRODUCTION BY SINGLE CELLS

Study of antibody formation at the cellular level has been very informative in several ways; it has identified the cells involved in this unique kind of protein synthesis, helped to estimate the time after antigen stimulation that antibody synthesis begins, aided in evaluating how adjuvants function at the cellular level, indicated how many different kinds of antibody can be synthesized by a single cell, and contributed to the solution of other immunobiologic problems.

Single cell techniques for studying antibody synthesis have come and gone, but the agar plaque technique of Jerne for identifying plaque-forming cells (PFCs) remains in use.

PFCs

The agar plaque technique devised by Jerne is the most widely applied single cell technique. In this method individual cells from lymphoid tissue or from the spleen of the immune animal are plated in a nutrient agar with erythrocytes of the type used in the immunization. The tissue culture medium supports the growth and excretion of antibody by the antibody-synthesizing cells. These antibodies diffuse radially from their originating cell and attach to the neighboring erythrocytes. Serum complement in the form of normal guinea pig serum is added; this promotes lysis of the red blood cells which have become coated with antibody. Consequently a clear area, or plaque, develops around the antibody-forming cell against the light red, erythrocyte-laden background (Fig. 8-4). The PFC is usually a plasmacyte, but lymphocytes sometimes are seen. Macrophages or other antibody-absorbing cells are rarely seen.

By the original Jerne procedure only IgM-forming cells are detected; this is because of the feeble complement-binding and lytic activity of IgG antibody. However, IgG PFCs can be observed by flooding the plate with an antibody to γ-globulin prior to the addition of complement. This antiglobulin procedure actually detects both IgM and IgG plaques, so duplicate plates must be prepared.

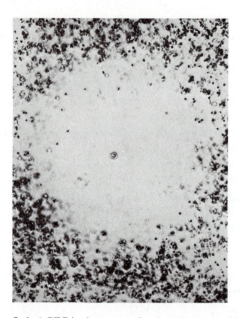

Fig. 8-4. A PFC in the center of a cleared area resulting from antibody from the PFC and complement lysis of the surrounding erythrocytes. (From Jerne, N.K. In Amos, B., and Kaprowski, H.: Cell-bound antibodies, Philadelphia, 1963, Wistar University Press.)

The IgG cells then must be calculated by difference.

Nonerythrocytic antigens can be used if they are adsorbed onto erythrocytes. There are many techniques for coupling soluble antigens to erythrocytes, so this is not a severe handicap. Bacterial cells of the gram-negative type can be used, since they too are lysed by antibody and complement. In one such study, after immunization of human subjects with *Salmonella typhi* vaccine, peripheral blood leukocytes produced 57 direct plaques and 570 indirect plaques per 10^6 leukocytes. From animal spleen cells 10 to 100 more plaques than this often are recovered.

The plaque-forming method has been used to determine the time that cells become primed for antibody formation. Within a few hours after the injection of polysaccharides rabbits have PFCs in abundance. The cytokinetics of PFC formation after primary and secondary immunization have shown that large quantities of antigen suppress antibody formation, very small quantities do not produce a good booster response, and the optimal quantity of antigen can elevate PFC counts several thousand above the counts following the primary response. The influence of immunosuppressant drugs can be examined at the cellular level by the PFC procedure. The opposite effect, that of adjuvanticity, especially by permeability-altering adjuvants, also has been studied. Kinetic studies of antibody-forming cells in culture indicate that spleen cells produce about 10 μg of antibody per gram of spleen per hour; this is roughly equivalent to two molecules per second per lymphoid cell.

Monoclonal hybridomas

In 1965 the first report of an immunoglobulin-secreting hybridoma was published. Since that time it has been recognized as one of the most significant advances in modern immunology. The improvements in creating hybridomas have relied primarily on the selection of the myeloma cells to be used; otherwise the procedure is much the same as originally described.

The hybridoma cells are created by a fusion of spleen cells from an immunized mouse with a mouse myeloma cell line (Fig. 8-5). The myeloma cells grow in normal culture media but fail to grow in a HAT (hypoxanthine, aminopterin, and thymidine) medium. The myeloma cells fail to grow in this medium because they lack the enzyme hypoxanthine phosphoribosyl transferase. The spleen cells fail to grow in HAT medium or other media because they are not a continuous cell line. Approximately equal numbers of spleen and meeloma cells are fused in the presence of PEG. This has replaced the viruses previously used as the fusing agent. PEG allows the cytoplasmic membranes of the two cell types to become more liquid. Contiguous cells may "melt," and when the PEG is removed, the membranes "freeze" again. The cell mixture is then plated on HAT medium. The spleen cells and any spleen-spleen doublets die a natural death. The myeloma cells (or myeloma-

myeloma doublets) fail to grow because they lack the hypoxanthine transferase needed to overcome the medium. The hybridomas have the needed hypoxanthine transferase derived from the spleen cells plus the growth capacity of the myeloma cell in continuous culture; consequently only the hybridoma cells grow. The clones that develop are screened for antibody production, and these may represent 10% of all the clones. Positive clones are propagated from single cell preparations and reexamined to ensure that they have not lost their immunoglobulin-producing capacity. During growth in culture approximately 10 to 100 μg/ml of specific antibody may be formed. The hybridoma cells will produce tumors in mice, since they are derived from plasmacytomas, and in the ascites fluid (or serum) 5 to 20 mg/ml of specific antibody may be present. These hybridomas may be perpetuated by transfers in mice or frozen as stock cultures.

In the original experiments both the spleen cells and myeloma cells were antibody producers, so it was necessary to examine the hybridoma not simply for the production of γ-globulin but also for the production of antibody-specific for the antigen used to immunize the mouse. Later it was possible to use mutant myeloma cells that had lost their immunoglobulin-synthesizing function. Hybrids produced from these cells secreted a single molecular form of antibody.

Hybridoma antibodies provide many advantages for immunologic research. Of major importance is the ability to get pure antibody from a crude antigen preparation. The hybridomas may even make antibodies to antigens that are not detectable by conventional means. Heretofore it was always necessary to purify the antigen to secure a pure antiserum. Moreover the hydriboma antibody is of a single immunoglobulin class and specific for a single epitope, since it arises from a single cell. Depending on the nature of the antigen and its use, an antiserum normally contains antibodies of many different classes and specificities. The class composition of an antiserum fluctuates with the intensity and time of immunization, whereas

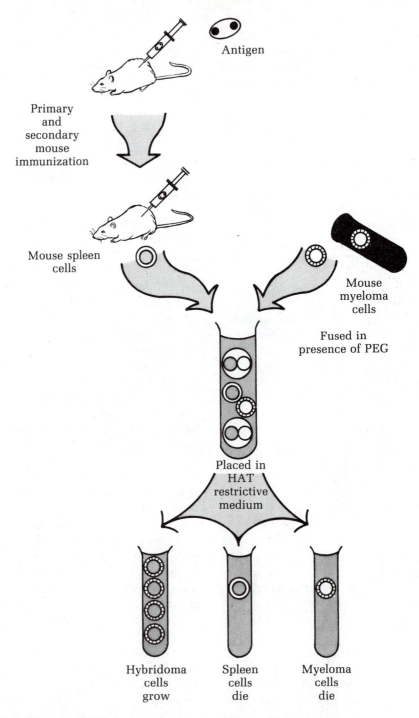

Fig. 8-5. The construction of a hybridoma begins with a primary immunization of a mouse, followed by a booster injection to ensure that a high density of antibody-forming cells will be present in the spleen. These are fused with nonsecreting myeloma cells and then plated in a restrictive medium. Only the hybridoma cells grow in this medium, where they synthesize and secrete a monoclonal immunoglobulin specific for a single determinant on the antigen.

the hybridoma product is constant. In addition, by selecting and analyzing the several hybridomas secured from one fusion it is possible to recover antibodies that are specific for different determinants of the antigen so that antigen mapping can be done. Since the hybridoma immunoglobulin is a monoclonal product, it is an extremely valuable asset for chemical and structural studies.

Another advantage of the hybridoma antibody is that it is always available from stock cells whenever needed, and it will be exactly the same as it was before. A new antiserum, even though prepared in the same species with the same immunization program, rarely will be the same as that produced in an earlier phase of the study.

Since the hybridoma cell line can be manipulated after pure cloning, one can study mutations in antibody-producing cells as they are expressed in terms of rate, antibody structure, antibody specificity, binding affinity, biologic activities such as cytotropism and complement activation, class switch, etc.

Human lymphoblastoid cell lines recently have been fused with mouse myeloma cells to produce human immunoglobulin-secreting hybridomas. By careful selection of the lymphoblastoid cell line and examination of the hybridoma for the expression of immunoglobulin synthesis coupled with chromosome analysis it has been demonstrated that human chromosome 14 contains the genes for μ-, γ-, and α-chain synthesis. The human κ-chain gene is on chromosome 2 and the λ-chain gene on chromosome 22. In mice the κ-chain genes are on chromosome 6 and the H chain genes on chromosome 12.

The hybridoma technique provides a novel avenue for investigating the antigenic nature of infectious agents, tumor antigens, histocompatibility antigens, and maturation of differentiation antigens and provides reagents of a purity never before available to immunologists for research and routine serology. It is also an excellent source of cells for immunogenetic studies. Hybridoma technology is still in its infancy, and one can but wonder at the marvels it promises based on the accomplishments already attributed to it.

THEORIES OF IMMUNOGLOBULIN FORMATION
The clonal selection theory

The current theories of antibody formation are modifications of either Ehrlich's original receptor theory or of the template theory. The template theory is an example of an instructive theory which assumes that the antigen can inform a cell in some way to make an antibody against that antigen. The contrasting assumption is that a cell is naturally endowed with the ability to make the specific antibody. This is a selective type of theory; its modern form is known as the clonal selection theory.

The earliest form of the selective theory, Ehrlich's receptor hypothesis, supposed that certain cells possess specific surface receptors for antigens. These are present in the normal, nonimmunized animal. When an antigen is injected and reaches the proper fitting receptor, it will combine with that receptor. The receptor then breaks off the cell, enters the blood, dissociates from the antigen, and exists as the free-circulating antibody molecule. A new receptor is formed in its place, and the process is repeated, the result of which is the appearance of antibody in the blood following the injection of antigen. This close fit of antigen and antibody, or lock and key hypothesis, so necessary here is also useful in explaining the serologic specificity of antigen and antibody reactions.

Burnet gradually evolved a modification of this selective theory of antibody formation, which became the modern clonal selection theory. (A clone is a population of cells arising from a single parent cell.) The present form of the clonal theory is essentially the following: in the mature animal the lymphocyte is genetically endowed with the capability of synthesizing immunoglobulins. At rest, unstimulated by antigen, only small amounts of immunoglobulin are made. This is found as surface IgM and IgD on the lymphocyte. On contact with the corresponding antigen, lymphocyte capping heralds a change of that lymphocyte to reproduce and differentiate into a clone of immunoglobulin-secreting plasma cells. The resulting clone of cells would consist of a large enough population that the antibody produced would become measurable in the blood.

What are the sources of support for the clonal theory? (1) Morphologically there is strong support. When antibody-forming cells are identified in highly stimulated animals, either by the fluorescent antibody or by plaque-forming center tests, the cells tend to be clustered in groups. By light microscopy these clones are seen as a part of typical germinal centers with dividing cells in the center and lymphocytes, immunoblasts, and plasma cells situated at the periphery (Fig. 8-6). (2) Clonal theories are harmonious with the kinetics of the immune response in both its primary and anamnestic phases. The latent period of the primary phase represents the time required for the transformation of lymphocytes into plasma cells and memory cells. Separate clones of cells corresponding to each type of antibody (IgG, IgA, and IgM) and for each determinant of the antigen must be generated. (3) Cell transition, so vitally a part of the clonal theory, explains the different effects of immunosuppressant drugs on the immune response before and after antigen stimulation and on the primary and secondary responses. The precursor cell is sensitive to these chemicals, but after contact with antigen it transforms to a resistant cell. The survival of this resistant cell until a subsequent antigenic exposure, followed

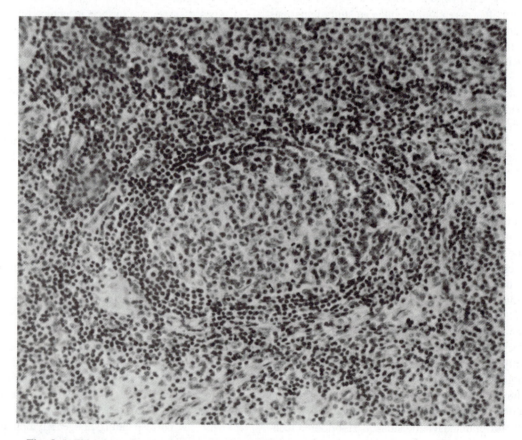

Fig. 8-6. This view of a germinal center clearly illustrates the self-containment of a clone of immunoglobulin-secreting cells within a perimeter of aligned cells.

by another reproductive spurt, would account for the known resistance of the anamnestic response to immunosuppression. (4) The recognition that B cells from normal, nonimmunized animals have IgM and IgD molecules scattered over their surface has been taken as physical evidence of the receptors first postulated by Ehrlich and incorporated into the selective theories of antibody formation. (5) A recent line of support for the clonal theory has been the discovery that embryonic cells do contain structural genes for immunoglobulins prior to exposure to antigen and that mature cells use the same biochemical processes to synthesize immunoglobulins which they use for the synthesis of other proteins.

The instructive theory

The principal contrasting theory to the clonal theory of antibody formation is the instructive, or template, theory. Several forms of this theory appeared almost simultaneously from 1930 to 1932. The basic tenet of all instructive theories is that the antigen enters a cell that is routinely engaged in normal γ-globulin synthesis. The antigen interferes with this process, possibly by complexing with mRNA in the polysome. The result is an adjustment in protein synthesis so that the globulin becomes molded into a complementary form with the antigen and therefore becomes an antibody globulin. The antibody dissociates from the antigen and is excreted into the blood. The antigen is retained and serves as the template for continued antibody synthesis.

Some of the arguments for and against instructive theories are the following.

1. How does each antigenic determinant have the same mRNA-binding ability when some 10^4 to 10^8 such determinants exist? Why fragments of all proteins and polysaccharides should bind to DNA or RNA and stimulate antibody formation cannot be readily explained by currently known biochemical reactions. On this basis template theories tend to be incompatible with biochemical knowledge.

2. Experimental immunologic tolerance is not explained by the template theory. In this condition an abundance of antigen is present. Thus one might expect that a prime immune response would follow, yet the opposite is the case; antibody synthesis is impaired.

GENETICS OF THE IMMUNOGLOBULIN RESPONSE

Among the dogmas of genetics, the concept that one gene codes for one protein has been one of the strongest. This became suspect when the amino acid sequence studies of immunoglobulins revealed that each had a series of identical C domains joined to a V domain in the L and in the H chain. In each immunoglobulin within a class, regardless of its specificity, the C domains were the same, but the V domains all differed. Thus for an L chain of the κ type the C_κ domain must be joined with a vast array of V sequences to construct globulins specific for the vast number of antigens that stimulate antibody synthesis. This logic also applies to the C_λ and C_H domains. A variation in the amino acid sequence of one portion of a molecule that is always joined to the same amino acid sequence in its remainder can be explained by several genetic hypotheses.

The germ line theory

The hypothesis known as the germ line theory, in harmony with the one gene–one protein dogma, envisioned one structural gene for each peptide in an immunoglobulin. This would consist of a V-C gene, and, to provide the variation in immunoglobulin structure that a cell can display, it would need a library of V-C genes. Each V region would differ, but the C region would be identical to the C regions in all other pairs. One problem with the hypothesis was in accounting for this supply of DNA in a single cell. The problem of DNA mass was resolved on the basis of a few assumptions and some mathematics. One early calculation suggested as little as 15% of the available nuclear DNA was needed to synthesize an antibody to each (potentially) existing antigenic determinant. More recent calculations indicate that

10^8 different antibodies could be generated from only 0.25% of the available DNA. Even so it seems uneconomic that a cell would carry so much excessive V-C gene baggage when it will only use one of these sets.

The somatic mutation theory

The uneconomic aspect of the germ line theory was met by the somatic mutation theory, which recognized the constancy of the amino acid sequences in the C domain as requiring but a single C gene and the demand for variations in the V gene as being met by a mutable behavior of this gene. Thus from any germ line V-C pair a series of gene pairs (V_1C, V_2C, V_3C . . . V_nC) would arise spontaneously. When the immunoglobulin corresponding to some antigen reacted with this antigen on the cell surface, capping, cell proliferation, and clone formation would follow. The probability that such an immunoglobulin would be present at any moment an antigen was injected is actually quite high even by normal mutation rates. Based on a population of 10^8 B lymphocytes in an animal, approximately 1,000 V gene mutants would emerge each day.

The somatic recombination theory

A modification of the germ line theory suggests that a series of V genes exists but not in an unlimited series as in the germ line theory. Recombinational events that occur during cell growth reorder the codons within the V genes to expand the library of V genes. These events would not transpire in the C genes, and the diversity of antibodies needed thus could be generated.

Because the existing models of one gene–one protein did not seem compatible with immunoglobulin structure, Dreyer and Bennett hypothesized that the V and C genes (whatever their origin) were not in tandem but were independent. A large series of V region genes could be joined to one or a few C region genes. Modern chemical and genetic techniques have been coupled to support this hypothesis.

Mapping immunoglobulin genes

Myeloma cells have the ability to grow readily in culture. Since these cells have focused on the production of a single immunoglobulin, it is possible to harvest their mRNA in substantial quantity with little contamination from mRNA contributing to the synthesis of other proteins. Immunoglobulin mRNA can be used in several ways as a probe for the structural immunoglobulin genes. By one method the mRNA is taken from cells grown in the presence of radiolabeled constituents. The mRNA is then fragmented and added to DNA taken from lymphocytes. Hybridization occurs between the complementary sequences in the mRNA and the DNA, and the isotope in the mRNA localizes the immunoglobulin gene sequences. These DNA sequences can be recovered, purified, and sequenced to confirm that they contain the correct triplet codons for the sequence of amino acids as they appear in the L or H chain. These DNA sequences then can be joined to a vector that will infect a bacterial cell, and multiple copies of the gene then can be recovered from the bacteria. This abundant DNA supply can be sequenced and either analyzed with probes that are specific for sectors of the immunoglobulin chain or be used as a probe itself.

Alternatively the mRNA can be used as a template for the enzyme reverse transcriptase to synthesize a copy DNA (cDNA). Fragmentation of the cDNA with restriction endonucleases will yield fragments that can be identified by sequencing to contain the codons for specific regions of the immunoglobulin molecule. Fragments of a radiolabeled cDNA fragment will bind to whole single-stranded DNA (ssDNA) from lymphocytes and localize the codons in the native DNA. By these methods specific probes for V_L, C_L, V_H, and C_H genes have been generated.

The use of probes for the mouse V_L and C_L domains has identified four to ten copies of the V_κ gene on chromosome 6 but only one copy of the C_κ gene. This finding eliminates the germ line theory as the basis for immunoglobulin diversity, since it predicted an equal number of V and C genes would be present.

There are actually much more than four to ten V_L genes in a mouse cell. First of all the probe used was a single V_κ probe. It is known that mice produce in excess of 50 V_κ chains, each differing slightly but regularly from the others in amino acid sequence. Thus there are 200 to 500 V_κ genes in the cell. Mouse V_λ chains are less variable, but adding some reasonable number of these to the V_κ genes would result in an excess of 500 or 600 V_L genes in mouse DNA.

The germ line theory also hypothesized that V and C genes would be adjacent to each other, and this was widely assumed to be the case, in harmony with the one gene–one protein dogma. However, the V_L probes applied to mouse embryo DNA were bound at several sites, each a definite distance from the C_L probes. When the same probes were applied to DNA from a mouse plasmacytoma, the V_L and C_L probes were positioned adjacent to each other.

The import of this discovery extends far beyond immunology. It indicates that clearly separated, multiple genes are required for the synthesis of a single peptide, and these genes are not expressed by a simple on-off switch but are expressed only after gene rearrangement. This space between the genes in the embryonic cell which has no known protein product is defined as an intron (intervening

sequence), whereas the expressed sequence is known as the exon.

When the DNA that had been identified to contain the exon for the C domain was sequenced, all the triplets needed to account for the 107 amino acids in the C_L domain seemed to be present. However, when the V_L gene sequence was completed, it was found to account for only the first 95 amino acids. This gap has been accounted for by locating a nucleotide sequence (in what was earlier thought to be an intron region) that accounts for the remaining amino acids. This is now referred to as the J (joining) gene. Thus the genes for the κ-chain consist of a DNA segment that codes for the first two HV regions—the V gene—a J gene segment that codes for the third HV region plus the first few amino acids of the C_L domain, and the C_L gene (Fig. 8-7). Antibody diversity is arranged by the selection of one of the several hundred V_L genes, one of the five different J genes that now have been identified, and the C_L gene. These are translocated, placed in a linear sequence, transcribed into mRNA, and translated into protein.

The mechanism of the translocation and excision of the introns and unification of the exons must be very complex. One recognition system for determining the location of introns may reside in the sequences known as palindromes. A palindrome is a base sequence in DNA that reads the same in both directions from a base pair when

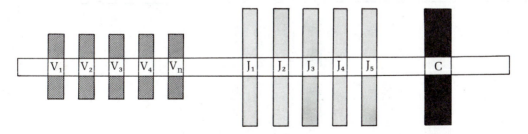

Fig. 8-7. Genetic analysis of the mouse κ-chains indicate the sixth chromosome contains a large library of V genes (V_1 to V_n), five J genes, and a single C gene. One of each gene set is translocated to place one V, one J, and the C gene in immediate sequence before being transcribed to form the mRNA.

read according to its respective 5' to 3' orientation. These palindromes create loops in the DNA strand. If an endonuclease breaks the DNA on both sides of the palindrome, when reannealing occurs, the intron is removed, and the exons are joined. Any error in this cleavage by the enzyme, at one or two bases away from its normal excision site, would cause a shift in the triplet reading frame. This would create deletions (or additions) in the amino acid sequence of the immunoglobulin chain and would be a mechanism for somatic mutation to occur.

The biogenetic analysis of H chains (which are located on mouse chromosome 12) has revealed several parallels to the conclusions about the L chains, with slight differences in terminology. A library of V_H genes is available that codes for the first two HV regions much like the V_L genes do for the L chain. These may be preceded by an L or leader sequence. The genetic unit coding for the third HV region is called the D (diversity) gene. The exact number of these on the chromosome is not yet known but probably would be large. A separate exon codes for the final framework region of the V_H domain. Thereafter a library of C genes are present in the sequence $C\mu$, $C\delta$, $C\gamma_3$, $C\gamma_1$, $C\gamma_{2b}$, $C\gamma_{2a}$, $C\epsilon$, and $C\alpha$. (Coding of the human H genes is incomplete but is believed to follow the sequence μ, δ, γ, ϵ, and α.) Thus in the construction of the H chain gene, introns between

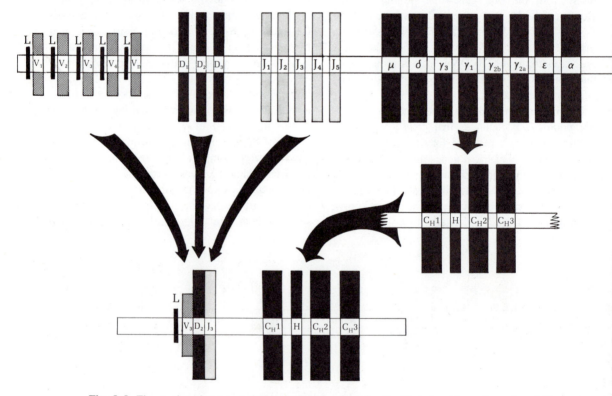

Fig. 8-8. The murine chromosome 12 contains the genes for the H chains. From the series of V genes one is selected and placed next to one D gene, which is placed next to a J gene. When one of the gene sets for an H chain class is chosen, the domain sequences are properly aligned. In this example the γ_1 H chain gene sequence is shown to contain individual genes for the C_H domains and the hinge *(H)* region.

these segments are excised to juxtapose the selected V_H, D, FR, and C_H domain genes (Fig. 8-8).

The present view is that each C_H gene actually consists of a large sequence encoding for the C_H1, the hinge region, the C_H2, and the C_H3 domains. An additional C_H4 sequence would be needed for certain immunoglobulins, for example, IgM. These subloci may be separated by short spacer introns, but this is uncertain.

It is interesting that the C_H domain genes are in the order which has been deciphered, since gene switching is in agreement with this order. The immature lymphocyte first has IgM on its surface, later often accompanied by IgD. Mature lymphocytes that synthesize IgM may later switch from IgM to IgG synthesis. The stimuli for such switching has not yet been identified, but a chemical basis for it has been suggested. Sequence analysis of the space between the H gene codons for μ, δ, γ, etc. has identified two sequences that are repeated. One of these is TGGGG, and the other is CAGCTG. These are hypothesized to represent switch sequences (S or SS) which, when recognized, cause the next H chain genome to be transcribed.

Progress in the mapping of human genes has trailed behind the studies in the laboratory mouse, but the data that are available follow the pattern of the earlier studies.

Allelic exclusion. Some of the data derived from immunoglobulin gene mapping has been used to explain the phenomenon known as allelic exclusion. When the immunoglobulin allotype of two parents is different, the immunoglobulin allotype of the F_1 is always that of one parent, never a blend of the two. One of the parental alleles is never expressed. This is unlike the inheritance of other characters, such as blood groups, where homozygous A and B parents produce AB children. Rabbit $a_1b_1 \times a_2b_2$ matings produce progeny that are a_1b_1 or a_2b_2 but never a_1b_2 or a_2b_1. Thus only one of the immunoglobulin genes is read. How this choice is made is uncertain. It is possible that, when gene translocations occur in one chromosome, genes in the other chromosome are in some way blocked from relocating. The genes in the other chromosome could persist but in a disconnected, nonexpressible configuration. Some data indicate that the unexpressed alleles are deleted or rearranged into a nonexpressible order. It will not be possible to decide whether stabilization of the original germ line configuration, rearrangement, or deletion is the end state of the excluded allele until further studies are reported.

IMMUNOSUPPRESSION

A reduction in the activities of macrophages and B and T lymphocytes, measured as a lowered capacity to phagocytose or to produce immunoglobulins or lymphokines, is the property of immunosuppressives. These functions can be limited by three types of action: by physical means such as x rays (γ-rays) and surgery, by chemical immunosuppressants, or by biologic means.

Physical immunosuppression

Radiation. Radiation immunology began in 1908 when it was discovered that the primary antibody response of rabbits to injections of whole serum was depressed by x rays. In the initial experiment irradiation was most effective if given prior to the antigen; irradiation given 4 days after antigenic exposure was ineffectual.

Many variations of the initial experiment have been performed to measure the effects of x rays on the primary immune response. The two immunosuppressing effects observed are an extended latent period, associated with a prolonged antigen elimination curve, and decreased antibody titers. B cells have proven to be more sensitive to irradiation than T cells. Sublethal doses of x rays, which amount to 400 to 500 R for most laboratory animals, impair the immune response when given not more than 4 days prior to the antigen. X rays are less effective if given with the antigen and have virtually no effect if given after the antigen. The irradiation is best given as a single dose rather than in fractionated doses. This impairment of antibody synthesis is transient; partial recovery is obvious after 1 week, and recovery is complete at 2 months. The IgG antibody response is more sensitive than the IgM response.

Small quantities of x ray, 10 to 25 R, given at about the same time as antigen, may stimulate the antibody response. The suggested explanation for this is that the depleted lymphoid cell population following low-level irradiation is repopulated disproportionately by the antigen-stimulated cells.

X rays have very little effect on the secondary response. This seems anomalous, since the secondary response is largely an IgG response, and the IgG portion of the primary response is more seriously affected than the IgM response. The cellular transformations that occur following antigenic exposure provide the best explanation for this apparent contradiction. Antigen contact with lymphoid cells stimulates differentiation to plasma and memory cells, which are more radioresistant than their parent.

The mechanism of action of an x ray is related to its effects on bone marrow and lymphoid cells. If lymphoid organs are shielded from irradiation, there is no effect on the immune capacity of the animal.

Surgery. Antibodies are produced by the joint action of macrophages and lymphoid tissues; the physical removal of these tissues from an animal will impair its response to antigen. Because macrophages are widely dispersed, it is physically impossible to locate and remove all these cells. Lymphoid tissue also is widely distributed throughout the body but tends to exist in concentrated packets in special organs: lymph nodes, bone marrow, tonsil, appendix, thymus, Peyer's patches, spleen, and elsewhere. As a consequence of this clustering it is more feasible to extirpate it, or sizable parts of it, than to remove phagocytic cells. When such removal is performed, an impairment of the immune response is noted.

Surgical extirpation of the mammalian thymus has a pronounced effect on the immune status of the animal, provided the surgery is properly timed with the maturation of the animal. In general, this means that surgery must be performed as soon after the birth of the animal as possible, although with slowly developing species (rabbits, hamsters) surgery after a few days will still illustrate the immunologic deficit. Care must be taken to remove the thymus without damaging the thyroid and parathyroid glands.

Among the most notable results of neonatal mammalian thymectomy is the wasting disease syndrome. This can be described simply as a failure to thrive. Young mice display a decreased growth rate and become listless, their hair becomes coarse and dirty, and premature death often associated with diarrhea ensues. Wasting disease reflects a novel and marked susceptibility to infectious disease, since germ-free mice do not exhibit wasting disease, and antibiotic treatment and good animal care procedures reduce the incidence of wasting disease. Thus thymectomy early in life reduces resistance to the T cell-dependent antigens of extraneous microorganisms.

Young bursectomized birds also develop wasting disease. This is clearly a result of the loss of B cells, which are the parents of the immunoglobulin-forming plasma cells. The earlier the bursa is removed from the chick or chick embryo, the greater is the deficit in the immunoglobulin response. If the developing chick embryo is treated with 19-nortestosterone, the bursa fails to develop during embryogenesis. Such hormonally bursectomized birds fail to develop an adequate immunoglobulin response. Bursectomy does not seriously affect any aspect of the immune response other than immunoglobulin synthesis.

Surgical or hormonal inhibition of the bursal equivalent centers is not possible in mammals as it is in birds, although a combination of x radiation and cyclophosphamide treatment is known for its central attack on B cell centers.

Chemical methods

A chemical that depresses any aspect of the immune response may be defined as an immunosuppressive. The application of the definition is not difficult when the activities of B and T lymphocytes are being examined but becomes confused when the influence of chemical substances on factors related to natural resistance such as iron concentration, action of ciliated cells in the respiratory tract, synthesis of the components of complement, motility of phagocytes (chemotaxis), and similar factors are considered. This conflict is avoided if the definition is restricted to the adaptive phases of the immune response. Even so immunosuppressives always must be clearly separated from antiinflammatory reagents. Inflammation is often a cardinal feature of the in vivo expression of the immune response, and often it is difficult to measure immunity without provoking its inflammatory expression. To separate the two, one must measure the immune response by methods less likely to induce a nonspecific inflammatory reaction.

Since immunosuppressive compounds are by nature cytotoxins, careful monitoring of their action is necessary to minimize their undesirable side effects. Pharmacologists use the term *therapeutic index,* the ratio of the toxic dose to the efficient dose, to express these relative activities. These dosages are very difficult to calculate in humans, but this can be done easily in animals. These figures are then used to estimate the immunosuppressive index in humans.

Many variables can influence the success of immunosuppressant therapy: the drug, the amount of the drug used, the route of administration, the schedule of administration, the time in relation to the exposure to antigen, the form of the antigen (soluble versus aggregated versus cellular), and the species of animal, to name a few. Even when the desired effect is reached, the general cytotoxic nature of many of the compounds demands the careful observation of the individual for the emergence of infectious disease or tumors, since host resistance to these decreases in the immunosuppressed condition.

An enhancement of antibody titers or adjuvant effect immediately following the administration of chemical immunosuppressants in low doses has been described. This response is fleeting and may be accounted for by three distinct mechanisms: (1) the release of preformed antibody in cells damaged by the drug, as has been suggested for the corticosteroids, (2) the release of nucleic acids from damaged cells, with these nucleic acids acting as adjuvants, and (3) a temporary overcompensatory hyperplasia of lymphoid tissue associated with antibody synthesis after the drug treatment. Continued administration or larger initial doses of the drugs will produce the more usual immunosuppressant activity.

By this time the question "What is the benefit of immunosuppressants?" often is posed. It is obvious that their use will provide no survival benefit to the normal animal; however, for the abnormal animal suffering from an autoimmune disease or undergoing a graft rejection reaction, immunodepressants are of considerable benefit. They may not be totally curative, but a clearer understanding of their action eventually may lead to the discovery of a totally effect and safe immunosuppressive therapy.

Corticosteroids. The glucocorticoids, so named because of their pronounced effect on glucose metabolism and their origin from the adrenal cortex, are more generally known as the corticosteroids because of their tissue of origin and typical steroidal chemical structure (Fig. 8-9). Cortisol is the major natural corticosteroid of humans and corticosterone that of rodents. These are the primary natural steroids which have been used in immunologic experimentation. A large number of synthetic or semisynthetic steroids, including prednisone, prednisolone, methylprednisolone, triamcinolone, and dexamethasone, has been used in immunologic experiments.

The immunosuppressive action of corticosteroids on lymphocytes may be related to several factors. One of these is lymphocytolysis, which can be demonstrated in vivo and in vitro with concentrations of the drugs that are used in immunologic experiments. This effect has been noted with human, guinea pig, mouse, and rat lymphocytes, although cells of the first two species were much more resistant than those of the latter two.

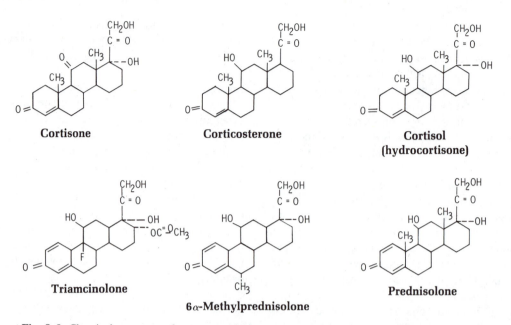

Fig. 8-9. Chemical structures of some steroidal immunosuppressants. The differences in structure reside primarily in the side chains and the oxidation state of carbon 11 in the C ring.

Evidence of in vivo lymphocytolysis is based on the development of a lymphopenia and a shrinkage of the thymus gland, both of which are evidence of an attack on T lymphocytes. The $T\mu$ cells are more sensitive to the steroids than the $T\gamma$ cells, but the effect on both is transient. B lymphocytes apparently also are attacked, although this is not conclusively proved; decreases in PFCs may be accounted for by the effect of these drugs on T–B cell interaction.

Even though lymphocytes may not be lysed by the steroids, their inhibition of DNA synthesis, RNA synthesis, and protein synthesis is sufficient to explain the capacity of these compounds to impair immunoglobulin and lymphokine synthesis.

Steroids also have pronounced effects on macrophages and neutrophils, probably more so than on lymphocytes. This would interrupt the normal processing of antigens. Steroids stabilize lysosomes, reducing their ability to release hydrolytic enzymes. A depression of oxidative metabolism, a feature of neutrophil metabolism closely related to intraphagocytic killing of bacteria, is characteristic of the steroids. A depression of neutrophil chemotaxis by steroids has been described in some experiments and denied in others, but an impairment of monocyte chemotaxis apparently is agreed on. Cytolysis of monocytes by steroids also is known to occur.

As a result of these multicellular effects, the corticosteroids have become useful immunosuppressants. They reduce the primary IgG response but have little effect on IgM or on the secondary IgG response. They prolong graft survival, minimize both immediate and delayed skin reactions, reduce lymphokine synthesis, and may predispose the patient to infection.

Purine and pyrimidine analogs. Purine analogs such as 6-mercaptopurine, 6-thioguanine, 8-azaguanine, 6-thioinosine, and azathioprine have been repeatedly confirmed as inhibitors of the immunoglobulin response in many species of animals ranging from chickens, mice, rabbits, dogs,

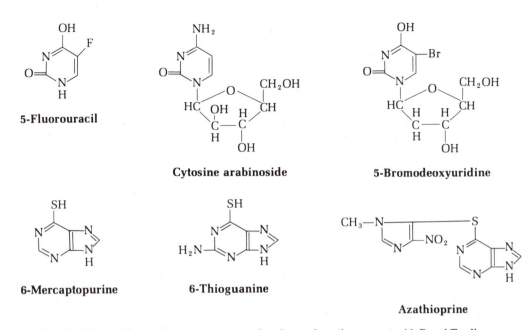

5-Fluorouracil

Cytosine arabinoside

5-Bromodeoxyuridine

6-Mercaptopurine

6-Thioguanine

Azathioprine

Fig. 8-10. Pyrimidine analogs *(upper row)* and purine analogs *(lower row)* with B and T cell–suppressing activity. A large number of similar compounds are available for human use.

and monkeys to humans. The activity of the purine analogs of course is based on their antimetabolite effect on the normal purines adenine, guanine, xanthine, and hypoxanthine. The analogs, including azathioprine, which bears the additional substituted imidazole ring, all have a close structural resemblance to the natural purines (Fig. 8-10). The addition of this moiety to 6-mercaptopurine to create azathioprine actually improves its immunosuppressive activity. This is rather surprising, since the side group is eliminated in vivo to liberate 6-mercaptopurine. One possible explanation is that the blocked sulfhydryl group alters cell permeability, allowing greater access of the drug to the immunoglobulin-synthesizing ribosomes. Another possibility is that detoxification may occur at the SH group, and, if temporarily blocked, the half-life of the inhibitor in vivo may be extended.

These purine analogs may function at more than one biochemical level: simple competitive inhibition of purine compounds in the biosynthetic pathway to other purine bases, inhibition of purine synthesis from low molecular weight precursors, and possibly analog incorporation into nucleotides as substitutes for the natural purine bases. Azathioprine and 6-mercaptopurine, the most widely used purine analogs, block the conversion of inosinic acid to adenylsuccinate and thus function directly via the first mechanism; however, their most important inhibitory effect is by way of its eventual incorporation into 6-methylthiopurine ribonucleotide, which is a potent inhibitor of purine synthesis. Incorporation of these purine analogs into mRNA to create a "nonsense messenger," which would result in the synthesis of defective proteins and antibodies, has not been conclusively demonstrated. The most "purine-sensitive" cell appears to be the immunoblast, an early cell in the sequence of cellular maturation of antibody-forming cells. This is consistent with the opinion that cells in the S phase, or phase of active DNA synthesis, are most susceptible to the purine analogs.

Pyrimidine analogs are structural mimics of uracil, thymine, cytosine, and other forms of cytosine such as 5-methylcytosine or 5-hydroxymethylcytosine, which have a more limited biologic distribution. Several of these pyrimidine compounds are halogen-substituted in the 5 position, 5-fluorouracil and 5-bromouracil being examples. Other cytotoxic chemicals based on the structure of pyrimidine are based on the nucleotides of the halogenated pyrimidine with D-ribose such as in 5-iodo-2-deoxyuridine, 5-iodo-2-deoxycytidine, and 5-trifluoromethyl-2-deoxyuridine. At least some of these halogenated compounds are incorporated into DNA and interrupt the basic genetic capabilities of the afflicted cell. False pyrimidine nucleotides such as cytosine arabinoside may function through their inhibition of DNA polymerase.

Folic acid antagonists. Aminopterin and amethopterin (methotrexate) are both antagonists of folic acid metabolism. Amethopterin is different from aminopterin by only one methyl group. These two antimetabolites are actually inhibitors of tetrahydrofolic acid, which is a carrier of one-carbon units essential to the synthesis of purines (Fig. 8-11). Folic acid antagonists interfere with this process and consequently impair DNA and protein synthesis. Cell division is halted at the S phase in the cell reproduction cycle—the period of DNA formation just prior to cell division. The mouse, rat, guinea pig, and human are all more sensitive to these compounds than is the rabbit, the animal most often used in these experiments. As with other suppressing chemicals, the IgG and primary antibody responses are more sensitive to folic acid analogs.

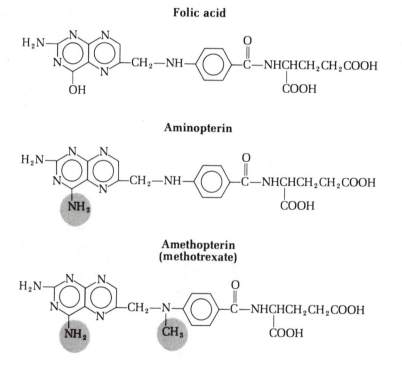

Fig. 8-11. Structural analogs of folic acid—aminopterin and methotrexate—differ from the vitamin by the substituents in the stippled circles. These differences confer an immunosuppressant function on the analogs.

Alkylating agents. Alkylating agents are compounds that have an affinity for nucleophilic (negatively charged) zones in other molecules. Typical nucleophilic centers in biomolecules include amino acid and sulfhydryl groups. Intracellularly the most critical point of attack for the alkylating agents is DNA, although obviously RNA and proteins also would be alkylated. Alkylation of the amino groups on guanine and adenine, of which guanine is probably the most sensitive, may result in several critical effects. The alkylated base may not be properly read in the transcription to RNA, forming fraudulent proteins. The same result occurs if the alkylated purine is excised and the depurinated DNA is falsely transcribed. Potentially the alkylated DNA can be repaired, but errors in the repair mechanism also could lead to the synthesis of nonfunctional proteins. Depurinization also is known to induce breaks in the DNA, and shortened DNA strands would result in the synthesis of incomplete proteins. The affected proteins may be the immunoglobulins or lymphokines themselves or enzymes responsible for their synthesis. Direct alkylation of the lymphokines and immunoglobulins easily could render them nonfunctional if their nucleophilic centers are required for combination with antigen or cell receptors.

Difunctional and polyfunctional alkylating compounds create bridges between natural biopolymers, thus rendering them inactive. In the case of DNA the two strands cannot separate as required in normal cell division (Fig. 8-12). As a result of this, the affected cells continue to enlarge but do not divide. Cell clones cannot form. Prolymphocytes, immunoblasts, or other cells in the maturation pathway of lymphocytes cannot escape their premitotic condition. This accounts for the severe lymphopenia that accompanies the administration of alkylating drugs.

The biologic effects of therapy with alkylating reagents so closely parallels the changes produced by x rays that these reagents are known as radiomimetic drugs. Like x rays, these drugs are more effective against the primary and IgG responses than against the secondary response or that of other immunoglobulin classes.

Although literally dozens of alkylating agents have been synthesized and tested for an immunosuppressive function, only a half dozen have had very widespread use. The relationship of the structure of these compounds to that of mustard gas is readily apparent except for triethylenemelamine and thiotepa. Most of the information about the immunosuppressive action of alkylating agents stems from experiments with cyclophosphamide.

A single injection of cyclophosphamide drastically reduces the number of lymphocytes in the spleen, thymus, and blood. Both B and T cells are reduced in number, but cyclophosphamide is especially active against B lymphocytes. When it is given to newly hatched chicks, an involution of the bursa resulting in an agammaglobulinemia is induced.

An important sidelight to the use of cyclophosphamide as opposed to other alkylating agents is its ability to enhance immunologic tolerance to several antigens. A specific protocol may need to be developed for specific antigens or certain animal species, but generally the antigen is given 1 or 2 days prior to the administration of the drug. This timing apparently is essential because it allows the antigen to induce immunoblast formation. The immunoblast is presumed to be more sensitive to cyclophosphamide than the unstimulated lymphocyte. Thus these cells are killed by the cyclophosphamide treatment, and normal lymphocytes are little affected, producing an antigen-specific immunologic tolerance.

Miscellaneous agents. A number of other cytotoxic agents display immunosuppressive activity, but because of uncertainties concerning their chemical structure or mode of action, they cannot always be pigeonholed into discrete classes. Several are antibiotics, others are enzymes, and still others are plant alkaloids. In the antibiotic category are actinomycin D, mitomycin C, puromycin, and chloramphenicol.

Puromycin, excreted by *Streptomyces alboniger*, functions at the RNA level and acts by im-

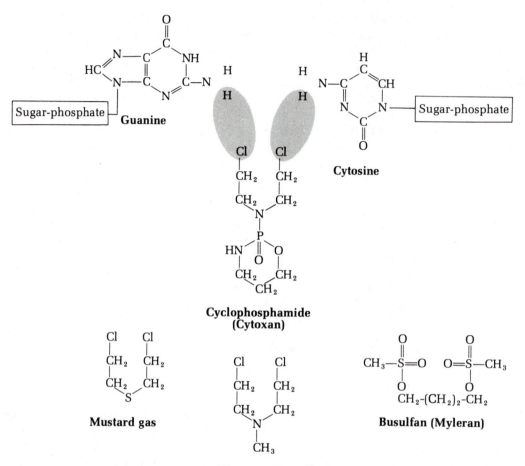

Fig. 8-12. Structures of cyclophosphamide and busulfan, which are alkylating immunosuppressants, clearly are related to the structure of mustard gas. The alkylating reaction of cyclophosphamide with nucleic acids also is illustrated.

pairing the transfer of the activated amino acids from transfer RNA (tRNA) to the ribosomal protein. *Streptomyces parvullus* is the source of actinomycin D, a third antibiotic operating on RNA, in this instance by preventing the movement of mRNA from the nucleolus to the cytoplasm, where the message for protein synthesis is "read." At doses lower than necessary for this effect RNA polymerase inhibition and DNA binding at guanine residues by actinomycin interfere with protein synthesis. Mitomycin C from *Streptomyces cae-*

spitosus acts as an alkylating agent and tends to depolymerize nucleic acid.

Two enzymes also have had immunosuppressive functions ascribed to them: ribonuclease and asparaginase. Mechanisms are not totally known, although ribonuclease could conceivably function on the RNA and RNA-antigen fragments from macrophages, should these ever exist free extracellularly on their way to "instruct" the lymphoid cells to initiate antibody formation. Asparaginase from *Escherichia coli* produces a marked lymphopenia and causes a reduction in the size of most lymphoid organs, which results in diminished immune responses. Colchicine, vincristine, and vinblastine are plant alkaloids that act on phagocytic cells and halt cell division, both of which are important in the sequence of events leading to antibody synthesis.

Biologic methods

There are five biologic means by which the production of antibodies can be hindered. One of these is nature's own experiment, a deficiency in the ability to synthesize γ-globulins: hypogammaglobulinemia or agammaglobulinemia. The other four methods are competition of antigens, antilymphocyte serum (ALS), feedback inhibition, and immunologic tolerance. The latter two of these techniques display immunologic specificity; that is, it is possible to predetermine on immunologic grounds which antibodies will be inhibited. With hypogammaglobulinemia and ALS, like the physical and chemical methods, there is a generalized diminution of the immunoglobulin response.

Immunologic tolerance. Immunologic tolerance is a state of specific nonreactivity to a normally effective antigenic challenge, induced by a prior exposure to the antigen concerned. As a consequence, immunologic tolerance is significantly different from other forms of immunosuppression, which are unlimited in spectrum and represent a nonspecific rupture of antibody-synthesizing systems against all antigens. The immunotolerant condition is restricted to one antigen and follows the rules of serologic specificity. The terms *immunologic paralysis* and *immunologic unresponsiveness* are interchangeable with *immunologic tolerance*.

The existence of immune tolerance was postulated by Burnet and Fenner in 1949 in the self-marker aspect of their theory on antibody formation. They hypothesized that there were recognition centers on self-antigens which caused them to be ignored as antigens by one's own antibody-making machinery. It was suggested that this self-identification occurred in embryonic life when the

antigens were first formed and at a time before the immune mechanism was functioning. This was logical and agreed fully with an example of natural tolerance that had just been postulated for cattle. Calves from the same dam and bull but from different pregnancies usually differ in their blood groups; twin calves, however, generally have identical blood groups. The most startling example of identical blood groups in twin calves is noted when calves have been sired by different bulls; such calves invariably have obvious phenotypic and genotypic differences. Why their red blood cell types should be the same was a mystery. It was then learned that all the different blood group antigens were not on the same erythrocytes but that identical blood groups in these dizygotic twins were the result of two entirely different populations of erythrocytes. One type of red blood cells contained half the antigens, and the other cell type contained the other half. These blood cell chimeras arise from anastomoses of the blood vessels and an exchange of hematopoietic tissues in the fetal calves. Hence the cells from one twin settle and produce their own kind of erythrocytes in the uterine partner. As a rule, this chimerism is reciprocal, that is, both calves are involved, but the proportions of the two cell populations may differ in each twin. This depends on the relative amounts of each type of erythroid tissue that is present. Qualitatively the mixtures are identical. It is noteworthy that this chimerism persists into adult life; this contrasts sharply with the survival of transplanted tissue in adult animals. Immunologically mature adults usually destroy transplants in 10 to 14 days unless the tissue is from a monozygotic twin. Survival of the erythropoietic tissue in dizygotic twin calves was explainable only by fetal recognition of the transplanted tissue as self and not as foreign (Reading 5).

The development of fetal immunologic tolerance in calves suggested that the introduction of any foreign antigen into a fetal animal would render the animal tolerant to a reexposure to the antigen in adulthood. Medawar and his colleagues performed just such tolerance experiments with skin transplants in CBA and A strain mice. The CBA line of mice is a brown-furred line, and the A line is an albino strain. Skin transplants exchanged between adults of these strains survive 10 to 11 days and then are sloughed. However, if CBA mouse embryos are exposed on the sixteenth or seventeenth day of fetal life and are injected intravenously with tissue from A line mice, most of the mice survive the manipulations and are delivered as healthy mice. When these mice are grafted with skin from white A line mice as adults, the graft survives. There is no more striking proof of the success of this experiment than seeing healthy white fur patches on the CBA (brown) mouse. Similar experiments have been performed in rats, rabbits, chickens, and other species with similar results: fetal exposure to antigens always promoted later tolerance to the antigen (Fig. 8-13). The tolerogenic state is measured by the survival of skin grafts and failure to make antibodies. Varying the choice of the antigen used for the intrauterine exposure makes the animal tolerant to other antigens such as erythrocytes, bacteria, and bovine serum albumin. Tolerance in these instances is defined as a failure (absolute tolerance) or diminished capacity (partial tolerance) to make antibody. There are certain limits to the experi-

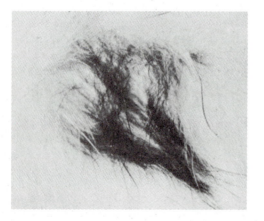

Fig. 8-13. Skin graft tolerance of a white rat for a black rat graft. (From Elves, M.W.: The lymphocytes, London, 1966, Lloyd-Luke Medical Books, Ltd.)

ment—for example, it is extremely difficult to get transplants of chicken skin to grow on a rat—but within those limits transplantation tolerance is a recognized immunologic phenomenon.

Induction of tolerance to skin grafts in fetal or juvenile animals can be accomplished by injection of skin or other tissues that have antigens in common with skin; however, the transfer of viable lymphoid tissues from an adult to a young animal should be avoided. The host, because of its immunologic immaturity, will be unable to reject the grafted immunocompetent tissue. The grafted lymphoid cells will respond immunologically to the host tissue, and the often fatal wasting syndrome known as runt disease, homologous disease, or graft-versus-host (GVH) reaction will ensue. In the mouse this is manifested by a failure to gain weight or a loss of weight, reddening of the skin, ruffling and loss of hair, diarrhea, general lethargy, and death within a few weeks. This GVH reaction does not occur when transplantation between syngeneic individuals is performed.

Other examples of immune tolerance can be found in the scientific literature. When adult mice are immunized with killed pneumococci or pneumococcal polysaccharide, the mice are resistant to subsequent experimental pneumococcal infection. This immunity can be developed when tiny quantities of the purified polysaccharide are used in the immunization; quantities ranging from 0.01 to 5 μg are quite adequate. But, surprisingly, if the mice are given a 500-μg dose of polysaccharide, they do not develop immunity; such mice will succumb quickly to the bacterial infection when challenged. This phenomenon was described as immune paralysis. Since it was clearly caused by excess antigen, it was thought to be the result of an antigen depot that "sponged up" the circulating antibody as it was formed.

A central failure in the immune response appears to be the mechanism of immune tolerance. The mechanism does not involve binding of antibody by antigen depots. Proof of a more central failure has come from two avenues of research, one involving PFCs and the other adoptive immunization. Of 17 rabbits treated with bovine serum albumin, only two contained higher numbers of plaque-forming centers in spleen than control rabbits. The other 15 were statistically deficient in plaque-producing cells. This is direct proof that antibody-forming cells simply are not formed in tolerant rabbits. Immunofluorescent studies confirmed this conclusion.

The PFC experiments in rabbits support the mechanism of tolerance known as clone inhibition or clone deletion. Other examples of clone deletion include the injection of highly radioactive antigen, which kills antigen-binding cells (antigen suicide), and the development of tolerance in utero.

Blocking or enhancing antibodies of various types are known to be immunosuppressive. Antiidiotypic or antiallotypic antibody passively administered will prevent the formation of antibodies containing those idiotypes or allotypes. Some antibodies may function through some form of feedback inhibition.

Specific suppressor factors produced by Ts cells and macrophages have been mentioned previously as another avenue to produce immune tolerance.

Tolerance is not necessarily permanent. Recovery from the tolerogenic condition takes time and appears to be related to the disappearance of antigen; repeated antigenic exposures promulgate continued tolerance. Low levels of irradiation and injection of cross-reactive antigens break tolerance. A known response to small quantities of x rays is a hyperplasia of lymphoid tissue. This may cause reproduction of the specifically antigenstunted, tolerant cell to a condition of responsiveness, or it may improve the chances for a mutant cell to arise that can respond to the antigen. Crossreactive antigens may function in the same way.

Antigen competition. The competition of antigens refers to an inhibition of the immune response to one antigen by the injection of a second antigen. Antigenic competition functions best when the inhibiting antigen is given prior to or concurrently with the primary antigen. There are virtually no criteria available to determine if an antigen is a good competitor or not. Although it is sometimes possible to exhibit a better competition of a "good" antigen on a "weak" antigen than the reverse, the frequently observed competition of a poor against a strong antigen is proof that no simple rules for antigenic competition can be established. This competition may take place at the level of the macrophage when large quantities of antigen are injected. Unfortunately little more can be stated about this phenomenon.

ALS. ALS, antilymphocyte globulin (ALG), or antithymocyte serum or globulin (ATS or ATG) is prepared by immunization of a heterologous species with cells from the lymph nodes, blood, thymus, or spleen of the donor. To produce its immunosuppressive effect, it is administered as a passive immunization of the donor species before, at, and after the exposure to antigen. Because the antigen preparation used to produce ALS is impure and contains cells of several types, ALS contains antibodies to these cells (granulocytes, erythrocytes, reticulum cells, and structural cells). Most of these antibodies can be removed by adsorption of ALS with homologous kidney or liver powder. More specific antisera can be prepared by using purified preparations of the antigen; for example, ATS or ATG can be prepared using thoracic duct lymphocytes.

ALS usually induces a transient lymphopenia. Repeated injections may extend this condition for several weeks; however, lymphocyte populations return to normal about 2 weeks after the last treatment. The size and structure of the thymus is not significantly altered by ALS but is by ATS. The white pulp of the spleen is reduced by ALS, and a similar cell loss is seen in lymph nodes and other peripheral lymphoid organs. In fowl, antibursa sera have a pronounced influence on the bursal lymphocyte population but little effect on thymocyte numbers. The reverse is true of antithymus sera administered to fowl.

The preferential elimination of lymphocytes from the blood and the thymus-dependent centers of peripheral lymphoid tissues appears to be a logical explanation for the capacity of ATG and even ALS to impair both the cell-mediated and immunoglobulin arms of the immune response. Lymphocytopenia is never total, and its degree does not always correlate with the extent of immunosuppression observed. This may be explained by the replacement of lost T cells by B lymphocytes or incompetent T lymphocytes.

Among the in vitro assays used to estimate the immunosuppressive property of ALS are leukoagglutination, cytotoxicity for lymphocytes in the presence of complement, mitogenic effect on lymphocytes, inhibition of the mitogenic effect of Con A or PHA on lymphocytes, inhibition of PFCs, and inhibition of rosette formation by lymphoid cells. There is no correlation of leukocyte agglutination with in vivo activity of ALS, possibly because impure antigen preparations of mixed granulocytes and agranulocytes have been used most often in the test and in the preparation of the ALS. Most immunosuppressive sera are lymphocytotoxic with complement, but the reverse is not always true. Little or no relationship between mitogenicity and ALS potency exists. ALS is not very inhibitory to the effect of mitogens on lymphocytes. ALS sera have relatively little effect on PFCs, probably because these are not the real target cells of ALS. The capacity of ATS to inhibit normal rosette formation correlates well with its immunosuppressive function, which is normally greater on T-dependent antigens than on T-independent antigens.

Several factors in nonimmune sera are known to suppress the immune response. An α-globulin fraction will prolong allograft survival and in vitro will reduce the lymphocyte response to PHA. The target cell appears to be the T cell. A low-density lipoprotein found in the sera of hepatitis patients binds to T cells and interferes with their ability to rosette with sheep erythrocytes but may not affect their response to antigen. The C-reactive protein found in the sera of certain patients also binds selectively to T cells and inhibits the generation of the CTC line but does not influence the activity of mature CTCs. The α-fetoprotein (AFP) found in the sera of certain cancer victims has been described as an immunosuppressant, although this claim has been challenged.

Feedback inhibition. It is almost an axiomatic part of modern biochemical thinking that the regulation of a biochemical pathway is partially controlled by the end product of that pathway. It is not surprising to find this idea of feedback inhibition applied to immunologic experiments, the results of which have paralleled those in other biochemical investigations.

Passively administered antibody depresses the synthesis of new antibody when injected just prior to, simultaneous to, or up to 5 days after the injection of the antigen. This inhibition is immunologically specific; that is, only the corresponding antibody against the antigen can suppress antibody formation against that antigen. Heterologous antibody is relatively ineffective. Injection of only that portion of the antibody molecule which combines with the antigen (Fab or $F(ab')_2$ fragments) is almost as inhibitory as injection of the entire molecule. Feedback inhibition of the primary response is much easier than for the secondary response; and even though the primary response is inhibited, the animal becomes primed for a secondary antibody response that can be demonstrated on reexposure to the antigen. IgG is a better suppressor than IgM. Feedback inhibition can be demonstrated at the cellular level by the PFC technique.

Careful attention to experimental design and technique is often essential before feedback inhibition can be regularly demonstrated because under certain conditions antibody may exhibit an adjuvant-like effect. This is often the result when antigen-antibody complexes are administered or when such complexes can be expected to form in vivo. The result of this complex formation is an increased phagocytosis of the antigen by the antigen-processing cells. This promotes rather than negates antibody formation.

The application of feedback inhibition has provided an effective means of preventing hemolytic disease of the newborn (HDN) caused by Rh incompatibility. This is discussed fully in Chapter 16. Briefly, most cases of HDN are caused by maternal antibodies to the Rh antigen present on fetal erythrocytes. These antibodies pass the placental barrier and combine with and promote destruction of the fetal red blood cells. The pregnant woman usually has these antibodies as the result of earlier pregnancies with Rh-positive children. With this information at hand it was rightly theorized that, if women were given anti-Rh sera at childbirth, by virtue of feedback inhibition they would be prevented from synthesizing the unwanted antibodies. This is such an effective procedure that it is considered a required part of perinatal care and, where practiced as described, essentially has eliminated Rh-dependent HDN.

Genetic immunodeficiencies. A primary genetic inability to form mature cells of the B, T, or phagocytic lineage can result in a permanently immunosuppressed condition unless corrected by medical intervention. These conditions are the subject of Chapter 22.

BIBLIOGRAPHY

Allison, A.C.: Mode of action of immunological adjuvants, J. Reticuloendothel. Soc. **26:**619, 1979.

Anderson, R.E., Lefkovits, I., and Troup, G.M.: Radiation-induced augmentation of the immune response, Contemp. Top. Immunobiol. **11:**245, 1980.

Bach, J.F.: The pharmacological and immunological basis for the use of immunosuppressive drugs, Drugs **11:**1, 1976.

Blann, A.D.: Cell hybrids: an important new source of antibody production, Med. Lab. Sci. **36:**329, 1979.

Bona, C.: Modulation of immune responses by *Nocardia* immunostimulants, Prog. Allergy **26:**97, 1979.

Chedid, L., Carelli, C., and Audibert, F.: Recent developments concerning muramyl dipeptide, a synthetic immunoregulating molecule, J. Reticuloendothel. Soc. (Suppl.) **26:**631, 1979.

deSaint Groth, S.F., and Scheidegger, D.: Production of monoclonal antibodies: strategy and tactics, J. Immunol. Methods **35:**1, 1980.

Dresser, D.W., editor: Immunological tolerance, Br. Med. Bull. **32:**99, 1976.

Fauci, A.S.: Immunosuppressive and anti-inflammatory effects of glucocorticoids, Monogr. Endocrinol. **12:**449, 1979.

Fitch, F.W.: Selective suppression of immune responses, Prog. Allergy **19:**195, 1975.

Geha, R.S.: Regulation of the immune response by idiotypic-antiidiotypic interactions, N. Engl. J. Med. **305:**25, 1981.

Gottlieb, P.D.: Immunoglobulin genes, Mol. Immunol. **17:**1423, 1980.

Howard, J.G., and Mitchison, N.A.: Immunological tolerance, Prog. Allergy **18:**43, 1975.

Kaplan, S.R.: Immunosuppressive agents, N. Engl. J. Med. **289:**952, 1234, 1976.

Kennett, R.G.: Monoclonal antibodies; hybrid myelomas—a revolution in serology and immunogenetics, Am. J. Hum. Genet. **31:**539, 1979.

Kennett, R.H., McKearn, R.J., and Bechtol, K.B., editors: Monoclonal antibodies, New York, 1980, Plenum Publishing Corp.

Milstein, C.: Monoclonal antibodies, Sci. Am. **243:**66, 1980.

Möller, G., editor: Mechanism of B lymphocyte tolerance, Immunol. Rev. **43:**1, 1979.

Morrison, D.C., and Ryan, J.L.: Bacterial endotoxins and host immune responses, Adv. Immunol. **28:**294, 1979.

Parillo, J.E., and Fauci, A.S.: Mechanisms of glucocorticoid action on immune processes, Ann. Rev. Pharmacol. Toxicol. **19:**179, 1979.

Parks, D.E., and Weigle, W.O.: New ideas about self-tolerance and auto-immunity, Clin. Exp. Immunol. **39:**257, 1980.

Pierce, C.W., and Kapp, J.A.: Regulation of immune responses by suppressor T cells, Contemp. Top. Immunobiol. **5:**91, 1976.

Pross, H.F., and Eidinger, D.: Antigenic competition: a review of nonspecific antigen induced suppression, Adv. Immunol. **18:**133, 1974.

Rabbits, T.H., and Milstein, C.: Quantitation of antibody genes by molecular hybridization, Contemp. Top. Mol. Immunol. **6:**117, 1977.

Rodkey, L.S.: Autoregulation of immune responses via idiotype network interactions, Microbiol. Rev. **44:**631, 1980.

Salaman, J.R., editor: Immunosuppressive therapy, Philadelphia, 1981, J.B. Lippincott Co.

Sercarz, E., and Cunningham, A.J., editors: Strategies of immune regulation, New York, 1980, Academic Press, Inc.

Tom, B.H., and Six, H.R., editors: Lysosomes and immunobiology, New York, 1980, Elsevier/North-Holland, Inc.

Urbain, J., Wuilmart, C., and Cazenave, P.A.: Idiotypic regulation in immune networks, Contemp. Top. Mol. Immunol. **8:**113, 1981.

Weigle, W.O.: Cyclic production of antibody as a regulatory mechanism in the immune response, Adv. Immunol. **21:**87, 1975.

World Health Organization Scientific Group: Immunological adjuvants, WHO Tech. Rep. Ser., 595, p. 1, 1976.

CHAPTER
9

THE COMPLEMENT SYSTEM

alexin An archaic term for complement.

alternate complement pathway A system for activating complement beginning at C3 and not involving a serologic reaction.

amboceptor An archaic term for antibody.

Ana INH Anaphylatoxin inhibitor.

anaphylatoxin Originally believed to be a substance that caused histamine release; now regarded as specific peptides from complement fractions 3 and 5, which release histamine from mast cells and basophils.

anaphylatoxin inhibitor An enzyme that destroys the biologic activity of C3a and C5a.

angioneurotic edema A sporadic edematous condition related to a genetic deficiency in C1 esterase inhibitor.

C1, C2, etc. Components of serum complement numbered sequentially from 1 through 9.

C1 esterase An esterase formed from activation of the C1s component of complement.

classic complement pathway A system for activating all nine components of complement that is initiated by a serologic reaction.

complement fixation Binding or use of serum complement in a reaction with antigen and antibody.

conglutination A type of complement fixation test incorporating bovine conglutinin that clumps sheep red blood cells in the presence of nonhemolytic complement.

conglutinin A protein normally present in bovine serum that reacts with C3.

C$\overline{1}$s INH The serum inhibitor of the activated first component of complement.

HANE Hereditary angioneurotic edema.

hemagglutination The agglutination of erythrocytes, especially by antiserum.

hemolysin An antibody with a specificity for erythrocytes, which in cooperation with serum complement will lyse the red blood cells.

hemolysis Lysis of erythrocytes by specific antibody and serum complement.

immune adherence The adhesive nature of antigen-antibody complexes to inert surfaces when complement is bound.

immunoconglutinin An antibody to antigenic sites of C3 revealed or created by antigen-antibody binding of complement.

kinins Peptides or polyamines released during anaphylaxis that possess vasodilating and muscle-contracting activity.

Despite the spectacular advances arising from the chemical study of immunoglobulins and their related proteins, recent immunochemical studies have markedly improved our understanding of serum complement. Because of the instability of certain complement components and the lack of suitable protein fractionation procedures, it was nearly impossible to characterize complement in chemical terms until recently. Intensive investigations have done much to illuminate the chemical and biologic nature of this important serologic reagent which contributes so dramatically to immunity through chemotaxis and opsonization, to inflammation through chemotaxins and anaphylatoxins, and to blood clotting, to cell lysis, to the dissolution of immune complexes, and to other immunologic phenomena.

COMPLEMENT: ITS DISCOVERY
The Pfeiffer phenomenon

The discovery of complement is credited to Pfeiffer and resulted from his studies in 1894 on experimental cholera infections in guinea pigs. Pfeiffer observed that a reinoculation of cholera bacilli *(Vibrio cholerae)* intraperitoneally into guinea pigs that had recovered from an earlier infection of the organism resulted in the rapid dissolution of the bacteria within the peritoneal cavity. Pfeiffer determined three facts from a further study of this system.

1. The immunity was specific and could not be induced by injections of antigenically unrelated bacteria, and the immunity could be transferred to normal guinea pigs with blood from the immune guinea pigs, that is, antibody was required.

2. Heated serum from immune animals, tested in vitro, was devoid of bactericidal power, but fresh serum was lethal to the cholera bacilli.

3. Heated immune serum would transfer the immunity between animals, and the cholera vibrios were lysed in the passively immunized animal.

It was concluded that heat-stable antibodies in blood could transfer cholera immunity to a living animal and that these antibodies cooperated with a heat-labile substance present in normal animals to create the immunity. When this substance in immune sera was destroyed by heating it at 56° C, antibody alone could not destroy the cholera organisms in vitro. Buchner had described earlier a

heat-labile protective activity of blood and had named it alexin.

In 1898 Bordet confirmed Pfeiffer's experiments by demonstrating that fresh normal serum contains a heat-sensitive substance which will dissolve bacteria (bacteriolysis) in the presence of specific antibodies in heat-inactivated antiserum. Bordet also described immune hemolysis following the mixture of red blood cells with specific antibody and alexin. Bordet continued his studies of the hemolytic activity of alexin and demonstrated that hemolytic assays were much simpler than bacteriolytic assays for detecting its presence in sera. At about this time Ehrlich proposed the term *complement* (something that completes or makes perfect) for alexin (to ward off), and this more meaningful term has persisted.

By 1901 Bordet and Gengou had formulated the complement fixation test, which they recognized could be very helpful in identifying antibodies to many different antigens, not just bacterial or erythrocyte antigens. This complicated serologic test is described in this chapter and has been an important test for the study of infectious disease. Until recently the complement fixation test for syphilis, known as the Wassermann test, was the standard serologic test for the diagnosis of this disease. Because of his many contributions to an understanding of complement and related studies of immunity, Bordet was awarded the Nobel Prize in 1919.

GENERAL PROPERTIES OF COMPLEMENT

Before considering the complicated chemistry of complement and its fractions it is advisable to consider some of the general properties of complement that serve to distinguish it from the immunoglobulins and other serum proteins and their activities.

1. Complement is required for the cytolytic destruction of cellular antigens by specific antibodies. Not all cellular antigens are susceptible to dissolution by complement and immunoglobulins. Yeasts, molds, many gram-positive bac-

teria, most plant cells, and even most mammalian cells resist complement-mediated cytolysis. The cells that are naturally most fragile—white blood cells of all types, erythrocytes, thrombocytes, and gram-negative bacteria—are the most susceptible to immune cytolysis.

2. The lytic activity of complement in antigen-antibody reactions is destroyed by heating sera at 56° C for 30 minutes. This is because of the heat sensitivity of some of the complement fractions and the lability of certain enzymes generated from these fractions during the activation of complement. The conditions traditionally used for the heat inactivation of complement do not affect the immunoglobulins that participate in serologic reactions with complement, although IgD and IgE are partially inactivated by these conditions.

3. Only immunoglobulins of the IgM and IgG classes react with complement, and the IgG subclasses are not equally potent in this regard. IgG4 is incapable of operating with the complement system, and of the remaining IgG subclasses, IgG3 is the most active. IgA, IgD, and IgE are incapable of functioning with complement.

4. Complement is bound into all antigen-antibody reactions, provided the immunoglobulin is of the proper class. This fixation of complement occurs even if complement is not required to display the serologic reaction being studied (for example, precipitation and agglutination). It is this characteristic of complement which allowed Bordet and Gengou to develop the complement fixation test. Binding or fixation of complement by complexes of antigen and antibody initiates the classic activation pathway of complement.

5. Complement is present in all normal mammalian sera and the sera of most lower animals, including birds, fish, amphibia, and sharks (elasmobranchs). The complement content of sera, which comprises about 10% of the total globulins, does not increase as a result of immunization.

6. Complement is a nonspecific serologic reagent in the sense that complement from one species of animal usually will react with immunoglobulins of another species from the same taxonomic order. The more distant the taxonomic position of the two species, the less interaction occurs. Avian complement or fish complement does not react as well with mammalian antibodies as does mammalian complement.

7. Portions of the complement system contribute importantly to chemotaxis, opsonization, immune adherence, anaphylatoxin formation, virus neutralization, and other physiologic functions.

8. Complement activation by nonserologic reactions is possible. The best known of these alternate pathways of complement activation is known as the properdin pathway. The alternate pathways are initiated by complex polysaccharides or enzymes.

9. Complement is not a single substance but a complex of nine major proteins that act in consort with one another. All nine are required for cytolytic reactions resulting from the classic pathway. In the properdin activation pathway the first three components of the classic pathway are not required.

The use of several different expressions to denote the participation of complement in a certain activity may lead to confusion until it is recognized that all the terms refer to essentially the same thing. "Complement binding" or "complement fixation" refers to the union of complement or one of its fractions with a substance, usually an immunoglobulin. Often this results in the expression of a new biologic activity and a change in that component of complement, known as "complement activation." Measurement of the residual complement activity in a serum after complement activation will determine that the complement level has been decreased. This is expressed as "complement consumption" or "complement inactivation," the latter of which is grammatically the exact opposite of complement activation, although the terms refer to basically the same reaction.

Early fractionation studies

The isolation and characterization procedures so conveniently applied to the study of other serum proteins and enzymes have now been applied to complement. One of the earliest discoveries was that dialysis of fresh normal serum against distilled water divided the activity of complement into two portions: a precipitated globulin fraction, which could be resolubilized, and a soluble, or albumin, fraction. Neither of these alone had complement activity, but a mixture of the two did. If the two fractions were added sequentially to sensitized (antibody coated) erythrocytes, lysis appeared sooner when the globulin was added before the albumin than under the reverse condition. This indicated that globulin attachment was necessary before albumin attachment, since the globulin was thought to attach to the antibody as a midpiece before the binding of the albumin endpiece (Fig. 9-1).

Further fractionation by simple chemical treatments showed that complement was a complex of at least four distinct proteins. C1 was precipitated by dialysis against distilled water. It is a heat-labile globulin. C2 is also heat labile but remains in solution on dialysis. C3 is a heat-stable protein found in the precipitate and adsorbs strongly to large polysaccharides. For this reason zymosan, a product from the cell walls of yeast, is used to remove C3. C4 is a heat-stable protein found in

endpiece that is destroyed by dilute solutions of alkali. All four fractions are required for lysis, and they attach to sensitized erythrocytes in the order C1, C4, C2, C3. That C3 was itself a complex of many components was soon determined from further fractionation efforts. These discoveries triggered even more intensive biochemical inquiry into the nature of complement.

CHEMISTRY OF THE COMPLEMENT COMPONENTS
Nomenclature

The components in the classic complement activation sequence, as stated previously, are nine in number, but since one of these exists as a trimolecular complex, it is also possible to consider that eleven proteins participate in the system. These molecules are numbered sequentially C1 through C9. The individual peptide chains of these proteins are designated by Greek letters in keeping with the biochemical system for identifying the subunit peptides of proteins that have a quaternary structure. Thus there is $C3\alpha$, $C3\beta$, $C4\beta$, $C4\gamma$, etc.

When a peptide chain is fragmented by proteolysis, the cleavage peptides are denoted by lower case Arabic letters, as in C3a and C3b. It is im-

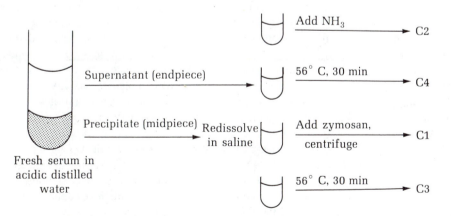

Fig. 9-1. The initial experiments that led to the description of complement midpiece and complement endpiece are depicted here, as are the further treatments of these, which produced C1, C2, C3, and C4.

portant to avoid confusion of the Greek and Arabic lettering systems; fragments C3a and C3b arise from C3α. If the fragment loses activity as the result of further proteolysis, the letter i is added as a subscript to indicate inactivation (for example, C3b$_i$).

When a complement protein acquires an enzymatic activity or is otherwise activated, a horizontal bar over the designation for the protein may be used, but this is a less common practice than previously. C1 becomes $\overline{C1}$ when it acquires its esterase activity. When it is desirable to identify the specific peptide fragments, then the appropriate letter designations are used, as in $\overline{C1s}$ or $\overline{C4b,2a}$.

Within the past decade attention has shifted away from the classic pathway for the activation of complement to a study of the alternate pathways by which complement can be activated. This has uncovered several additional serum proteins which function with the late-acting components of complement (those which follow C3 in the classic system). At least five additional proteins participate in the properdin alternate pathway. A new nomenclature system recently has been advanced for these proteins. These are properdin, factor B (formerly known as C3 proactivator), factor D (formerly C3 proactivator convertase), C3b,Bb (the C3 activator), and an as yet uncharacterized initiating factor. This raises the number of proteins in the complement system to 14—nine classic pathway molecules plus five alternate pathway molecules.

To these 14 molecules, all of which are present in normal serum, additional serum proteins that modulate complement-derived activities must be added. At the present time five such proteins are recognized: $\overline{C1s}$ inhibitor ($\overline{C1s}$ INH), C3b · C4b inactivator (C3b · C4b INAC, or factor I), C3a and C5a anaphylatoxin inactivator (Ana INH), C6 inactivator (C6 INAC), and C5b inactivator. C3b · C4b INAC is identical to conglutinogen-activating factor (KAF, from the German abbreviation).

The total number of proteins in serum that participate in the complement system can be extended beyond these 19 if plasmin, Hageman's factor, Hagemen's factor fragments, and other molecules are included. The complement system is thus a highly complex system that may involve as many as two dozen molecules whose biologic activities are numerous and closely coordinated.

Components of the classic activation pathway

The nine originally described molecules of the complement series, C1 through C9, act in consort with one another when the C1 molecule is activated by certain antigen-antibody reactions. Since C1 is the first component to participate in the reaction, it is referred to as the recognition unit. When this recognition unit becomes activated, the next three components to participate are C4, C2, and C3, in that order rather than in a straight numeric sequence. These three molecules compose the activation unit, so named because important enzyme activities appear during their participation in the sequence. The remaining molecules, C5 through C9, are referred to as the membrane attack group or unit, which terminates in cytolysis of certain cellular antigens that initiated the complement sequence.

The recognition unit: C1. The first component of the complement cascade is a true macromolecule with a molecular weight of approximately 600,000 and a sedimentation coefficient of 18 (Table 9-1). C1, in its associated form, is a trimolecular complex held together by calcium ions. (Since the alternate pathway does not require Ca^{2+}, a loss of complement activity in the presence of buffers that bind Ca^{2+} indicates use of the alternate pathway.) When the calcium is removed by the use of chelating compounds like ethylenediaminetetraacetic acid (EDTA), C1 dissociates into its three subunits. Restoration of calcium to the system permits the reassociation of C1 into its trimeric form. The three subunits of C1 are designated C1q, C1r, and C1s, which, because of differences in their size and chemical properties, can be separated from each other easily by gel filtration (in calcium-free buffers).

Table 9-1. Characteristics of the complement components

Component	Serum concentration (μg/ml)	Sedimentation coefficient ($S_{20,w}$)	Molecular weight	Number of peptide chains	Electrophoretic position
C1q	150	11.2	410,000	18	γ_2
C1r	50	7.5	83,000	2	β
C1s	50	4.5	83,000	1	α
C2	15	4.5	110,000		β_1
C3	1,250	9.5	180,000	2	β_2
C4	400	10.0	206,000	3	β_1
C5	80	8.7	180,000	2	β_1
C6	60	5.5	130,000	1	β_2
C7	55	6.0	120,000	1	β_2
C8	55	8.0	150,000	3	γ_1
C9	60	4.5	79,000	1	α

C1q is the largest of the C1 subunits and has a molecular weight of essentially 410,000 and an $S_{20,w}$ value of 11.2. It has the electrophoretic mobility of a γ_2-globulin, which is notable because most components of complement behave as β-globulins. Normal human serum contains 150 μg/ml of C1q.

Chemically C1q is a novel molecule because of its high content of hydroxyproline, hydroxylysine, and glycine at frequencies of nearly 5%, 2%, and 18%, respectively. Since these three amino acids are so common in collagen, C1q can justifiably be described as a collagen-like molecule. However, this description must be tempered somewhat, since both the amino and carboxyl terminal ends of C1q are typically globular in structure. C1q also can be considered a glycoprotein because it contains about 9.8% of its weight in the form of carbohydrate. This carbohydrate is divided almost equally among glucose (3.4%), galactose (3.1%), and a cluster of remaining monosaccharides.

C1q is composed of 18 separate polypeptide chains, each with a molecular weight of approximately 23,000. Although these small proteins are similar in amino acid composition and size, they differ in the amount of carbohydrate that they carry and in electrophoretic mobility. Thus there are six A chains, six B chains, and six C chains.

These appear to be associated as six A-B subunits and three C-C subunits, each held together by disulfide bonds but not covalently linked to the other subunits.

The C1q molecule is so large that it can be viewed in the electron microscope, where it gives the appearance of six globes held on slender shafts that fuse into a common base (Fig. 9-2). The globes serve as the recognition unit and bind to the Fc region of the complement-activating IgM and IgG immunoglobulins. This occurs in the C_H4 domain of IgM but in the C_H2 domain of IgG. All subclasses of IgG are not equally effective receptors for C1q. In descending order of effectiveness they are IgG3, IgG1, IgG2, and IgG4. IgG4 dissociates so readily that it is not described as a complement-activating globulin. For C1q to initiate the complement cascade it must attach to two immunoglobulin molecules. Since these are adjacent in IgM, IgM is described as a better complement-binding antibody than IgG. IgA, IgD, and IgE do not bind C1q and cannot catalyze the complement cascade.

C1r and C1s are similar molecules, each composed of a single peptide chain approaching 83,000 mol wt and containing about 7% to 9% of its protein weight in polysaccharide. In their native state C1r and C1s exist as proteolytic zymo-

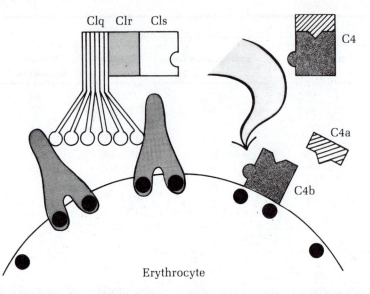

Fig. 9-2. The C1 triad of C1q, C1r, and C1s is held together by calcium ions. When the C1q receptors for the Fc region of complement-activating immunoglobulins bridge two Fc units, its C1s portion becomes activated so that it can cleave C4. The C4b product attaches to the antigen surface, and the C4a peptide is left free.

gens, or proenzymes, with C1r self-associating to form a dimer. This explains the frequent listing of C1r as having a molecular weight of about 180,000.

Exactly how C1r and C1s are activated is uncertain; perhaps their incorporation into antigen-antibody complexes creates a susceptibility to a naturally existing serum protease such as plasmin or thrombin. The result of their activation is the formation of proteases consisting of two peptide chains of 56,000 and 27,000 molecular weight joined by a disulfide bond. C1r̄ has a very feeble proteolytic activity associated with its smaller b chain, but the C1s̄ b chain is active on peptide bonds (or ester bonds) in which arginine, lysine, or tyrosine become the carboxyl terminal unit after cleavage. This is exactly the same substrate specificity displayed by trypsin, chymotrypsin, plasmin, and other serine proteases. These enzymes were so labeled because alteration of an active site serine destroys their enzymatic activity. Amino acid sequencing of the b chains of C1r̄ and C1s̄ has revealed a remarkable homology with

the serine esterases, with which they now are classified.

The activation unit: C4. The next molecule to participate in the complement sequence is C4 (Table 9-1). The discrepancy of binding order and sequential numbering is described in the opening section of this chapter.

C4 has a molecular weight of 206,000 and an $S_{20,w}$ value of 10. It originates from a pro C4 (210,000 mol wt), synthesized by macrophages. It positions itself electrophoretically with the β-globulins. Its concentration in human serum is 400 μg/ml, which makes it second only to C3 in serum concentration. C4 consists of three peptide chains, C4α, C4β, and C4γ, with molecular weights of 95,000, 78,000, and 33,000, respectively. These three chains are joined by disulfide bonds (Fig. 9-3). The attack of C1s̄ on C4 takes place in the α-chain and releases C4a, which has a molecular weight of about 9,000. The remainder of the molecule, known as C4b, has a molecular weight of about 198,000.

C4b will attach to erythrocyte surfaces, bacterial

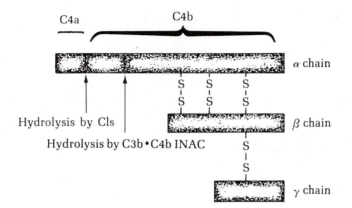

Fig. 9-3. C4 consists of three peptide chains. Hydrolysis of the α-chain by C1s activates the C4 molecule by releasing the C4a peptide.

cell membranes, and other antigens. It does not attach to C1 on the antigen-antibody complex. C4b, the portion of the α-chain remaining after the release of C4a, can be cleaved by the serum C3b · C4b INAC. This scission of C4b produces C4c (150,000 mol wt) and C4d (49,000 mol wt) concomitant with the destruction of C4b activity.

The C4a molecule consists of 77 amino acids and does not possess any carbohydrate side chains. This small molecule now has been recognized as an anaphylatoxin. Anaphylatoxins are able to bind to mast cells and basophils and cause them to discharge their cytoplasmic granules. (See Chapter 18.) When freed from these cells, the contents of these granules contract smooth muscles, causing edema and shortness of breath.

The activation unit: C2. Fraction C2 of complement is a β_1-globulin, with a molecular weight of 110,000 and $S_{20,w}$ of 4.5. It is rather scant in serum, with 15 μg/ml being recorded as the average level. The amino acid composition of C2 is nearly identical to that of factor B of the alternate pathway. The activity of C2 is destroyed when it is combined with p-chloromercuribenzoate or iodoacetamide in a molar ratio of 1:2. This indicates that C2 possesses two sulfhydryl groups necessary for its activity. It is not essential for these — SH moieties to be in the reduced condition to measure C2 activity. In fact the treatment of C2 with iodine, which oxidizes the — SH groups to

the disulfide or — S — S — forms, results in a tenfold to twentyfold increase in C2 activity.

The alteration of C2 during the complement sequence has been analyzed, with the discovery that it binds to C4b (Fig. 9-4) and is cleaved by C1s into C2a and C2b. These proteins have molecular weights of 70,000 and 30,000, respectively. The role of C2b is unclear at this time, but C2a functions with C4b to activate C3 and C5 and may be the critical catalytic portion of the enzyme known as C3 convertase, written C4b,2a.

The activation unit: C3. The substrate for C3 convertase, or C4b,2a, is C3, that protein of the complement system which is the most abundant in serum, at 1,250 μg/ml (Table 9-1). C3 is a β_2-globulin with an $S_{20,w}$ of 9.5 and a molecular weight of 180,000; it originates from a pro C3 secreted by macrophages. C3 consist of an α-chain with a molecular weight of 105,000 and a β-chain with a molecular weight of 75,000 joined by disulfide bonds (Fig. 9-5). C3 convertase hydrolyzes a peptide bond at positions 77 and 78 in the α-chain to produce C3a, a peptide with a molecular weight of 8,900, which is an anaphylatoxin. The remainder of the molecule is known as C3b, and it attaches to C4b,2a. C3b is subject to inactivation by a serum C3b · C4b INAC, which removes a further peptide, C3d, from the α-chain. This means that C3d is the receptor for the late-acting components of complement. The residuum after

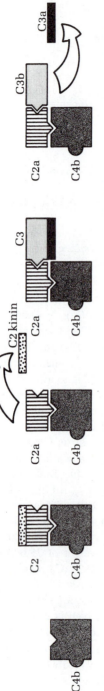

Fig. 9-4. After C4b is produced and attaches to the antigen surface, it is able to combine with C2. C2 kinin is released, leaving the C4b, C2a complex, which is now able to receive C3. C3 then is degraded to release the anaphylatoxin C3a, and its residue remains attached to the C4b, 2a complex.

C3d release is C3c. Both free C3d and C3e can be further degraded by the serum enzyme plasmin.

The new complex $C\overline{4b,2a,3b}$ is known as C5 convertase, which, like the C3 convertase, relies heavily on C2a for its enzymatic activity.

The membrane attack unit: C5. In several respects C5 is much like C3 (Table 9-1). C5 is a β_1-globulin; its molecular weight is 180,000, and its $S_{20,w}$ value is 8.7. These figures are similar to those for C3. Like C3, C5 also is derived from a precursor molecule, in this case pro C5 from macrophages, which has a molecular weight of 220,000. Structurally C5 is also like C3, being composed of two peptide chains, C5α, and C5β, linked by disulfide bonds (Fig. 9-6). C5α has a molecular weight of 105,000 and C5β, 75,000. In parallel with C3a, a C5 convertase removes a fragment C5a with a molecular weight of about 11,000 from the α-chain of C5. C5a is an anaphylatoxin and a chemotaxin for granulocytes. It is larger than C3a partially because of its polysaccharide content. The C5 convertase is represented by $C\overline{4b,2a,3b}$. C5b, which remains after the removal of C5a, can be further degraded to C5c and C5d. The biologic roles of C5c and C5d are not known, but intact C5b, which attaches to the earlier complement components, serves as the receptor for C6 and C7 and is the first element of the membrane attack complex.

The membrane attack unit: C6 and C7. Very little is known about C6 and C7 except that both are β_2-globulins with molecular weights near 125,000 (Table 9-1). C6 is reported to have a molecular weight of 130,000 and C7 one of 120,000. The $S_{20,w}$ values for C6 and C7 are 5.5 and 6, respectively. C6 is available in human serum at a level of 60 μg/ml and C7 at 55 μg/ml. The difficulties in securing further information about these molecules are attributed to the ease with which they associate with C5 in a trimolecular complex.

The membrane attack unit: C8 and C9. The next molecule to combine in the complement sequence is C8, an unusual molecule consisting of three peptide chains, two of which are covalently

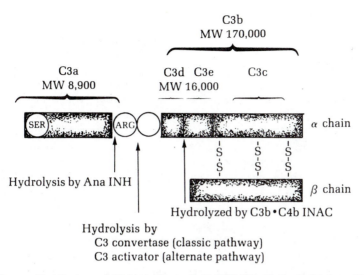

Fig. 9-5. The peptide structure of C3 is similar to that of C5 (Fig. 9-6). Activation of C3 follows peptide bond cleavage in the α-chain by C3 convertase or C3 activator. The anaphylatoxic split product, C3a, is inactivated by removal of its carboxyl terminal arginine by Ana INH. C3b is converted to $C3_i$ by C3b · C4b INAC hydrolysis and removal of C3d.

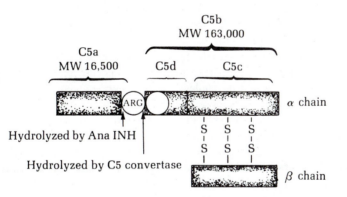

Fig. 9-6. The peptide structure of C5 is reminiscent of that of C3 (Fig. 9-5). C5 convertase cleaves the α-chain next to an arginine residue in C5a. Removal of this arginine by Ana INH inactivates the C5a and C3a anaphylatoxins.

linked to each other and a third that is not covalently joined to the other two (Table 9-1). After treatment of C8 with detergents and reducing agents three peptide chains, C8α (69,000 mol wt), C8β (64,000 mol wt), and C8γ (22,000 mol wt), can be isolated. C8γ and C8α are linked by disulfide bonds, and C8β is noncovalently joined to them.

These figures indicate that C8 has a total weight of 150,000. C8 is a γ_2-globulin with an $S_{20,w}$ of 8 and is present in human serum at concentrations of 55 μg/ml.

The last of the complement molecules to interact is C9 (Table 9-1), an α-globulin like C1s, which is identical to it in $S_{20,w}$ value of 4.5 and similar in molecular weight (79,000 versus 83,000 for C1s). The level of C9 in human serum is 60 μg/ml.

The aggregation of all these complement molecules on sensitized erythrocytes (erythrocytes combined with specific antibody) or sensitized gram-negative bacteria results in cytolysis of the antigen. The exact causative force for this lysis continues to escape identification. The C5 to C9 complex inserts into the lipid bilayer membrane, where it forms a transmembrane protein channel. This channel is funnel shaped, being larger in diameter on the exterior surface. The membrane attack complex of C5 to C9 can be eluted from the lysed cells, where it is found in company with a hitherto unidentified molecule X, which has a molecular weight of 88,000. This molecule may be the lytic agent. Complement reagents C1 through C3 can be eluted from the red cell surface, and lysis still will follow when only the membrane attack complex is adsorbed to the cell surface.

Even in the absence of C9 the cells will undergo lysis at a slow rate. These ''leaky'' cells, which have bound C1 through C8, lyse more readily when 1,10-phenanthroline or 2,2′-bipyridine, which are bivalent cation chelators, are added to the reaction mixture. When C9 is added, ''holes'' about 80 to 100 μm in diameter can be observed on the surface of the sensitized red blood cell (Fig. 9-7). These holes do not penetrate the cell membrane and are more accurately described as etched areas or erosions on the membrane. These erosions can be erased with lipid solvents. How they contribute to rapid cell lysis may be clarified when the role of molecule X is better understood.

Components of the alternate activation pathway

It is perfectly correct to refer to alternate pathways of complement activation in the plural. One of these pathways begins with the nonserologic activation of C1 by tissue enzymes with the same substrate specificities as trypsin and chymotrypsin. Other enzymes such as plasmin can initiate the alternate pathway. A number of acidic mole-cules—heparin, DNA, LPS, or lipid A—can bind to C1 and activate the classic pathway without the intervention of immunoglobulin.

The original description of an alternate complement pathway was made in 1954 by Pillemer and his associates, who found that cell wall preparations from yeast, or zymosan, would activate complement. This activation was related to a newly discovered serum globulin, properdin, and became known as the properdin pathway. Since then it has been found that many complex polysaccharides will active the properdin pathway. Among these are LPS, bacterial capsules, teichoic acids from bacterial cell walls, inulin, dextran, fungal cell walls, and aggregated globulins which are high in carbohydrate content. At least four serum proteins function in the properdin alternate pathway of complement activation that do not contribute to the classic pathway: factor B, factor D, C3b,Bb, and properdin (factor P) (Table 9-2).

An initiating factor for the properdin pathway has not yet been clearly identified, but it is not properdin, as was earlier believed. Neither is it the C3 nephritis factor (C3 NeF), which has now been identified as an immunoglobulin. The first molecule of the alternate pathway that can be accurately described is C3. It is acted on by an enzyme complex formed in the alternate pathway (C3 activator), which has the same enzymatic activity as C3 convertase of the classic pathway. The formation of the complex in the alternate complement pathway that generates C3b (and C3a) from C3 is a multistage process which involves several molecules. The participation of these molecules is no longer questioned, although several uncertainties remain as to exactly how they participate. Fortunately research in this area is progressing rapidly and is encouraging.

Factor B. Factor B, the C3 proactivator, is a normal serum protein with a molecular weight of 93,000. As such, it has an $S_{20,w}$ of about 6. It is a β-globulin found at a level of 200 μg/ml of serum. Factor B shares several features with C2, such as size, sedimentation rate, single peptide structure, and proenzyme nature. The enzyme

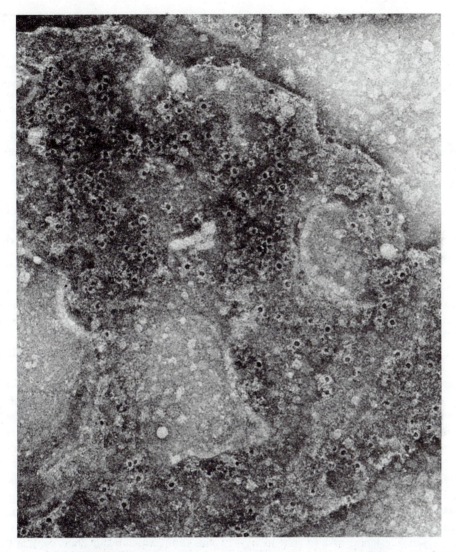

Fig. 9-7. The "holes" in these erythrocytes caused by the erythrocyte-antierythrocyte-complement interaction do not penetrate entirely through the cell membrane. All the holes are about 80 to 100 μm in diameter. (Courtesy R. Dourmashkin and J. Humphrey.)

nature of factor B is not released until it is bound to C3b and acted on by a protease.

The question usually posed is, "Where does the C3b originate that is needed for factor B activation?" It generally is assumed that there is an endogenous generation of C3b from the classic pathway (Fig. 9-8). The actual amount of C3b needed

for alternate pathway activation may be trivial. Certainly the complement pathways do not flow unchecked, since inhibitors block the cascade and prevent complement depletion except under conditions of intense stimulation. The endogenous C3b normally would be degraded by C3b · C4b INAC, but this may be prevented if the complex poly-

Table 9-2. Characteristics of proteins in the alternate complement activation pathway

Component	Abbreviation	Serum concentration (μg/ml)	Sedimentation coefficient ($S_{20,w}$)	Molecular weight	Electrophoretic position	Comment
Properdin	P	25	5.4	184,000	γ_2	Exists as tetramer
C3 (factor A)	C3	1,250	9.5	180,000	β_2	Also intermediate in classic pathway
C3 proactivator convertase (factor D)	C3 PAse	2	3	24,000	α	Trypsinlike enzyme
C3 proactivator (factor B)	C3 PA	200	5 to 6	93,000	β	Proenzyme
C3 activator	C3 A	Unknown	4	63,000	γ	Cleaves C3 at bond 77-78
Cobra venom factor	CoF, CVF	Not found in serum	6.7	144,000		May be cobra C3b

saccharides which catalyze the alternate pathway combine with and stabilize this C3b.

Factor D. Factor B in the C3b,B complex (possibly in association with some polysaccharide factor that could generate or stabilize C3b) becomes the substrate for factor D. Factor D is more descriptively referred to as C3 proactivator convertase, since it enzymatically converts the C3 proactivator (factor B) to a state where it too can express an enzymatic activity as the C3 activator. This cleavage of factor B generates two fragments: Ba, an α-globulin with a molecular weight near 33,000 and Bb, a γ-globulin of 60,000 mol wt. Ba is released, but Bb remains bound to C3b, The complex of C3b,Bb now displays the typical features of a serine esterase and is able to hydrolyze C3.

Properdin. The C3b,Bb enzyme, or C3 activator, also is known as the C3 convertase of the alternate activation pathway. It hydrolyzes C3 at the same peptide bond cleaved by the C4b,2a enzyme of the classic pathway. However, the alternate pathway C3 convertase is labile and decays rapidly. It is stabilized by the addition of properdin. The addition of more C3b to C3b,Bb generates a labile C5 convertase C3b$_n$,Bb, which also is unstable but becomes stabilized by the addition of properdin. Thus properdin, once thought to be the initial compound of the alternate pathway, now is believed to be its terminal component and to function as a stabilizer for the labile C3 and C5 activating enzymes.

Properdin, with an $S_{20,w}$ value of 5.4, is a γ_2-globulin with a molecular weight of 184,000. Properdin contains about 9.8% polysaccharide. Its concentration in normal human serum is 25 μg/ml. Properdin is composed of four peptide subunits, each with a molecular weight of 46,000, held together by hydrogen and ionic bonds. These subunits separate from each other in high-molarity solutions of urea or guanidine. When the dissociating reagents are removed, dimers of the subunits form, which regain about 50% of the activity of intact properdin.

With the generation of stable C3 and C5 convertases the remainder of the pathway from C6 through C9 is ensured.

Cobra venom factor. Cobra venom factor (or CVF) is a protein found in cobra venom that is capable of combining with factor B to form a complex which can activate C3 via Bb. For complete activation of C3, factor D also is required. The chemical mechanism for cobra venom factor activation of the alternate pathway is founded in its

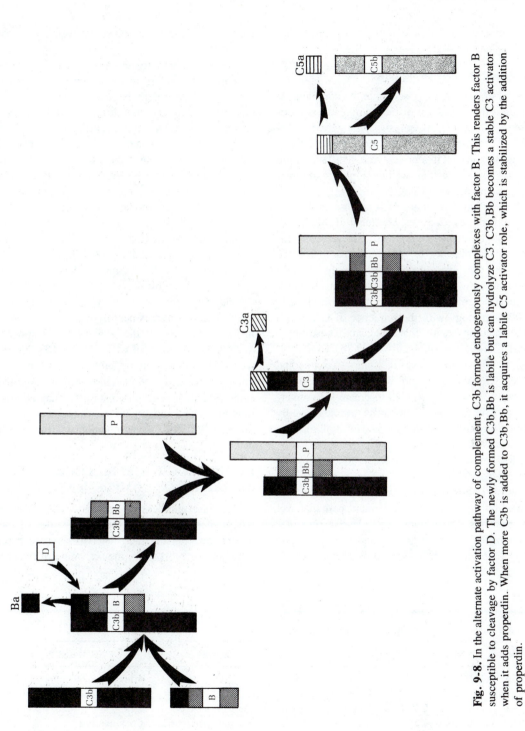

Fig. 9-8. In the alternate activation pathway of complement, C3b formed endogenously complexes with factor B. This renders factor B susceptible to cleavage by factor D. The newly formed C3b,Bb is labile but can hydrolyze C3. C3b,Bb becomes a stable C3 activator when it adds properdin. When more C3b is added to C3b,Bb, it acquires a labile C5 activator role, which is stabilized by the addition of properdin.

behavior as cobra C3b and ability to complex with mammalian factor B.

Complement-derived peptides

At several of the early stages in the complement sequence the activation of the component is associated with limited proteolysis. This generally results in the expression of an enzymatic activity previously masked in a proenzyme. This activation releases low molecular weight peptides of great biologic importance (Table 9-3).

C4a. When $\overline{C1s}$ attacks C4, a low molecular weight peptide, C4a, is liberated (Table 9-3). The C4b remnant acquires an adhesiveness for antigen and attaches to it rather than to the C1 complex. C4a has a molecular weight of only 9,000 and now has been identified as an anaphylatoxin. C4a contains 77 amino acids, which have a 30% homology with the sequence of C3a and a 39% homology with that of C5a. These three peptides are not serologically cross-reactive.

C2b. $\overline{C1s}$ also cleaves C2 into two unequal halves: C2a of 70,000 mol wt and C2b of 30,000 mol wt. C2a binds with C4b to create C3 convertase or $\overline{C4b,2a}$ and is probably the catalytically active portion of that complex. The biologic significance of C2b is unknown.

C3a. To release C3a, $\overline{C4b,2a}$ hydrolyzes C3 between residues 77 and 78 of its α-chain. This is the same bond ruptured by the C3 convertase formed by the alternate complement pathway, yet the enzymes themselves are clearly separate. Amino acid 77 is an arginine, and this is the carboxyl terminus of C3a. C3a thus consists of 77

amino acids and has a molecular weight of 8,900 (Table 9-3).

C3a is anaphylatoxic. Anaphylatoxic activity of a molecule refers to its ability to release histamine and basic peptides from mast cells. Since histamine contracts smooth muscle and causes an edema and wheal reaction in skin, these techniques are used to measure anaphylatoxins. At concentrations as low as 10^{-8}M, C3a is still effective in producing these responses. Removal of the carboxyl terminal arginine by serum carboxypeptidase B, also known as anaphylatoxin inhibitor (anaphylatoxin INH, or Ana INH), completely destroys the biologic activity of C3a. Ana INH, an α-globulin with a molecular weight of 300,000, is susceptible to inhibition by ϵ-aminocaproic acid, a compound that also will inhibit $\overline{C1s}$.

C5a. C5 convertase, the $\overline{C4b,2a,3b}$ complex, like C3 convertase, is peptolytic for a single bond in the amino end of the α-chain of C5 and produces C5a (11,000 mol wt) and C5b (163,000 mol wt). C5a also has an arginine as a carboxyl terminal amino acid, and its removal by the Ana INH carboxypeptidase B eliminates its anaphylatoxic function. C5a is anaphylatoxic at levels approaching 10^{-10}M. C5a is also chemotaxic for granulocytes.

IMMUNOLOGIC AND BIOLOGIC ACTIVITIES OF COMPLEMENT

The vast number of proteins involved in the complement system and the complexities of their interaction plus the fact that two separate mechanisms have evolved for the activation of the com-

Table 9-3. Properties of the complement-derived peptides

Protein	Source	Molecular weight	Biologic activity	Released by
C2b	C2	37,000	Unknown	$\overline{C1s}$
C3a	α-Chain of C3	8,900	Anaphylatoxic	C3 convertase and C3 activator
C4a	α-Chain of C4	9,000	Anaphylatoxic	$\overline{C1s}$
C5a	α-Chain of C5	11,000	Anaphylatoxic and chemotactic	C5 convertase

plement system almost dictate that several important biologic activities would originate from this system. Although all these activities may not be known yet, a rather large number of them are known (Fig. 9-9). Those activities arising from C1, C4, and C2 are expressed only when complement is activated through the classic pathway; those arising from C3 through C9 are expressed after either the classic or alternate pathway activation.

Cytolysis

The classic pathway of complement activation is opened by a serologic reaction between an antigen and immunoglobulin of the IgM or IgG isotypes, and only IgG3, 1, and 2 (in order of activity) of the latter.

There seems to be very little restriction on the nature of the antigens that will inaugurate (with antibody) the complement sequence. Proteins, polysaccharides, protein or polysaccharide complexes, and hapten-antigen conjugates are all effective, although an occasional antigen that fails to activate complement can be found in any biochemical class. Haptens alone do not initiate the complement cascade, presumably because there is no locus for C4 attachment.

Aggregation of the membrane attack components C5 through C9 on the surface of sensitive cellular antigens bearing C4, C2, and C3 results in cytolysis. The number of antibody molecules required for this differs with the immunoglobulin class. By a mathematic correlation of the number of lesions produced in the cell membrane and the number of antibody molecules bound, it was estimated that one IgM molecule and 2,000 to 3,000

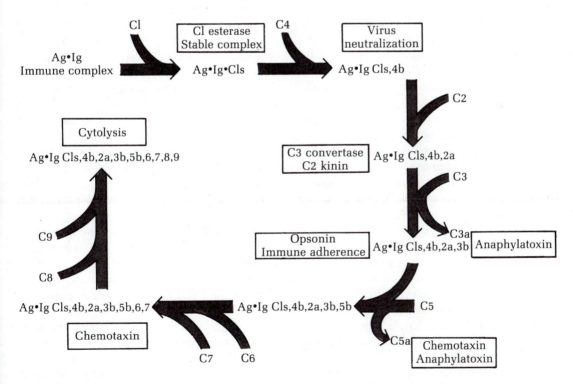

Fig. 9-9. In the classic pathway of complement activation a new biologic activity appears (in *blocks*) at virtually every step of the pathway.

IgG molecules were needed to produce a lesion. It has been suggested that two IgG molecules must be bridged by C1 for lysis to ensue. This requirement for multiple molecules is not necessary for IgM because it has within its own pentameric structure an abundance of complement fixation sites. It has been calculated that 90,000 IgM and 60,000 IgG molecules can attach to a single erythrocyte.

Cytolysis by the alternate pathway is possible. If sufficient C3 through C9 molecules are generated, these molecules may attach to neighboring cells and lyse them as bystander cells. Rabbit erythrocytes, especially when treated with reducing agents, are highly sensitive to lysis by the alternate pathway. Liposomes also are lysed by the complement system.

Enzyme formation

In the classic complement activation pathway three new enzyme activities appear. These are C$\overline{1s}$ esterase and the C3 and C5 convertases. Several enzyme stages may exist in the alternate pathway.

C$\overline{1s}$ esterase is derived from its catalytically inert proenzyme precursor on fixation of the C1 complex to the antigen-antibody pair. The manner by which this activation occurs is as yet unknown but could be caused by a molecular rearrangement of C1s or a heretofore undetected proteolysis.

C3 convertase activity develops after attachment of C2a and C4b to activated C1. Because this activity does not appear until C2a is bound, C2a is believed to play a critical role in the enzyme. This may be the case with C5 convertase also, since no new enzyme activity has been associated with C3. Moreover, the cleavages of C3 and C5 have so many parallels (for example, substrate size and nature of the peptide bond split) that it is likely that C3 convertase and C5 convertase activities reside in the same portion of the C$\overline{4b,2a}$ and C$\overline{4b,2a,3b}$ complexes, respectively.

Factor D (C3 proactivator convertase) is a serine protease normally present in serum. It converts factor B complexed with C3b to an enzyme that then activates C3 and C5. Other enzymes associated with the complement system serve as regulators of the classic and alternate pathway and are described later in this chapter.

Anaphylatoxins

An anaphylatoxin is any low molecular weight substance of natural origin which will generate a permeability-increasing factor that is inhibited by antihistamines. This is essentially synonymous with a definition of anaphylatoxin as any substance that degranulates mast cells and/or basophils because these cells are the primary source of histamine, which is stored in intracellular granules. Because of the generality of this definition, many substances can be considered as anaphylatoxic. The three known anaphylatoxins generated from complement are C4a (9,000 mol wt), C3a (8,900 mol wt), which is formed by the action of C3 convertase and C3 activator on C3, and C5a (11,000 mol wt), produced by C5 convertase and C5 activator. Of these, C4a is the least active. A synthetic octapeptide representing residues 70 through 77 of C3a mimics the complete molecule. A pentapeptide (amino acids 73 through 77) of C4a mimics it. When arginine 77 is removed from either of these, they are no longer anaphylatoxic, whereas C5a loses its anaphylatoxic but retains its chemotactic activity even when the last arginine is removed. A kinin is liberated from C2, but this is apparently different from the vasoactive peptides (kinins) released by anaphylatoxins. (See Chapter 18.)

Since anaphylatoxins result in the degranulation of mast cells, and since mast cell degranulation has become a hallmark of anaphylaxis, hay fever, and other allergies, the tendency to categorize the C3a, C4a, and C5a anaphylatoxins as undesirable expressions of complement is inescapable. Mast cell degranulation releases several bioactive amines, which cause tissue edema, smooth muscle contraction, and changes in blood clotting. These functions can contribute to immunity when an offensive antigen such as a pathogenic bacterium or toxin is involved and are undesirable only when the antigen is intrinsically noninfectious or nontoxic.

The local edema caused by these peptides results from a flow of fluid from the vascular system into the tissue. This causes a continued flux of antibodies from the blood into the tissue, where potential pathogens may have activated the complement system, and facilitates the emigration of phagocytic cells into the tissue. These actions plus the accompanying dilution of any toxins elaborated by the bacteria are clearly protective functions of the inflammatory response initiated by anaphylatoxins.

Chemotaxins

Chemotaxins are substances that induce the migration of leukocytes from an area of lesser concentration to an area of higher concentration of the agent. Chemotaxigens are substances that create chemotaxins from chemotactically inert precursors. In the sense of these definitions C5a is a chemotaxin, and C5 convertase is a chemotaxinogen. Another chemotaxin less directly related to the complement cascade is ECF-A. ECF-A originates from mast cell granules where the anaphylatoxic property of C3a and C5a would ensure its release.

C3a once was described as a chemotaxin, but this was an error and has been identified as resulting from trace contamination of C3a preparations with C5a.

The biochemical changes that develop in leukocytes after exposure to chemotaxins are considered the clue to the expression of their directional motility. Many chemotactic agents induce new esterase activities in leukocytes, but it has not been possible to connect this with the new kinetic potential of the cell. This problem and the methods used to measure chemotaxis are described in Chapter 4.

Opsonization

To detect the direct sensitization of a particle for phagocytic engulfment, it is necessary to have an excess of phagocytic cells in the proximity of the subject particle. Otherwise one might measure the combined action of chemotaxins and opsonins and falsely attribute increased phagocytosis to the latter alone. Opsonins are described in Chapter 4.

Attachment of the C3b to antigen-immunoglobulin complexes improves phagocytosis. Receptors for C3b are found on phagocytic cells, and it is by binding the complex to these receptors that C3b behaves as an opsonin.

Immune adherence

In the traditional serologic agglutination reaction extraneous cells or particulate matter usually are avoided. However, when such particles are present, they are included in the agglutinate in a reaction known as immune adherence or serologic adhesion. This reaction was first described by Levaditi (in 1901), who noted bacterial adhesion to platelets in the presence of antibacterial sera. The reaction has been rediscovered and renamed several times since then.

Immune adherence is visually detectable when a particulate antigen, homologous antibody, complement, and indicator particle are present. The indicator particle may be a platelet, erythrocyte, leukocyte, yeast, heterologous bacterium, starch granule, or other. In the course of the reaction the antigen-antibody-complement complex is extended to include the heterologous particle. Analyses with functionally purified components of complement affirm that C3 is the last in the complement series needed for immune adherence. When 50 to 100 C3 molecules are attached to the erythrocyte antigen, adhesion of the indicator particle is just detectable. A maximal reaction requires the fixation of about 1,000 C3 molecules per erythrocyte. Since 10,000 or more C3 molecules per erythrocyte are needed for hemolysis, it is clear that immune adherence is the more sensitive measure of C3. The part of C3 responsible for this activity is C3b.

Immune adherence occurs indiscriminately on any surface. This includes the in vivo attachment of particles to blood vessel walls, which makes them easier prey for phagocytes and must be considered as a protective influence of antibody and complement.

Immunoconglutinins

Lachmann has defined immunoconglutinins as antibodies that display a specificity toward antigenic determinants that are exposed by fixed complement but which are unavailable in free complement. Immunoconglutinin is produced by an animal against its own complement, that is, it is an autoantibody, and arises during ordinary immunization or infections. In the course of the complement fixation the new antigenic determinants are exposed. These new sites appear to be in C3b, although some experiments have suggested C4b. The chemistry of the antigenic determinant is not known.

Autostimulated immunoconglutinins are frequently IgM in nature, although this is not absolute. The serologic method for the detection of immunoconglutinin is based on the agglutination of complement-bound cellular antigen-antibody complexes.

Immunoconglutinin formation has been associated with an increased protection of laboratory animals against challenges with infectious bacteria. This is perhaps one of the few instances in which an autoantibody has a protective influence.

Conglutinin and conglutination

Bovine conglutinin is a β-globulin with a molecular weight of approximately 750,000 and an $S_{20,w}$ value estimated at 6.6 to 7.8. It is present in normal bovine serum at a concentration of 50 μg/ml. It is an unusual protein on two accounts: it is composed of 18% glycine, and it reacts rather nonspecifically with complex polysaccharides. It is on the basis of this latter activity that conglutinin is able to combine with complement component C3b and to agglutinate antigen-antibody-complement complexes. In this sense conglutinin and immunoconglutinin have an identical serologic activity, and it is this attribute of conglutinin which has permitted the development of the conglutinating complement fixation or absorption test.

The basis of the conglutinating complement fixation test is that no lysis occurs when sheep red blood cells are mixed with antibody and horse complement because of the sublytic quantities of C2 in equine sera. Mixture of the sensitized sheep cells with normal bovine serum containing conglutinin causes agglutination of the erythrocytes. Thereby an alternative indicator system to the standard lytic complement fixation test is provided.

In the complete conglutinating complement fixation test an unknown serum and known antigen are incubated with horse complement. Thereafter sheep erythrocytes and bovine serum are added. The bovine serum contains conglutinin and a natural, low-titer antibody against sheep red blood cells. If hemagglutination occurs after a second incubation period, there is no antibody in the test serum. Horse complement is left free to bind with the sheep red blood cells and its nonhemagglutinating antibody in bovine serum. The presence of conglutinin in the bovine serum promotes the hemagglutination. In the opposite way a failure of hemagglutination to develop is an indication of antibody in the test serum. The conglutinating complement fixation test is slightly more sensitive than complement fixation tests based on red cell hemolysis (Fig. 9-10).

It is known that conglutinin reacts only with altered C3b. In fact the combination of conglutinin with sensitized sheep erythrocytes bearing nonhemolytic complement cannot take place until after a further normal serum component originally termed KAF has acted on C3b. KAF is a β-globulin with a molecular weight of 100,000 and an $S_{20,w}$ value of 5.5 to 6. It is present in serum at a concentration of only 25 μg/ml. KAF is now better known as C3b · C4b INAC, an enzyme that hydrolyzes C3b, thus interrupting the complement cascade.

MODULATION OF COMPLEMENT-MEDIATED FUNCTIONS

As described in the preceding section, a multitude of biologic functions are associated with

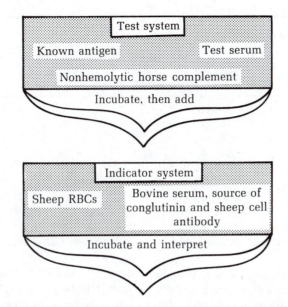

No hemagglutination = C fixed in test system = positive test
Hemagglutination = C fixed in indicator system = negative test

Fig. 9-10. In the conglutinating complement (C) fixation test the test serum is incubated with the known antigen and a source of nonhemolytic complement. Then bovine serum, which contains conglutinin and a natural agglutinin for sheep red blood cells, is added simultaneously with the addition of sheep red blood cells. The test is interpreted as indicated. The natural sheep red blood cell agglutinin needs conglutinin before it can cause hemagglutination.

complement and complement-derived peptides. Obviously biologic control devices have evolved to regulate these activities; otherwise, once initiated, they would continue until the complement system was exhausted. Two principal control systems are known: inactivators, mostly enzymes that destroy the primary structure of the complement protein thus rendering it inactive, and inhibitors, compounds that combine with the complement molecule to halt its further function (Table 9-4). A third, unrelated method by which complement is regulated is partial or total genetic loss of a component, inactivator, or inhibitor.

Complement inactivators

C3b · C4b INAC. C3b · C4b INAC is an enzyme found in normal sera of several species, including human, guinea pig, and rabbit. C3b · C4b

INAC splits C3b in the α-chain to form C3c and C3d. C3c and C3d may be further degraded by serum plasmin. C4b also is hydrolyzed by C3b · C4b INAC.

C3b · C4b INAC is a β-globulin with a molecular weight of 90,000, and it is found in serum at a level of 25 μg/ml. C3b · C4b INAC is synonymous with KAF. In its role as KAF, C3b · C4b INAC alters C3b on antigen-antibody complexes so that the activity of conglutinin can be detected.

C3b · C4b INAC accelerator. A recently identified modulator of the complement system is serologically identical to a human blood serum protein originally known as βIH because of its immunoelectrophoretic mobility in the β-globulin region. The term *C3b · C4b INAC* was proposed on the basis that this protein increases the rate at which C3b and C4b are inactivated by C3b ·

Table 9-4. Modulators of the complement system

Modulator	Molecular weight	Electro-phoretic mobility	Concentration (μg/ml serum)	Comment
C1s INH	90,000	α_2	100	α_2-Neuraminoglycoprotein
C3b · C4b INAC	90,000	β	25	Synonym of KAF
C3b · C4b INAC accelerator	150,000	β	500	
Ana INH	300,000	α	35	Carboxypeptidase; acts on C3a and C5a
C4 binding proteins	60,000	β	Unknown	Complexes with C4
C6 INAC	Unknown	β	Unknown	$S_{20,w}$ is 6.6

C4b INAC; that is, it serves as an accelerator of C3b INAC.

C3b · C4b INAC accelerator is a β-globulin present in human serum at a concentration of 500 μg/ml. Its molecular weight is 150,000. This molecule, in conjunction with C3b · C4b INAC and C3a Ana INH, must be considered a key regulator of the complement system, since C3 is the pivotal molecule linking the classic and alternate pathways of complement activation.

Ana INH. A single enzyme that removes the carboxyl terminal arginine from C4a, C3a, and C5a is inappropriately referred to as an inhibitor. In keeping with a system in which enzymes are called inactivators, it really should be termed Ana INAC rather than Ana INH, since it is a carboxypeptidase. Ana INH is a macroglobulin normally present in serum. It is an α-globulin and has a molecular weight of 300,000.

C4 binding protein. Both human and mouse sera contain a β-globulin of 60,000 mol wt that binds to C4, thereby preventing its participation in the complement cascade.

C6 INAC. An inactivator of C6, C6 INAC, is not yet well characterized. It is a β-globulin with an $S_{20,w}$ value of 6.6 and acts on bound, but not on free, C6.

Complement inhibitors

C$\overline{1}$s inhibitor (C$\overline{1}$s INH). The first molecule described with a known complement-modulating

activity was C$\overline{1}$s INH, a normal component of the α_2-globulin fraction of human serum. The normal level of C$\overline{1}$s INH in human blood is 180 μg/ml. C$\overline{1}$s INH is an acid-labile, heat-labile α_2-neuraminoglycoprotein, which is inactivated below pH 6 and above 60° C. Of its molecular weight of 90,000, 17% is in the form of neuraminic acid, and 14% is represented by other carbohydrates. Other glycoproteins, including those from egg white, soybean, pancreas, and blood, are also C$\overline{1}$s inhibitors. C$\overline{1}$s INH will not combine with C1, only C$\overline{1}$s, and inhibition is achieved at unit stoichiometry, that is, a 1 : 1 molar ratio. Deficiency of C$\overline{1}$s INH results in hereditary angioneurotic edema (HANE), a disease characterized by episodic bouts of edema.

COMPLEMENT PHYLOGENY AND ONTOGENY

Comparative studies on the distribution of the complement components in the sera of animals at several levels of the animal kingdom now have been performed. These studies have been hampered somewhat by the specificities of complement from various species for antibodies of their own or closely related species, even though it is well known that complement does have a rather broad specificity.

Invertebrates do not have a classic complement system. The horseshoe crab and the sepunculid worm have a lytic activity inducible after treatment of their hemolymph with cobra venom factor, which suggests that some of the terminal complement components are present. Lampreys, which are capable of antibody formation, do not produce complement. All higher life forms have a complement system: elasmobranchs, fishes, amphibia, avians, and mammals. All nine components have been identified only in mammals, however.

Complement polymorphism

All complement molecules are not identical in the different species nor within a single species. Indeed allotypic variations already have been described for human C3, C4, C6, and factor B and proposed for C2 and C7. A dozen polymorphic forms of C3 have been identified by simple electrophoresis in agarose or starch gels, in which C3 can be detected easily because of its relatively high concentration in sera. In agarose gels three variants were found in C3. One was an electrophoretically slow (S) variant, and the other two were fast (F) variants, all detected in company with normal C3. Phenotypically a person may be FF, FS, or SS. Subscripts have been used to indicate how fast or how slow a C3 component may be, $F_{1.0}$, $F_{0.8}$, and $F_{0.5}$ being examples. Analysis for S and F gene distribution has revealed the following frequencies for S/F: whites, 0.75/0.25; blacks, 0.90/10; and Orientals, 0.98/0.02. No significant differences in antigenicity, sedimentation properties, or hemolytic activities have been detected yet in these C3 allotypes.

Polymorphism of human C4 has been noted, with at least 10 different patterns being detected in the immunodiffusion test. Two of these bind to erythrocytes and were erroneously believed to be red blood cell antigens. The human blood groups Chido and Rogers were created as a result of this confusion. Two relatively frequent allotypes and several less common variants of C6 are known. A double pattern of C2 bands has been observed on electrophoresis, and one variant of C7 is known. Both factors B and D of the alternate complement pathway have several electrophoretic variants, which probably are allotypic variants.

All complement components are synthesized early in fetal development, considerably before the appearance of immunoglobulins. C1 has been identified in human fetal intestinal tissue by the nineteenth week of gestation. Tissue cultures of cells taken from human fetal liver at 8 weeks of gestation will synthesize both C4 and C2. Fetal liver, lung, and peritoneal cells taken from fetuses at 14 weeks can be stained successfully with fluorescent anti-C4 and anti-C3. Circulating C4 can be recovered from all fetuses older than 18 weeks and C3 from all those older than 15 weeks.

Determinations of hemolytic complement titers of 44 pairs of maternal and cord sera have revealed that maternal blood contains approximately twice as much complement as cord blood. The complement level of the newborn child reaches the adult level within 3 to 6 months after birth, and the bulk of this recovery occurs within the first 1 or 2 weeks of life. The amount of each individual component of complement in the blood of newborn infants has not been determined, but analyses of C3, C4, and C5 have been accomplished; cord blood contains 38%, 60%, and 50%, respectively, of the maternal level of these three components. Maternal C1q titers average about four times those of the newborn infant. Newborn lambs, calves, and pigs are also deficient in complement but repair this defect within the first few weeks of life.

The sources of the complement components in human tissues have been identified. It might be expected that since there are nine major proteins to be considered, several different organs might be involved in the synthesis of these molecules, each organ or tissue being specific for a certain component, but this is not the case.

Tissues of the small and large intestine are the source of all three components of C1. The major intestinal source is the columnar epithelial cell. Monocytes and fibroblasts are also sources of C1q, and C1r and C1s also are produced by cultured cells from several organs. Biosynthesis of C2 can be detected in several organs, and eventually cells of the monocyte-macrophage lineage were identified as the cell source. Macrophages are also the source of other components of the classic activation pathway, including C4 and C5, for which the evidence is quite good, and of C6, C7, and C8, where the evidence is less satisfactory. Both C3 and C9 arise from parenchymal cells of the liver.

It should be remembered that C3, C4, and C5 all are derived from precursor molecules that are slightly larger than the active complement component.

Macrophages are the source of factor B, factor D, and properdin, but this is based on studies in different rather than a single species.

Complement genetics

In 1963 serologic studies with a rabbit antiserum to mouse serum globulins distinguished several mouse strains by the ability of the serum from only a few of the strains to precipitate with the antiserum. The variation was designated as due to differences in the quantity of Ss (serum serologic variant) protein in their blood. The gene that regulates Ss formation is situated between the Ir and H-2D regions of the mouse chromosome 6.

Subsequently another mouse protein originally believed to be present only in the sera of males and thus tagged Slp (sex-linked protein) was found in the high producers of Ss. Now it is accepted that female mice of some strains produce Slp; so mice may be Ss+, Slp−, or Ss+, Slp+. Purification of Ss and Slp accompanied by immunologic and biochemical characterization now has revealed that Slp is an antigen determinant of Ss, since double immunodiffusion tests produce reactions of partial identity. The molecules are identical or very nearly so in terms of the biochemical characteristics: both are globulins with molecular weights of 180,000, and mercaptoethanol reduces them to units of 70,000 to 80,000 mol wt.

The Ss protein is serologically cross-reactive with human C4 and may function as either C4 or C2 in the mouse.

The structural genes for the mouse Ss and Slp proteins are adjacently situated on chromosome 6 near the Ir genes. In the human system the genes for C2 and C4 (and factor B) also neighbor each other on chromosome 17 adjacent to the human Ir genes D/DR. (See Fig. 11-2.) Thus in the mouse and human systems the genes for some complement components are placed with the genes of the MHC—H-2 and HLA, respectively.

DEFICIENCIES OF THE COMPLEMENT COMPONENTS

Inadequate amounts of the various components of the complement system, including the inhibitors and inactivators that regulate the activation cascade, may arise from genetic conditions in which the component is not synthesized at all or is produced at subnormal levels. It is also possible that the molecule may be synthesized in the normal amount, but it may be structurally defective and functionally inert. Hypercatabolism also may produce a deficiency of one of the complement proteins, and this may be difficult to distinguish from activation of the molecule, especially if only a late-acting component is involved. Before it is possible to establish that a deficiency of some complement molecule exists, it is necessary to have a reliable method for quantitating the individual component or the whole complement system.

Quantitation of complement activity

Hemolytic titration. The total complement level of a serum is determined in a hemolytic assay system. In the titration of complement sheep red blood cells that have been preincubated with a slight excess of antisheep hemolysin are added to varying amounts of the complement source. Such erythrocytes are known as sensitized sheep cells because they are susceptible to lysis in the presence of complement. The exact volumes used in the test will vary according to whether it is a macroscopic tube test (final volume 3 to 7.5 ml) or a microtiter test (final volume 0.2 to 0.5 ml). The erythrocyte suspension also is adjusted according to the dimensions of the test, with its final concentration ranging from 1% to 0.25%. After a suitable incubation period at 37° C the tubes or wells containing the several complement dilutions are examined for hemolysis. The amount of complement present in the test material usually is expressed as the dilution of complement necessary to achieve lysis of half the red cells added, that is, the CH50 dilution. This can be determined very accurately by a spectrophotometric determination of the amount of hemoglobin released in different tubes in the complement dilution series compared with a standard containing half the amount of cells used in the titration that have been lysed with distilled water.

Complement components. Quantitation of the individual components of the complement system is possible by serologic means or by hemolytic assays. It should be remembered that the latter method measures the functional capacity of the molecule, whereas the former measures only the antigenic integrity of the molecule. For example, it is known that the activation of C3 removes such a small peptide, C3a, from the parent molecule that nearly all the serologic activity of the parent molecule is left with C3b. When C3b is acted on by C3 · C4 INAC, another low molecular weight peptide, C3d, is freed. The remainder is hemolytically inactive but serologically identical (with respect to most antisera) to total C3. Thus, if one recovers C3 as an antigen, it could be C3, C3b, or C3c that is being measured, but if C3 is measured by hemolytic assays, only C3 (C3b) is being determined.

Measuring each of the components in sera is a useful way to determine if a classic or alternate pathway of complement activation is in progress. If levels of C1, C4, and C2 are normal in company with low C3 levels and a low hemolytic activity of the serum, then it can be assumed that the complement level of the serum was lowered by activation of the alternate pathway.

Commercially available Mancini plates with the specific antiserum incorporated into agarose are used for the quantitative immunodiffusion determination of C3 and C5. Standards are provided with the test kits. Mancini plates can be prepared for C4, C8, C9, and properdin from commeric ally available antisera. Other antisera undoubtedly will be available soon.

To measure the biologic activity of human or other sources of the individual complement components, special serum reagents are available that are devoid of the component to be quantitated. A sample containing an unknown quantity of the component to be measured is added to sensitized sheep erythrocytes; this is incubated to allow lysis to take place. The amount of lysis that occurs is relatable to the quantity of the component being measured, since an excess of all the other components is present in the mixture.

Genetic complement deficiency

C1q and C1r. Human deficiency of C1q initially was reported in 1961, and several examples have been added since that time. Most of these cases have been associated with a sex-linked agammaglobulinemia or a combined immuno-deficiency disease. The C1q level is reduced to about half that of normal levels. In 5 patients in one study the average C1q concentration was 6.4 μgN/ml, compared with 20.2 for control subjects. Bone marrow grafting was performed to repair the immune deficit and was successful, restoring the C1q levels to normal. The basis for the C1q loss is uncertain. In some persons a hypercatabolism of the molecules has been suggested as the cause, although restoration of C1q blood levels by marrow transplants indicates that the cellular origin of the molecule is lacking in these persons. Since C1q deficiency is regularly associated with a loss of B and T lymphocytes, it is difficult to recognize any single defect associated with the C1q deficiency.

Normal C1q levels were noted in those few persons in whom C1r levels were markedly depressed. It is striking that all patients with the C1r deficiency had an extensive medical history, including multiple episodes of upper respiratory tract disease, chronic kidney disease, or a lupus erythematosus (LE)–like syndrome. Genetic studies indicate that the C1r loss is transmitted as an autosomal recessive trait.

C1s and C̄1s̄ INH. Patients with C1r deficiency may have a loss of nearly 50% of their C1s. Little is known about the relationship of C1s deficiency and human health, although several of the individuals studied had an LE-like syndrome. This is not the case with $\overline{C1s}$ INH deficiency, which is clearly associated with HANE, also known as hereditary giant edema or giant edema. This disease is transmitted as an autosomal dominant deficiency in which the afflicted individuals average but 31 μg/ml of $\overline{C1s}$ INH, compared with 180 μg/ml for normal persons. A second form of $\overline{C1s}$ INH deficiency should be classified as a dysfunction or paraproteinemia, since a protein antigenically identical to the α_2-neuraminoglycoprotein is present in serum but is functionally inert.

The importance of α_2-neuraminoglycoprotein in homeostasis is best represented by its genetic deficiency disease, HANE. Persons with this disease suffer sporadic attacks of subcutaneous edema, which may be more or less localized, often associated with minor trauma of the affected part. In extensive reactions, edema of the face, neck, and joints may develop. The edema usually resolves within 72 hours, is not especially bothersome, and may not be associated with extensive pain, itching, or marked erythema. However, edema in the throat may make breathing difficult, and abdominal pain of considerable intensity is associated with edema of the viscera. The pathogenesis of the disease is not entirely known but may ultimately reside in a kinin released from C2. It is possible that Hageman's factor becomes activated by tissue enzymes released by the local trauma, and this is followed by the formation of plasmin from plasminogen and the activation of C1. In the absence of $\overline{C1}$ INH, C2 kinin may be released. Patients with HANE have depleted plasma levels of C4 and C2 (and of $\overline{C1}$ INH) consistent with this hypothesis. Injection of C1s into the skin of these patients produces a local edema. Prevention of this edema or attacks of angioneurotic edema with antihistamines or adrenergic drugs is not successful, suggesting little, if any, contribution of C3a or C5a to the disease. Infusion of plasma that contains the normal level of $\overline{C1s}$ INH and treatment with ϵ-aminocaproic acid, which inhibits plasmin

formation from plasminogen, are both therapeutic.

C4. An autosomal recessive deficiency of C4 first was recognized in an inbred strain of guinea pigs. In the homozygous condition absolutely no C4 could be detected, whereas in the heterozygous state up to 30% of normal values were observed. Homozygotes could be successfully immunized with guinea pig C4. The C4-deficient guinea pigs developed feeble immune responses to egg or bovine serum albumin but developed normal Arthus and passive cutaneous anaphylactic reactions. The alternate complement pathway is intact and may be the major source of protection for these animals against bacterial and viral infections.

Two human examples of C4 deficiency have been reported, and one of the victims had a pronounced skin rash of uncertain cause.

C2. The C4-deficient guinea pigs just mentioned have about 40% of the normal C2 levels, and this has been attributed to a decreased synthetic rate of this protein and is not directly related to the C4 loss as such.

Human C2 deficiencies of both homozygous and heterozygous origin have been described on numerous occasions. Over 40 cases have been recognized, making this the most common of the human complement deficiencies. The heterozygous individuals have 30% to 70% of the normal C2 serum level, whereas the homozygous deficient persons range below 4% of normal values, based on hemolytic assays. Immune adherence assays for C2 are normal for both classes of individuals, probably because only 100 molecules of C3 need to be fixed for immune adherence to occur, whereas many thousand C3 molecules must be bound before hemolysis can occur. The frequency of hypersensitive disease such as LE and dermatomyositis and repeated infectious disease in C2-deficient persons exceeds what would be expected on the basis of random distribution. The basis for these relationships is not known.

C3. Over 20 separate hospital admissions for multiple bouts of middle ear infections, meningitis, pneumonia, etc. are in the medical history of the one known human with total C3 deficiency

(2.5 μg/ml of serum, compared with a normal level of 1,250 μg/ml). Five other children in the same family plus the mother had about half-normal C3 levels. The preponderance of infections by the patient emphasizes the critical role of C3 not only in linking the classic and alternate pathways but also in immune adherence, opsonization, and chemotaxis, all of which are important defense functions. Approximately a half dozen C3-deficient persons are recorded in the medical literature.

C5. About 40% of inbred mice lack a functional C5 but produce a unique protein termed *MuB1*. Because of antigenic similarities between MuB1 and C5, the former is considered an inactive form of the normal complement component. The hemolytic deficiency of C5-deficient mouse serum is totally replaced by fresh whole mouse serum or by pure C5. These mice are apparently as healthy as other mice, although there is provisional evidence that they are more susceptible to infection with *Corynebacterium kutscheri* and *Candida albicans*.

Human dysfunction of C5, unlike that of mice, is more clearly relatable to recurrent infectious disease. Only three human examples are known, and in these the C5 level as determined immunochemically was normal, but hemolytic titrations of complement could detect no C5. Phagocytosis was depressed and could not be restored to normal with C5-deficient mouse sera but could be with human C5. This loss of the expected phagocytic activity accounts for the higher incidence of infectious disease in these patients.

C6 and C7. A strain of rabbits with a genetic deficiency of C6 is known. This is apparently only part of a more generalized fault in the immunologic functions of complement, since serum of the affected individuals is not chemotactic, a property related to C5 but not to C6. These rabbits also develop only a feeble delayed hypersensitivity to tuberculin and retain skin grafts longer than is typical, phenomena that are quite unrelated to complement function and indicate a broad immunodepressed condition in these animals. Sera of these rabbits are devoid of bacteriolytic as well as hemolytic properties, both ascribable to their complement deficit. These latter defects were correctable with addition of purified C6. The deficiency was inherited as a single autosomal recessive characteristic. A C6 deficiency in hamsters also has been recognized.

Human C6 deficiency has been described in four individuals who lacked hemolytically or immunochemically active C6. The parents and siblings of the individuals had half-normal serum levels of C6. C6 deficiency appears to be associated with a heightened susceptibility to *Neisseria* infections. Several patients have been described who are deficient in C7, and another group lacking C8 also has been identified.

COMPLEMENT FIXATION TESTS
Standard complement fixation test

The complement fixation test takes advantage of two of the properties of complement: its combination in all antigen-antibody reactions, whether or not it is required for that reaction, and the requirement of complement in immunolytic reactions. The complement fixation test is divided into the test system and the indicator system (Fig. 9-11). The test system contains an antigen and a serum believed to contain antibody to that antigen. This serum is heat treated prior to the test to destroy its complement. To these two is added a measured amount of complement in the form of normal guinea pig serum, and an incubation period is allowed. Following this incubation the indicator system, consisting of sheep red blood cells and hemolysin (antibody against sheep red blood cells), is added, and another incubation period is allowed. Hemolysin is identical to hemagglutinin but has been renamed to more aptly describe its activity in the presence of serum complement.

Interpretation of the complement fixation test is based on the presence or absence of hemolysis in the indicator system. When there is antibody present in the test serum, it combines with the antigen, and complement is fixed into the test system. No erythrocyte lysis occurs. This is re-

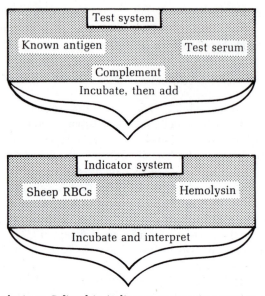

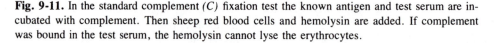

Hemolysis = C fixed in indicator system = negative test

No hemolysis = C fixed in test system = positive test

Fig. 9-11. In the standard complement *(C)* fixation test the known antigen and test serum are incubated with complement. Then sheep red blood cells and hemolysin are added. If complement was bound in the test serum, the hemolysin cannot lyse the erythrocytes.

ferred to as a positive complement fixation test. When there is no antibody in the test serum, complement remains free to be bound later in the indicator system. Erythrocyte lysis is then observed; this is a negative complement fixation test. Complement is always fixed in the complement fixation test, either in the test system or in the indicator system. Where it is fixed determines whether the test is positive or negative.

Hemagglutination is not observed in the complement fixation test for the following reason: the antibody to sheep red blood cells is active in a much greater dilution in hemolytic tests than in hemagglutination tests. The amount of antibody required to produce hemagglutination is about 0.01 μg of antibody nitrogen per milliliter of antiserum; only about 0.001 μg of antibody nitrogen per milliliter of antiserum is required for hemolysis. The quantity of hemolysin used for complement fixation is simply too little to cause hemagglutination.

The dilution of hemolysin used is so great that it is hardly necessary to heat inactivate it before use, since its complement activity at that dilution is negligible.

The complement fixation test is a delicate test, depending as it does on several serologic reagents, one of which is heat labile. For this reason the quantity of each reagent must be carefully titrated just prior to use, and adequate controls must be applied. For example, the quantity of hemolysin used is determined first by a hemolysin titration. This is performed by making a dilution series of hemolysin in buffer, adding a constant, excess amount of guinea pig complement to each tube, and observing for hemolysis after a suitable incubation period. The hemolysin dilution series should be carried out until dilutions of several thousand are achieved. The extent of hemolysis is either estimated visually, based on an end point of 100% hemolysis, or measured in a colorimeter for an exact reading of the 50% hemolytic end point. From this assay the exact amount of hemolysin needed to produce lysis of 50% of the erythrocytes is determined, and in the complement titration test a multiple of two to five times this amount is used to ensure sufficient reagent in that titration.

To determine the hemolytic activity of complement, different quantities of fresh complement are added to tubes containing sheep red blood cells and hemolysin. After incubation the degree of lysis is read colorimetrically, and the amount of complement required for 50% hemolysis is determined. This is referred to as the CH50 unit, and in the complete complement fixation test two CH50 units of complement are the minimum amount employed. Four to five CH50 units of complement may be used. This means that in a positive complement fixation test as many as five CH50 units of complement must be fixed in the test system; otherwise some complement will be left free to interact in the indicator system.

Separate anticomplementary controls on the antigen are necessary. This includes antigen, complement, sheep red blood cells, and hemolysin (the latter two sometimes premixed and referred to as sensitized erythrocytes). If this tube does not exhibit lysis, it is because of an anticomplementary activity of the antigen. A separate anticomplementary control of the serum also is performed as proof that the serum did not contain nonspecific complement-inactivating substances. If the antigen or serum were anticomplementary and such controls were not included, false positive complement fixation test results of a serious nature could be reported. Since complement is heat labile, a positive lytic control containing only complement and sensitized red blood cells also is included.

The titer of a complement-fixing antiserum is determined in the same way as the titer in most other serologic tests, that is, by testing dilutions of the antiserum.

The complement fixation test can be applied to virtually any antigen-antibody system. It is especially useful when only small quantities of antigen or antibody are available because it is a very sensitive serologic procedure. Moreover certain serologic tests are difficult to demonstrate by other means. For example, antibodies to viruses can be identified much more quickly and less expensively by complement fixation than by animal neutralization tests. If one has a known antiserum, it can be used in complement fixation assays for the antigen. Thus the complement fixation test can be used to determine either antigen or antibody.

The complement fixation test has been used to detect and quantitate antibodies of patients infected with viruses of poliomyelitis, mumps, smallpox, influenza, St. Louis encephalitis, measles, herpes, and adenovirus; bacteria such as *Treponema, Mycobacterium, Neisseria,* and *Hemophilus* organisms; fungi such as *Histoplasma, Blastomyces,* and *Coccidioides* organisms; and many others. Antigens of all varieties have been used in complement fixation tests: enzymes, serum proteins, those of viral, bacterial, rickettsial, and fungal origin, thyroid tissue, blood group substances, etc. Theoretically there is no limit to the antigens or antisera that can be used in this test; this is what has made the complement fixation test so widely appreciated.

The Wassermann test

The most extensive use of the complement fixation test has been in the serologic diagnosis of syphilis by the Wassermann test and its variations. In this test, as originally designed, extracts of the liver of fetuses, stillborn because of syphilis and teeming with *Treponema pallidum,* were used as the antigen. The antibody in a patient's serum, combining with this antigen and fixing complement in the test system, was thought to be a specific antitreponemal antibody. It subsequently was discovered that this antibody would fix complement when alcoholic extracts of normal human or animal tissues were used as the antigen. The antigen now used is a purified alcoholic extract of beef heart to which lecithin and cholesterol have been added. This is known as cardiolipin. The lecithin is added to reduce the anticomplementary activity of the antigen and to replace the lecithin that is removed in the purification procedure. The antigen will not fix complement if cholesterol is omitted.

Since the Wassermann antibody reacts with nonspecific antigen, it is clear that it is not an antibody of the usual type. This view is fortified by the rapid disappearance of this antibody during successful therapy. For these reasons the terms *syphilitic reagin* or *Wassermann reagin* have been applied to this antibody. Caution must be taken not to confuse this with allergic reagin, now known as IgE. Syphilitic reagin may be an unusual autoantibody that reacts with tissue. This ''antibody'' could be formed originally against treponemal altered autoantigens.

Truly specific serologic tests for syphilis have been developed using antigens prepared from *T. pallidum* spirochetes taken from experimental lesions in rabbits or cultured in vitro. These procedures have replaced the Wassermann test as a diagnostic device for syphilis. In these instances immunologically specific antibody is measured; the titer of this antibody remains high during and after successful therapy.

The Rice indirect test

When the sera of various animal species are being examined for their complement-fixing ability with a certain antigen, negative results of a spurious type may arise from the failure of antisera from some species to bind guinea pig complement. Such a result, if overlooked or if assumed to be caused by the lack of antibody, would provide erroneous data. This possibility can be obviated by employing the Rice indirect complement fixation test as a control. In this procedure the test serum, antigen, and complement are incubated as usual, but thereafter a second antiserum, one of known ability to fix complement, is added, and a second incubation is permitted before the hemolytic system is added. If the result of the ordinary test is positive, the results of the Rice test may be ignored. If the standard test is negative (hemolysis) and the Rice test shows no hemolysis,

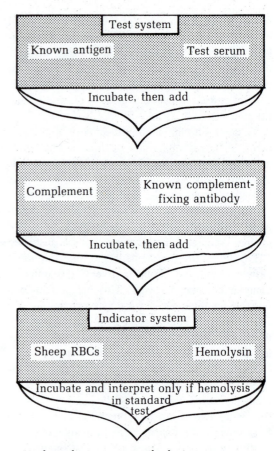

No hemolysis = no antibody in test serum

Hemolysis = antibody in test serum

Fig. 9-12. In the Rice modification of the complement fixation test a known antigen is incubated with the test serum prior to an incubation with complement and a proved complement-fixing antibody. After a second incubation sheep red blood cells and hemolysin are added. The test is used only when the standard complement fixation test is negative.

then the negative test is the result of a lack of antibodies in the test serum. Since no antibodies were in the test serum, the standard antiserum added in the Rice control reacts with the antigen, binds complement, and precludes lysis in the indicator system. If the Rice test results in hemolysis, then the unknown serum contained an antibody that bound antigen, but not complement, and the complement was left free to function in the indicator portion of the test. The indirect complement fixation test thus uses the fact that antigen fixation by antibody can occur without complement fixation. Disappearance of antigen in such a reaction removes the possibility of complement fixation by the standard antiserum (Fig. 9-12.)

Conglutinating complement fixation test

The conglutinating complement fixation test is described earlier in the chapter in the discussion on conglutinin.

BIBLIOGRAPHY

Alper, C.A., and Rosen, F.S.: Genetics of the complement system, Adv. Hum. Genet. **7:**141, 1976.

Alper, C.A., and others: Nomenclature of the alternative activating pathway of complement, J. Immunol. **127:**1261, 1981.

Bianco, C., and Nussenzweig, V.: Complement receptors, Contemp. Top. Mol. Immunol. **6:**145, 1977.

Colten, H.R.: Biosynthesis of complement, Adv. Immunol. **22:**67, 1976.

Fearon, D.T.: Activation of the alternative complement pathway, CRC Crit. Rev. Immunol. **1:**1, 1979.

Frank, M.M., and Atkinson, J.P.: Complement in clinical medicine, Disease-A-Month, January 1975, p. 1.

Hugli, T.E.: Chemical aspects of the serum anaphylatoxins, Contemp. Top. Mol. Immunol. **7:**181, 1978.

Hugli, T.E.: The structural basis for anaphylaxtoxin and chemotactic functions of C3a, C4a, and C5a, CRC Crit. Rev. Immunol. **1:**321, 1981.

Hugli, T.E., and Müller-Eberhard, H.J.: Anaphylatoxins: C3a and C5a, Adv. Immunol. **26:**1, 1978.

Lachmann, P.J.: Complement, Antigens **5:**284, 1979.

Lachmann, P.J., and Rosen, F.S.: Genetic defects of complement in man, Springer Semin. Immunopathol. **1:**339, 1978.

Mayer, M.M., and others: Membrane damage by complement, CRC Crit. Rev. Immunol. **2:**133, 1981.

Minta, J.O., and Movat, H.Z.: The complement system and inflammation, Curr. Top. Pathol. **68:**135, 1979.

Möller, G., editor: Biology of complement and complement receptors, Transplant. Rev. **32:**1, 1976.

Movat, H.Z., editor: Inflammatory reaction, New York, 1979, Springer-Verlag New York, Inc.

Müller-Eberhard, H.J.: Complement, Annu. Rev. Biochem. **44:**697, 1975.

Müller-Eberhard, H.J., and Schreiber, R.D.: Molecular biology and chemistry of the alternative pathway of complement, Adv. Immunol. **29:**1, 1980.

Opferkuch, W., Rother, K., and Schultz, D.R., editors: Clinical aspects of the complement system, Littleton, Mass., 1978, PSG Publishing Co.

Osler, A.G.: Complement: mechanisms and functions, Englewood Cliffs, N.J., 1976, Prentice-Hall, Inc.

Porter, R.R., and Reid, K.B.M.: Activation of the complement system by antibody-antigen complexes: the classical pathway, Adv. Protein Chem. **33:**1, 1979.

Rosse, W.F.: Interactions of complement with the red-cell membrane, Semin. Hematol. **16:**128, 1979.

Takahashi, M., Takahashi, S., and Hirose, S.: Solubilization of antigen-antibody complexes: a new function of complement as a regulator of immune reactions, Prog. Allergy **27:**134, 1980.

Weissmann, G., Samuelsson, B., and Paoletti, R., editors: Advances in inflammation research, New York, 1979, Raven Press.

SITUATION: HANE

Barbara, a 16-year-old white girl, was admitted to the hospital because of repeated attacks of abdominal pain that she had experienced since early childhood. Although early childhood recurrences seldom exceeded 2 or 3 per year, since puberty the attacks had become more frequent and seemed to coincide with the menses. She also complained that severe facial edema, especially of the lips and eyelids, was interfering with her social life. The symptoms usually persisted for 2 or 3 days and then were repeated a month later. Intervening bouts seemed to be associated with mild physical exercise; she had given up guitar lessons because they caused her fingers to swell.

Questions

1. How is the immunologic and clinical diagnosis of HANE established?
2. How does $C\overline{1s}$ INH regulate this disease?
3. In what way is the complement cascade regulated by current therapeutic programs?

Solution

A definitive diagnosis of $C\overline{1s}$ INH deficiency on immunologic grounds cannot be made in the usual hospital or clinic. Assays for $C\overline{1s}$ INH depend on the activity of the patient's serum in neutralizing the action of C1 esterase on synthetic substrates. Traditionally N-acetyl-L-tyrosine ethyl ester (ATEE) is used as the substrate for C1 esterase, which removes the ethyl ester group, liberating the carboxyl group of tyrosine that is titrated with dilute alkali. The C1 esterase inhibitor, incubated with a sample of the esterase, would depress hydrolysis of the substrate. Neither this test nor immunodiffusion tests for the inhibitor are performed in the routine laboratory. This means that the diagnosis is established on indirect laboratory evidence and clinical grounds. The former depends on low complement activity in diluted sera of patients with HANE compared with those of normal persons. Diagnostic features include familial distribution of the disease, anatomic distribution, frequency of the episodes, and response to therapy.

Transfusion of normal plasma to reconstitute the patient's level of $C\overline{1s}$ INH is one of the most direct means of therapy. It may be the content of plasmin inhibitors in transfused plasma, more than its content of $C\overline{1s}$ INH, that is therapeutic. Angioneurotic edema frequently is treated just as any acute urticarial condition—with epinephrine and antihistamines. ϵ-Aminocaproic acid is a more specific drug because it is a specific esterase inhibitor.

References

Donaldson, V.H., and Evans, R.A.: A biochemical abnormality in hereditary angioneurotic edema, Am. J. Med. **35:** 37, 1963.

Fong, J.S.C., Good, R.A., and Gewurz, H.: A simple diagnostic test for hereditary angioneurotic edema, J. Lab. Clin. Med. **76:**836, 1970.

SECTION TWO

IMMUNITY

NATURAL RESISTANCE
AND ACQUIRED IMMUNITY

The defense of an animal against infectious organisms or their toxic products can be considered from several viewpoints: (1) whether it is local or systemic, (2) whether it is caused by cellular or humoral factors, (3) whether it is external or internal in location, and (4) whether it is a naturally existent or acquired characteristic. No matter where one begins, most of these subjects eventually are encompassed when immunity is studied. Since natural resistance or immunity appears to be somewhat broader in scope than acquired immunity, this chapter discusses natural resistance first.

NATURAL RESISTANCE

Natural resistance or natural immunity, known also as innate immunity, native immunity, or inherited immunity, should not be confused with naturally *acquired* immunity. Innate immunity refers to that type of resistance which each individual has by virtue of being the individual he or she is in terms of species, race, sex, or other factors associated with genetically controlled resistance. Natural immunity, unlike acquired immunity, commonly is thought of as a nonspecific barrier that is effective against many different kinds of infectious agents. Because of this, some prefer the term *natural resistance* to *natural immunity*, the word *immunity* often connoting specificity.

Examples of natural resistance

Species. Fowl malaria, dog tapeworm, avian tuberculosis, canine distemper, mouse pox (but not chickenpox), fowl typhoid, and many similar terms indicate the host range or species specificity certain pathogens possess. This also indicates that other species of animals are resistant to the infectious agent mentioned. This fact is easily supported by simple observation; humans get mumps, but dogs and cats do not; mammals may contract anthrax, but birds do not; amphibia are resistant to tetanus and diphtheria. Exactly *why* one species contracts a certain disease when other species are resistant is not always explainable. In certain cases the body temperature of the animal will not permit growth of the pathogen; for example, if the body temperature of chickens is lowered from 39° to 37° C, they become susceptible to anthrax. Avian tuberculosis germs prefer the higher body temperature of fowl and seldom infect mammals. Some species of mycobacteria grow optimally at 25° C and cause only superficial lesions on the skin of mammals, where the temperature is near 25° C.

Race or strain. It always has been difficult to evaluate differences that the human races seem to have in susceptibility or resistance to certain diseases. Unequal economic and social opportunities almost always have resulted in gross variations in exposure to most infectious agents. Only in limited segments of our population in which all persons share the same environment (for example, military installations, prisons, and mental hospitals) do we find that exposure for all individuals has been nearly the same. Under these conditions, racial differences can be detected. It appears that blacks are more susceptible than whites to tuberculosis. Conversely, blacks appear more resistant than whites to diphtheria, influenza, and gonorrhea.

Natural resistance of several mouse strains to the immune pathogen *Corynebacterium kutscheri* has been genetically analyzed. The $\log_{10}$ of the number of organisms consisting of the LD_{50} (lethal dose for 50% of the mice) varied from 3.8 to 5.8 (Fig. 10-1). When the C57BL/6 resistant mice were bred with the susceptible Swiss Lynch strains, the LD_{50} of the F_1 hybrids and back crosses agreed

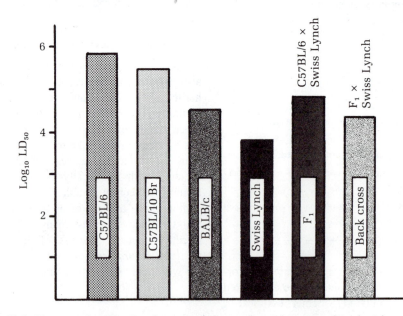

Fig. 10-1. The natural resistance of mouse strains to *Corynebacterium kutscheri* is genetically controlled. Mating of C57BL/6 and Swiss Lynch mice produced offspring with the expected susceptibility.

with the predicted values. For example, the calculation for the C57BL/6 × Swiss Lynch mating is

$$F_1 = \frac{5.8 \times 3.8}{2} = 4.8$$

which was the observed value.

Sex. As mentioned for racial differences, apparent differences in susceptibility of the two human sexes have been clouded by the improbability of equal exposure; in laboratory animals, however, such differences have been demonstrated repeatedly. BALB/c female mice are more resistant to *Listeria monocytogenes* infection than males, but male and female C57BL/6 mice are equally susceptible.

Nutrition. Another quality that influences resistance and susceptibility is an individual's nutritional status. Protein-calorie malnutrition lowers the level of C3 and factor B of the complement system, decreases the IFN response, penalizes the neutrophil's activities, and seems to stress the T cell more than the B cell system. Low-protein diets alone are not invariably detrimental; the NZB mouse on a 6% protein diet may develop lower IgG1 and IgM levels but maintains its IgA level. The lymphocytes of these mice actually responded better to Con A and PHA than the cells of control mice on ad libitum diets. The lethal autoimmune disease that typically develops in NZB mice was slowed or prevented by low-intake diets.

Vitamin deficiencies often exhibit significant effects on host defense. Vitamin A deficiency affects epithelial cell integrity and allows more skin infections to develop. Folic acid deficiencies lower T cell numbers, whereas vitamin B_2 and B_1 deficiencies lower B cell activities. Vitamin C deficiencies have been related to increased or more severe bacterial infections in a number of studies. Zinc deficiency recently has been related to thymus and thus T cell insufficiency.

Overnutrition also may be harmful. Many bacteria must scavenge iron from the body fluids in which they grow. When transferrin and lactoferrin, the body's natural iron transport compounds, are saturated by an excess of this metal, free iron is available for bacterial growth. When iron is in short supply, bacterial growth is restricted. Limited overnutrition may increase susceptibility to viral diseases. The logic used to explain this is that more virus is produced (and hence more disease) when a virus invades a healthy cell than when it infects a cell whose metabolic rate has been slowed by malnutrition.

Hormone-related resistance. Hormone imbalance (such as insulin diabetes) has a direct effect on susceptibility to a number of infectious diseases. Staphylococcal, streptococcal, and certain fungal diseases definitely occur more frequently in diabetics. The hormonal changes that occur in females at the time of puberty are responsible for a thickening of the vaginal epithelium and for the production of more intracellular glycogen and lactic acid in the adult vagina. Therefore the adult woman is more resistant than the young girl to local vaginal infections. Pregnancy is associated with marked hormonal alterations and an increase in urinary tract infections and poliomyelitis. The latter seems not to be related to any direct effect pregnancy might have on the female genitourinary system. Hormone balance may be related to different sexual susceptibilities to pathogens.

Miscellaneous. The age of an individual has a marked effect on innate immunity also. The very young and the very aged always have more infectious diseases than the middle-aged groups, possibly because of less phagocytic activity. Likewise, fatigue, climate, including simply climatic variation, and numerous other factors can significantly alter host resistance.

Mechanisms of natural resistance

The host defense system is built on chemical, cellular, and structural properties. As described in the following paragraphs, specific macromolecules are antiviral, antibacterial, or antifungal, depending on their nature. Cellular defense rests most obviously with phagocytic cells but also with the direct action of T cells, K cells, and NK cells on invading pathogens. The basis for physical defense is not so much in individual cells as it is in the fetaures of their physical arrangement into keratinized epithelial structures, in their peristaltic action, etc. To these we can add passive features which provide an unattractive environment for pathogens; features such as lack of oxygen, too much oxygen, or the wrong temperature could be listed here (Fig. 10-2).

External defense factors. The first barrier that most microbes encounter against their successful invasion is the intact skin or mucous membranes. Intact skin represents a formidable mechanical barrier than can be penetrated by only a few organisms, such as the *Treponema* organisms of syphilis, *Francisella (Pasteurella) tularensis,* and certain fungi that enter at the hair roots. While being held outside the body, the microorganisms are exposed to drying, which alone may be enough to cause their death. In addition, lactic acid, caproic acid, and caprylic acid of the sebaceous glands have a proven antibacterial effect. Especially on the scalp and possibly other hairy parts of the human body, saturated C7, C9, and C11 fatty acids are present in the skin secretions (Table 10-1). These are distinctly fungistatic and are important in the elimination of fungi that cause superficial skin and hair infections. Fungal infections more often begin on areas of the body devoid of sebaceous glands, for example, between the toes.

The upper respiratory tract may be considered as no more than a major invagination into the body and as such does not represent a truly internal environment. Although it is true that the very uppermost portion of the respiratory tract is lined with visible hairs to exclude particles of great size, it is obvious that these will not remove particles the size of ordinary microbes. As a consequence, droplets in the range of 0.5 to 2 μm in diameter are inhaled somewhat more deeply than larger particles. Fortunately the entire respiratory

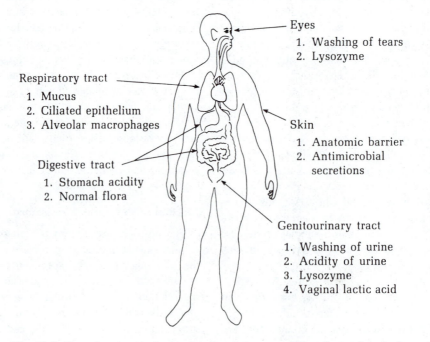

Fig. 10-2. Natural resistance factors that function on external surfaces of the body.

tract is bathed with a mucus secretion that acts as a glue and holds particles coming into contact with it directly on the membrane's surface. The mucus is swept upward at a rate of 10 to 20 mm/minute by the action of the ciliated epithelial cells lining the respiratory tree and usually is swallowed. In a healthy person this mucous coat clears 90% of the deposited material every hour. A recent description of four patients who had abnormal cilia has emphasized the importance of these structures to normal health. All four patients suffered from recurrent episodes of bronchitis and sinusitis as well as frequent pneumonias and ear infections. No ciliary action could be noted in biopsy specimens, nor could mucociliary clearance of inhaled, aerosolized particles 6 μm in diameter be detected within a 2-hour test period. All evidence pointed toward a failure to form complete cilia, a fault that rendered the cilia immobile.

Unfortunately the mucous membranes do not trap all droplet nuclei; those less than 0.5 μm in diameter may be inhaled deeply into the pulmonary alveoli and there initiate an infection, provided that the pathogens can escape the alveolar macrophages. These macrophages roam over the respiratory mucosae and phagocytose inhaled particles. Alveolar macrophages of the rat can kill 99% of a dose of microorganisms that is reduced only 50% by blood phagocytes. These phagocytes killed 88% of pathogens such as *Streptococcus pneumoniae* and *fecalis* within a 3-hour test period.

The microbes in the mucus that are swallowed or which enter the digestive system through food or water find very little in the upper alimentary canal that is detrimental to their growth. A number of nonpathogenic and potentially pathogenic bacteria reside in the mouth and throat. Lower in the digestive system the microorganisms encounter the tremendous acidity of the stomach, bordering on pH 1 because of the hydrochloric acid secreted from the parietal cells. Only markedly aciduric organisms or those embedded deeply in food particles can escape the protein-precipitating capacity of this acidity. As the microbes pass into the small intestine, an alteration in pH to the slightly alkaline side occurs because of the pH of the entering pancreatic and biliary fluids. In this section of the digestive system the microbial population is still rather low. A remarkable increase in this population takes place in the large intestine. The tremendous numbers of nonpathogens are undoubtedly of great importance in regulating the population of any pathogens or potential pathogens which have survived this far. If this population is suppressed, as by broad-spectrum antibiotic therapy, intestinal yeast infections may ensue. This classic example of iatrogenic illness emphasizes the role of the natural flora in maintaining body health.

Little is known about any protective functions other than the slight acidity, lysozyme content, and flushing action of urine, all of which help cleanse the urinary system. Those urine samples most lethal to the gonococcus were also the most acidic. The exterior portions of the female reproductive system also are held at a low pH because of the lactic acid in the secretions.

It may seem unusual to consider the lungs and intestinal and reproductive tracts as portions of the

Table 10-1. The relationship of carbon length on the antimicrobial activity of fatty acids for *Neisseria meningitidis*

Carbon length	Concentration for 50% growth inhibitor (mM)
C1	90
C2	40
C3	9
C4	20
C11	0.1
C13	0.02
C16	0.001
C14:1*	About 0.007
C16:1	About 0.007
C18:1	About 0.007
C20:1	About 0.007

*:1, One unsaturated bond.

external rather than the internal defense system. Justification for this is that any microbe residing in these locations has not yet penetrated the most exterior of the body's anatomic barriers, the skin or mucous membranes. Although infectious parasites dwelling in the respiratory, digestive, or reproductive tract may be warmed and nurtured by their host, they actually are residing in major invaginations into the body and are not within the body per se. Thus the fluids and cellular and enzymatic activities which contribute to the resistance of these tissues to invasions by infectious microbes are considered a part of the external body defense.

The human eye is not protected by a third eyelid, or nictitating membrane, like that of certain lower animals, but it is blessed with a defensive mechanism many lower animals lack: the ability to cry. Crying has a simple mechanical benefit: it washes both small and large particles from the eye. A selective and very active antibacterial substance, lysozyme, in tears is of much greater value. Lysozyme is a bactericidal enzyme first found in tears by Sir Alexander Fleming in 1922. Fleming is much better known for his discovery of penicillin some 7 years later, but the scientific world is keenly aware of his important early studies of natural immunity with lysozyme and with phagocytosis. Today lysozyme is one of our best-understood proteins. Lysozyme has an isoelectric point at about pH 11. It has been suggested that it is this alkaline isoelectric point which permits the firm combination of lysozyme with bacteria, which have acid isoelectric points. After this combination occurs, lysozyme begins a hydrolytic digestion of the bacterial cell wall. The cell walls of both gram-positive and, to a lesser extent, gram-negative bacteria are susceptible to this enzymatic erosion. In strict biochemical terms, lysozyme is a muramidase and cleaves the β-1,4-glycoside bond that unites N-acetylglucosamine and muramic acid, the backbone of the bacterial cell wall. Lipids in the cell walls of gram-negative bacteria tend to mask the substrate from lysozyme, but a combination of lysozyme and complement is lytic for these cells, too.

Internal defense factors. Phagocytosis is probably the most vital of the internal defense factors of the immune animal (Table 10-2). This is equally true of the nonimmunized animal.

The major phagocytic cells are the neutrophils (Fig. 10-3) and the monocytes of blood and the monocytes and macrophages in tissues. The neutrophils also may enter tissues as part of the inflammatory response. These cells are drawn to areas of inflammation by various leukotactic substances and lymphokines. Opsonins such as C3b and immunoglobulin molecules, both humoral and cytophilic, augment phagocytosis. Rats depleted of C3 by cobra venom factor suffered a greater mortality from *Hemophilus influenzae* than did normal rats.

Basic polyamines, polypeptides, and proteins display antibacterial activity. Histones, protamines, spermine, and spermidine are examples; these function by combining electrostatically with negatively charged bacterial cells and altering in some unknown way the vital cellular functions of the bacteria. The mechanism of action and nature of β-lysins (probably identical to plakins, from platelets) are unclear, but it is known that their action is primarily against gram-positive bacteria. Unsaturated lactoferrin in milk is one of its key

Table 10-2. Natural internal defense systems

Phagocytosis	Neutrophils
	Monocytes
	Macrophages
Leukotaxis	C5a
	C(5,6,7)
Opsonins	C3b
	Miscellaneous proteins
Complement activation	Alternate pathway (polysaccharides)
	C1, enzymatic activation
	C3, enzymatic activation
Macromolecules	Glycoproteins
	Transferrin
	Lysozyme
	Various polyamines

protective agents. Several glycoproteins of serum, of which fetuin, tranferrin, and α-1-glycoprotein are examples, inhibit attachment of viruses to susceptible cells and thus aid in termination of viral infections. A number of different viral inhibitors are present in serum and tissue fluids. Most of these have not been adequately characterized, but some are known to be glycoproteins.

ACQUIRED IMMUNITY

Acquired immunity refers to that immunity which a person develops during a lifetime. It is antigen (pathogen) specific and may be based on humoral or circulating substances such as IFN or antibodies or may be cellular in origin and more closely associated with the activities of macrophages and T lymphocytes.

Antibody-mediated immunity

Immunity based on antibodies is probably the most efficient and the single most formidable type of immunity. This form of immunity is conve-

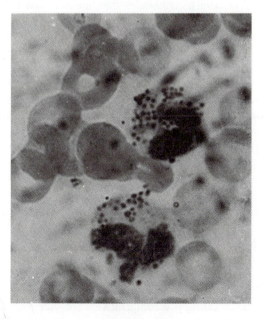

Fig. 10-3. The two phagocytic cells have engulfed numerous *Staphylococcus aureus* cells.

niently subdivided into that which is actively acquired and that which is passively acquired.

  I. Innate or natural resistance
 II. Acquired immunity
    A. Actively acquired
      1. Natural
      2. Artificial
    B. Passively acquired
      1. Natural
      2. Artificial

In active immunity the individual synthesizes his or her own antibodies, whereas in passive immunity the individual receives these antibodies from some other individual, either a human or a lower animal. Both active and passive immunity are subdivisible into two categories, depending on whether the immunity is acquired by natural or artificial means. Naturally acquired immunity should not be confused with natural immunity.

Actively acquired immunity. A degree of naturally acquired active immunity results from any infection from which a person recovers, whether the illness is serious or subclinical. During the illness the individual receives an antigenic stimulus which initiates antibody production against that specific pathogen. On a subsequent visitation by this same or an antigenically related pathogen, these antibodies will assist in the body's defenses. Because many microbes produce diseases with a high mortality, this is not a very satisfactory way of developing immunity.

A major goal of immunologists interested in preventing infectious diseases has been the development of vaccines or toxoids that can be used in immunization. The immunity resulting from the injection of these immunogens is said to be of the artificially acquired type, since it is a man-made procedure. Killed and attenuated strains of bacteria and viruses now are used widely for immunization against many diseases, for example, typhoid fever, smallpox, poliomyelitis, yellow fever, and measles. Attenuated vaccines contain viable but weakened organisms and will produce a mild infection of little danger to the host. It has the advantage, however, of producing a much more permanent form of immunity than killed vaccines.

Toxoids, that is, the detoxified but still antigenically active poisons excreted by certain bacteria, are also excellent antigens. Antibodies against toxoids are fully reactive with the native toxin and provide an excellent immunity against diseases caused by toxigenic bacteria (tetanus and diphtheria).

Passively acquired immunity. Passive immunity also may be acquired by natural means or by artificial means. Naturally acquired passive immunity at least in the human being, usually refers to the transplacental passage of antibodies from the mother to her unborn child during the latter part of pregnancy. This is caused almost entirely by IgG, since IgM, IgD, and IgA do not pass the placental barrier. Colostrum contains secretory IgA and secretory IgM but very little IgG. Since the digestive system of the newborn infant is poorly developed, breast-fed babies can absorb these immunoglobulins directly from the gastrointestinal system. Even is not absorbed, these antibodies may passively coat the infant's digestive tract and ward off intestinal infections. Naturally this system cannot operate in bottle-fed babies.

Artificial passive immunity refers to the original production of antibodies in some other individual (either human or lower mammal) and the acquisition of these antibodies through a needle and syringe. Injections of hyperimmune serum, of antiserum, of γ-globulin, or of immune serum are this type of immunization. Several pharmaceutical companies are involved in the production of antibodies in horses and cows by active immunization so that these antibodies may be used later to modify or prevent human diseases by passive immunization. A more limited program of hyperimmunization of humans is used for this same purpose.

A special form of antibody-related immunity is exemplified by adoptive immunity with B lymphocytes. If such cells or (more commonly) bone marrow is successfully grafted into a B cell–deficient person, the recipient will form antibodies that he or she previously could not. (See Chapter 11.) This usually is not done in human medicine, since the simpler injections of pooled human γ-globulin serve the same purpose. Such bone marrow grafts are useful in experimental immunology

in lower animals solely deficient in B cells or in human victims of combined B and T cell immunodeficiency. Adoptive immunity is a special form of passive immunity.

Comparison of active and passive immunity. Active and passive immunity must be compared on a broader basis than whether a person makes his or her own antibodies. There are other important and sometimes subtle differences between the two, most of which are summarized in Table 10-3.

The comparative effectiveness of active and passive immunity is heavily weighted in favor of the former. This is related to several factors, one of which is the duration of the immunity. Active immunity is known to persist for relatively long periods, usually years, without reactivation through booster immunization. This is true because, once the plasma cells of the animal are activated to produce antibodies, they, or perhaps their progeny, continue to do so for the lifetime of the cell. In passive immunization this does not happen. The injected antibodies are removed from the circulation without internal replacement, and the immunity then can be directly correlated with the amount of antibodies injected and their half-life. The half-life of human antibodies in a human is about 25 days, but the half-life of equine or bovine antibodies in a human is nearer 7 days. It must be remembered that foreign serum proteins, including γ-globulins, are antigenic to the human being. Consequently the human recipient will make antibodies against the administered foreign antibodies, which results in their rather speedy elimination.

Passive immunity can be quickly restored or maintained by repeated injections of the antiserum. This is satisfactory when a human antiserum is employed but not when a foreign species antiserum is used. In this instance the possibility of anaphylaxis or serum sickness is great, anaphylaxis itself being a life-threatening proposition. (See Chapter 18.) On the other hand, the reactivation of active immunity by booster injections of the vaccine or toxoid is a comparatively risk-free method and one that is commonly used.

It must be pointed out that active immunity of

Table 10-3. Comparison of active and passive antibody-mediated immunity

	Active immunity	Passive immunity
Source	Self	Some other human or lower animal
Effectiveness	High	Moderate to low
Method	1. Disease itself, clinical or subclinical	Administration of antibody by
	2. Immunization	1. Maternal transplacental transfer
	a. Vaccines: killed or attenuated	2. Injection
	b. Toxoids	
Time to develop	5 to 14 days	Immediate on injection
Duration	Relatively long, perhaps years	Relatively short, a few days to several weeks
Ease of reactivation	Easy (by booster)	Dangerous, possible anaphylaxis
Use	Prophylactic	Prophylactic and therapeutic

high efficiency requires 5 to 14 days to develop after the primary immunization. This is the time it takes for protective quantities of antibodies to appear in the serum. After booster injections of antigen only 1 to 3 days are required. On passive immunization, protection is provided immediately on completion of the injection.

Active immunization usually is restricted to prophylactic (preventive) applications, by which the person receives the immunization far in advance of the exposure to the infectious agent. Under special conditions (rabies or smallpox), when the incubation time of the disease is longer than the time required for antibody formation, it is possible for the individual to be immunized after exposure. Passive immunization also can be used prophylactically, that is, prior to or immediately after exposure, in individuals who have not been actively immunized. Passive immunization (but not active immunization) also can be used therapeutically. Unfortunately this is a relatively inefficient process because the organisms or their toxins may have created considerable undetected cell damage prior to the administration of the antiserum. None of this damage is reparable by antiserum alone.

Cell-mediated immunity (CMI)

The classic example of CMI as a mechanism of acquired immunity is the Koch phenomenon. Koch observed that the responses of normal guinea pigs

and tuberculous guinea pigs to an injection of tubercle bacilli were grossly different. In the former there is a gradual swelling of the lymph nodes near the site of a subcutaneous injection. These nodes may become caseous within about 2 weeks, and the animal usually will die after 6 to 8 weeks. If during the course of this infection a second injection of tubercle bacilli is given, the injection site will appear red and indurated within a few days. This area will necrose, and the dead tissue and injected bacilli will be sloughed. The elimination of the bacilli is clear evidence of a developing resistance. This acquired resistance is not caused by circulating antibodies and cannot be transferred to other animals with immune serum. It is instead a cell-mediated type of immunity. It is also referred to as an expression of delayed hypersensitivity because the tuberculous guinea pig will exhibit a hypersensitive skin reaction that develops over about 2 days if injected with growth products of the tubercle bacillus such as old tuberculin (OT) or PPD. (See Chapter 20.)

The term *cell-mediated immunity* usually is taken to refer to T cell–mediated immunity, but others extend it to include nonantibody-mediated functions of phagocytes. Because of their clearly different chemical and physical activities, perhaps it is satisfactory to consider T cells and phagocytes as two separate compartments of the CMI response. At the same time it must be recognized that the most aggressive phagocyte, the activated macrophage, becomes so after exposure to a T cell lymphokine.

The kinetic interdigitation of CMI and humoral immunity is noteworthy. Lymphokine production (represented by IFN in Fig. 10-4) begins within hours after the antigen stimulus but wanes within a few days. Within a few hours after the lymphokines are secreted, their effects on host cells—chemotaxis, activation of macrophages, etc.—become observable. These activities gradually fade as lymphokine synthesis ceases. By this time immunoglobulins appear in the blood and shortly thereafter reach protective levels.

Cell-mediated hypersensitivity and cell-mediated immunity are not identical. The cellular hypersensitivity seen in the Koch phenomenon is highly specific and relatable only to tubercle bacilli. The sensitized guinea pigs have a delayed skin reaction only to tuberculin and not to the products of antigenically unrelated bacteria. Cellular immunity, on the other hand, is partially nonspecific. In the development of cellular immunity activated macrophages appear. Mouse liver macrophages cleared 80% of a 1.2×10^9 dose of *Salmonella typhimurium* within 30 minutes and 70% in a single pass of blood through isolated, perfused liver. Through this the body is better able to handle other, even antigenically unrelated, organisms. An increased phagocytic capacity is thus one, if not the only, expression of cellular immunity that can be distinguished from antigen-specific cellular hypersensitivity.

The antigen-specific aspect of CMI resides with the T lymphocyte. The antigen-exposed T lymphocyte readjusts its pattern of nucleic acid and protein synthesis. This is reflected by the appearance of a macromolecule dominated by a RNA chemistry known as transfer factor and the synthesis of lymphokines, all of which are proteins. Whereas the lymphokines all are excreted by the T cells, transfer factor tends to remain intracellular except under contrived conditions (such as massive exposures to the antigen or lysis of the T cells). It is important to note that it is only the induction of lymphokine synthesis and secretion which is antigen specific. For the most part lymphokines operate on other host cells, and the changes in these host cells are reflected by their reaction to many different types of invading pathogens (antigens). Both the induction and activity of transfer factor are antigen specific.

Transfer factor is a ribonucleopeptide from T cells, which has a molecular weight of about 4,000. Its function is similar to that of mRNA in

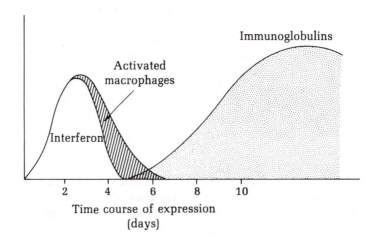

Fig. 10-4. Prior to the time immunoglobulins appear in the blood, protective interferons and activated macrophages have been engaged in host defense.

the sense that transfer factor taken from T cells of an animal with a good T cell–dependent immunity to a pathogen will transfer that immunity to a normal animal. Transfer factor seems to imprint the recipient cell with the capacity to synthesis lymphokines following contact with that particular pathogen but not other pathogens. Transfer factor is not antigenic, so it is possible to give repeated injections of transfer factor to maintain this immunity. This has been practiced with some success in human diseases such as chronic mucocutaneous candidiasis and vaccinia gangrenosa and has been tested in human cancer. Injections of transfer factor are a special form of passive immunity.

It is always a little difficult to entirely separate the protective role of antibodies and cellular immunity under natural circumstances. The acid test for identifying antibodies as the cause of an immune condition is to prove that antiserum can transfer the immunity to a normal recipient. This requires that the passively immunized animal be challenged to see if it is immune, something that simply cannot be done in human immunology. Since both cellular immunity and humoral immunity usually develop in the primarily or actively immunized animal, no concrete conclusion can be made about their relative role in that animal. The failure of serum transfer experiments suggests that cellular immunity may be an important aspect of acquired immunity against some bacterial diseases and against several fungal and viral illnesses.

IMMUNITY TO INFECTIOUS DISEASES
Viral diseases

Before considering specific instances of viral disease and their immunologic prevention, a number of special features of viral disease first should be considered. Certain viruses possess attributes that have caused difficulties in developing satisfactory vaccines or immunoprophylactic measures; shifts in antigenicity and latency are two examples. In addition, the general public is unaware that certain viral diseases can be produced by a wide array of antigenically diverse strains. This creates a different set of problems than that presented

by diphtheria or tetanus, each of which has a single, constant cause.

A factor known as antigenic shift of viruses is exemplified most frequently by the influenza virus. There are three serotypes of human influenza virus, and only two of them, types A and B, are involved with any great incidence in respiratory tract disease. Actually very effective vaccines can be made against each of these, but new antigenic subtypes, especially of influenza A virus, continually arise. It has been calculated that there are a limited number of possible antigenic variations of influenza A virus and that a single major antigenic form will reoriginate and recirculate every half century. Although this may be of great epidemiologic interest, it indicates that a large unexposed, nonimmune population will be available for practically every intervening cycle so that we can expect a series of flu epidemics periodically, perhaps every 5 to 10 years. The only creditable solution to this constant antigenic shift is to monitor each outbreak of influenza for new antigenic variations and, if significant, to prepare a special vaccine for that strain. The logistics of flu vaccine production allows mass production of vaccine in sufficient time to stave off epidemics, but there is as yet no way to forecast what antigenic form of virus will cause the next epidemic so that proper vaccine can be prepared for the occasion.

The mechanism of virus infection is a second important factor to be considered. Many viruses produce only local infections that tend to shield them from the full play of the host's defense system. Many of the respiratory viruses are of this type, causing infection only of the superficial tissues of the lung. Reinfection with identical virus serotypes indicates that the earlier infections promoted only a very shallow antigenic stimulus.

A second type of evasion by viruses is by their intracellular latency. Herpes simplex virus (cold sores, fever blisters) invades host cells and remains dormant and protected there from host immunity. High levels of circulating antibody may be present, but these antibodies cannot enter the virus-containing cells. Many virus particles may be neutralized by these antibodies when the virus erupts and spreads to new cells, but every person with recurrent herpes is witness to the success of intracellular hibernation by the virus. After some appropriate shock—sunburn, fever, abrasion— the virus erupts into activity, invading and destroying cells.

Another distinction that must be made concerning viral diseases is the difference between producing active immunity to a specific virus and producing immunity to a type of viral disease. In general, there are few novel problems encountered in making effective vaccines against a specific virus; most of the problems have been encountered before, although not always solved to perfection. The problems of virus production, purification, preservation, and attenuation, theoretically at least, can be solved for any virus. These procedures are of no avail in disease prevention when the disease is produced by a multiplicity of distantly related viruses and are often unsuitable even when closely related viruses are involved. More than 90 serotypes of rhinovirus and three coronaviruses are involved in the common cold, and more than 10 Coxsackie viruses cause pharyngitis in children and young adults. To halt the common cold by immunoprophylaxis would require a polyvalent vaccine containing 100 different viruses, a problem of considerable magnitude.

Immunity to reinfection after a viral disease or successful immunization often can be correlated with the development of specific circulating immunoglobulins. The protection afforded by these antibodies against viruses that must pass through the blood to their target tissue is the whole key to immunity. On the other hand, there are many illustrations that circulating antibodies are only indirectly related to viral immunity and simply arise as one index of an immune response to the virus. In herpes simplex and herpes zoster recurrent disease takes place in the presence of high levels of neutralizing antibody. CMI may be more critical to the resistant state than antibodies of the blood (Table 10-4). Agammaglobulinemic children develop and recover from most childhood viral diseases with the same sequence of events depicted by normal children. These two illustrations support the contention that CMI is extremely important to virus immunity.

Smallpox. Jenner's historic experiment revealed that smallpox virus was closely related to cowpox virus. Indeed the names of these viruses, *variola* for human smallpox and *variola vaccinea* or *vaccinia* for cowpox virus, show their close relationships. After Jenner's time person-to-person transmission of infectious vaccinia virus was the method for vaccinating against smallpox for nearly a century. By that time the possibility of transferring syphilis, leprosy, malaria, or other diseases was sufficiently recognized that domestic animals were selected as the source of the virus. The method of preparing smallpox vaccine has not changed appreciably in the past 75 years. Healthy calves are vaccinated several times over a large area of fresh-

Table 10-4. Immunity to various pathogens provided by B and T lymphocytes

Source of infection	B lymphocyte	T lymphocyte
Bacterial	Streptococcal, staphylococcal, neisserial, hemophilus infections	Tuberculosis, leprosy, treponematosis
Viral	Enteroviruses, poliomyelitis	Herpes viruses, measles, vaccinia, cytomegalovirus
Fungal	Few, if any	Candidiasis, cryptococcosis, histoplasmosis, etc.
Parasitic	Trypanosomiasis, malaria(?)	Leishmaniasis, pneumocystic disease, Chagas' disease

ly shaved, scrubbed flank. After 4 to 6 days the area is washed, and the animal is sacrificed. The infectious lymph is scraped from the skin and usually treated with a disinfectant. In most modern production schemes the virus is partially purified and preserved by the addition of glycerol. Such preparations must be stored in the cold, so for tropical use lyophilized virus vaccines are prepared. The vaccine is administered by multiple skin punctures; the virus grows locally and develops a systemic immunity.

Because of the success of jennerian vaccination, the world has been declared free of natural smallpox. Repository samples of the virus now are held in several research institutes throughout the world, and laboratory accidents have caused smallpox infections and death. Yet for more than 2 years no natural cases of the disease have been discovered, culminating from a heroic effort of many physicians and scientists coordinated through the efforts of the World Health Organization (WHO). For this reason smallpox vaccination is not required in many countries but is for travel from the former endemic regions of smallpox in Africa, India, and Pakistan.

Rubella. The rubella virus causes a mild infection in children and adolescents known as the German measles. The agent is not as transmissible as regular (hard) measles virus; this results in a large population who escape the disease as children and remain susceptible as adults. Immunization against this seemingly benign disease assumed importance when it was recognized that rubella infections of women in the first trimester of pregnancy produced congenital defects in the fetus. The fetus of a nonimmune mother is highly susceptible to the virus, and any and all tissues may be infected. Infants who acquire the virus in utero are totally lacking in any defensive system to eliminate it. The virus continues to reproduce and invade new tissues. If the infant is not stillborn, one or more of the following conditions may be noted: cataract, deafness, heart abnormalities, microcephaly, hepatomegaly, splenomegaly, and anemia, caused by virus alteration of tissue during

development. These children excrete rubella virus at birth and may continue to shed viruses for as long as 2 years.

Since between 15% and 35% of pregnant women are not immune to rubella, considerable need exists for vaccination. After it was recognized that serious fetal deformities arose from rubella and before a vaccine became available, rubella parties were held for young girls prior to puberty. It was hoped that close contact of the girls with the person who had rubella would overcome the low infectivity of the virus and cause the disease necessary to protect them and their future children. Now an attenuated vaccine is available for the same purpose. It is recommended for females but is not recommended after puberty because of the risk of unknown pregnancy and the possibility of fetal infection with the vaccine strain.

Poliomyelitis. Successful active immunization against poliomyelitis was based first on formaldehyde-inactivated virus developed by Salk. A polyvalent vaccine containing a representative from each of the three antigenic types was administered in three intramuscular injections over a 3-month period to develop high levels of humoral antibody. These antibodies afford complete protection against paralytic or systemic poliomyelitis, but protection against polio virus infection is not achieved by this vaccination scheme. The polio virus is basically an enteric virus; it gains entrance to the body by the oral route and infects and multiplies in the mucosa of the intestinal tract. From its intestinal phase it enters into the viremic or blood phase, from which it progresses to the central nervous system. By developing high levels of neutralizing antibody in the bloodstream the vaccine halts the virus at the blood level, which ably prevents the dreadful paralytic threat of poliomyelitis.

Immunization with active attenuated polio vaccine by the oral route is presumed to provide better protection, since both an intestinal and humoral immunity are developed. The intestinal immunity may serve very little additional benefit to the immunized person compared with the Salk vaccine, but this immunity probably removes that person as a potential carrier of virulent virus. This influence is known as group or herd immunity and is the result of removing carriers or persons with active disease from the local environment and eliminating them as potential initiators of an epidemic. This type of herd immunity—by virus vaccination of only a few persons—is magnified by that which occurs through dissemination of the active virus from the immunized person to close associates, with subsequent development of their immunity. Such transmission of the virus does occur and may be a benefit of live virus immunization. Since continued transfer of the virus provides a better opportunity for reversion to virulence, this is also a hazard of active virus immunization.

Statistics reveal the success of both the Salk and Sabin live vaccines. In 1955, the first year of inactive virus vaccination, 28,985 cases of polio were reported in the United States. In 1961 live virus vaccination was approved, and in 1964 there were only 121 cases of polio reported. Since polio is exclusively a human ailment, it is theoretically susceptible to total eradication; however, public apathy and failure to be immunized prevent the realization of this goal.

Hepatitis B. A hepatitis B virus vaccine was approved in the United States in 1981. This virus, described as the Australia antigen in 1965, when it was found to be common in the blood of Australian aborigines, causes a long-term carrier state in about 10% of the infected persons. In Africa, Asia, and certain populations in Australia the endemicity of the disease can reach 60% to 80% of the population. Chronic hepatitis B infections are known to increase susceptibility to hepatocellular carcinoma.

The major hurdle to vaccine production was the inability to perpetuate hepatitis B virus in tissue culture. Several forms of the virus are present in the blood of its victims, and these were separated, purified, treated with formaldehyde, and tested for efficacy. The surface antigen, which consists of spherical and tubular structures only 20 nm in diameter, will convert virtually 100% of all vaccinates given three doses of the vaccine with adjuvant.

Rabies. All rabies viruses are of a single antigenic type, which was very critical to the success of Pasteur's experiments in 1885 and always simplifies the production of vaccines. This antigenic constancy of rabies virus is clouded by the terms *street virus* and *fixed virus,* which refer not to changes in antigenicity but to changes in infectivity. Street virus is rabies virus freshly isolated from natural infections. When first transferred to laboratory animals, street virus will have a long incubation time, will be more apt to produce furious rabies infections, and will produce numerous Negri inclusion bodies. As it is transferred, its incubation time shortens to a fixed period (hence the name fixed virus). Negri bodies are less often produced, and infectivity by the subcutaneous route is diminished.

Pasteur's vaccine was from spinal cords of rabbits infected with fixed rabies virus, considered as a live or active attenuated strain. Cords dried for 1 week are normally noninfective and presumably contain no active virus. Infected cords dried for shorter periods contain active virus, the quantity being inversely proportional to the length of the drying period. The early Pasteur immunization schedules required 11 subcutaneous injections of vaccine, one injection daily, beginning with vaccine dried for 2 weeks. The drying period was gradually shortened until the last injection was of infected cord dried for only 1 day. This method was obviously inexact, since there was no standardization of virus potency, but it was effective, if not without hazard.

The primary hazard of the Pasteur vaccine is the production of postvaccinal encephalitis. This is an allergic reaction, of the cell-mediated type, to the rabbit neural tissue of the vaccine. The lengthy immunization schedule and the high content of rabbit spinal cord antigens in the vaccine induce an allergic encephalitis that is easily reproduced experimentally. The incidence may be as low as 1 in 8,500 uses of vaccine. Unfortunately the Semple vaccine, which followed the Pasteur vaccine, did not eliminate the possibility of neural complications following immunization. Rabies virus vaccines prepared from chicken or duck eggs were less involved but did not totally eliminate neurologic symptoms. Now a vaccine from virus grown in nerve tissue–free human diploid fibroblast cell culture is the preferred vaccine.

Immunity to rabies is based on a high content of humoral antibody. The pathogenesis of rabies virus is based on its entrance and spread through neural tissue until involvement of the central nervous system occurs. After rabies virus enters the spinal cord, it is protected from antibody, but if high levels of antibody are present before this stage of disease, immunity is the result. On this basis prophylactic immunization for veterinarians, kennel employees, and others at high risk is recommended. Rabies immunization after exposure is practiced successfully, apparently because the long incubation time of street virus allows time for immunoglobulin synthesis before virus invasion of the central nervous system occurs. IFN induction by vaccine also may contribute to this protection, but this has not yet been proved.

Measles. Attenuated strains of active measles virus produce protective antibodies in approximately 95% of all 1-year-old children receiving the vaccine. The Edmonston B strain vaccine now has been replaced by more attenuated strains. This has reduced the incidence and extent of the febrile episodes typically following measles vaccination and eliminated the need for the accompanying injection of measles globulin (0.02 ml/kg body weight). Measles vaccination of all children is recommended. During the first decade of use measles virus is believed to have prevented 2,400 deaths. The disease is far more serious than generally recognized; it can produce encephalitis with permanent brain damage or death.

Mumps. Attenuated mumps virus vaccine has been available in the United States since 1967. An important aspect of mumps prophylaxis is that it obviates mumps orchitis, which occurs in 20% of postpubertal males who develop natural mumps. A single dose of the vaccine will confer protection on 95% of the vaccinates and has few complications. The mumps vaccine can be adminis-

tered successfully in combination with measles and rubella vaccines in a single injection.

Hazards. Immunologists and virologists are often prone to hail the advantages of immunization without citing the hazards, which *do* exist and include the reversion of active attenuated viruses to virulent forms, the spread of attenuated viruses to undesired parts of the body, and allergic reactions to contaminating antigens in the vaccine. An additional illustration is provided by mice infected as adults with lymphocytic choriomeningitis (LCM) virus. This infection usually is acquired by newborn mice from their mothers or other adult carriers, and the disease in this instance is mild. The mice survive the infection, which passes quickly, but they become chronic carriers of the virus. LCM virus can be isolated from any tissue of the mouse. The mice are devoid of humoral antibodies and cannot be induced to make antibodies against the virus; they are in a state of complete tolerance to the virus.

Healthy adult mice, who never have been exposed to LCM virus, develop a serious disease if virus is administered intracerebrally or intraperitoneally. Central nervous system disorder, pleural effusions that are predominantly lymphocytic in nature, and dense viral burdens in the associated tissues are typical, with death ensuing in about a week. This all can be prevented if the mice are treated with immunosuppressive drugs. The virus is present and continues to reproduce, and the animals develop into chronic carriers like infant mice, but the drug totally prevents any outward signs of the disease, and the mice survive the infection. Immunosuppression apparently has halted an immune (allergic) response necessary for manifestation of the disease. This is truly a startling example of how the immune response can serve as a detriment rather than a benefit to health.

Bacterial diseases

Immunity to bacterial diseases is based on circulating antibodies to bacterial toxins or specific cellular antigens, and except for mycobacterial diseases and a few others the contribution of CMI has been debatable (Table 10-4).

Tetanus and diphtheria. Tetanus and diphtheria are two bacterial diseases clearly caused by potent exotoxins that the bacteria excrete. Tetanospasmin, the exotoxin of *Clostridium tetani* that is responsible for muscular contraction, is a neurotoxic protein with a molecular weight of 67,000. The exotoxin of *Corynebacterium diphtheriae* has a similar molecular weight, 72,000, but its action is on the protein-synthesizing machinery of host cells. Both toxins were studied in the golden era of medical bacteriology between 1880 and 1900 and were identified as the basis for the diseases tetanus and diphtheria. Resistance was definitely proved to depend on the antitoxic content of sera in immune animals, and Behring and Erhlich received Nobel prizes in part for their study of these toxins and their antitoxins. Although it was learned about this same time that formaldehyde treatment of toxins would destroy their toxicity while preserving their antigenicity, it was not until 1923 that toxoids produced in this fashion were used in human immunization. In the first World War the United States' rate of tetanus was 16 in 100,000 wounds. In World War II it was 0.44 in 100,000, or 12 cases in 2.5 million injuries. Of these 12, eight has not been properly immunized.

Currently in the United States a combined diphtheria and tetanus toxoid preparation absorbed to an adjuvant is used for routine immunization against these two diseases. The usual adjuvant is an aluminum hydroxide or aluminum phosphate gel; such preparations are unequivocally superior to fluid preparations. An antitoxin level of 0.01 to 0.1 unit per milliliter of serum is regarded as protective and usually develops after exposure to about 10 Lf units of toxoid. One Lf unit of toxoid is the amount that precipitates most rapidly with 1 unit of antitoxin. This can be determined by precipitation tests with fluid toxoid or toxin, but in regard to diphtheria this is unnecessary. Normal human skin reacts slowly to injections of diphtheria toxin with the development of a tender erythematous area, the positive Shick test. If a person has a sufficient level of antitoxin (more than 0.03 unit of antitoxin per milliliter of serum),

the test is negative. The Schick test is exceptionally valuable in assaying the efficacy of immunization and in screening large populations for those who are susceptible to diphtheria. Interpretation of the test can be hindered in those persons who have developed a cell-mediated hypersensivity to the toxin, since the delayed hypersensive skin reaction and the positive Shick test closely mimic one another in appearance. Persons who are allergic to the toxin can be detected by the injection of toxoid, which is innocuous to normal skin (the Moloney test).

Pertussis. Immunization against diphtheria and tetanus usually is accomplished with a single preparation, which also is used for whooping cough vaccination because it contains killed *Bordetella pertussis* organisms. Bacteria that possess a capsule must be selected for this vaccine, since capsule presence correlates highly with virulence. Protection after vaccination correlates well with the titer of circulating antibody.

Tuberculosis. BCG vaccination against tuberculosis is the only example of an attenuated bacterial vaccine that has stood the test of time. As is widely known, BCG is the abbreviation for Bacille Calmette Guérin, a strain of *Mycobacterium tuberculosis* variety *bovis,* attenuated by 13 years of cultivation on media containing bile salts by Calmette and Guérin. Since its initial trial in 1921 it has received widespread adoption throughout the world except in the United States. Under the auspices of WHO and UNICEF more than 300 million vaccinations have been given in the past 25 years. The vaccine is a lyophilized culture that is given intradermally only to tuberculin (OT or PPD)-negative individuals. Immunization of persons who already display a positive tuberculin skin reaction is not only needless but may activate old, healed lesions. The injected bacteria multiply feebly at the point of inoculation, frequently causing a small ulcer that does not heal completely for 4 to 6 weeks and leaves a small scar. On successful immunization the recipient is converted to a tuberculin-positive skin reactor. This is taken as external proof of a specific CMI.

Numerous statistical analyses have proved the

effectiveness of the vaccine, and new uses are being found in immunization against leprosy, dermal infections caused by *M. ulcerans,* and cancer. The first two examples may be based on cross-immunity resulting from shared antigens, but the last appears to function through a nonspecific mobilization of macrophages. Leprosy has been reduced by 87%, and *M. ulcerans* infections have been reduced by 18% to 74%, depending on the trial. BCG vaccination near melanomas has been known to totally clear the skin of tumor cells.

Pneumococcal and meningococcal vaccines. A polyvalent vaccine containing the capsular polysaccharide of 14 different antigenic strains of *Streptococcus pneumoniae* has been commercially available in the United States for the past 3 years. This vaccine is recommended for the elderly, who represent a very susceptible age group for infection by this organism. Use of the vaccine has reduced the attack rate by 76% to 92% in separate trials.

The success of the polyvalent pneumococcal polysaccharide capsular vaccine has not been echoed in the polyvalent meningococcal polysaccharide vaccine. *Neisseria meningitidis,* a serious pathogen of young children, exists in three major antigenic groups, A, B, and C. Young children respond well to the A and C polysaccharides but not to the B, an unexpected finding that has seriously hampered the efforts to prevent childhood meningitis.

IMMUNIZATIONS

Since most active immunizations are begun and completed in childhood, the American Academy of Pediatrics has established a schedule of such immunizations for normal infants and children dwelling in the United States.

Active immunization

The Academy advises protection against the following diseases through a prophylactic immunization program: diphtheria, tetanus, whooping cough (pertussis), poliomyelitis, measles, rubella, and mumps (Table 10-5). Routine smallpox vaccination is no longer recommended.

Bacterial diseases. The first vaccination given

Table 10-5. Recommended active immunizations*

Vaccine	Time administered
DPT	At 2, 4, and 6 months with boosters at 1½ years and at entrance to school; tetanus booster at 16 years
Oral polio	As with DPT
Measles†	At 1 year
Rubella	After 1 year, before puberty in females
Mumps	After 1 year

*Smallpox, BCG, and other vaccinations recommended for international travel, medical personnel, and other conditions.
†May be given with rubella and mumps.

the young child is the DPT (diphtheria, pertussis, and tetanus) vaccine administered at 2, 4, and 6 months of age with later booster injections. DPT preparations contain the toxoids of *Clostridium tetani* and *Corynebacterium diphtheriae* and killed cells of *Bordetella pertussis*. The amount of diphtheria antitoxin required for protection is between 0.01 and 0.1 unit per milliliter, and such quantities in the blood can be determined very simply by the Schick test. If a person has greater than 0.03 unit of antitoxin per milliliter of blood, this test is negative. Since tetanus toxin has no effect on human skin, no simple appraisal of immunity like the Schick test can be used, but it is well known that the present toxoid will confer protection (after the series of injections) for 12 years.

The killed *B. pertussis* organisms in the DPT preparation consist of the phase I capsular type. These bacteria play two important roles in this triple vaccine: the induction of specific antipertussis immunity and a pronounced adjuvant effect on the other two antigens. Most DPT preparations containing additional adjuvants—aluminum hydroxide or aluminum phosphate gels—are clearly superior to fluid preparations.

It is interesting that no other vaccines against bacterial diseases are recommended by the American Academy of Pediatrics. In the case of the vaccines for several enteric diseases this is understandable; the vaccine for typhoid and paratyphoid fevers is of dubious value, and modern sanitation probably has done as much to reduce the incidence of typhoid fever in the United States, as has immunization. The risk for cholera is low, and its vaccine confers only a tenuous immunity, and even that has an expected duration of only 3 to 6 months. However, these features do not apply to BCG vaccination, which, under the auspices of WHO and UNICEF, has been administered to over 300 million individuals since 1950. Considerable proof of the success of this vaccine is available in the immunologic literature, not only for protection against tuberculosis but also suggesting an important role in the control of leprosy, dermal infections by *Mycobacterium ulcerans,* and most recently certain forms of cancer.

Viral diseases. Poliomyelitis vaccination with the oral, attenuated strain is recommended on the same schedule as the DPT vaccine. The measles vaccine is composed of an attenuated strain derived from the more virulent Edmonston strain. It is given at approximately 1 year of age, about the same age recommended for the attenuated mumps vaccine. The live, attenuated rubella vaccine can be administered any time prior to puberty.

Passive immunization

Passive immunization continues to play a significant role in infectious disease control, but there have been obvious adjustments in its application in the last two decades. Prior to recent times passive immunization was limited almost exclusively to tetanus and diphtheria with occasional uses in cases of botulism or gas gangrene.

Newer developments in immunoglobulin therapy include the preparation of human hyperimmune sera and the consequent decrease in allergic reactions from their use. A second development is the use of hyperimmune sera against measles, mumps, vaccinia, and rubella viruses to modify the severity of the responses to attenuated vaccines or to modify the severity of disease in very young infants exposed to or developing these infections (Table 10-6). The recognition of hypo-

Table 10-6. Passive immunizations

Disease	Immunization
Measles	Hyperimmune globulin immediately after exposure or with weakly attenuated vaccines
Rubella	Pregnant women exposed to rubella
Infectious hepatitis	Immediately after exposure
Tetanus	Immediately after injury if not immunized or if immunization is outdated
Rh disease	Within 72 hours after delivery
Hypogammaglobulinemia	Pooled human γ-globulin

gammaglobulinemic persons has created a continued need for antiserum therapy. Perhaps most dramatic of all, since it is outside the realm of infectious disease, is the use of human anti-Rh sera to prevent the development of Rh antibodies in women delivering Rh-positive babies. This is an expected part of perinatal medical care and should greatly reduce HDN caused by maternal-fetal Rh incompatibility.

BIBLIOGRAPHY

Allen, J.C., editor: Infection and the compromised host, ed. 2, Baltimore, 1981, Williams & Wilkins Co.

Amos, D.B., Schwartz, R.S., and Janicki, B.W., editors: Immune mechanisms and disease, New York, 1979, Academic Press, Inc.

Barringa, O.O.: The immunology of parasitic infections, Baltimore, 1981, University Park Press.

Basu, R.N., Jezek, Z., and Ward, N.A.: The eradication of smallpox from India, New Delhi, 1979, World Health Organization.

Campbell, P.A.: Immunocompetent cells in resistance to bacterial infections, Bacteriol. Rev. **40:**284, 1976.

Chandra, R.K.: Immunology of nutritional disorders, London, 1980, Edward Arnold (Publishers), Ltd.

Dick, G., editor: Immunological aspects of infectious diseases, Baltimore, 1979, University Park Press.

Doria, G., and Eshkol, A., editors: The immune system: functions and therapy of dysfunction, New York, 1980, Academic Press, Inc.

Edebo, L.B., Enerbäck, L., and Stendahl, O.I.: Endocytosis and exocytosis in host defense, Monogr. Allergy **17**:1, 1981.

Falkner, F., Kretchmer, N., and Rossi, E., editors: Advances in vaccination against virus diseases, Basel, 1979, S. Karger AG, Medical and Scientific Publishers.

Ganguly, R., and Waldman, R.H.: Local immunity and local immune responses, Prog. Allergy **27**:1, 1980.

Gershwin, M.E., and Cooper, E.L., editors: Animal models of comparative and developmental aspects of immunity and disease, Elmsford, N.Y., 1978, Pergamon Press, Inc.

Gross, R.L., and Newberne, P.M.: Role of nutrition in immunologic function, Physiol. Rev. **60**:188, 1980.

Hennessen, W., and vanWezel, A.L.: editors: Reassessment of inactivated poliomyelitis virus, Basel, 1981, S. Karger AG, Medical and Scientific Publishers.

Lambert, H.P., and Wood, C.B.S., editors: Immunological aspects of infection in the fetus and newborn, London, 1981, Academic Press, Inc. (London), Ltd.

Larralde, C., and others, editors: Molecules, cells, and parasites in immunology, New York, 1980, Academic Press, Inc.

Makinodan, T., and Kay, M.M.B.: Age influence on the immune system, Adv. Immunol. **29**:287, 1980.

Mansfield, J.M., editor: Parasitic diseases, vol. 1, Immunology, New York, 1981, Marcel Dekker, Inc.

Nahmias, A.J., and O'Reilly, R.J., editors: Immunology of human infection, New York, 1981, Plenum Publishing Corp.

Roberts, N.J., Jr.: Temperature and host defense, Microbiol. Rev. **43**:241, 1979.

Schiff, G.M.: Active immunization for adults, Annu. Rev. Med. **31**:441, 1980.

Singhal, S.K., Sinclair, N.R., and Stiller, C.R., editors: Aging and immunity, New York, 1979, Elsevier/North-Holland, Inc.

Sissons, J.G.P., and Oldstone, M.B.A.: Antibody mediated destruction of virus-infected cells, Adv. Immunol. **29**:209, 1980.

Skamene, E., Kongshavn, P.A.L., and Landy, M., editors: Genetic control of natural resistance to infection and malignancy, New York, 1980, Academic Press, Inc.

SITUATION: INTERNATIONAL IMMUNIZATIONS

J.B., a 45-year-old archeologist, was invited on a "dig" in central Nigeria. His previous travel abroad had been limited to excavations in 1964, 1965, and 1966 near Roskilde, Denmark. He was excited about the possibility of opening an African chapter in his career; however, he was concerned about the need for immunizations and consulted his family physician. His International Certificate of Vaccination revealed only smallpox immunization in 1964. He had been in the U.S. Army in 1945 and 1946 but was uncertain about the immunizations he had received either in the service or in civilian life. Accordingly his physician scheduled the following immunizations: smallpox, typhoid fever, tetanus, poliomyelitis, yellow fever, and cholera.

Questions

1. What is the current status of smallpox immunization in the United States, and what is the recommendation for international travel?

2. Will a full immunization course or only a tetanus booster be required for protection against that disease?

3. What is the need for poliomyelitis vaccination in middle-aged adults with an unknown history of polio immunization?

4. What geographic areas of the world are at risk for yellow fever?

5. Why are typhoid and cholera immunizations recommended when it is known that they are of dubious, short-term value?

Solution

Smallpox. The American Academy of Pediatrics no longer recommends routine smallpox vaccinations for children. The rationale for this is the estimated cost of $150,000,000 per year for smallpox surveillance and control in the United States, where the last confirmed case was diagnosed in 1949. The U.S. Public Health Service no longer requires a validated smallpox certificate for those entering the United States from smallpox-free areas.

In terms of this specific case it is believed that Nigeria has been free of smallpox since 1972. However, international traffic between central African nations is increasing, and the possibility of a nonimmune person being exposed is sufficiently great to advise vaccination. Although J.B. was vaccinated in 1964, the policy of a revaccination every 10 years (if needed, as described previously) would necessitate his immunization at this time.

Tetanus. Fluid tetanus toxoid boosters are recommended every 12 years. Persons engaged in dangerous occupations where wound contamination with soil is probable are obviously at a greater risk than the average individual and are doubly advised to maintain their tetanus immunization program. Because of his military tetanus immunization, only the fluid booster needed to be given to J.B.

Poliomyelitis. J.B. was not certain about his polio vaccinations but hesitantly recalled receiving at least a portion of the Salk injection series. In the United States adults like J.B. are unlikely to be exposed to polio. Although the incidence is rising slightly, there were only 19 cases in 1971. Medical personnel and travelers to nations with limited control of polio should receive the oral polio vaccine. This is given as three separate immunizations—one for each antigenic type of virus—over a period of about 3 months, that is, 6 to 8 weeks between immunizations.

Yellow fever. The yellow fever attenuated vaccine was developed by Max Theiler, and he received the Nobel Prize for this in 1951. In the United States the 17D, chick embryo–grown vaccine is used. It must be administered by a WHO-approved Yellow Fever Vaccination Center, and it is a rare physician who has actually given the vaccination. It consists of a 0.5-ml dose administered subcutaneously. Immunity following vaccination persists for 10 years.

In Africa serologic studies have indicated that exposure to yellow fever occurs in the tropical and subtropical regions from the Sahara to Northern Rhodesia. This zone extends from the Atlantic to the Indian Ocean and includes central Nigeria.

The Dakar or French strain vaccine is more neurotropic than the 17D strain, and its use is complicated by a 5% incidence of meningoencephalitis. Complications following the administration of the 17D strain are unusual, but since the vaccine is egg-derived, persons who are highly allergic to eggs may develop an immediate hypersensitive reaction.

Cholera. Cholera vaccines are of very limited efficacy. No more than 50% of the vaccinates are protected and then only for a period of 3 to 6 months. Consequently vaccination within a month of departure for foreign travel is advised. The International Certificate of Vaccination (international health card) confirming cholera vaccination is invalid after 6 months. The vaccine is given twice within a period of about a month and may provoke considerable local discomfort, generalized fever, and headache because of the high endotoxin content of the vaccine.

References

Cvjetanovic, B., and Uemura, K.: The present status of field and laboratory studies of typhoid and paratyphoid vaccine, Bull. WHO **32:**29, 1965.

Gangarosa, E.J., and Faich, G.A.: Cholera, the risk to American travelers, Ann. Intern. Med. **74:**412, 1971.

Regamey, R.H., and Cohen, H., editors: International symposium on smallpox vaccination, Basel, 1973, S. Karger AG, Medical and Scientific Publishers.

Scheibel, I., and others: Duration of immunity to diphtheria and tetanus after active immunization, Acta Pathol. Microbiol. Scand. **67:**380, 1966.

TRANSPLANTATION IMMUNOLOGY

GLOSSARY

allogeneic Of different genetic and thus antigenic type within one species.

allograft A graft that contains antigens different from those in the graft recipient, as considered within a single species; replaces *homograft*.

autograft A graft of tissue in which the donor and recipient are the same individual or genetically identical.

congeneic (congenic) A strain of animal identical to another strain except at one allele.

first set rejection A normal rejection of a graft containing antigens not present in the recipient.

graft-versus-host (GVH) reaction A reaction resulting from the attack of immunocompetent tissue in a graft against an immunologically compromised host.

H-2 The major histocompatibility antigen system of mice; H-2K, H-2D, and H-2L.

haplotype That half of the histocompatibility genes which is situated on one chromosome and received from one parent.

histocompatibility antigen The antigen on the surface of a cell that, when the cell is transplanted in a different host, induces the response leading to graft rejection; synonymous with *transplantation antigen*.

HLA The major histocompatibility antigen system in humans (human leukocyte antigen).

homograft An archaic term for allograft.

host-versus-graft (HVG) rejection The usual cause of graft rejection; the loss of grafted tissue by immunologic responses of the grafted individual toward foreign antigens of the graft.

hyperacute rejection An accelerated rejection of a graft because of the presence of preformed antibodies specific for the grafted tissue.

isogeneic Of the same genetic and thus antigenic constitution; synonym of *syngeneic*.

isograft A graft from another individual within the same species; preferred usage is now *allograft* or *syngraft*, as appropriate.

isologous Referring to the same species; preferred usage is now *allogeneic* or *syngeneic*, as appropriate.

MHC Major histocompatibility complex.

microcytotoxicity test A test used to identify HLA antigens by the toxicity of anti-HLA sera for lymphocytes.

microglobulin A 12,000 mol wt β-globulin associated with H-2 and HLA antigens.

mixed leukocyte reaction (MLR) The transformation of leukocytes in cultures with foreign leukocytes and believed to indicate the histoincompatibility of their donors.

mixed lymphocyte culture (MLC) Synonym for *mixed leukocyte reaction*.

orthotopic graft A graft placed in its usual anatomic position.

transplantation antigens Antigens on tissue that, when grafted, induce the immune responses critical to tissue rejection.

xenogeneic Being totally different in genetic composition, as between different species.

xenograft A graft between different species.

The transplantation of tissues from a healthy donor to a recipient who has suffered irreparable damage to some tissue or organ or who has a deformity of an arm or leg is such a logical experiment it is not surprising that it was attempted many times in ancient medical history. In virtually every instance the grafted tissue failed to survive more than a few days. There is no doubt that many of the early failures resulted from lack of surgical expertise or from bacterial infections, but the bulk of these medical adventures were doomed to fail because the laws regulating tissue transplantation immunity were being transgressed. Even today all the immunologic and genetic principles that govern successful tissue transplantation probably are not known, but admirable progress has been made in the past two decades.

The scientific history of transplantation immunology really did not begin until the 1950s, although organ grafting was studied extensively by Carrel and others prior to 1920. Even blood transfusions, which can be considered a form of tissue transplantation, were not practiced extensively until after 1940, although much of the immunologic basis, at least for the ABO blood group system, was well delineated prior to this time. During World War II the benefits of successful tissue transplantation were outlined against a tragic background. In the 1950s the rebirth of genetics and the availability of inbred mouse lines opened tissue transplantation as a new subject for immunologic investigation, which itself was undergoing a renaissance.

Another force that has favored a more diligent study of transplantation is the subject of tumor immunity. Although at first glance tissue transplantation and tumor immunity seem to be at opposite poles, they share many characteristics. In the development of tumors the host often is exposed to new antigens in the malignant tissue that do not exist in the host's normal cells. If the host's immune system permits the continued reproduction and growth of the neoplastic tissue, then in effect the host is accepting foreign tissue. This does not differ in immunologic principle from the acceptance of tissue from a second antigenically unrelated individual. Those individuals who can marshal their defense system to reject malignant cells when they arise in the body are likewise similar in immunologic activities to those who reject graft tissue; it is therefore appropriate that tissue transplantation and tumor immunity be considered as adjuncts and in consecutive chapters.

TERMINOLOGY

The nomenclature of tissue transplantation has its origins in three different sciences: surgery, immunology, and genetics. The result of this has been the emergence of a multiple nomenclature system, which now is able to include terms based on the genetic relationship of tissues (Table 11-1).

When tissue is transplanted from one location to another within or on the same individual, the prefix *auto-* is used, as in the terms *autograft, autologous graft, autochthonous graft,* and *autogenous graft*. The tissue is said to be autogeneic, meaning that it is genetically identical to that of the recipient, who, as defined by auto- (self), is also the donor.

When tissue is transplanted between two genetically identical individuals, the tissue is described as syngeneic or congeneic. The prefix *syn-* means with or together, and congenic or congeneic means of the same kind. In many genetic studies congenic means identical except for the gene or gene set under investigation. The graft is referred to as a syngraft or congraft, although the latter term is not in widespread use, and these and other terms with the *syn-* or *con-* prefix are replacing terms such as *isograft, isogeneic,* and *isologous*. The reason for this is that, in terms such as *isoantibody* and *isoimmunization,* the prefix *iso-* has come to mean same, in terms of species origin, rather than same in terms of genetic composition.

In grafting terminology the preferred terms for same, in referring to species origin, are *allograft* and *allogeneic*. These words supplant earlier terms

Table 11-1. Tissue transplantation nomenclature

Type of transplantation	Type of tissue	Older term	Genetic and antigenic relationships
Autograft	Autogeneic	Autologous	Identical: donor and recipient are same individual
Syngraft	Syngeneic, congeneic	Isologous	Identical, but between different individuals
Allograft	Allogeneic	Homologous	Different: genetically different individuals within one species are involved
Xenograft	Xenogeneic	Heterologous	Different: individuals from different species are involved

such as *homograft, homologous,* and *homogeneic,* in which the prefix *homo-* means similar or like. It is clear that words based on the prefix *iso-* or *homo-* could be easily confused. The use of *allogeneic* and similarly derived terms should minimize this confusion, since *allo-* means other, and *-geneic* means race or strain. Thus an allograft is a graft made between two genetically different individuals within one species.

To complete the nomenclature system, we find that terms such as *heterograft* and *heterologous* (with *hetero-* meaning other) are replaced by *xenograft* and *xenogeneic,* in which *xeno-* serves to identify the graft or tissue as being from a foreign source.

To these, the surgical terms *orthotopic* and *heterotopic* must be added. When tissue is grafted orthotopically, it is relocated in its normal anatomic position in the recipient; otherwise the tissue is placed heterotopically.

All these terms are applicable when the graft is of tissue that must remain alive, even grow, in the recipient. This is not true of homostatic grafts, in which the tissue merely serves as a structural support on which or through which host tissue grows to reestablish the original structure. Among homostatic grafts, transplantations of blood vessels, bone, and cornea are examples. The following discussion is concerned primarily with homovital transplants, in which tissue viability is demanded.

GRAFT REJECTION
Acute rejection

If skin is transferred from one individual to a recipient who is destined to reject the transplant, one of three sequences may be observed. The first of these is the hyperacute or acute rejection reaction, caused by the presence of preformed antibodies with a specificity for the transplanted tissue (Fig. 11-1). This can be the case when the donor and the recipient have not been matched for the ABO blood group antigens. These antigens are present on all cells of the body, and if cells bearing the A antigen are transferred to a group O or B individual, the anti-A hemagglutinin initiates cytotoxic destruction of the transplanted tissue. Or the recipient may have developed a resistance to the new tissue from prior grafts. In either case the reaction involves the components of the complement system, polymorphonuclear phagocytes, and macrophages which function so quickly in tissue destruction that the tissue never really "takes." In the case of skin the transferred tissue remains as a "white graft"—one in which revascularization never occurs. In the case of organs in which the major vascular connections are achieved surgically, stasis of blood flow, engorgement of the organ with blood, and even coagulation of blood in the donor organ may occur so rapidly that it is obvious the graft will fail, and the organ is transplanted and removed in the same surgical procedure.

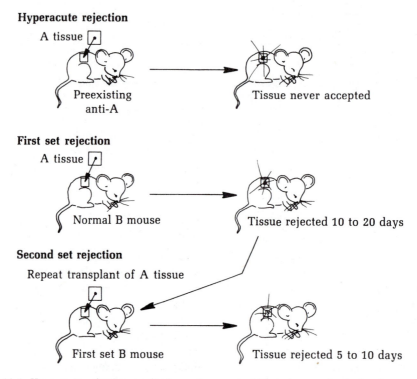

Fig. 11-1. Hyperacute rejection results from placement of tissue in an animal already possessing antibodies to antigens of grafted tissue. Second set rejection is an accelerated first set reaction and is seen in animals that have already rejected tissue at least once.

First set rejection

The usual sequence of events seen in the unsensitized recipient is less rapid and is known as the first set rejection or first set reaction. Within the first few hours or days after relocation of the allograft all outward signs belie the knowledge that the graft will be rejected. Revascularization appears to proceed normally, and skin assumes its normal healthy color. Solid tissues or organs assume their typical functions of hormone production, urine excretion, pumping of blood, etc. But within a few days skin takes on a darker, purplish hue that proceeds in the ensuing days to absolute necrosis, and by the end of the eleventh to seventeenth day, depending on the animal species and other factors, the graft will be rejected. In the case of solid organs, signs of tissue rejection will include loss of vital function of the organ, fever, and malaise. Histologically the tissue becomes heavily infiltrated with mononuclear cells of several varieties: macrophages, lymphocytes, and plasma cells. By the end of the first week fibrin accumulation and loss of blood flow and/or vascular integrity foreshadow the eventual complete loss of nutritive supply to the tissue and its death.

The actual time of graft survival varies with the species, size of the graft, tissue, and other variables. Rats reject very small skin grafts in about 21 days, but larger grafts are rejected in 8 days. Extremely large grafts may induce tolerance and survive for weeks. Kidneys often survive longer than skin.

Second set rejection

If a graft of this same sort with the same donor and recipient is repeated, the first set sequence is repeated at an accelerated pace (Fig. 11-1). This second set rejection reflects the previous exposure and sensitization to the donor antigens. Skin is sloughed in 3 to 4 days as the result of the rapid infiltration of macrophages, lymphocytes, and plasma cells. If regrafting is performed within a few days after a first set rejection, rejection of the second graft may assume the kinetics of a hyperacute rejection.

The evidence is now unassailable that graft rejection or acceptance relies on immunogenetic principles, as attested by the following:

1. Antigen specificity. Tissue transplanted between antigenically identical individuals (syngraft) or autografted tissue does not undergo rejection if surgical and septic procedures meet the accepted standards. In these two situations there is no exposure to new antigens and therefore no new immune response.

2. Immunosuppression. In the case of allografts the onset of first set and second set rejection can be prolonged by suitable immunosuppressive treatments.

3. Immunologic memory. The accelerated second set rejection applies to a repeated transplant from the same donor but does not apply to tissues from a second donor who is antigenically unrelated to the first.

4. Immunopathology. The histologic responses occurring during rejection are typical of immune crises, involving macrophages, lymphocytes, and plasma cells.

5. Transfer. Adoptive immunization with presensitized T cells will cause the rejection of tissues matched between donor and recipient.

6. Tolerance. Grafts between monozygotic twins or antigen-tolerized persons are not rejected.

Privileged sites and privileged tissues

Although allografts of tissues are routinely lost through the rejection process when they are placed orthotopically, they may persist almost indefinitely in certain heterotopic locations. Heterotopic grafting is a convenient method in experimental transplantation studies, since the transferred tissue may be placed where its survival can be easily monitored by external observation. Through experimental studies in laboratory animals and from corneal grafting in humans several immunologically privileged sites, that is, sites where allografted tissue is protected from the rejection process, have been detected. The best known of these sites is the hamster cheek pouch, although the brain and anterior chamber of the eye also have been described as privileged sites.

The hamster cheek pouch is exactly what its name indicates, a saclike cavity running along each cheek or jaw line of the hamster for approximately 5 cm. The length of the pouch places its distal end over the shoulder of the hamster. These pouches are used by the animal for food storage or transport. The inner surface of the pouch is well endowed with vascular tissue and has a layer of connective tissue, which is its privileged site. Implantation of normal or neoplastic tissues from other hamsters or even from foreign species, including humans, into the pouch is followed by their long-term survival. The tissues become vascularized and grow rapidly, whereas the same tissues placed orthotopically are quickly destroyed. The striking anatomic feature of the hamster cheek pouch, and of other immunologically privileged tissues, is its paucity of a lymphatic drainage system. This fact, coupled with the known abundance of T lymphocytes in lymph, was useful in developing our present concept that CMI is responsible for first set allograft rejection. The absence of lymphoid tissue in the hamster cheek pouch is the key to long-term graft survival.

The anterior chamber of the eye is a second and more generally available immunologically protected site. Grafts placed in the eye chamber may not become vascularized unless placed near the iris. Only in the latter situation does good tissue growth ensue; however, prolonged survival may follow in the absence of tissue growth. There is no uniform agreement that the eye chamber is a truly protected tissue. Some experimenters are very successful in demonstrating prolonged tissue survival in the eye; others are not. The reasons for this may be related to the surgical techniques employed.

The cornea is one of the best-described privileged sites. When transferred from one host to another, under ideal surgical conditions when the vascular bed is not damaged, the cornea is accepted and can successfully restore vision lost from corneal defects. This standard ophthalmologic surgical procedure is almost invariably successful. If the cornea is placed heterotopically in vascularized tissue, it is rejected in the usual fashion. This seems sufficient evidence to negate the presumption that the cornea is nonantigenic or resistant to the allograft rejection process, ideas that were forwarded to explain the easy success of corneal transplants. However, the secret to success of corneal grafts is that the cornea customarily is situated where it is protected from the host's lymphatic system.

Tissues from a variety of anatomic locations that appear to escape the usual allograft rejection process have been described as immunologically privileged tissues. These, in contrast to privileged sites, are tissues which are not rejected, regardless of where they are relocated. Among these are bone, cartilage, heart valves, sections of the aorta or other major blood vessels, and tendon; the developing fetus also can be added to this list. The first mentioned group of tissues—bone, cartilage, etc.—can be preserved indefinitely in the lyophilized state or frozen, and when needed, they can be rehydrated or thawed and are immediately ready for use. Chemical sterilization of these tissues is also practical, even with solutions that contain as much as 4% formalin. It is obvious that these procedures are lethal to the living constituents of these tissues, and this makes it essential to consider them for what they really are: physical structures with little if any cellular vitality that, when allografted, provide a matrix of the size

and shape desired about which new host tissue can form during its regeneration. This type of repair has little if any real advantage over the use of steel pins, plastic tubes or valves, or other synthetic parts for the replacement or repair of vital tissue. In fact the use of artificial devices will avoid the possibility of sensitizing the recipient to antigens of the natural tissue, which might interfere with a later medical procedure.

The developing fetus is considered the example par excellence of an immunologically privileged tissue. With the exception of completely syngeneic laboratory animals, natural fertilization demands that each cell of the developing embryo contain antigens unique to the male. In outbred animals potent antigenic differences between the male and female should hazard the success of the pregnancy on the grounds of histoincompatibility, but it is known that even females preimmunized with tissues of the male will still bear that male's offspring without incident. From this one could reason that the usual rejection process, although present, cannot reach the fetus, that is, the uterus is an immunologically protected site. Transplantation of other tissues to the uterine wall results in graft rejection, however, and this clearly indicates that the nonpregnant uterus behaves the same as other tissues in its permeability to sensitized lymphocytes and immunoglobulins. Thus there must be some other specific property of the pregnant uterus to account for protection of the fetus aside from lack of antigenicity of fetal tissues or loss of immune responsiveness by the mother. This special property is believed to reside in the trophoblast. The trophoblast is a layer of tissue that physically separates the uterine wall from the tissues of the fetus. Each cell in this membrane appears to surround itself with a mucoprotein, and the amount of this substance formed is proportional to the antigenic distance of the mother and fetus. In syngeneic relationships very little of the mucoprotein is formed. Consequently a general impermeability of the trophoblastic layer is credited with the protective role that is provided the fetus. This is operationally the same condition which exists in the hamster cheek pouch.

Immunologic tolerance and immunologic enhancement

The prolongation of transplant viability may occur as the result of a host failure to respond to antigens of the tissue (immunologic tolerance) or from the production of enhancing antibodies (immunologic enhancement or immunologic blockade). Although immunologic tolerance customarily has been examined through the use of purified antigens, its principles also apply to transplantation and tumor immunology. Immunologic enhancement has been studied primarily in the domain of tumor immunology but can be applied equally as well to the study of tissue rejection or survival.

Immunologic tolerance is described in Chapters 5 and 8, so only brief attention will be given to this subject in this section. A state of tolerance to foreign histocompatibility antigens is developed easily in fetal or newborn animals by an exposure to tissue (nonlymphoid tissue will avoid GVH reactions) containing foreign antigens. The unresponsive condition can best be detected by reexposure to the antigens in the form of a skin graft. Such grafts persist almost indefinitely in the recipient. This state is related primarily to an induction of Ts cells and down regulation of the immune response. This procedure has been applied to human transplantation successfully by giving the recipient a large-volume blood transfusion (of the donor's blood type) prior to the transplantation of tissue.

Immunologic enhancement refers to the active prolongation of tissue life by antibodies to antigens of the tissue. This has been so intimately connected with tumor immunology that it is discussed in the following chapter.

Mechanism of graft rejection

The relative role of immunoglobulins and sensitized lymphocytes in graft rejection differs considerably according to the circumstances. In the rejection of dispersed cellular grafts humoral immunity may dominate the rejection process. In such instances the donated cells—erythrocytes, leukocytes, platelets, etc.—are fully exposed to the developing immunoglobulin response. These cells are highly susceptible to membrane damage by complement activated by the initial serologic reaction. If cytolysis does not occur immediately, the immunoglobulins may function as opsonins to encourage the phagocytic destruction of the transfused cells. Erythrophagocytosis is known to occur when immune elimination of red blood cells is part of the transfusion reaction or hemolytic disease. Humoral immunity also is suspected of playing a major role in the rejection of xenografts and in hyperacute rejection of transplanted tissue. Xenografts possess a large number of antigens not shared between donor and recipient. Frequently one species will possess agglutinins for cells of distantly related species, which can attack the xenogeneic tissue as soon as it is transplanted. However, as described more fully later, under certain circumstances immunoglobulins directed toward the grafted tissue may favor graft acceptance.

In contrast to these circumstances, the activation of cellular immunity by the T lymphocytes is the predominant cause of the first set allograft rejection. As described in several earlier chapters, such lymphocytes may directly attack cellular antigens to which they are sensitized by previous exposure, or they may attack these cells by extracellular products grouped under the generic term *lymphokines*. The first few days after grafting, when the tissue may appear perfectly normal, is a sufficient time period for sensitization to occur. Thereafter the effector phase follows, causing loss of the tissue in 10 to 20 days. When sensitized lymphocytes are already present in an animal from a prior graft rejection, an accelerated rejection of tissue results from regrafting—the second set rejection. Lymphoid cells from a sensitized animal transferred by adoptive immunization to a first graft recipient will accelerate rejection of the graft. Thus graft rejection is primarily a T cell function with some assistance from immunoglobulins. The responsible T cell is the Tc. The role of NK, or null, cells in graft rejection is deserving of further study.

Immunosuppression

By January of 1973, 200 heart transplants had been performed in the world, but only 27 of these patients were still alive in 1974. Even these would not have survived were it not for significant developments in immunosuppression made since the beginning of kidney transplantation in the 1950s. In the early 1950s transplantation of kidneys from cadavers into patients with renal failure was initiated. Some of these patients lived as long as 6 months without treatment with cytotoxic drugs, but low dosages of steroids, probably too low to be effective immunosuppressants, were used for some patients. By 1960 it was documented that 6-mercaptopurine would prolong rabbit and dog renal allografts, and since that time virtually all human transplant patients have received some form of suppressant therapy.

Radiation. The status of radiation in prolonging allograft survival can be summarized by stating that, as a single agent, it is relatively ineffective, but when combined with chemical and ALG treatment it is beneficial. Local graft irradiation and extracorporeal radiation of tissue to be grafted and of the recipient's blood are preferred to total body irradiation, which has not been successful. Irradiation suffers the handicap of being totally nonspecific and may lead to prolonged paralysis of nearly all aspects of the patient's immune response. Its utility is closely related to the success of newer cytotoxic chemical agents, which have essentially replaced radiation treatments.

Chemical. In practical terms it is necessary to know if a compound is most effective when used prior to surgical grafting, at the approximate time of grafting and immediately thereafter, or both before and after, so that the treatment can be designed for the maximum benefit. In the first group

of compounds are included mitomycin C, a few but certainly not all alkylating agents, cortisone and other steroids, and mitogens such as PHA. Those compounds most active just after transplantation are additional alkylating agents (nitrogen mustards), purine and pyrimidine analogs, folic acid analogs, and the alkaloids. Specific compounds that can be mentioned, excluding the alkylating agents, are 6-mercaptopurine, 6-thioguanine, 5-fluorouracil, cytosine arabinoside, methotrexate and aminopterin, and vinblastine and vincristine. Activity before or after transplantation is exhibited by cyclophosphamide, a potent alkylating agent, and to a much lesser degree by steroids and a few other agents.

The immunosuppressant therapy given recipients of transplanted tissue will vary according to the surgical unit, the patient's well-being, the tissue transplanted, and other factors. Among the chemical immunosuppressants, azathioprine and methylprednisolone frequently are used in combination with ALG and/or radiation.

ATG. ALS and ALG are discussed previously, especially the problems encountered in determining the source of the lymphocyte, choice of animal to be used, choice of assay for activity, and mechanism of action. From the present literature it appears that ATG is enjoying widespread use in transplantation surgery, but patient records reveal that treatment with ATG often is terminated after about 2 weeks. By this time a large percentage of patients develop severe local reactions in the form of edema, induration, erythema, and pain when the ATG is given intramuscularly. When it is given intravenously, fever and mild anaphylactic shock have been recorded as distinct hazards. Many patients produce precipitating antibodies to ATG or ATS preparations, which may contribute to allergic reactions and neutralize their effectiveness. These factors plus the more general hazards of suppressant therapy contribute to its withdrawal from the treatment regimen of most patients after a few weeks.

A prime hazard of all immunosuppressant treatments is their general depressive activity on the immune system. The incidence of infections by all classes of organisms is increased in patients receiving this type of therapy. Among the bacteria, the pyogenic cocci and *Pseudomonas* infections become more frequent. Intracellular protozoa, including *Pneumocystis* and *Toxoplasma* organisms, emerge as important pathogens. Among the viruses, whose defense relies heavily on an intact CTC system, increased herpes simplex, herpes zoster, Epstein-Barr virus (EBV), and cytomegalovirus infections are noted. Among the fungi, *Candida, Cryptococcus,* and *Aspergillus* infections are more common in the immunosuppressed patient. More startling has been the discovery that about 2% of immunosuppressed human patients develop oncogenic complications. When the immune surveillance system for neoplastic cells is thwarted by these treatments, these aberrant cells find the compromised host an ideal tissue culture incubator for proliferation. The seriousness of this fact hardly needs further discussion.

GVH reactions

When tissue is transplanted from one individual to another, there are actually two rejection processes to be considered. The first and traditionally most studied is the host rejection of grafted tissue, but the reverse of this is also a distinct possibility and is known as the graft-versus-host (GVH) reaction. GVH reactions may develop when immunocompetent tissues are transferred to an immunologically handicapped host. This form of adoptive immunization results in a host-directed rejection process. This has been recognized to occur under natural circumstances when maternal lymphoid tissues are transferred to the fetus during pregnancy. Artificially these reactions may develop when adult tissues are injected into unborn or newborn animals or when lymphoid tissue is transferred to adults who have been irradiated or heavily immunosuppressed with chemical agents.

The situation in the newborn or fetal animal develops into the condition known as runt disease (homologous disease); the animal fails to grow, develops a distinct splenomegaly, diarrhea, and

anemia, and often dies. All young animals with runt disease do not die, however; those which survive may progress through a transitory period of only a few days in which splenomegaly and hepatomegaly, an erythematous skin, and fever are the major signs that a reaction is taking place. Human examples of maternally acquired runt disease are known. Mild, reversible GVH reactions are more frequent when the donor and host share a good degree of histocompatibility but are not syngeneic. It is this fact which gave courage to those pediatricians and surgeons who transplanted bone marrow and/or thymus tissue into young children with proved genetic immunodeficiencies. Some of these children did progress through a GVH reaction, but both tissues survived the reaction with the desired repopulation of the host with immunocompetent cells. Adult GVH reaction may be seen when the host's lymphoid system has been depleted by ALG treatment, x-irradiation, or chemical immunosuppression. GVH reactions are not seen when skin or other tissue lacking mature lymphoid cells is transferred, for example, transfer of fetal cells to adult animals or the transfer of tissues that have been treated with x rays to destroy immunologically capable cells.

In experimental animals simple and suitable indexes of GVH reactions have been developed that are not adaptable to the human. The first of these is the spleen index. The spleen weight of normal animals is directely related to body weight, and any deviation from the known ratio is evidence of splenic change in response to the grafted tissue. The phagocytic index is also a parameter of GVH reactions and is applicable to human studies. Clearance of colloidal carbon from the blood is accelerated in an individual undergoing a GVH reaction. This is a nonspecific expression of hyperreactivity of the immune system and is easily detected with a small sample of blood.

THE MOUSE MHC
Discovery of the H-2 system

The MHC of mice was described serologically in 1936 by Gorer, who was studying mouse blood

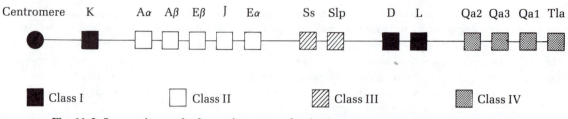

Fig. 11-2. Structural genes for four major groups of antigens are present on mouse chromosome 17: the histocompatibility *(Class I)*, the immune response *(Class II)*, complement *(Class III)*, and cell surface antigens *(Class IV)*.

group antigens. Of the four antigens under investigation, Gorer noted that antigen II was related to transplant survival; grafts between animals that had antigen II were usually successful. Snell suggested that such antigens be called histocompatibility antigens, and the nomenclature system was born. H-2 antigens in mice and the genetic basis for their inheritance were clarified by the use of inbred, congeneic mouse strains developed by Snell. Ultimately more than 50 alloantigens were described that controlled graft rejection, and the genes determining these antigens were linked to other traits such as the regulation of the immune response, the complement system, and antigens of lymphocytes (Fig. 11-2).

Class I genes and their products

In the mouse three genes or gene clusters, the H-2K, H-2D, and H-2L genes, situated on chromosome 17 are the structural genes that determine the composition of the histocompatibility antigens. The K gene locus is separated from the juxtaposed D and L loci by the Ir genes and genes associated with the complement system. The K, D, and L loci are very polymorphic and have been identified to result in the production of more than 50 proteins that are antigenically distinct. Allogeneic immunization and adsorption experiments have yielded highly purified sera, which can be used to identify these antigens on cells. Xenosera and hybridoma antibodies are available for this same purpose.

These histocompatibility antigens have been identified on the surface of all nucleated cells. It is the immune response of a transplant recipient against these antigens which dominates the graft rejection process; hence these are defined as the major transplantation antigens. Less potent or minor histocompatibility antigens also may contribute to graft rejection.

The H-2 antigens can be removed from cell membranes by detergents or potassium chloride salt extraction procedures, which disturb the lipid bilayer of the membrane. The free H-2 antigens have been identified as glycoproteins with a molecular weight near 44,000 (Fig. 11-3). The polysaccharide portion of the H-2 molecule is subdivided into two subunits, each of which contains galactose, mannose, glucosamine, and fucose. Sialic acid may be present in only one of the saccharide side chains. These polysaccharide side chains appear to be identical on all H-2 proteins and thus do not contribute to their antigenic specificity. The specificity of the transplantation antigens resides within the amino acid sequences 30 to 40, 60 to 80, and 105 to 114, all of which are located external to the plasma membrane. The extracellular sequence encompasses amino acids 1 to 281, the membrane-bound segment, 282 to 308, and the cytoplasmic segment residues, 309 to 346. Just external to the membrane-bound segment a papain cleavage site exists, and exposure of cells to this protease will release the external 281 amino acid unit.

β_2-Microglobulin. Noncovalently bonded to the H-2 protein is the β_2-microglobulin, a unique

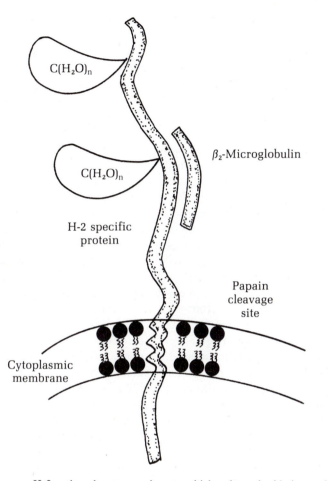

C(H₂O)ₙ

β₂-Microglobulin

C(H₂O)ₙ

H-2 specific
protein

Papain
cleavage
site

Cytoplasmic
membrane

Fig. 11-3. The mouse H-2 antigen has two regions to which polysaccharide is attached: a hydrophobic region in the cytoplasmic membrane and an anchor in the cytoplasm. The β_2-microglobulin (12,000 mol wt) is noncovalently associated with the antigen-specific protein (44,000 mol wt).

protein containing 99 amino acids with a molecular weight of approximately 12,000 (Fig. 11-3). This identical β_2-microglobulin is ionically associated with all the antigenically diverse H-2 proteins. Structural genes on mouse chromosome 2 encode for this protein. The β_2-globulin is of interest because it was recognized early in the study of the human histocompatibility antigens that they functioned as cross-reactive antigens with antisera to IgG. This now has been related to the close amino acid sequence homology of the C_H domains with the β_2-globulin and a disulfide loop of 57 amino

acids in the microglobulin which is similar to those seen in IgG.

Class II genes and their products

Situated between the H-2K and H-2D genes are a cluster of structural genes known as the Ir genes. (See Chapters 3 and 5.) The exact number of these genes is uncertain, but the I-A, I-C, and I-J genes are generally agreed on. The I-A and I-C genes are associated with helping the immune response and the I-J gene with hindering the immune response. Proteins encoded by these genes are present on B cells and macrophages. Th cells have receptors for the I-A or I-E proteins that, through unidentified mechanisms, stimulate the immune response. The contrary role is played by the Ts cells by virtue of their interaction with I-J proteins.

The chemistry of the I-A and I-E proteins has been partially determined and is presumed to be a model for the I-J proteins as well. The I-A and I-E proteins consist of two noncovalently joined peptides, one of about 32,000 mol wt and the other slightly smaller, near 28,000 mol wt. (See Fig. 3-1.) The larger protein has been designated as the α-protein and the smaller as the β-protein. Each is encoded by subloci of the A or E gene on the seventeenth chromosome to produce Aα, Aβ and Eα, Eβ, respectively. Both the α- and β-proteins are embedded into the cytoplasmic membrane of B cells and macrophages by hydrophobic regions that hold the proteins close to one another despite the absence of covalent bonding. Structural variations in α-chains have been detected, and these may confer the antigen-recognition specificity needed for the proper interplay of B cells, T cells, and macrophages to regulate the response to the T cell–dependent antigens.

Class III genes and their products

On the mouse chromosome 17 two genes (Ss and Slp) are present between the Ir region and the D gene locus. These and their gene products in the complement system are described in Chapter 9.

Class IV genes and their products

To the right of the L gene locus as one progresses from the centromere of chromosome 17 are situated a set of three genes of the Qa series plus the T1a gene. The T1a locus is the structural gene for antigens found on T cells present in leukemia and on immature T cells in the mouse thymus. As normal T cells are prepared for release into the circulation, the T1a antigen is lost, but the antigen is retained on the primitive leukemic cells. The Qa proteins also are found on

lymphocytes. The exact function of these proteins is uncertain. The gross chemical characteristics of the Qa and T1a proteins resembles the H-2 proteins in consisting of the β_2-microglobulin noncovalently associated with a 44,000 mol wt protein that is embedded in the cell membrane.

THE HUMAN MHC
Discovery of the HLA system

The human histocompatibility antigens are present on all nucleated cells of the body, including leukocytes. Antibodies to human leukocytes were discovered in persons who had undergone several transfusions and were found to function independently of the ABO antigens. Beginning in about 1958 several groups of workers began a serious study of the HLAs, each adopting its own nomenclature system and in some instances reporting some observations about the transmission or grouping of these antigens. For example, Dausset indicated in 1958 that monozygotic (identical) twins had identical leukocyte agglutination patterns and that dizygotic twins did not. By 1962 van Rood and van Leeuwen arranged a simple leukocyte antigen grouping system from the examination of the agglutinating susceptibility of leukocytes from 100 individuals tested against a panel of antisera. By 1967 it was obvious that many antigens existed on the white blood cell surface; a special workship of experimenters on this subject accepted HL-A1, HL-A2, etc. as the symbols to refer to human leukocyte antigen 1, 2, and so on (Reading 7). At the same time studies of transplantation antigens of mice revealed that they were located on the surface of leukocytes, and by the early 1960s it was learned that injections of human leukocytes resulted in accelerated graft rejection. Thus the HLA antigens came to be synonymous with the human transplantation or histocompatibility antigens.

Class I genes and their products

Three gene sets of the HLA systems have been identified on human chromosome 6 and are desig-

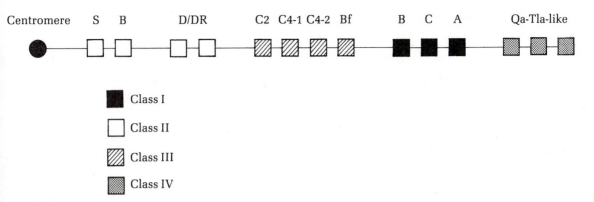

Centromere   S   B   D/DR   C2   C4-1 C4-2   Bf   B   C   A   Qa-Tla-like

■ Class I

☐ Class II

▨ Class III

▧ Class IV

Fig. 11-4. The human histocompatibility *(Class I)* genes HLA-A, HLA-B, and HLA-C are grouped between the complement *(Class III)* and cell surface marker *(Class IV)* genes. The class III genes are imprecisely located toward the centromere from the D/DR *(Class II)* genes.

nated as HLA-A, HLA-B, and HLA-C (Fig. 11-4). These gene regions are clustered, as is the case in all species studied except the mouse. Each gene is highly polymorphic, and currently A, B, and C are recognized to have 19, 42, and 8 alleles, respectively. Each allele is associated with an antigenically unique protein with a molecular weight of 44,000. This is the human transplantation or histocompatibility antigen, which is noncovalently associated with the β_2-microglobulin. The HLA specific protein is embedded in the cytoplasmic membrane by a hydrophobic region that precedes its base in the cell cytoplasm. Studies of the HLA proteins indicate an exact parallel with our knowledge of the mouse H-2 system.

Class II genes and their products

The D region (D or DR) of the human parallels the mouse Ir region. The studies in humans are incomplete, but all evidence to the present is supportive of this conclusion. The DR proteins are found on B cells and macrophages but are absent from T cells. These DR proteins consist of a larger and smaller peptide, noncovalently joined, but both embedded in the cytoplasmic membrane. The D region is believed to control the helper and suppressor functions of the immune system.

Class III and IV genes and their products

Four gene loci situated between the HLA and the D/DR loci on chromosome 6 are associated with the complement system. These Class III genes and their products are described in Chapter 9.

Qa-T1a-like loci have not been fully characterized in humans, but the available evidence indicates, as with other MHC genes, a close parallel with the mouse system.

Genetic relationships and their application

In humans the HLA-A, B, and C genes exist as multiply varied alleles of a paired chromosome system. Because one antigen of each set is transmitted through the germ cells, the genetic composition of progeny can be described in terms of their paternal and maternal haplotypes. The gene products of each A, B, and C gene set are numbered (Table 11-2). These numbers are not sequential within the A, B, or C series because they were numbered prior to knowledge of their gene association.

Because so many different antigens are involved (19 A, 42 B, and 8 C), most haplotypes are rare except within a specific line of inheritance. Mathematically the chance for two persons to have a

Table 11-2. Human HLA antigen specificities and frequencies*

HLA-A	Frequency (percent)	HLA-B	Frequency (percent)	HLA-C	Frequency (percent)
A1	15.8	B5	5.9	Cw1	4.8
A2	27.0	B7	10.4	Cw2	5.4
A3	12.6	B8	9.2	Cw3	9.2
A9	11.2	B12	16.6	Cw4	12.6
A11	5.1	B13	3.2	Cw5	8.4
A25	2.0	B14	2.4	Cw6	12.6
A26	3.9	B15	4.8	Cw7	Unknown
A28	4.4	B17	5.7	Cw8	Unknown
A29	5.8	B18	6.2		
Plus 10 Aw antigens		B27	4.6		
		B37	1.1		
		B40	8.1		
		Plus 30 Bw antigens			

*Includes antigens not precisely identified, as designated by the gene letter plus *w* (for workshop).

common phenotype is less than 1 in 20 million. As a consequence of this, any haplotype that is common between a child and a putative father is nearly absolute evidence of parentage (Table 11-3). Because of its mathematic superiority, HLA typing is destined to replace blood grouping to identify individuals in cases of disputed parentage, unidentified infants, violent death, etc. The major application of the HLA system at the current time is in histocompatibility testing preparatory to tissue transplantation.

HLA and disease

Since the genes that regulate the synthesis of the HLA antigens and those which govern the immune response are positioned so close to one another on the chromosome, it has been interesting to examine the relationship of HLA antigens to various forms of disease. The diseases investigated have been for the most part those with some presumed immunologic origin: neoplastic disease, autoimmune disease, and allergies. These are described in Chapter 21 and summarized in Table 21-2.

Histocompatibility testing

There are two basic procedures employed to determine the suitability of tissue for grafting purposes. In one system the histocompatibility antigens of both the donor and recipient are determined by microcytotoxicity testing, and only tissues that share common histocompatibility antigens are considered suitable for use in transplantation. In the other method lymphocytes of the donor and recipient are placed together in culture (MLC) and observed for antagonistic reactions. When these are not noticed, the tissues are considered histocompatible. Some investigators prefer the second system, since it is a ''natural'' system and may measure antigenic disparities for which no antisera are yet known, but microcytotoxicity testing is a far more common procedure.

Cytotoxicity assay. Although agglutination tests and complement fixation tests have been used to detect histocompatibility antigens on leukocytes or to quantitate HLA, H-2, or other antisera, the lymphocyte toxicity test is now the most widely applied method for this purpose. To identify the HLA antigens, a reasonably pure prepara-

Table 11-3. Genetic transmission of HLA antigens and haplotypes

	A antigens						B antigens					
	1	2	3	9	11	25	5	7	8	12	13	14
Father	+	−	+	−	−	−	−	+	+	−	−	−
Mother	−	+	−	+	−	−	+	−	−	+	−	−
Children												
First	+	+	−	−	−	−	+	−	+	−	−	−
Second	+	−	−	+	−	−	−	−	+	+	−	−
Third	−	+	+	−	−	−	+	+	−	−	−	−
Fourth	−	+	+	−	−	−	+	+	−	−	−	−

	Interpretation	
	Phenotypes	Haplotypes
Father	A1, 3/ B7, 8	A1, B8/ A3, B7
Mother	A2, 9/ B5, 12	A2, B5/ A9, B12
Children		
First	A1, 2/ B5, 8	A1, B8/ A2, B5
Second	A1, 9/ B8, 12	A1, B8/ A9, B12
Third	A2, 3/ B5, 7	A3, B7/ A2, B5
Fourth	A2, 3/ B5, 7	A3, B7/ A2, B5

tion of lymphocytes is prepared from heparinized blood. The blood may be centrifuged to remove the bulk of the erythrocytes, and the buffy coat, or white blood cell film resting on top of the erythrocytes, is further purified. The buffy coat or whole blood may be added to commercially available solutions, which on standing or light centrifugation will stratify the lymphocytes in an isolated band. The lymphocytes are then adjusted to 10^6 cells per milliliter. A few microliters of the cell suspension are added to each of many histocompatibility antisera that have been dispensed in microliter droplets in a multiconcavity test tray. Serum complement is added, and incubation, usually for 1 hour at room temperature or 37° C, is allowed before staining the dead cells with eosin or trypan blue. Living cells do not take up these dyes; so by microscopic evaluation one can determine if a certain antiserum-complement combination was cytotoxic for the lymphocytes (Fig. 11-5). When this is the case, then the antigen corresponding to that antiserum was present on the lymphocyte surface. By performing this test on lymphocytes of both donor and recipient with a battery of antisera, one can determine their histocompatibility antigen composition.

Naturally there are many subtle variations to the microcytotoxicity test. The lymphocytes may be labeled with ^{51}Cr by incubating them briefly with Na_2 $^{51}CrO_4$, followed by a centrifuge washing to remove the excess isotope. This ^{51}Cr is released by cells undergoing membrane damage and is a rapid and sensitive test for cytotoxicity. Viable lymphocytes also can be labeled with a fluorescein dye; when the integrity of their cell membrane is lost, the dye leaks out. In this test the presence of unstained cells is an index of cytotoxicity. Regardless of the system employed, the cytotoxic assays are the most generally used of the histocompatibility tests.

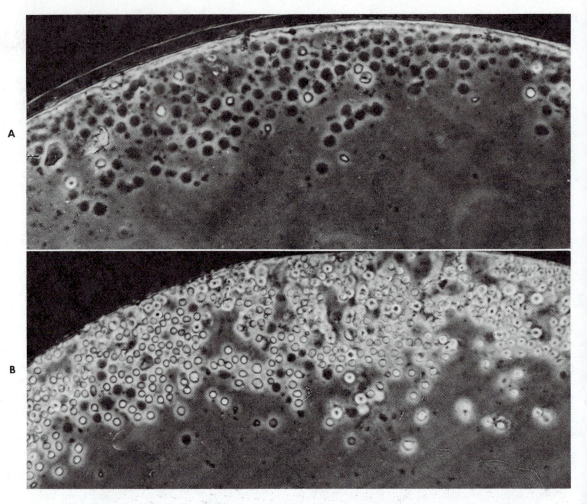

Fig. 11-5. A, The dark stained lymphocytes represent a positive microcytotoxicity test. **B,** A negative test in which the refractile living lymphocytes remained unstained. (Courtesy Dr. A. Luger.)

Data collected over the past decade clearly demonstrate the relationship of HLA antigen matching with transplantation success. Even as early as 1971, before all HLA antigens could be identified, it was found that bone marrow transplants were successful in 6 of 11 instances in HLA-matched persons but in only 2 of 16 instances in nonmatched persons. Skin grafts between siblings with two haplotype differences survived 11.6 days, but when one parental haplotype was matched, the grafts were not rejected for 14.4 days. With HLA identical at the A and B antigens, skin grafts survived an average of 24.9 days. Kidney transplants between fully matched A and B persons have a record of 70% success over a 2-year span in one study as opposed to 35% when only one antigen was matched. In a Scandinavian study of 4 years 83% of HLA-A- and HLA-B-matched renal grafts survived compared with 65% if only one haplotype was common. Because of the gene

Normal mixed lymphocyte culture

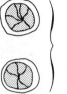

Donor lymphocytes
haplotypes 1,5 × 2,7

Recipient lymphocytes
haplotypes 1,5 × 3,9

Lymphocyte transformation

But whose?

One-way mixed lymphocyte culture

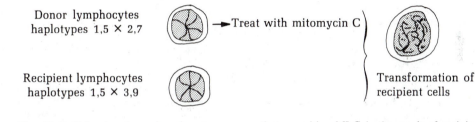

Donor lymphocytes
haplotypes 1,5 × 2,7

Treat with mitomycin C

Recipient lymphocytes
haplotypes 1,5 × 3,9

Transformation of
recipient cells

Fig. 11-6. Poisoning donor lymphocytes ensures that a positive MLC is the result of recipient lymphocyte transformation.

(and antigen) frequencies, it is extremely difficult to establish a perfect HLA-A, B, and C match. Siblings are obviously the best source, but the size of the modern family renders this possibility slight.

MLC. From studies conducted in the early 1960s it was realized that the in vitro culturing of peripheral blood leukocytes from two separate donors was an assay for histocompatibility differences between the two individuals. The test does not attempt to measure the antigenic composition of donor and recipient, only their compatibility. Individual cultures of cells from either donor or mixed cells from monozygotic twins retain their basic structure throughout a 5-day incubation period, with some expected loss in vitality of the cells. Cells from unrelated donors undergo lymphocyte transformation, as evidenced by intensive nucleic acid metabolism, enlargement of the cell nucleus with an accompanying increase in mitotic figures, and an increase in cell size before division. Such is the result of an MLC or MLR. These changes can be detected cytologically (Fig.

11-6), but because this requires tedious microscopic observation, resort to radioassay has been necessary to expedite data collecting. The basis of the radioassay is that tritiated thymidine added to the cultures is incorporated into the nuclear DNA of rapidly proliferating cells but not into unstimulated control cultures. Fixation of the radiolabel by the cultures can be determined by scintillation counting and used as an index of histocompatibility difference between the two persons.

The MLC reaction is a response of T cells to antigens on B cells. When the HLA-A, B, and C antigens are identical, the MLC is a measure of D/DR disparity between the donor and recipient cells. Antisera which inhibit the MLC in these instances are sources of antibodies to the D/DR antigens.

The MLC reflects primarily incompatibilities of the major transplantation antigens; the "weak" antigens often go undetected. The peak reaction may not require the full 5-day incubation period, and often the results can be read within 2 days.

Results of MLC tests agree closely with those of cytotoxicity studies for nonidentity of the major HLA antigens but may detect some antigens missed by the cytotoxicity test because of the lack of antisera for all antigens. Most experimenters agree that the MLC does predict graft survival between donor and recipient. Since circumstances could exist in which only the lymphocytes of a donor could react to antigens of the recipient and thus give a false view of potential grafting success, the one-way MLC was developed. In this modification the lymphocytes of the donor are poisoned with mitomycin C (20 μg/ml) or irradiation (4,000 rad for 6½ minutes) before mixing them with the recipient's cells. Such donor cells are incapable of incorporating tritiated thymidine after these treatments and thus cannot contribute to positive tests. Under these circumstances the test becomes solely a measure of the recipient's response to the donor's transplantation antigens and a predictor of transplant success.

Normal lymphocyte transfer reaction. What the MLR attempts to do in culture the normal lymphocyte transfer reaction attempts to determine in vivo with somewhat less reliance on sophisticated technology. To perform the normal lymphocyte transfer test, lymphocytes are collected and purified from the peripheral blood of a person needing a transplant. These lymphocytes are injected into the skin of a potential donor or a series of donors. After 24 to 48 hours areas of pronounced inflammation may be seen at the inoculation site; however, donors who share the major histocompatibility antigens with the recipient will display only a mild erythema at the site. Thus from the size and intensity of the reaction graft success can be estimated.

This method has been in use since 1963, and, although it does predict graft survival times accurately in experimental animals of normal health, it is not adaptable to certain classes of humans who, by virtue of certain diseases, have lymphocytes that are unreactive in this test. Patients with severe kidney disease, the very ones who need kidney transplants, have lymphocytes that are largely inert in this test. There is also some risk when using lymphocytes from patients with diagnosed or potential malignancies. This test is basically a test of recipient tissue for its ability to respond to donor antigens, which is the direction of reactivity that should be measured in histocompatibility testing, but this can be done in vitro and quantitated more precisely than by the lymphocyte transfer reaction. This probably explains why the cytotoxicity test is the preferred histocompatibility testing method at the present time.

BIBLIOGRAPHY

Anonymous: Transplantation and clinical immunology, Amsterdam, 1979, Excerpta Medica.

Bach, F.H., and Sondel, P.F.: Cellular immunogenetics—definition of HLA-D region encoded antigens by T lymphocyte reactivities, Clin. Immunobiol. **4:**123, 1980.

Bach, F.H., and van Rood, J.J.: The major histocompatibility complex—genetics and biology, N. Engl. J. Med. **295:**806, 872, 927, 1976.

Ballantyne, D.L.: Experimental skin grafts and transplantation immunity: a recapitulation, New York, 1979, Springer-Verlag New York, Inc.

Ballantyne, D.L., and Converse, J.M.: Experimental skin grafts and transplantation immunity, New York, 1979, Springer-Verlag New York, Inc.

Braun, W.E.: HLA and disease: a comprehensive review, Boca Raton, Fla., 1979, CRC Press, Inc.

Carpenter, C.B., d'Apice, A.J.F., and Abbas, A.K.: The role of antibodies in the rejection and enhancement of organ allografts, Adv. Immunol. **22:**1, 1976.

Dick, H.M., and Kissmeyer-Nielsen, F., editors: Histocompatibility techniques, Amsterdam, 1979, Elsevier/North Holland Biomedical Press.

Dorf, M.E., editor: The role of the major histocompatibility complex in immunobiology, New York, 1980, Garland STPM Press.

Ferrone, S., Curtoni, E.S., and Gorini, S., editors: HLA antigens in clinical medicine and biology, New York, 1979, Garland STPM Press.

Festenstein, H., and Demont, P.: HLA and H-2 basic immunogenetics, biology and clinical relevance, London, 1978, Edward Arnold (Publishers), Ltd.

Grebe, S.C., and Streilein, J.W.: Graft-versus-host reactions: a review, Adv. Immunol. **22:**120, 1976.

Herberman, R.B.: editor: Natural cell-mediated immunity against tumors, New York, 1980, Academic Press, Inc.

Herberman, R.B.: Natural killer cells and cells mediating

antibody-dependent cytotoxicity against tumors, Clin. Immunobiol. **4:**73, 1980.

Katz, D.H., and Benacerraf, B., editors: The role of products of the histocompatibility gene complex in immune responses, New York, 1976, Academic Press, Inc.

Kissmeyer-Nielsen, F.: The serology of HLA-A, B and C, Clin. Immunobiol. **4:**99, 1980.

Klein, J.: Biology of the mouse histocompatibility-2 complex, New York, 1975, Springer-Verlag New York, Inc.

Klein, J.: H-2 mutations: their genetics and effect on immune functions, Adv. Immunol. **26:**56, 1978.

Lange, C.F.: HL-A histocompatibility antigens and their relation to disease, Prog. Clin. Pathol. **6:**137, 1976.

Law, L.W., and Appella, E.: Biological and biochemical properties of solubilized histocompatibility-2 (H-2) allo-antigens, Contemp. Top. Mol. Immunol. **5:**69, 1976.

Morris, P.J., editor: Kidney transplantation, principles and practice, London, 1979, Academic Press, Inc. (London), Ltd.

Morris, P.J.: Suppression of rejection of organ allografts by alloantibody, Immunol. Rev. **49:**93, 1980.

Rose, N.R., Bigazzi, P.E., and Warner, N.L., editors: Genetic control of autoimmune diseases, New York, 1978, Elsevier/North-Holland.

Rubinstein, P.: Other markers in the HLA linkage group, Clin. Immunobiol. **4:**183, 1980.

Sachs, D.H.: The Ia antigens, Contemp. Top. Mol. Immunol. **5:**1, 1976.

Selwood, N., and Hedges, A.: Transplantation antigens—a study in serological data analysis, Chichester, England, 1978, John Wiley & Sons, Ltd.

Shreffler, D.C., and David, C.S.: The H-2 major histocompatibility complex and the I immune response region: genetic variation, function, and organization, Adv. Immunol. **20:** 125, 1975.

Skamene, E., Kongshavn, P.A.L., and Landy, M., editors: Genetic control of natural resistance to infection and malignancy, New York, 1980, Academic Press, Inc.

Snell, G.D., Dausset, J., and Nathenson, S.: Histocompatibility, New York, 1976, Academic Press, Inc.

Svejgaard, A., and Ryder, L.P.: HLA and disease, Clin. Immunobiol. **4:**173, 1980.

van Rood, J.J., and Persijn, G.G.: HLA and graft survival, Clin. Immunobiol. **4:**113, 1980.

van Rood, J.J., and van Leeuwen, A.: The serology of HLA-DR, Clin. Immunobiol. **4:**113, 1980.

Winchester, R.J., and Kunkel, H.G.: The human Ia system, Adv. Immunol. **28:**222, 1979.

Zinkernagel, R.M.: Associations between major histocompatibility antigens and susceptibility to disease, Annu. Rev. Microbiol. **33:**201, 1979.

CHAPTER
12

TUMOR IMMUNOLOGY

The similarities of transplantation immunology and tumor immunology are truly astounding. In each instance a host is confronted with a set of tissue cells similar, although not identical, in antigenic composition to the autologous cells. Through the normal events of transplant rejection the histoincompatible cells activate the immune response in the graft recipient. This embodies all aspects of the defense system—macrophages, B cells, and T cells, of which the macrophages and T cells are the most effective. In transplantation immunology every effort is made to suppress this immune response so that the grafted tissue can survive. This includes physical and chemical immunosuppression as well as the use of ALS. Studies of privileged tissues, privileged graft sites, and antigenic tolerance all have been important in the campaign to escape the graft rejection phenomenon.

In neoplastic disease, tumor cells appear spontaneously in the host, probably from only a single or a few transformed cells. The accidental transfer of tumors simultaneous with organ grafts would be an exception to this. These tumor cells, like allografts, have some antigenic similarity to host cells but are not antigenically identical to them. For reasons that still escape a precise delineation, the host's immune response is either not fully activated and fails to reject the tumor tissue or develops in such an imbalanced pattern (enhancing or blocking antibody) that growth of the tumor not only is permitted, it is even encouraged.

It is apparent from this capsule presentation that common immunologic events are shared by tumor immunology and transplantation immunology. Why the outcomes of these events are so distantly polarized from each other—the sur-

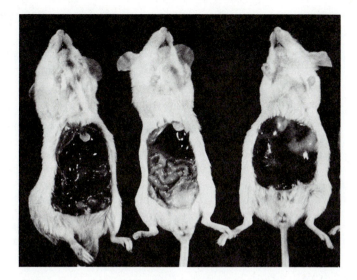

Fig. 12-1. Normal mouse in the center is flanked on the left by a mouse with a large subcutaneous plasmacytoma (IgA type) seen as a large, dark mass. The mouse on the right has an ascites, a dispersed cell tumor distributed throughout the peritoneal cavity. (Courtesy H. Gebel and M. Daley.)

vival of oncogenic tissues on one hand versus the death and rejection of transplanted cells on the other—is the mystery that immunologists must try to solve.

TUMOR TERMINOLOGY

The word *tumor* actually means swelling, and this can develop as a result of neoplasia (new cell growth) or edema (leakage of fluid into the tissues). By common practice the use of the word *tumor* is largely restricted to the first meaning. The Greek stem word for tumor is *oncos;* hence the study of tumors is oncology, the development of tumors is oncogenesis, etc. A benign tumor is relatively slow growing, restricted in anatomic location, and not considered life threatening. These features are not shared by malignant tumors, which are life threatening, easily metastasize (disseminate), and may have either a slow or rapid growth rate. *Cancer* is the standard term for all malignant tumors, but benign tumors also may be referred to as cancers. Nonmalignant tumors are named by adding the suffix *-oma* to the type of tissue from which they originate or are

composed (Fig. 12-1). Malignant tumors of mesenchymal origin are sarcomas; those of epithelial origin are carcinomas. There are many exceptions to this nomenclature, especially for malignancies of blood cells and for diseases that were not recognized as malignant in their early description (Table 12-1).

TUMOR ANTIGENS

As the neoplastic cell arises from the normal cell, antigens not previously recognized or not produced become detectable on the cell surface. Tumors of lower animals that have been carefully studied can be placed into one of two categories in regard to these antigens. In the case of chemically induced tumors the new antigens are different for each tumor. For example, a tumor induced on a mouse by painting its skin with methylcholanthrene will have a different antigenic composition than the tumor of a partner mouse treated with the same carcinogen. In fact two anatomically distinct tumors induced on a single mouse by the same chemical carcinogen will be antigenically distinct. Exceptions do occur, but the antigen-

Table 12-1. An abbreviated classification of tumors

Tissue origin	Benign	Malignant
Mesenychymal		
Connective tissue		
Fibrous	Fibroma	Fibrosarcoma
Fatty	Lipoma	Liposarcoma
Bone	Osteoma	Osteogenic sarcoma
Endothelial and blood		
Lymph vessels	Lymphangioma	Lymphangiosarcoma
Brain covering	Meningioma	
Granulocytes		Granulocytic leukemia
Monocytes		Monocytic leukemia
Lymphocytes		Lymphocytic leukemia
Lymphoid tissue		Lymphoma, plasmacytoma, Hodgkin's disease(?)
Epithelial		
Squamous	Squamous cell papilloma	Epidermoid carcinoma
Gland lining	Adenoma	Adenocarcinoma
Respiratory tract		Bronchogenic carcinoma
Placenta	Hydatidiform mole	Choriocarcinoma

ic cross-reactions between chemically provoked cancers arise by chance and are mathematically unpredictable.

In the same way viral induced tumors express unique antigens, but these tumors are antigenically constant from specimen to specimen. This is true even though the tissue origin or even the species origin of the tumor may differ. These constant antigens are known as tumor-specific antigens (TSA) or tumor-specific transplantation antigens (TSTA). The constant expression of an identifiable antigen is a useful diagnostic aid and has been used to suggest that a tumor of unknown cause is of viral origin. Either DNA or RNA viruses may induce these antigen-specific tumors.

Among the DNA viruses that can code for new antigens in host cells are herpesviruses, adenoviruses, and the papovaviruses, formerly known as the polyoma and papilloma viruses (Table 12-2). Specific examples of the herpesvirus group are Marek's disease of chickens, Lucké's carcinoma of frogs, and Burkitt's lymphoma of humans, the most convincing candidate to be the first proved virus-induced tumor of humans. Adenoviruses from humans, notably types 12 and 18, will cause cancers in laboratory mice. Simian virus SV40 and Shope papilloma virus are examples from the papovavirus group. These DNA viruses are tiny and can carry only sufficient genetic information to code for approximately a half dozen proteins. Most of these are involved with virus replication, but at least one of them is the TSA.

RNA viruses are usually larger and can code for a variety of proteins. Here again at least one is a TSA of the cell surface, unique to each virus. It seems that the leukemia viruses of practically every species have this property, as does the Rous sarcoma virus and mouse mammary tumor virus. In addition, the RNA viruses also must code for their special viral synthesizing enzymes.

Tumor and TSAs

The antigens associated with viral transformed cells are of three types: (1) those which are asso-

Table 12-2. Oncogenic viruses

Type of virus	Animal involved
RNA	
Leukemia: sarcoma viruses	Bird, mouse, cat, rat, guinea pig, hamster, cattle, monkey, and possibly human
Mammary tumor viruses	Mouse, monkey, and possibly human
DNA	
Herpesviruses	Frog: Lucké's kidney carcinoma; bird: Marek's lymphomatosis; monkey: malignant lymphoma; human*: nasopharyngeal carcinoma and Burkitt's lymphoma
Adenoviruses	Monkey, avian, and human viruses in cell cultures; hamsters
Papovaviruses	Rabbit: Shope papilloma; mouse: polyoma, monkey SV40, bovine papilloma, human wart

*Evidence very good but circumstantial.

ciated with the infective virion, (2) the tumor (T), or nuclear, antigens, and (3) the TSA, or cytoplasmic membrane antigens. A discussion of the viral antigens is beyond the scope of this chapter; however, it is clear that the presence of antibodies or T cell responses to known oncogenic viruses could bear importantly on the diagnosis of the cancerous condition they cause.

The T antigens first detected in transformed cells following viral infection are located in the nucleus. These antigens are specific for the inducing virus and not for the malignant cell. These antigens are detectable in all cells infected by the virus even though the cell may not become transformed, but the T antigens persist in malignant cells. These antigens are not identical with antigens of the virus particle, and some of them may be virus-induced enzymes. These T antigens are immunogenic for the tumor-bearing animal, and high levels of circulating anti-T globulins follow oncogenic conversion by adenoviruses, polyoma, and SV40 viruses. Because of the intracellular location of the T antigen, these antibodies are not able to react with the antigens in vivo and thus cannot contribute to tumor immunity, only to tumor diagnosis.

The most important antigens from the standpoint of availability as targets for the immune response are the TSAs of the cytoplasmic membrane. The TSAs have been recognized in the adenovirus, papovavirus, herpesvirus, and leukemia-sarcoma

virus systems. Antibodies to these antigens are found in the circulation of tumor-bearing animals; however, the titer of these antibodies does not correlate well with resistance to the tumor or regression of the tumor. How tumor cells with specific TSA escape the rejection process, which to all purposes should be identical to an HVG rejection, is not yet clear. T cells that are responsive to these TSAs also are generated by infections with these viruses.

Burkitt's lymphoma. Natural regression of Burkitt's lymphoma and chemotherapeutic cures of this malignancy have been of great interest to immunologists and tumor biologists. Burkitt's lymphoma is presumed to have a viral origin, a suggestion made in 1958 when Burkitt noted a high incidence of this cancer across the mosquito belt of central Africa. This disease is predominantly a malignancy of the jaw and associated facial bones and the abdominal tissues of children. Histologic examination of the tissue allows it to be classified as a lymphoma. The disease may run a fatal course, although spontaneous cures have been noted. Treatment with the alkylating agent cyclophosphamide will produce long-term remission.

Interest in Burkitt's lymphoma stems from several features of the disease: its cause, its cytology, and its immunology. The epidemiologic pattern of Burkitt's lymphoma indicated a potential arthropod vector in its cause. The disease has its highest incidence in the malarial regions of Africa where the mosquito population is highest. Examination of Burkitt's cells in culture with the electron microscope has revealed that some of the cells contain viruslike particles which are indistinguishable from those of the herpes group (DNA viruses). Nearly 90% of African Burkitt's patients have these viral particles in their tumor cells. Some cells produce and release these viral particles, which are known as Epstein-Barr virus (EBV). Several EBV antigens have been identified in these cells, including the nuclear antigen (EBNA) and viral capsid antigens. Many investigators are now willing to accept EBV as the first proved viral agent to cause human cancer, but much of the data to support this is circumstantial and based on immunologic analyses.

Before considering the serologic status of Burkitt's lymphoma it is important to emphasize that the tumor cells represent an immunoproliferative activity of the immune system. Lymphomas are malignancies of lymphocytes or their precursor cells. If the cell line producing the lymphoma is sufficiently differentiated toward the T or B cell line, it can be classified as such. Waldenström's macroglobulinemia, for example, is often classified as a B cell immunoproliferative disease because the cells involved are morphologically distinct from plasma cells, and their IgM product is easily demonstrated. Burkitt's lymphoma is classified as a proliferative disease of B cells that are at an early stage in the maturation sequence, that is, lymphoblastoid cells; thus no immunoglobulin product in blood is associated with the disorder. These cells often will produce antibodies in culture. As aberrant B cells, Burkitt's lymphoma cells would be expected to contain unique or unusual antigens.

One of the novel antigens in Burkitt's cells is the EBV agent. Patients with the lymphoma have higher than normal levels of antibody to EBV capsid antigens and to cell membrane antigens of the lymphoma cells. They also possess high titers of EBV-neutralizing antibodies. In the examination of sera for EBV antibodies it was discovered that

persons recently recovered from infectious mononucleosis were those with the highest titers. In fact 80% of Africans have EBV antibodies, although only a few have Burkitt's lymphoma. These antibodies do not differ from those found in patients with Burkitt's lymphoma. The links between infectious mononucleosis, Burkitt's lymphoma, and EBV are not yet completely understood, but their association is unique in viral oncogenesis. It may be that persons who develop infectious mononucleosis do so as the normal course of EBV virus infection. An unfortunate few are unable to respond in this normal way to the infection, and they develop Burkitt's lymphoma. Fortunately Burkitt's lymphoma is treatable with cytotoxic drugs, and spontaneous cures, evidence of a self-generated immunity, are known.

Nasopharyngeal carcinoma. Another neoplastic disease associated with the EBV particle is nasopharyngeal carcinoma. This cancer is common in southern China but rare in other parts of the world, including central and northern China. Serologic studies of these patients have revealed that they more frequently have elevated titers to the EBV particle than do Burkitt's lymphoma patients. Unlike Burkitt's lymphoma, viral particles have not been observed in cells of patients with nasopharyngeal carcinoma, but viral DNA has been identified in these cells. The expression of EBV antigens, including EBNA and capsid and membrane antigens, occurs in the tumor cells.

Nasopharyngeal carcinoma and Burkitt's lymphoma are thus ideal candidates for the first human cancers to be induced by a virus, but the associations thus far established are not critical proof despite the knowledge that EBV is oncogeneic for some laboratory animals. EBV could be an innocent passenger virus needed for the oncogenic expression of some as yet unidentified virus. In addition, environmental and genetic factors may be involved. This is suggested by the geographic distribution of the EBV-associated tumors and by the recognition of damage to chromosome 14 in Burkitt's lymphoma. This chromosome is the locus for the structural gene of immunoglobulin H chain synthesis in B cells, of which the lympho-blastoid cell of Burkitt's disease, at least, is an example.

Carcinofetal antigens

A second type of TSA exists in the form of antigens known as carcinofetal, carcinoembryonic, or regression proteins. The synthesis of these proteins is unrelated to viral oncogenesis and is an expression of the metabolic shift of cancerous cells from an adult to an "immature" pathway of protein synthesis. The carcinofetal proteins are synthesized by normal fetal tissues and by tumors of these same tissues in adults. Whereas the TSAs are specific for a particular oncogenic virus, the carcinofetal proteins are not. Although once thought specific for anatomic locations of cancers, the carcinofetal antigens now are believed to be general expressions of cell reversion to a more primitive metabolic pathway (Table 12-3).

Carcinoembryonic antigen. In 1965 Gold and his co-workers began a series of investigations of an antigen they isolated from a human cancer of the colon. This antigen was not present in the normal tissue surrounding the tumor, but it was found in tumors of the digestive tract, including the small intestine, liver, pancreas, stomach, and rectum, in addition to the colon. This antigen also was found in human embryonic gut and gut-associated organs during the first two trimesters in utero, after which the antigen became more difficult to demonstrate. These facts led to the description of the antigen as the carcinoembryonic antigen (CEA).

Since the first descriptions of CEA based on immunodiffusion studies more and more sensitive serologic tests have been used to identify it. The current method of choice is radioimmunoassay (RIA). This test can identify nanogram quantities per milliliter of this antigen. One of the results is that a greater percentage of patients with gastrointestinal tumors can be identified as CEA positive, as follows: rectal and colonic, 56%; stomach, 67%; and liver and pancreas, 73%. At the same time it became evident that persons with other carcinomas were positive for CEA in significant percentages; breast cancer, 47%; prostate, 40%; lung, 77%; and gynecologic tumors as a group, 65%. These figures vary from study to study but reveal the nonspecificity of CEA for colonic tumors and for gastrointestinal tumors and that CEA titrations might indicate cancer of a more expansive group of tissues. Unfortunately the use of CEA was further clouded by the finding that many nonmalignant conditions produced RIA-positive tests for CEA. These conditions include cigarette smoking (19% compared with 3% nonsmokers), chronic lung disease (57%), cirrhosis of the liver (45%), and ulcerative colitis (32%). Even 21% of healthy donors were positive in one report.

These data have not denied an important use of CEA in human medicine. It is now accepted that CEA titrations must be evaluated carefully in cancer diagnosis, and such tests may be a very useful prognostic index of the success of surgery or chemotherapy of cancer. If preoperative CEA titers persist after surgery, it can be presumed that the surgery was incomplete. Perhaps significant metastases precluded a surgical cure of the patient. If the CEA titers fall and then rise, this

---

Table 12-3. Characteristics of carcinofetal antigens

Synthesis	By embryonic and fetal tissues and cancers in adult tissues; fetal synthesis ceases near birth
Source	Embryonic organs, cancerous organs, blood
Specificity	Slight specificity for organ system producing them
Chemistry	Proteins or glycoproteins; some are enzymes
Identification	Immunoassay with antisera rendered specific by adsorption with normal tissues
Value	Possibly in cancer diagnosis; definitely in prognosis

would indicate a failure to completely remove the tumor, followed by its regrowth, CEA production, and an increase in titer. Similar evaluations would apply to the treatment of cancer with cytotoxic drugs.

The CEA antigen is a β-globulin with an $S_{20,w}$ of 7 to 8. It has a molecular weight near 200,000 and exists as a β-glycoprotein with its major saccharide being N-acetylglucosamine. It is an unusual protein, since it contains 40% to 80% carbohydrate by weight. Its normal function in the fetus and the signal to halt or to renew synthesis in the malignant state are unknown.

AFP. An α-globulin found in fetal serum but not in the adult serum of several species is known as the α-fetoprotein (AFP). The organ source of AFP is the liver. In fetal plasma AFP may reach a concentration of 3,000 ng/ml. Pregnancy sera levels may reach 500 ng/ml.

It now is recognized that nearly all primary hepatomas result in a metabolic shift of liver tissue to the fetal state and the synthesis of AFP. The detection of AFP, like that of CEA, is of potential diagnostic and prognostic significance in human oncology.

The history of AFP parallels closely that of CEA. At first relatively insensitive serologic procedures such as gel diffusion were used for its identification. This meant that rather significant quantities of the antigen had to be present in sera to produce a positive test. Such persons usually had hepatomas of substantial size so that positive tests for AFP correlated nicely with the incidence of hepatocarcinoma. With the development of RIA and the capacity to detect AFP in nanogram quantities per milliliter of serum it was found that AFP persisted in small quantities into adult life. Normal adult serum levels are only 1 to 2 ng/ml. AFP levels above 10 ng/ml, considered a diagnostic level, are reached in 94% of patients with hepatoma and in 68% with teratoma. The diagnostic range is exceeded 12% of the time in patients with acute hepatitis, 67% with chronic hepatitis, and 49% with alcoholic cirrhosis. AFP also was detected above the normal level in some patients

with extrahepatic tumors such as those of the stomach, lung, and pancreas and in patients with ataxia telangiectasia. AFP determinations as an aid to the diagnosis of liver cancer must be used in company with diagnostic aids for other forms of liver disease and for cancers of other organs.

AFP is a glycoprotein that behaves electrophoretically like an α_1-globulin. It has a molecular weight near 70,000, of which about 4% is carbohydrate. It is so similar in its biophysical properties to albumin that is has been difficult to secure the highly purified preparations needed to develop antisera for RIA.

The normal biologic function of AFP is unknown. The globulin fraction of serum is immunosuppressive, and this may have some importance to the maternal-fetal relationship and to the cancerous state. T lymphocytes bind AFP, and this may block proper recognition of antigen by T cells, thus allowing the cancer to grow.

A very successful use of AFP is in the monitoring of neural tube malformations (spina bifida) in fetuses by measuring the AFP level in amniotic fluid, which is normally 1.5 to 26 μg/ml at the fifteenth week of gestation. Excesses of this concentration correlate well with serious defects, including anencephaly.

Other carcinofetal proteins. The α_2-hepatic protein (AHP), a globulin with a high iron content and synonymous with α_2-hepatic globulin or α_2-ferroglycoprotein, first was associated with cancer of the liver in 1965, when it was extracted from the hepatomas. AHP also is extractable from liver tissue of persons with tumors in other anatomic locations. Although 50% of adult cancer patients have positive RIA tests for α_2-hepatic ferroprotein in their serum, 20% of patients with nonmalignant disease are also positive. The figures are more impressive in juveniles with cancer: 80% of children with cancer have positive RIA tests for AHP versus an incidence of only 8% in healthy children. AHP and ferritin are closely related proteins. Both are found in liver, and both are rich in iron, with AHP containing 15% to 25% iron in the ferrous state. Ferritin also contains about 23%

iron, but this is in the ferric state. The molecular weight of AHP is estimated at 600,000, and ferritin has a molecular weight of 465,000. The normal physiologic function, if any, of AHP is unknown, but it is believed to be identical to β-ferritin, a carcinofetal form of ferritin. A γ-ferroprotein also has been identified in fetal serum and in the serum of adults with malignancies.

A sulfated glycoprotein antigen that can be isolated with a high frequency from stomach cancers is a TSA also found in fetal tissues. This fetal sulfoglycoprotein is antigenically related to CEA.

Several enzymes described as carcinoplacental or carcinoembryonic enzymes and originating from trophoblastic tissues have been associated with a broad range of cancers. The best known of these are the isozymes of alkaline phosphatase, particularly the Regan isozyme. This enzyme is present in the sera of persons with various forms of cancer and is not restricted to those with placental or trophoblastic tissue tumors, although the enzyme from all these sources is indistinguishable from the enzyme produced by normal placenta. The enzyme is present in about 20% of persons with cancer. Other isozymes associated with cancerous states include aldolase, glycogen phosphorylase, glucosamine 6-phosphate synthetase, and amino acid transaminase. Virtually all these have been studied in relation to hepatomas. As the hepatoma develops, there is an expression of altered gene behavior in the excretion of the fetal isozyme form of each of the isozymes just mentioned. The adult or mature isozyme is produced by the remaining normal liver tissue, but when electrophoretic and immunologic studies are performed, the shift toward the immature carcinofetal type of enzyme is detectable.

TUMOR IMMUNITY
Natural immunity

Spontaneous remissions of cancer may occur and have been recognized in isolated instances involving nearly every variety of carcinoma. Immunologists naturally have assumed that the rejection of tumors was based on the same events, possibly plus other mechanisms, which were responsible for graft rejection. This has focused attention on Tc cells and their relatives, the K and NK cells. To these, macrophages and possibly antibodies can be added as additional tumor defense forces.

The cytotoxic T lymphocyte (CTL) is the CTC, the cell identified by unique antigens on its surface (Lyt 2,3 in the mouse) and its biologic activity. These cells are described in Chapter 5, and some of the activities are described in Chapters 10 and 11. CTCs have no inherent cytocidal activity; this is developed as a result of exposure to antigens. These antigens may include the histocompatibility antigens, viral antigens, or TSAs. In human oncology this exposure occurs naturally, and in experimental oncology it occurs by injecting sublethal quantities of a tumor into the animal. The CTC is MHC restricted and antigen specific, a phenomenon first conclusively demonstrated by a CTL effect on virus-infected cells. Thus the CTC exposed to target cells in culture will destroy only tumor cells bearing its own transplantation antigen and the tumor antigen to which it is programmed. It has been generally accepted that CTLs were effective by virtue of the lymphotoxins they excrete. These lymphokines are more fully described in Chapter 7 as a collection of molecules of descending molecular weight all derived from a common precursor macromolecule, thus accounting for lymphotoxins α, β, and γ and their electrophoretic subclasses. Some experimental results, notably the inability of certain antisera against the lymphotoxins to neutralize their cytotoxic role, have suggested the CTC may use other avenues to cause cell death. Cytoplasmic shedding by a CTC in contact with target tumor cells has indicated a particulate substance may be involved, but the identity of this substance has not been seriously examined.

The cytotoxic activity of specific antibody acting with any of several cell types has been labeled antibody-dependent cell cytotoxicity (ADCC). The antibody is usually, if not always, an IgG and may be of any subclass. Complement is often present in the assay but is not required. The major source of confusion about the ADCC test is in deciding which cells contribute to target cell lysis. It is generally agreed that the effector cell must have receptors for Fc regions of IgG. Macrophages and granulocytes, especially neutrophils, have these receptors and are accepted as participants in ADCC; platelets and B cells do not participate even though they have Fc receptors. Macrophages and neutrophils do not phagocytose the target cell during ADCC and must be cytocidal by other means. Since these cells undergo the oxidative burst typical of activated phagocytes when they contact the target cell, ADCC may result from the secretion of toxic forms of oxygen.

Certain lymphocytes that cannot be identified as T or B cells are active in ADCC. These cells lack the Thy 1 antigens typical of T cells and are devoid of surface immunoglobulin characteristic of B cells. These cells have been described as null cells to reflect their independence from both B and T cells. (See Chapter 5.) They also have been designated as K cells to reflect their killer activity on foreign cells.

K, or null, cells must be distinguished from the NK cells, which also display a target cell destructive activity. NK cells are present in nude mice, which are T cell deficient, and unlike T cells, NK cells need no previous exposure to antigens of the target cell before they become active. NK cells are not target cell or antigen specific, although their indiscriminate activity could result from the combined activity of several NK subsets, each of which has a restricted target cell specificity. Another distinguishing feature is that target cells are more quickly destroyed by NK cells than by CTC or K cells. K cells are more resistant to corticosteroids than NK cells but more sensitive to inhibition by the incorporation of protein A in the assay. NK cell activation by lectins and IFN converts them to more aggressive cells, and this plus their natural presence indicates a role both in early and late recognition and destruction of tumors.

Among the criteria supporting a tumoricidal role for NK cells is (1) their presence in nude mice and the surprising resistance of nude mice to transplantable tumors in view of their lack of T cells, (2) the decreased numbers of NK cells in the beige mouse line coupled with its heightened sensitivity to tumors, (3) the loss of NK cells as mice age concomitant with an increased incidence of tumors, and (4) the protection against transplantable tumors afforded by adoptive immunization with an enriched population of NK cells.

Phagocytic cells have long been accorded a protective role against foreign cells, and there is substantial evidence that macrophages, especially when activated, engulf and kill tumor cells.

Tumor vaccines

There are many problems associated with the use of vaccines of tumor origin in human oncology. It is clearly impossible to prepare prophylactic vaccines because there is no assurance that any one individual eventually will develop cancer. Although epidemiologic studies point to an increasing incidence of cancer, it still is not possible to predict the antigenic form this cancer will take, especially since many cancers are chemically induced. This prevents a rational choice of the vaccine for immunoprophylaxis.

The use of tumor vaccines in immunotherapy is clouded by several uncertainties. If the patient already has a cancer and is being exposed to tumor antigens, the rationale for additional antigen exposure demands clarification. Among the hypotheses favoring the use of autogenous tumor vaccines is that the existing tumor may be saturated with blocking antibody. Injections of additional antigen could adsorb this antibody and leave a remnant of free antigen sufficient for an advantageous stimulation of T cells needed to develop a protective immunity. A second possibility is that alteration of the tumor cells by an in vitro exposure to enzymes such as neuraminidase or trypsin, which peel their outer surface, might expose important antigens that are shielded from the normal in vitro immune response. Or the reinjection of dead tumor cells or cell fractions might create the antigen load necessary to escape the generalized immunosuppressed condition of most cancer victims. The additional use of adjuvants with these preparations might result in a protective immunity that cannot be arranged through natural immunization.

One type of cancer vaccine that has produced favorable results is the neuraminidase-treated tumor cell. Treatment of mammalian tissue cells with neuraminidase from *Vibrio cholerae* increases their antigenic potency far beyond what might be expected from the known chemical effect—the removal of *N*-acetylneuraminic acid from the cell surface. The cells are not killed by this process. DBA/2 Ha mice repeatedly immunized with neuraminidase-treated mouse leukemia L1210 cells subsequently were able to resist 10^7 untreated tumor cells. C3H/f mice treated with a similar preparation of 6C3HED lymphosarcoma cells resisted 10^6 normal tumor cells. This resistance was associated with a marked increase in T cell–based immunity and complement-fixing antitumor globulins. Spontaneous leukemia was treated successfully in AKR mice with a combination of chemotherapy and neuraminidase-treated E2G cells.

The effect of neuraminidase-treated human tumors as vaccines has been evaluated in several trials. Patients with acute myelocytic leukemia remained in remission for 79 to 132 weeks if they received a combination of enzyme-treated vaccine and chemotherapy, versus 19 weeks when only chemotherapy was applied. Neuraminidase-treated tumors may be used advantageously in other human cancers, including breast cancer, skin cancer, and gastrointestinal tumors, but further trials are needed. This type of immunotherapy, combined with Con A as a T cell stimulant and surgery, shows great promise in the treatment of bronchogenic carcinoma.

Adoptive immunity

The repeated descriptions of cancer sufferers as victims of a faulty immune surveillance system suggests that their macrophages and T cell functions are depressed. Such T cell functions may be stimulated by transfer factor or be supplemented by adoptive immunization. In the latter

case it could be hypothesized that only histocompatible cells would be beneficial, but this is not necessarily true. GVH reactions may be tumoricidal.

Adoptive experiments in laboratory animals that have avoided both HVG and GVH reactions have been successful in many systems. Survival rates of 75% versus expected mortality of 100% have been observed in leukemic mice that received lymphoid tissue from syngeneic donors. Transfer of immune lymphoid cells has a more dramatic effect than transfer of normal lymphoid cells in producing tumor regression or cures. Unfortunately this is a difficult experiment to reconstruct in the human, but these experimental studies have demonstrated the significance of the T cell in tumor immunity (Figs. 12-2 to 12-4).

Acute leukemia and malignant lymphoma in humans can be treated successfully with bone marrow grafts and active immunization. Although the recurrence of leukemia was noted, the survival rate was extended.

Adjuvant therapy

Potentially one of the most promising of the new immunologic approaches to the control of neoplasms is the use of IFN. IFN has the capacity to slow cell growth and to stimulate NK cells, macrophages, and possibly other antigen-responsive cells. A major restriction in the use of IFN for cancer therapy has been its impurity and expense. Molecular cloning of IFN genes into bacteria and yeasts has minimized these handicaps, and human trials with IFN of bacterial origin already have been conducted with partial success.

Transfer factor and immune RNA also have been used in human trials, but the results have been inconsistent. Clearly futher experience is necessary with these products and IFN before significant conclusions can be reached.

One of the most promising avenues in tumor immunotherapy is the catalysis of natural resistance through nonspecific immunization with BCG vaccine (an attenuated strain of *Mycobacterium tuberculosis* variety *bovis*). Cell fractions of the

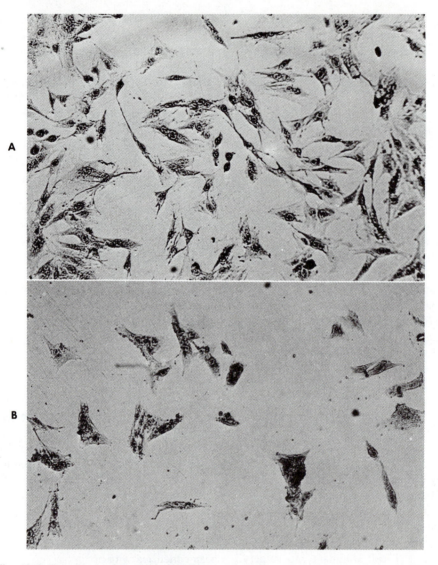

Fig. 12-2. The effects of cytotoxic lymphocytes on tumor cells can be seen here. **A,** The tumor cells prior to contact with the immune lymphocytes. **B,** The tumor cells after this contact. Notice that many cells have detached from the surface, some cells are swollen, and few cells show the morphology of the normal cells. (Courtesy Dr. J. Berkelhammer.)

BCG organism and other potentiators of non-specific resistance such as *Propionibacterium acnes* also can be used successfully. The greatest success with these vaccines applied as nonspecific adjuvants has been observed when the vaccine is deposited in the immediate vicinity of the tumor.

Within a few weeks the tumor can be observed to diminish in size, and this regression continues in some instances until the tumor is no longer detectable. Intradermal BCG vaccination near melanomas on the skin has proved successful in both experimental animals and humans. This thera-

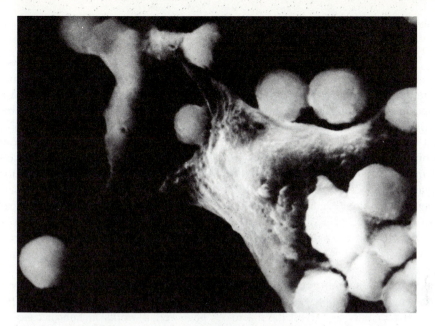

Fig. 12-3. The white spheres seen in this scanning electron microscope view are T lymphocytes attacking a much larger Walker carcinoma cell. T lymphocytes are a significant part of our defense against foreign, including cancer, cells. (Courtesy Dr. E. Adelstein.)

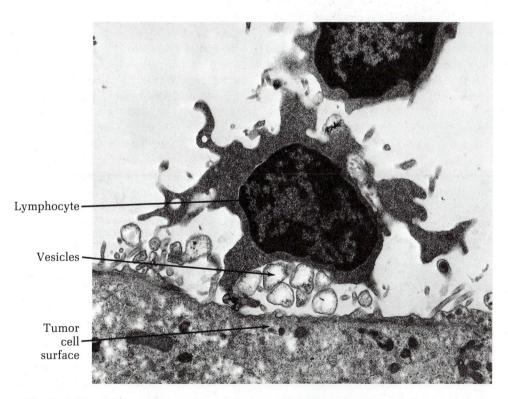

Lymphocyte

Vesicles

Tumor
cell
surface

Fig. 12-4. Transmission electron microscopy reveals the initial stages of the attack of a cytotoxic lymphocyte on a tumor cell, only a portion of which is seen. Notice the vesicles and blebs of cytoplasm that are being shed by the lymphocyte. (Courtesy Dr. E. Adelstein.)

peutic mode is unsuccessful for disseminated or internally located tumors.

Five separate mechanisms have been advanced to explain the immunopotentiation of tumor immunity by BCG vaccine. These include (1) the enhancement of macrophage cytotoxicity, (2) a stimulation of lymphocyte trapping, (3) an activation of T lymphocytes, (4) a direct influence on B lymphocytes, and (5) the existence of shared antigens between the mycobacteria and certain tumors. There is evidence to support each of these. When the ability of macrophages from BCG-vaccinated, tumor-bearing animals to release ^{51}Cr from isotopically labeled cells was compared with the same activity of normal macrophages, it was found that the immune macrophages were twice as active. It was necessary to harvest the macrophages at 14 days after BCG immunization to show this effect, which was very time dependent.

When ^{51}Cr lymphocytes were infused into BCG-treated and normal animals, the amount of radioactivity in lymph nodes in the region of the subcutaneous injection of BCG increased sharply for up to 35 days after immunization until it reached three times the values observed in the normal animals. No such effect was noted in the contralateral lymph nodes or when the BCG vaccine was given intravenously. Local trapping of lymphocytes is presumed to ensure their exposure to tumor antigens that drain into the lymphatic system near the tumor.

The possibility that BCG acts nonspecifically on T cells is supported by the observation that the vaccine nearly doubles the delayed hypersensitive reaction of mice to picryl chloride. Stimulation of mice to produce IgM (a T cell–independent immunoglobulin) and antibody to TNP-flagellin (a T cell–independent antigen) has been cited to support the direct action of BCG on B cells without a helper effect of T cells.

A surprising amount of evidence has been accumulated to defend the hypothesis that BCG shares antigens with many tumors and causes their regression through a specific form of immunostimulation. Guinea pig line 10 hepatocarcinoma, mouse EaG2 cells, avian Rous sarcoma, human malignant melanoma, human myeloid leukemia, and human neuroblastoma will bind radiolabeled or ferritin-labeled anti-BCG. No serologic cross-reaction was noted with mouse plasmacytoma, mouse EL4 cells, or human acute or chronic lymphatic leukemia cells. It is noteworthy in this regard that BCG offers no protection to mouse EL4 tumor cells but does to its cross-reactive EaG2 cell line. BCG cell wall preparations produced cures in 60% of guinea pigs carrying the line 10 hepatoma. Removal of the protein and free lipid from the BCG cell wall preparation sharply reduced its curative activity.

Although the experimental efficacy of BCG vaccination as an antitumor agent is well established, how well it works in human cancers other than melanoma is still to be determined. Two approaches have indicated limited success. One of these was a retrospective comparison of a large population of blacks in Chicago for their incidence of death from cancer and leukemia and their status as BCG vaccinates. Of 83,356 subjects who had received BCG, 13 deaths were attributed to leukemia and other forms of cancer, for a rate of 1.2 per 100,000. The "non-BCG group" consisted of 534,820 persons. Their cancer mortality was 4.4 per 100,000, or a total of 306 deaths. Although environmental factors were beyond control, both groups were of the same race, encompassed the same socioeconomic groups, and were from the same area of the city.

BCG vaccination of patients with active malignant lymphoma or acute myelogenous leukemia was not helpful. However, in one study of 100 patients with acute lymphoid leukemia no relapses were observed in a 48-month follow-up period after BCG and chemotherapy. With the chemotherapy alone the relapse rate was 35% in the same period.

TUMOR SURVIVAL AND IMMUNE ENHANCEMENT

There is no single satisfactory explanation for the success of tumors in escaping the allograft rejection process. Many theories have been forwarded, practically all of which have been based on immunologic observations surrounding the development of a limited number of neoplastic conditions. Many of the earlier hypotheses were naive and have been discarded. For example, it was suggested that cancerous tissue was nonantigenic and that tumors lost their antigens, thereby escaping the host's immunologic defense system. Certain tumors do definitely lose some of their antigenic components, for example, tumors of endocrine tissue often lose their ability to produce hormones. It is also known that the normal histocompatibility antigens may be more diluted on the surface of tumor cells as they are replaced or crowded out by TSA, but these are examples of antigenic drift and not of total nonantigenicity. Antigenic drift also has been suggested as an escape mechanism for tumors, but it is doubtful that this antigenic change is sufficiently rapid to protect the cancer cells from the host's immune response.

In transfer experiments it is known that the quantity of tumor tissue injected is very instrumental in predicting cancer development. Low doses of tumor cells are easily eliminated; larger doses are not. When an animal acquires the ability to reject a small dose of tumor cells, it usually is equipped to reject continually larger and larger doses. This information has been used to support the concept of specific immunologic tolerance as the means for graft survival. The hypothesis is that a sufficiently large dose of tumor cells inoculated into an animal, by continuous direct antigen exposure of the T and B cell population, deletes the normally expected rejection response. These is good evidence that tumor patients do not respond to their tumor antigens. Only a low percentage of these patients produce circulating antibodies in any quantity to the tumor antigens, and their lymphocytes tend not to be cytotoxic to tumor tissue in vitro. This may not be an expression of specific tumor antigen tolerance, however, since many of these patients do not respond to other antigens either. These patients are probably best classified among those persons who have a borderline, previously unnoticed, immunodeficiency disease.

The emergence of tumors is regularly cited as evidence of a failure of the immune surveillance system. Immunologists are reluctant to accept this and cite the possibility that the body may be producing oncogenic cells every day. For weeks, months, or years the immune surveillance system successfully contains these aggressive cells. Then on a later single occasion when this does not occur, the immune surveillance system is described as faulty.

Recent evidence with hybridoma antibodies originally believed to be specific for tumor antigens has revealed an unexpected incidence of cross-reactions with normal tissues. This has raised the question as to whether true TSAs actually exist. Perhaps tumors have only an uneven distrubution of normal antigens, with greater concentrations of some and lower concentrations of others, which has given the appearance of a unique antigenic composition. This cannot be answered until more definitive studies of the specificity of these anti-tumor hybridomas are completed, but if these indicators prove true, then the immune surveillance system cannot be expected to control cancer.

The recognized anergic state of many T cell–dependent responses in cancer patients, some of which can be overcome with adoptive immunization and transfer factor treatment, indicates that tumors themselves may be immunosuppressive. The chemically induced fibrosarcoma in the A/J mouse strain elicits a potent Ts response that, when negated by anti-J protein serum, decreases the rate of tumor growth. Even alterations of macrophage metabolism may abet rather than hinder tumor growth. Activated macrophages release argininase, an enzyme with a long history as an immunosuppressant because of its degradation of arginine, which is required by lymphocytes. Oxidation of free amino groups of protein or of amino acids by macrophage polyamine oxidase creates aldehyde groups that possess a cytostatic effect by reacting with nucleic acids.

To these suggestions, we also can add immunologic enhancement as a means of encouraging tumor survival. Immune enhancement can be defined as the enhancement of tumor growth by specific antibodies. This phenomenon stands in contrast to immunologic tolerance, in which specific antibodies and sensitized T lymphocytes simply are not formed in response to an antigen. Although immune enhancement could be applied to many situations such as the fetus as an allograft and to normal graft rejection or survival, it is considered here only as it may be applied to tumor immunology.

Immune enhancement was discovered through the transplantation of tumors to recipients that had been preimmunized to produce circulating antibodies to the tumor tissue. Rather than observing a hastened rejection and elimination of the tumor, it was noted that the tumor had an increased growth rate. Further experiments of this type in laboratory animals have been supported by human studies which have demonstrated conclusively that certain immunoglobulins were not cytotoxic but were growth promoting instead. These antibodies have been purified and have the following characteristics: (1) sedimentation values and molecular size consistent with their inclusion among the IgG antibodies, (2) an enhancing activity when in low titer or when transferred in small quantities to a recipient, but a cytotoxic activity when present in high titer, (3) a failure to appear in the circulation until several days or a few weeks after exposure to tumor antigens (this is typical of IgG), (4) an antigenic specificity typical of all antibodies that can be measured by fluorescent antibody studies which detect the enhancing antibody bound to tumor cells, and (5) a high avidity for antigens on the tumor cell surface.

Several of these features have been incorporated into a theory that does much to explain the immune enhancement phenomenon. First, the enhancing antibody may be considered as an immunosuppressor via the mechanism of feedback inhibition, which prevents the formation of more actively cytolytic antibodies. Second, it may attach to the tumor cells, and because of its high avidity, it may create a firm antigen-antibody complex, which serves as a physical blockade to prevent the attachment of cytolytic antibodies. In this sense enhancing antibodies can be listed among the blocking antibodies. If the host response to tumor antigens is dictated by genetic control mechanisms to produce large amounts of cytolytic antibody and low amounts of enhancing antibody, the tumor regresses. In the opposite circumstance the tumor growth is enhanced. In an effort to establish the proper protective balance of these immunoglobulins in a cancer victim, plasmapheresis has been attempted. In this process the patient's plasma is passed over a column of immunoglobulin-adsorbing material, such as protein A, and reinfused into the patient.

BIBLIOGRAPHY

Adinolfi, M.: Human alpha fetoprotein 1956-1978, Adv. Hum. Genet. **9:**165, 1979.

Blasecki, J.W.: Mechanisms of immunity to virus-induced tumors, New York, 1981, Marcel Dekker, Inc.

Chirigos, M.A., and others, editors: Mediation of cellular immunity in cancer by immune modifiers, New York, 1981, Raven Press.

Clark, R.L., Hickey, R.C., and Hersh, E.M., editors: Immunotherapy of human cancer, New York, 1978, Raven Press.

Ferrone, S., and others: Current trends in tumor immunology, New York, 1979, Garland Publishing, Inc.

Friedman, H., and Southam, C., editors: International conference of immunobiology of cancer, Ann. N.Y., Acad. Sci. **276:**1, 1976.

Green, I., Cohen, S., and McCluskey, R.T., editors: Mechanisms of tumor immunity, New York, 1977, John Wiley & Sons, Inc.

Haller, O., editor: Natural resistance to tumors and viruses, Curr. Top. Microbiol. Immunol. **92:**1, 1981.

Harris, J.E., and Sinkovics, J.S.: The immunology of malignant disease, ed. 2, St. Louis, 1976, The C.V. Mosby Co.

Herberman, R.B., editor: Compendium of assays for immunodiagnosis of cancer, New York, 1978, Elsevier/North-Holland, Inc.

Herberman, R.B., editor: Natural cell-mediated immunity against tumors, New York, 1980, Academic Press, Inc.

Hirai, H., and Alpert, E., editors: Carcinofetal proteins: biology and chemistry, Ann. N.Y. Acad. Sci. **259:**5, 1975.

Jones, S.E., and Salmon, S.E., editors: Adjuvant therapy of cancer II, New York, 1979, Grune & Stratton, Inc.

Kaplan, H.S.: Hodgkins disease, ed. 2, Cambridge, 1980, Harvard University Press.

Kirkpatrick, A.M., and Nakamura, R.M.: Alpha-fetoprotein; laboratory procedures and clinical applications, New York, 1981, Masson Publishing USA, Inc.

LoBuglio, A.F., editor: Clinical immunotherapy, New York, 1980, Marcel Dekker, Inc.

Reif, A.E., editor: Immunity and cancer in man, New York, 1975, Marcel Dekker, Inc.

Richards, V.: Cancer immunology—an overview, Prog. Exp. Tumor Res. **25**:1, 1980.

Rosenberg, S.A., editor: Serologic analysis of human cancer antigens, New York, 1980, Academic Press, Inc.

Sela, M., editor: The role of non-specific immunity in the prevention and treatment of cancer, Amsterdam, 1979, Elsevier/North Holland Biomedical Press.

Sell, S., editor: Cancer markers: diagnostic and developmental significance, Clifton, N.J., 1980, Humana Press.

Schultz, J., and Leif, R.C., editors: Critical factors in cancer immunology, New York, 1975, Academic Press, Inc.

Shuster, J., and others: Immunologic approaches to diagnosis of malignancy, Prog. Exp. Tumor Res. **25**:89, 1980.

Siskin, G.W., Christian, C.L., and Litwin, S.D., editors: Immune depression and cancer, New York, 1975, Grune & Stratton, Inc.

Skamene, E., Kongshavn, P.A.L., and Landy, M., editors: Genetic control of natural resistance to infection and malignancy, New York, 1980, Academic Press, Inc.

Terry, W., editor: Tumor immunology, New York, 1979, Elsevier/North-Holland, Inc.

Waters, H., editor: The handbook of cancer immunology, vols. 1-9, New York, 1978-1981, Garland STPM Press.

Weitzel, H.K., and Schneider, J., editor: Alpha-fetoprotein in clinical medicine, Stuttgart, 1979, Georg Thieme Verlag.

Wolf, P.L., editor: Tumor associated markers, New York, 1979, Masson Publishing USA, Inc.

Woodruff, M.F.A.: The interaction of cancer and host; its therapeutic significance, New York, 1980, Grune & Stratton, Inc.

Wybran, J., and Staquet, M.J., editors: Clinical tumor immunology, Elmsford, N.Y., 1976, Pergamon Press, Inc.

Ziegler, J.L.: Burkitt's lymphoma, N. Engl. J. Med. **305**:735, 1981.

SECTION THREE

SEROLOGY

INTRODUCTION TO
SEROLOGIC REACTIONS

GLOSSARY

Danysz's phenomenon A phenomenon involving toxin and antitoxin that demonstrates the dissociability of antigen-antibody complexes and the formation of such complexes with variable proportions of the reactants.

equivalence point That dilution in a serologic reaction when all the antigen and antibody are mutually involved in complexes.

optimal proportions That dilution in a serologic reaction which becomes positive first.

postzone Failure of a serologic reaction to occur in extreme dilutions of antibody.

prozone Failure of a serologic reaction to occur in a high concentration of antibody.

titer The greatest dilution of a substance used in a serologic reaction that will produce the desired result.

The presence of antibodies in an antiserum is demonstrated by performing a serologic reaction. The end result of the reaction may be a clumping or agglutination of particulate antigens, a precipitation of fluid antigens, a binding of the antigen without any outward evidence of the reaction, or some other type of reaction, depending on the physical nature of the antigen and the conditions imposed on it. Regardless of the exact physical nature of the end result, the basic steps in preparing the test and the events that occur during it are very similar. A general description of these events and their mathematic interpretation is presented in this introductory chapter prior to a consideration of the individual, specific reactions in the later chapters of this section.

SEROLOGIC BEHAVIOR OF THE IMMUNOGLOBULINS

In the usual serologic test a dilution series of the antiserum is prepared, and to this an appropriate quantity of antigen is added. Additional tubes lacking antigen or antiserum are prepared as controls for the stability of the two serologic reagents. After a suitable incubation time at a specified temperature the test is examined for the evidence of a serologic reaction. This always is done by comparing the experimental tubes with the control tubes. The dilution of the serum in the last tube to exhibit a positive test is the titer of the antiserum. Sera with different titers thus can be compared roughly as to their antibody content.

In such a dilution series several zones of the serologic reaction may be noted. In the first few tubes, where the antiserum concentration is greatest, a positive test may not be apparent; this is the prozone. Prozone can be caused by an excess of antibody, as is clarified in the following discussion. In the last tubes in the dilution series a negative result always should be observed; otherwise the final titer cannot be determined. This obviously is caused by dilution of the antiserum to the point at which there are too few antibody molecules present to produce a positive test.

The dilution of optimal proportions is that dilution in which the serologic reaction is visible in the shortest time. This usually occurs in and near the center of the equivalence zone. Therefore the optimal proportions dilution is a useful test prior to quantitative precipitation tests because is indicates the zone within which antigen dilutions should be made for the most precise estimation of the equivalence point. When different dilutions of antiserum are used and the optimal proportion for each is calculated, it is observed that the ratio of antigen to antibody is nearly constant. Thus an antigen diluted $1:100$ that precipitates with antibody at a $1:5$ dilution for optimal proportions will do so at dilutions of $1:200$ and $1:400$ with antibody diluted to $1:10$ and $1:20$, respectively; the optimal proportions ratio is constant at $40:1$ (antigen:antibody).

MECHANISM OF THE SEROLOGIC REACTION

Bordet proposed that the serologic reaction takes place in two phases. In the first phase combination of the reactants occurs; this is followed by the second phase, aggregation. The first stage takes place almost instantaneously, although there is no external evidence that combination has occurred. Proof that combination takes only a few moments is seen in the experiment in which bacteria and specific antibody are mixed and immediately pelleted in a centrifuge. Examination of the supernatant fluid will reveal that it is now devoid of specific immunoglobulin. Antigen and antibody can combine in the absence of electrolytes. Combination is the portion of the reaction wherein the major change in free energy occurs.

In the second stage of the reaction aggregation of antigen-immunoglobulin complexes occurs. This phase takes time, requires electrolytes, and involves very little change in free energy. This phase does not occur when monovalent antibodies or monovalent haptens are involved in the reaction. Marrack has explained, in his lattice hypothesis of serologic reactions, how aggregation develops the reaction into a visibly detectable complex. Moreover, Marrack's hypothesis convincingly portrays why aggregation fails when monovalent reactants are used. The lattice hypothesis, which is based on multivalent antigens and antibodies, is also useful in explaining the zone phenomena—prozone, equivalence zone, and postzone—that so often are noted in antibody titration tests.

Marrack developed his theory of serologic reactions on the assumption that antigen and antibody molecules unite through their specific determinant groups and that these groups have a special affinity for each other. This union of antigen with antibody is assumed to be a firm but dissociable combination. Aggregate formation consists of the dissociation and recombination of these molecules with each other until a reasonably stable network of alternating antigen and antibody molecules is formed. At the equivalence point all the antigen and all the antibody molecules are consumed in lattice formation. It should be noted that lattice formation with simple antigens, which do not contain more than 1 mole of a specific antigenic determinant per molecule, requires the presence of two different species of antibody in the antiserum, each directed against different antigenic sites (Fig. 13-1). When there is an excess of antibody (prozone), aggregation is not observed because, as an antibody dissociates from the antigen, there is a better chance for one of the free antibody molecules than for an antibody that already is attached to an antigen to combine with the original molecule of antigen (Fig. 13-2). Essentially the reverse situation occurs in postzone, where too little antibody is present to produce a complete reaction (Fig. 13-3).

In Marrack's hypothesis one can visualize how antigen-antibody complexes of unequal composition (varying proportion or multiple proportion) could occur, since aggregation of a multivalent antigen molecule would be possible when only

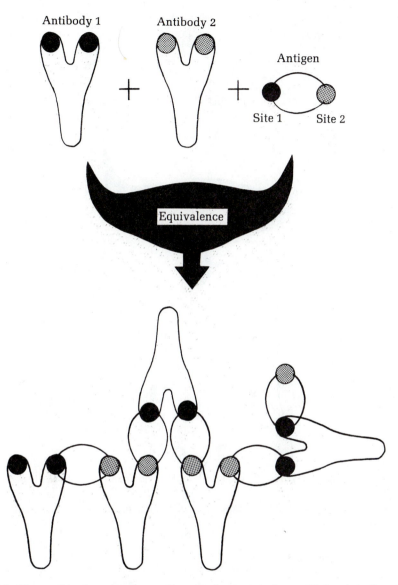

Fig. 13-1. The combination of antigen with antibody at equivalence. Notice that all molecules of both reactants are combined in the lattice and that, when an antigenic determinant occurs only once on an antigen molecule, two species of antibody are required for the reaction.

two or three of its valence sites are combined with antibody. The inability of monovalent haptens or antibodies to produce aggregation is also self-evident. Furthermore, if antibody is reacted with an excess of hapten so that all combining sites are saturated, there is no possibility for a hapten-conjugated antigen to combine and form a lattice with the antibody. This is the basis for the hapten inhibition reaction.

The use of antibody digests, especially Fab and $F(ab')_2$ fragments, has made it clear that it is the HV regions within these fragments which

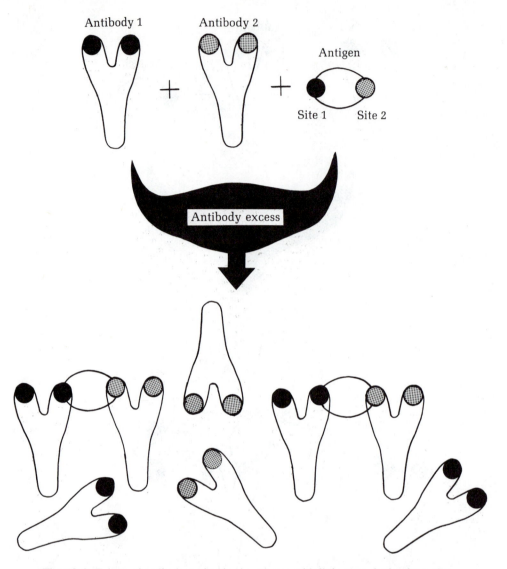

Fig. 13-2. Excess of antibody molecules in prozone with little or no lattice formation.

contain the antigen-binding activity. Indeed it is the unique amino acid sequences of these HV regions which provide antigen specificity to the immunoglobulins. These HV regions provide the physical and electrostatic notch in the Fab unit that conforms with the structure of an antigenic determinant in an antigen.

Although the combination of antigen or hapten with antibody may be firm, it is still dissociable and reversible. This is true of essentially all chemical reactions, but it is sometimes difficult to demonstrate for a specific chemical reaction in which the equilibrium constant is in favor of product formation. This is not true of serologic reactions, in which dissociation and recombination are fairly easy to demonstrate.

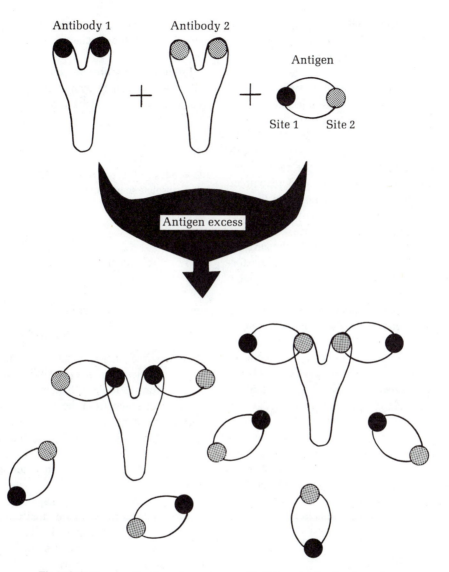

Fig. 13-3. Excess of antigen in postzone with little or no lattice formation.

The Danysz phenomenon illustrates the reversibility of serologic reactions. In 1902 Danysz established that certain proportions of toxin and antitoxin produced a neutral mixture under experimental conditions. Let us assume a neutral mixture consisted of 10 parts of toxin mixed with 10 parts of antitoxin held 10 minutes at room temperature before inoculating a test animal. Danysz found that, if he placed seven parts of toxin and three parts of antitoxin in one tube and three parts of toxin and seven parts of antitoxin in a second tube, held each at room temperature for 10 minutes, mixed the two tubes, and then immediately injected the experimental animal, the animal succumbed. If he waited an additional 10 minutes after mixing the tubes, the animal survived. To

Danysz and to immunologists since his time, this has meant that the antigen in the second tube bound with more antibody than needed to make a just neutral mixture, whereas in the first tube there was insufficient antitoxin to neutralize the toxin. A quickly prepared and injected mixture was toxic; this was a measure of the unfavorable balance in the first tube. But let an additional 10 minutes of incubation occur, and some of the antitoxin that saturated the toxin in the second tube had an opportunity to dissociate and recombine with the unneutralized toxin arising from the first tube. The result of this antitoxin shift was the formation of a neutral complex. Hence the Danysz phenomenon illustrates dissociation of the antigen-antibody complex and also demonstrates the formation of antigen-antibody complexes in variable proportions.

A more modern illustration of the reversibility of serologic reactions involves the addition of sheep red blood cells to hemolysin in proportions that bind all the hemolytic antibody. Complement, required for lysis of the erythrocytes by hemolysin, must be absent. Then ^{51}Cr-labeled sheep red blood cells are added, and incubation is continued. Complement then is added to initiate the lytic reaction. Only those cells coated with antibody will rupture. The unlysed cells are sedimented by centrifugation, and ^{51}Cr in the supernatant fluid is measured. This is evidence of the antibody shift to the labeled red cells added after all antibody had been bound initially to the unlabeled cells.

MATHEMATIC TREATMENT OF SEROLOGIC REACTIONS

The equilibrium constant for the reaction of a hapten with an antibody (or complete antigen with its antibody) can be handled mathematically like the calculation for the equilibrium constant in ordinary chemical reactions: hapten + antibody $\rightleftharpoons$ hapten — antibody complex (H + ABY $\rightleftharpoons$ H—ABY).
Therefore

$$K_H = \frac{(H—ABY)}{(H)(ABY)} \qquad (1)$$

where the parentheses refer to the actual concentrations of the reactants and product in moles per liter.

From the equilibrium constant one can also calculate the change in free energy ($\Delta F°$) of the reaction by the following formula

$$\Delta F° = -RT \ln K_H \qquad (2)$$

where

R = the standard gas constant (2.0 cal/mol/degree)
T = absolute temperature

Since

$$\ln K = 2.3 \times \log_b K$$

at 37° C this formula reduces to

$$\Delta F° = -1420 \log_{10} K_H$$

and at 5° C the formula is

$$\Delta F° = 1280 \log_{10} K_H$$

Thus the free energy made available by the reaction of 1 mole of hapten with 1 mole of antibody to form 1 mole of hapten-antibody complex can be calculated from measurement of the equilibrium constant. If the $\Delta F°$ value is negative, the reaction will proceed spontaneously to the right, and if $\Delta F°$ is positive, the reaction will proceed only if energy from an external source is applied.

Calculations of $\Delta F°$ for hapten-antibody reactions usually produce figures that range from -5 kcal/mole to -8.5 kcal/mole. The agreement of several studies that produced figures in this limited range suggests that these values will be typical of all antibodies. These $\Delta F°$ numbers are quite small compared with ordinary chemical reactions, which may be 10 times greater. This means only that the serologic reaction will proceed slowly, but spontaneously, to completion.

Comparison of the affinity of two different haptens for an antibody can be made on the basis of the $\Delta F°$ values of the separate reactions. Since these figures invariably will be very close to each other, the true similarity or difference of the two

Δ F° values (and thus of the haptens) is not always immediately obvious. These Δ F° values can be compared on a broader scale if Δ F$_{relative}$ is calculated from the following equation

$$\Delta F_{relative} = -RT \ln K_{relative} \qquad (3)$$

where R and T are as in formula 2 and K$_{relative}$ is the relative dissociation constant of the two separate hapten-antibody reactions. This is calculated from

$$K_{relative} = \frac{\text{Concentration of reference}}{\text{Concentration of hapten}} \qquad (4)$$
$$\frac{\text{hapten for a 50\% effect}}{\text{for a 50\% effect}}$$

Formula 4 represents an acceptable approximation of the true K$_{relative}$ based on the assumption that the concentration of total antibody is small compared with the concentration of total hapten in the serologic reaction. K$_{relative}$ is actually equal to $\frac{K_H}{K_{relative}}$, but formula 4 is a good approximation. The 50% effect may refer to inhibition by the hapten of precipitation by some antibody to a hapten-antigen conjugate, or it may refer to the quenching of 50% of an antibody's fluorescence by the hapten. The interpretation of K$_{relative}$ values is, of course, that numbers close to each other indicate that the two haptens are very closely related and that one can effectively replace the other. For example, an antibody to the *p*-azobenzoate group reacts with benzoate with K$_{relative}$ of 1.00. (This is the homologous reaction and is simultaneously the reference and experimental hapten.) K$_{relative}$ for the reaction when benzenearsonate is used as the hapten is less than 0.001; there is thus 1,000 times less binding of the arsonate to the benzoate antibody than benzoate itself. K$_{relative}$ for *p*-nitrobenzoate with the *p*-azobenzoate antibody is 11.5, indicating that it binds 11.5 times better with the azobenzoate antibody than does benzoate itself. This is considered evidence that the antibody-binding site recognizes the para NO$_2$ group as a reasonable facsimile of the diazo linkage of the immunizing hapten with its antigen carrier and that

some antibody was actually directed against that linkage group. In benzoic acid no substituent is present in the "attachment position," so the antibody does not bind quite so fully with it. Table 13-1 presents additional data for the *p*-azobenzoate antibody reactions with haptens.

From formula 1 one can derive the formula r/c = nK − rK, if it is assumed that all hapten-combining sites of the antibody have the same dissociation constant and each is uninfluenced by the combination of another site with hapten. In this formula, *r* = moles of hapten bound/mole of antibody, *c* = concentration of free hapten, and *n* = valence of antibody. This formula is that of a straight line whose intercept on the abscissa is n and whose intercept on the ordinate in nK. Deviations from linearity are known to occur. One of the causes for this is the heterogeneity of hapten-binding sites in antibodies. When representative data are plotted (Fig. 13-4), a straight line does not result, but extrapolation indicates an antibody valence of 2. This is the value obtained for IgG from many experiments. IgA has a valence of 2, and IgM has a valence of 10.

According to Fig. 13-4 the average dissociation constant, K$_0$, is taken as equal to the reciprocal of the hapten concentration where r = 1, that is, where there is an average of one hapten molecule per antibody molecule. At this point r/c = 1/c, and the reciprocal = c. For most hapten-antibody

Table 13-1. Combination of the *p*-azobenzoate antibody with various haptens

	K$_{relative}$	Δ F$_{relative}$ (cal)
Benzoate	1.0	0
p-Nitrobenzoate	11.5	
Benzenearsonate	<0.001	>13,800
Benzenesulfonate	<0.001	>13,800
p-Chlorobenzoate	2.8	−550
Phenylacetate	0.002	3,500

Data from Pressman, D., and Grossberg, A.L.: The structural basis of antibody specificity, New York, 1968, W.A. Benjamin, Inc.

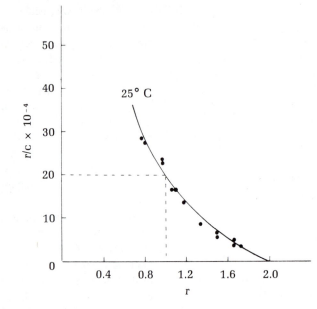

Fig. 13-4. Binding data indicate $r = 2$ (antibody valence of 2) and K_0, average dissociation constant of 20×10^{-4}. (Redrawn from Karush, F.: Immunologic specificity and molecular structure, Adv. Immunol. **2:**1, 1962.)

reactions K_0 approximates 10^5 liter/mole. This means that, at a hapten concentration of 1×10^{-5} M, the antibody is half saturated with hapten. This molar number is an indication of the avidity of the antibody. If an antibody were half-saturated by 10^{-10} M hapten, the hapten-antibody contact would be very permanent. If K_0 were 10^{-2} liter/mole, the antibody would not be very avid, and the antibody-hapten complex would dissociate very easily. In other words, a high concentration of free hapten is required to keep the antibody half saturated with hapten.

SEROLOGIC HETEROGENEITY OF THE IMMUNOGLOBULINS

The immunoglobulins do not participate with equal effectiveness in the several serologic reactions that are possible in vitro and in vivo. This has been determined by testing purified immunoglobulins and whole antisera with known immunoglobulin content in the different tests.

Table 13-2 summarizes the results of these studies.

IgG precipitates more rapidly and somewhat more efficiently than IgM or IgA. As might be expected from its valence, antigen excess is less apt to inhibit IgM precipitation than IgG precipitation. Several investigators have reported very little precipitating ability of IgM, and generally it is accepted that IgM is capable of, but is inefficient in, precipitation.

IgM is an excellent complement-fixing antibody. This is because of the fact that the first component of complement must attach to two Fc units to initiate the complement cascade. In IgM five Fc units are available in a single molecule. Fixation of complement by IgG molecules varies perceptibly with the subclass and is, in descending order, IgG3, IgG1, IgG2, and IgG4, with IgG4 binding but not activating the complement system. IgA and IgE do not fix complement.

IgM is a more efficient agglutinating antibody

Table 13-2. Serologic heterogeneity of the immunoglobulins

Serologic reaction	IgG	IgM	IgA
Precipitation	Strong	Weak	Variable
Agglutination	Weak	Strong	Positive
Hemagglutination	Weak	Strong	Positive
Complement fixation	Varies with subclass	Strong	No activity
Hemolysis and bacteriolysis	Weak	Strong	No activity
Virus neutralization	Positive	Positive	Positive
Toxin neutralization	Positive	Negative	Unknown

than IgG or IgA. It has been calculated that only 25 molecules of IgM are required for 50% erythrocyte agglutination, whereas over 19,000 IgG molecules are required. Quantitative agglutination tests have produced a range of values for the actual microgram quantities of these two immunoglobulins needed for bacterial agglutination, but consistently less IgM than IgG is required.

Lysis of erythrocytes by antibody, since it requires complement, would seem to favor that antibody which is most capable of fixing complement. It has been calculated that only two or three molecules of IgM are required for lysis of a red cell, and 200 to 300 molecules of IgG are needed for the same event. The differences in hemolytic activity of these two immunoglobulins are indicated earlier in the discussion of the Jerne plaque-forming center test.

Both IgG and IgM are capable of neutralizing the infectivity of viruses, but the toxicity of bacterial exotoxins is only feebly neutralized in the presence of IgM. Both IgG and IgM can participate in the Arthus reaction; however, since this is an in vivo precipitation reaction, one can presume that IgG is more active in this regard.

RELATIVE SENSITIVITY OF SEROLOGIC REACTIONS

Several in vitro and in vivo serologic reactions are available and useful in identifying antigens or antibodies. These reactions differ in their physical conditions and the requirement for external reagents such as white blood cells, serum complement, conglutinin, and test animals. Furthermore these tests may measure different molecular species of antibodies. Thus it is not surprising that these tests should differ significantly in their sensitivity for detecting antibody (Table 13-3).

One of the least sensitive tests is precipitation, and the fluid and gel tests are of approximately the same insensitivity. For a positive precipitation reaction 3 to 15 μg of antibody nitrogen per milliliter of serum is usually necessary, but some tests may require more. Several tests require only 0.01 to 1.0 μg of antibody nitrogen per milliliter; these include bacterial agglutination, toxin neutralization, complement fixation, passive cutaneous anaphylaxis, Schultz-Dale reaction, Prausnitz-Küstner (P-K) reaction, and flocculation tests for syphilis. Tests that require only 0.001 to 0.01 μg of antibody nitrogen per milliliter include hemolysis, RIA, enzyme immunoassay, conglutinating complement adsorption, bacteriolysis, and passive hemagglutination. Of these, passive hemagglutination, RIA, enzyme immunoassay, virus neutralization, hemolytic, and bacteriolytic tests often are cited as the most delicate. Naturally there is much variation with the exact procedure used, but under the most optimal conditions as little as 0.00001 μg of antibody nitrogen in 1 ml of antiserum may suffice to produce a positive reaction in these tests.

Table 13-3. Comparative sensitivity
of serologic tests

Serologic test	Positive test requires
Fluid precipitation	
Interfacial (ring) test	20 to 30 μg anti-body nitrogen/ml
Quantitative, colorimetric	3 to 10
Quantitative, nephelometric	0.5 to 3
Gel precipitation	
Double diffusion (Ouchterlony)	3 to 15
Single diffusion (Oudin)	12 to 110
Radial diffusion (Mancini)	3 to 10
Immunoelectrophoresis	50 to 200
Bacterial agglutination	0.01
Hemagglutination	
Direct	0.5 to 1.0
Passive (indirect)	0.001 to 0.03
Hemolysis	0.001 to 0.003
Complement fixation	0.01 to 0.1
Toxin neutralization (diphtheria)	0.01
Anaphylaxis, passive cutaneous	0.01 to 0.03
RIA, enzyme immunoassay	0.001 or less
Bacteriophage or virus neutralization	1 molecule of antibody
Immunocyte adherence	1 antibody-producing cell
Fluorescent antibody	1 antibody-producing cell
Jerne PFC	1 antibody-producing cell

SEROLOGIC REACTIONS IN VIVO

Students of medicine, dentistry, nursing, and related health sciences often are dismayed to find that very few of the serologic reactions which occur in vitro are known to occur in vivo. From this information these students often assume a negative attitude toward the importance of serology to immunity. It is true that bacterial agglutination, capsular swelling, passive agglutination, bacterial immobilization, precipitation, and other reactions occur only rarely in the animal body.

Those serologic reactions which do occur in vivo include bacteriolysis, neutralization, opsonization, and phagocytosis; these are all highly contributory to the well-being of the individual when the antigen is a pathogenic microbe or its toxic products. Although it must be admitted that immunity is not caused by these functions alone, these activities of the immunoglobulins are very important in immunity.

BIBLIOGRAPHY

Aloisi, R.M.: Principles of immunodiagnostics, St. Louis, 1979, The C.V. Mosby Co.

Chase, M.W., and Williams, C.A., editors: Methods in immunology and immunochemistry, vols. 1-5, New York, 1967-1975, Academic Press, Inc.

Friedman, H., Linna, T.J., and Prier, J.E., editors: Immunoserology in the diagnosis of infectious diseases, Baltimore, 1979, University Park Press.

Froese, A., and Sehon, A.H.: Kinetics of antibody-hapten reactions, Contemp. Top. Mol. Immunol. **4:**23, 1975.

Garvey, J.S., Cremer, N.E., and Sussdorf, D.H.: Methods in immunology, ed. 3, Reading, Mass., 1977, W.A. Benjamin, Inc.

Hudson, L., and Hay, F.C.: Practical immunology, ed. 2, Oxford, 1980, Blackwell Scientific Publications, Ltd.

Karush, F.: Multivalent binding and functional affinity, Contemp. Top. Mol. Immunol. **5:**217, 1976.

Lefkovits, I., and Pernis, B., editors: Immunological methods, vols. 1 and 2, New York, 1979 and 1981, Academic Press, Inc.

Macario, A.J.L., and de Macario, E.C.: Antigen-binding properties of antibody molecules; time-course dynamics and biological significance, Curr. Top. Microbiol. Immunol. **71:** 125, 1975.

Mayer, R.J., and Walker, J.H.: Immunochemical methods in the biological sciences: enzymes and proteins, London, 1980, Academic Press, Inc. (London), Ltd.

Metzger, H.: The effect of antigen on antibodies: recent studies, Contemp. Top. Mol. Immunol. **7:**119, 1978.

Milgrom, F., Abeyounis, C.J., and Kano, K., editors: Principles of immunological diagnosis in medicine, Philadelphia, 1981, Lea & Febiger.

Mishell, B.B., and Shiigi, S.M., editors: Selected methods in cellular immunology, San Francisco, 1980, W.H. Freeman & Co., Publishers.

Nakamura, R.M., Dito, W.R., and Tucker, E.S., III, editors: Immunoassays in the clinical laboratory, New York, 1979, Alan R. Liss, Inc.

Peacock, J.E., and Tomar, R.H.: Manual of laboratory immunology, Philadelphia, 1980, Lea & Febiger.

Rose, N.R., and Bigazzi, P.E.: Methods in immunodiagnosis, ed. 2, New York, 1980, John Wiley & Sons, Inc.

Rose, N.R., and Friedman, H., editors: Manual of clinical immunology, ed. 2, Washington, D.C., 1981, American Society for Microbiology.

Stansfield, W.D.: Serology and immunology: a clinical approach, New York, 1981, Macmillan, Inc.

Thompson, R.A., editor: Techniques in clinical immunology, ed. 2, Oxford, 1981, Blackwell Scientific Publications, Ltd.

Van Vunakis, H., and Langone, J.J., editors: Immunochemical techniques, parts A and B. In Colowick, S.P., and Kaplan, N.O., editors: Methods in enzymology, vol. 70, New York, 1980, Academic Press, Inc.

Vollmer, A., Bartlett, A., and Bidwell, D., editors: Immunoassays for the 80s, Baltimore, 1981, University Park Press.

Ward, A.M., and Whicher, J.T., editors: Immunochemistry in clinical laboratory medicine, Baltimore, 1979, University Park Press.

Weir, D.M., editor: Handbook of experimental immunology, ed. 3, Oxford, 1978, Blackwell Scientific Publications, Ltd.

RADIOIMMUNOASSAY, ENZYME IMMUNOASSAY, AND OTHER BINDING REACTIONS

GLOSSARY

antiglobulin test A test to determine the presence of a globulin with an antibody to that globulin, as by fluorescent antibody to γ-globulin.

EIA Enzyme immunoassay.

ELISA Enzyme-linked immunosorbent assay.

Enzyme-linked immunosorbent assay A serologic test in which one reagent is labeled with an enzyme.

FAB Fluorescent antibody.

ferritin-labeled antibody An immunoglobulin conjugated to ferritin for use in electron microscopy.

fluorescence quenching Reduction in fluorescence of an antibody molecule when combined with a hapten or antigen.

fluorescent antibody An immunoglobulin conjugated to a fluorescent dye for use in ultraviolet microscopy.

immune complex A complex of antigen with antibody, perhaps including complement, which may be soluble or deposit on tissues.

protein A A protein on the surface of *Staphylococcus aureus* that binds IgG.

radioimmunoassay An immunologic test using radio-labeled antigen, antibody, complement, or other reactants; may be adapted to radioimmunodiffusion, radioprecipitation, etc.

RIA Radioimmunoassay.

solid phase radioimmunoassay A radioimmunoassay in which one of the reactants is bound to a surface.

In certain systems the serologic reaction cannot proceed to its second, or aggregative, phase, as, for example, when haptens are used. Haptens by definition consist of but a single antigenic determinant and, since they lack a multivalent character, do not fulfill the conditions of serologic valence needed to establish the serologic lattice work. On the other hand, some antisera contain high levels of antibodies, referred to as monovalent, incomplete, or blocking antibodies, which fail to aggregate with antigen, and this is typical of normal IgE molecules. It is a known property of IgE to combine with antigens or haptens in vitro but to be unable to continue into agglutination, precipitation, complement fixation, etc. Even though the reasons for this remain enigmatic, the presence of high levels of IgE or IgE-like immunoglobulins in a serum does much to explain the prozone phenomenon and the blocking antibody effect. Blocking antibodies are those which, by binding to an antigen, block the attachment of other antibodies or cells with the antigen receptors. Blocking antibody used in this sense is an incomplete antibody and in unable to aggregate the antigen.

Under certain circumstances deliberate efforts to prevent development of the aggregative portion of the serologic reaction can be rewarding. When expensive reagents are used, it is obviously economic to use the reactants at the greatest dilution possible. When this is the case, the reaction is rarely detectable with the unaided eye. Reliance must be placed on sophisticated instrumentation or serologic procedures to note that the reaction has occurred. Frequently this involves the use of labeled haptens, antigens, or antibodies. Methods used to detect antigen or antibody binding in the absence of aggregation are described in this chapter.

TRADITIONAL HAPTEN REACTIONS

Since the reaction of a hapten with its antibody cannot progress through the aggregation phase and become directly visible, serologic tests for hapten-antibody interaction are dependent entirely on changes that occur in the first, or combination, phase of the serologic reaction. Fortunately this combination can be measured accurately and sensitively by several methods. Classically this has been done by measuring the influence the hapten may have on the aggregation of the antihapten with the hapten-antigen conjugate, that is, the hapten inhibition test. The hapten inhibition test has been superceded by other more sensitive tests such as equilibrium dialysis, fluorescence quenching, and labeled hapten binding; also, other procedures such as electron spin resonance and fluorescence polarization are being developed.

In the hapten inhibition test increasing quantities of hapten are mixed with an appropriate (constant) amount of antibody or antiserum and incubated prior to the addition of a fixed amount of hapten-antigen conjugate. After a second incubation the extent of the inhibition by hapten can be calculated. The hapten inhibition reaction has been criticized on several grounds, including the

difference in the composition of the aggregate in the presence of hapten and the conversion of the system to one of great antigen excess when sufficient hapten has combined with antibody. Although this technique permitted Landsteiner and others to originate many ideas about hapten-immunoglobulin interactions that are still valid today, methods that quantitate the hapten-antibody reaction in the absence of complete antigen are preferred.

One of the most widely applied alternative reactions is equilibrium dialysis, from which the equilibrium constant of the hapten-antibody system can be determined. The experimental arrangement for equilibrium dialysis requires the placement of the antibody (antiserum or its globulin fraction) within a dialysis membrane. This filled dialysis bag is placed in a container filled with a solution of the hapten. The concentration of the hapten in this solution must be known. During the incubation that follows the hapten is able to diffuse freely across the dialysis membrane, but the antibody, because of its larger size, cannot. When equilibrium has been reached, the concentration of hapten inside and outside the dialysis bag is determined. These measurements are corrected for nonspecific binding by the dialysis membrane and normal γ-globulin solutions; the binding is determined by simultaneously conducting appropriate controls. The increase in the concentration of hapten inside the dialysis tube, compared with its concentration outside the tube, is a measure of the hapten actually bound by the antibody and held inside the dialysis membrane. Relatively simple calculations allow this information to be converted into K_0, the average dissociation constant, and provide direct proof that a hapten-antibody reaction has occurred.

A simpler and more rapid procedure that will yield the same information is the fluorescence-quenching technique. Nearly all proteins fluoresce when activated by ultraviolet light at or near the absorption maximum of phenylalanine, tyrosine, and tryptophan—between 280 and 350 nm. However, the fluorescent light emitted is at 350 nm;

so the preferred choice of excitation light is at or near 280 nm. When an antibody molecule combines with a hapten, its fluorescence is quenched, presumably by a transfer of its excitation energy to the hapten rather than into light energy. This quenching of fluorescence is easily quantitated in a spectrofluorometer. The extent of this quenching is mathematically relatable to the quantity of hapten bound and thus can be treated to derive an association constant of the antibody. One distinct limitation to this method is the requirement for purified antibody solutions. Certain haptens do not absorb the excitation energy very easily and thus are poor quenchers.

RADIOIMMUNOASSAY (RIA)

One of the most active areas of immunologic research in the recent past has been the development of RIAs. The impetus for this stemmed from the pioneer work of Berson and Yalow in the middle 1950s. These investigators were interested in diabetes and believed that diabetic individuals might eliminate insulin too rapidly from their bodies, thus creating a hormonal insufficiency. To test this, they injected radiolabeled insulin into normal and diabetic subjects. Contrary to their hypothesis they observed that the insulin was retained longer in the blood of diabetics. Further studies revealed that this was caused by the presence of insulin antibodies in diabetics as a result of insulin injections used in the treatment of their disease. When a combination of radiolabeled and unlabeled insulin was injected, it was noted that the unlabeled hormone competitively inhibited antibody binding by the labeled hormone. When this information was translated from those in vivo experiments to in vitro conditions, the basis for the development of RIA tests for many antigens and haptens was founded.

The arrangement of most RIAs establishes a competition of a known amount of radiolabeled antigen (or hapten) and an unknown amount of the same unlabeled antigen with a limited, standard amount of antibody. The amount of antibody used is determined by an earlier titration with

labeled antigen and is usually the amount of antibody or antiserum that will bind 70% of the antigen; however, a simpler mathematic explanation of the reaction based on 100% binding is used here. If it is assumed that only the IgG class of antibody is involved in the reaction, then 100 molecules of immunoglobulin will bind 200 molecules of antigen (hapten), since each IgG molecule has two binding sites. If a mixture of 200 molecules of radiolabeled antigen and 200 molecules of unlabeled antigen is incubated with the 100 molecules of IgG, it is obvious that half the radiolabeled antigen will be displaced from the antibody, creating a bound:free ratio of 1:1 (Fig. 14-1). Thus in any experimental determination that results in a 50% diminution in binding of the radiolabeled antigen, the concentration of the unknown sample is exactly the same as that of the known. It follows logically that other bound-versus-free ratios of antigen could be used to determine other concentrations of the unknown antigen.

A critical part of any RIA is clearly the problem of distinguishing between the bound and free portions of the labeled antigen (hapten). If the antigen precipitates with the antibody, the unbound molecules can be removed simply by washing the precipitate. The difference in the amount of radiolabel added and that recovered in the precipitate is then the amount of free antigen. As a matter of practical application, RIA tests of this type usually are not performed. RIA tests are conducted more frequently with nonprecipitating haptens, or for reasons of economy, with antigen or antibody solutions diluted beyond their capacity to form a visible reaction. Under these conditions some physicochemical method must be used to separate the bound and free haptens.

There are at least a dozen different methods that can be used to separate antibody-bound antigens and free antigens, some of which are applicable only to certain antigens and some of which are wasteful, offer poor recovery of the antigen, or have other disadvantages.

When the antigen is of low molecular weight, or when a hapten is used, advantage can be taken

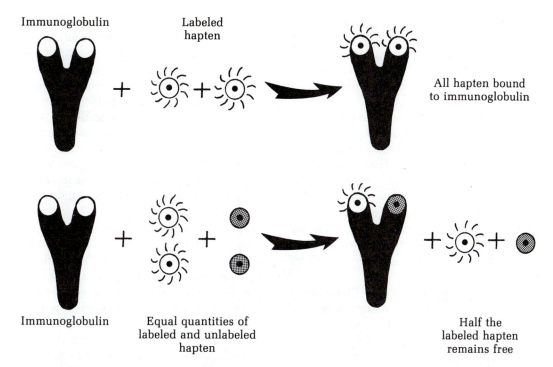

Fig. 14-1. In a preliminary titration prior to the RIA test the amount of radiolabeled hapten (or antigen) that will react with a standard amount of antibody is determined. In this example two parts of hapten saturate one part of immunoglobulin. To determine the amount of hapten in a solution of unknown concentration, it is added to two parts of labeled hapten and one part of immunoglobulin. After the reaction is complete, if one finds that half the labeled hapten is bound to the antibody and half is free, then the unknown solution contained two parts of hapten.

of the insolubility of immunoglobulins in 50% saturated ammonium sulfate to separate the free from the immunoglobulin-bound hapten. After the competition between a known amount of labeled and an unknown amount of unlabeled antigen has reached equilibrium, the mixture is adjusted to 50% saturation with ammonium sulfate. This precipitates the antibody and its bound antigen but leaves the unbound antigen in solution. Counting the radioisotope content of the precipitate and subtracting this from the amount of isotope added indicates how much labeled antigen was displaced, which is the amount of unlabeled antigen present in the unknown. Precipitants other than ammonium sulfate may be used; other sulfate salts and ethanol are examples. The only restriction is that

they must not precipitate the free antigen nor affect any dissociation of the bound antigen from the antibody.

A second method of precipitating soluble antibody-antigen complexes is by the double antibody procedure, or antiglobulin method, sometimes referred to as an "immunologic sandwich." In this form of RIA testing it is necessary to know the species origin of the primary antibody being used in the assay and to have a secondary antibody that will precipitate that species of γ-globulin. If the competitive binding portion of the assay uses a rabbit antibody, the experimenter needs an antibody against rabbit γ-globulin to complete the test. If the original antiserum is of goat origin, then an antibody against goat γ-globulin is needed. The primary antibody and its bound antigen are precipitated by the antiglobulin. The primary immunoglobulin serves both as an antibody and as an antigen and is the "meat" of the sandwich. Unbound antigen is not affected by the secondary antibody and remains in solution.

There is nothing mysterious about the ability of a γ-globulin to serve as an antigen. It meets all the criteria of an antigen when injected into a foreign species. γ-Globulins contain antigenic determinants in their Fab and Fc portions, and the combination of the Fab portions with an antigen does not sterically block the attachment of antibodies to the Fc determinants. Advantage of this is taken in other double antibody procedures, in the Coombs tests, and in histochemical precipitation.

An innovative approach to the harvesting of soluble antigen-antibody complexes has been the use of protein A. This protein is present on the surface of certain strains of *Staphylococcus aureus,* where it is covalently linked with the peptidoglycan support structure of the cell wall. Protein A has been isolated from lysed preparations of *S. aureus* and identified as a single peptide of 42,000 mol wt that contains several regions of internal amino acid homology. A unique biologic characteristic of protein A is its ability to combine and precipitate with IgG from several species. This reaction is specific for human IgG subclasses 1, 2, and 4, with two molecules of immunoglobulin binding to one molecule of protein A. This binding occurs in the Fc domain of the IgG molecule, which enables protein A to bind with IgG that already has combined with antigen. Since protein A does not bind with free antigens, soluble protein A, protein A attached to insoluble particles, or even intact *S. aureus* can be used to insolubilize antigen-antibody complexes as a substitute for an antiglobulin technique.

A third method of RIA is the one used most frequently and generally is referred to as a solid phase RIA. In this variation the antibody already is provided or converted to an insoluble form. In one form of the test the antibody is allowed to attach by physical adsorption to the inner surface of polystyrene assay tubes or wells in a plate. A known amount of the labeled antigen and an unknown quantity of unlabeled antigen are added. After an incubation period the unreacted reagents are rinsed from the wells, and the amount of isotope bound to the well is determined. Any decrease from the amount expected (added) is an index of the quantity of antigen in the unknown. Titrations with known quantities of the competing unlabeled antigen should be conducted to establish a standard curve and simplify subsequent calculations.

Covalent linkage of the antibody to an insoluble carrier might be preferred, since this precludes dissociation of the antibody from the carrier. This is accomplished by coupling the antibody to cellulose, Sepharose, or Sephadex or embedding it in porous glass beads or polyacrylamide particles as the solid phase support. The cross-linked dextrans (Sephadex or Sepharose) and porous glass entrap the large antibody molecules within their matrix yet still permit the entry and exit of smaller molecules by simple diffusion. After equilibrium is reached, centrifugation separates the bound antigen from the free.

Regardless of the exact RIA procedure used, the great advantage of all RIAs is their sensitivity. Commercially available RIA kits may detect as little as one nanogram (a billionth of a gram) or a picogram (10^{-12} gram, or a trillionth of a gram) of antigen. This is obviously of great significance in monitoring or determining the blood level of certain hormones or therapeutic agents that seldom exceed a few micrograms per milliliter. RIA procedures have the disadvantage of relatively great expense in terms of both the reagents and radioisotope-counting equipment and the unavoidable hazards associated with radioisotopes. These features obviously have not been a serious handicap to the clinical application of RIA. RIA procedures are currently in use for monitoring cardiovascular function, reproductive functions, hematopoietic function, and various other metabolic functions and are available for the quantitation of opiates, barbiturates, amphetamines, and other abused drugs (Table 14-1). Detection of hepatitis-associated antigen is another important application of RIA (Reading 4).

For RIA tests not all radioisotopes are of equal utility. Many isotopes have a half-life of only a few days, and any serologic reagent incorporating

Table 14-1. A partial list of biologically important substances measured by RIA

Follicle-stimulating hormone (FSH)	Digoxin
Adrenocorticotropic hormone (ACTH)	Digitoxin
Human chorionic gonadotropin (HCG)	Renin
Pituitary human growth hormone (HGH)	Vitamin A
Luteinizing hormone (LH)	Folic acid
Luteinizing hormone release factor (LHRF)	Hageman factor
Thyroid-stimulating hormone (TSH)	cAMP
Human placental lactogen (HPL)	cGMP
Melanocyte-stimulating hormone (MSH)	Plasmin
Parathyroid hormone (PTH)	Trypsin
Calcitonin (CT)	Chymotrypsin
Insulin	Carboxypeptidase
Glucagon	Elastase
Oxytocin	Hepatitis virus
Vasopressin	Mouse leukemia virus
Prolactin	CEA
Gastrin	AFP
Secretin	AHP
Bradykinin	Properdin
Cholecystokinin (CCK)	C1 esterase
Thyroxine (T_4)	C1q
Triiodothyronine (T_3)	Fibrinogen
Corticosteroids	IgG
Estrogens	IgE
Androgens	Myelin basic protein (MBP)
Prostaglandin	Cholera toxin

them would have too brief a shelf life to be of much use. Isotopes of iodine—^{125}I (half-life, 57.5 days) and ^{131}I (half-life, 8 days)—are the two most frequently used isotopes in immunology. Advantages of their use include the ease of in vitro labeling, which allows for labeling of a predetermined activity, and, in the case of ^{131}I, the emission of γ-rays of relatively high energy. ^{125}I and tritium labels are preferred for autoradiography because of the lower energy of their emission, which permits a more exact identification of the isotopes' location.

ENZYME-LINKED IMMUNOSORBENT ASSAYS (ELISA)

The expense, intrinsic hazards, and instability of the reagents used in RIAs have spurred a search for other labels that could be used with serologic reagents—haptens, antigens, and antibodies. Several nonisotopic labels have been employed, including active bacteriophage, free radical, or spin labels, fluorescent dyes, and enzymes. The advantages offered by enzyme-linked immunosorbent assays (ELISA) are those of most antibody-labeled reactions and include specificity, sensitivity, rapidity, inexpensiveness, and safety. These advantages suggest that ELISA may replace RIA for many analyses.

Since the enzyme label is the critical portion of enzyme immunoassay methods, its selection is very important. The primary criteria are that the enzyme be stable under the conditions used for storage, cross-linking, and assay, have a high specific activity or substrate turnover number, and be inexpensive. Equally important is that the enzyme must be absent from the antigen or antiserum preparation to be used in the serologic tests; otherwise false positive tests would result. False negative results could stem from the presence of enzyme inhibitors or inactivators in the serologic reagents. Appropriate controls must be incorporated into the tests to identify these potential problems in ELISA.

At least nine different enzymes have been used in ELISA (Table 14-2). These are horseradish

Table 14-2. Enzymes employed in enzyme immunoassay

Enzyme	Source	Molecular weight
Peroxidase	Horseradish	40,000
Alkaline phosphatase	*Escherichia coli*	80,000
Glucose oxidase	*Aspergillus niger*	160,000
Lysozyme	Egg white	14,400
Malate dehydrogenase	Pig heart	70,000
β-Galactosidase	*Escherichia coli*	540,000
G6PD	*Leuconostoc mesenteroides*	104,000
Acetylcholinesterase	*Electrophorus electricus* (electric eel)	260,000

peroxidase, alkaline phosphatase from *Escherichia coli* or calf intestinal mucosa, glucose oxidase and glucoamylase from fungal sources, egg white lysozyme, malate dehydrogenase from pig heart mitochondria, β-galactosidase from *E. coli*, glucose-6-phosphate dehydrogenase (G6PD) from *Leuconostoc mesenteroides,* and acetylcholinesterase from the electric eel. Peroxidase and alkaline phosphatase have been the most widely used, but lysozyme and G6PD are available in commercial preparations. Certain preparations of peroxidase seem not to cross-link well or to dimerize spontaneously, with a resultant low recovery of enzyme activity in the labeled antibody molecule. One advantage of lysozyme, in addition to its stability, is its low molecular weight (14,400); so several molecules can be attached to each immunoglobulin molecule without fear of problems related to steric hindrance. This also minimizes steric hindrance of the antigen-antibody reaction by enzyme, since its size is small compared with that of the antibody molecule.

Glutaraldehyde is a common cross-linker used to join the enzyme to the antigen or antibody. The reaction proceeds through the dialdehyde portion of the molecule and amino groups on the reactants. A unique and valuable aspect of the glutaraldehyde-peroxidase reaction is that only one aldehyde group attaches to the enzyme so that peroxidase-peroxidase dimers are rarely formed. Dimaleimide, another cross-linker, bridges proteins through their — SH groups, and

even though the native structure of the antigen may lack this group, it often can be introduced into the antigen. Other bifunctional reagents used are toluene 2,4-diisocyanate, tetrazotized *o*-dianisidine, difluorodinitrophenyl derivatives, and substituted carbodiimides (Fig. 14-2). Several enzyme conjugates have proved stable for at least a year. Here it must be remembered that the half-life of ^{131}I is only 8 days.

The conjugate of enzyme with antigen or of enzyme with antibody must be separated from unreacted molecules or from the homodimers formed during the cross-linking step. This depends almost entirely on size differences among the reaction products and is accomplished by filtration through membranes of selected pore size or by molecular sieving chromatography. For example, lysozyme labeling of a purified immunoglobulin preparation would produce free lysozyme, lysozyme-lysozyme, lysozyme-immunoglobulin, immunoglobulin-immunoglobulin, and free immunoglobulin as the hypothetical end products. The use of an excess of lysozyme and cross-linking reagents would be expected to reduce the amount of immunoglobulin left unreacted. Filtration through a membrane with a pore size of 50,000 would allow the excess lysozyme and lysozyme-lysozyme dimers to pass but would retain the larger molecules. Then a filter with a pore size near 200,000 could be used to allow the desired conjugate to pass and to retain the immunoglobulin-immunoglobulin dimers. By collecting those fractions with

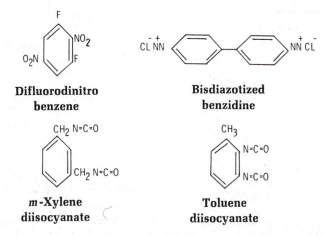

Fig. 14-2. Divalent coupling reagents used for ELISA and ferritin-labeled antibody procedures. Under ideal conditions one molecule of coupling reagent is simultaneously attached to one molecule of enzyme or ferritin and one molecule of antibody.

enzyme activity which are eluted from a molecular sieving column and selecting only that one with antibody activity, one can separate the enzyme-linked antibody from the unwanted molecules.

Enzyme activity generally is determined spectrophotometrically. Alkaline phosphatase is easily determined by the color change associated with cleavage of p-nitrophenylphosphate as the substrate. The oxidizing activity of the H_2O_2 formed by glucose oxidase is its measure of concentration. Peroxidase is measured by its ability to change the color of o-dianisidine. Other enzymes have equally simple colorimetric or spectrophotometric quantitation methods. Thus, if an enzyme-labeled antibody is bound serologically to a solid phase antigen contained in a tube, it is only necessary to add the enzyme substrate in a suitable buffer and follow spectrophotometrically the appearance of the enzyme end product within a specific time period. This quantitates the amount of enzyme present and the amount of antigen. A decrease in the amount of bound enzyme activity created by preincubation of free antigen with the labeled antibody is then a reflection of the amount of free antigen in an unknown solution.

ELISA methods may be even more sensitive than RIA methods (Table 14-3). In the latter, when the radionuclide emits the γ or β particle, it is then less radioactive or inactive and cannot be measured again as a radioisotope. In ELISA the enzyme catalyzes a change in a substrate molecule, but the enzyme itself is not consumed in this process. The enzyme molecule continues to act on more substrate molecules and in the form of the end products produced can give off literally thousands of signals of its presence. Thus in ELISA antigens and haptens are detectable when present in only nanogram and picogram quantities.

Four forms of enzyme immunoassay have been developed: the competitive binding test, the immunoenzymometric test, the sandwich method for antigen or antibody, and the homogeneous enzyme immunoassay. Only the competitive binding test is properly referred to as the ELISA procedure. The ELISA test was the first to be developed and is patterned exactly after the standard competitive RIA procedure. Labeled and unlabeled antigens compete for attachment to a limited quantity of solid phase antibody. The enzyme label that is displaced is quantitated, and the calculations that follow are essentially the same as in RIA procedures.

Table 14-3. A partial list of biologically important substances measured by enzyme immunoassay

Antigen or hapten	Enzyme label
Human serum albumin	Glucose oxidase
CEA	Alkaline phosphatase
AFP	Alkaline phosphatase, glucose oxidase, peroxidase
Haptoglobin	Alkaline phosphatase
IgE	Alkaline phosphatase
IgG	Alkaline phosphatase, glucose oxidase, peroxidase, β-galactosidase
Insulin	Alkaline phosphatase, peroxidase, β-galactosidase
Human placental lactogen	Peroxidase
Estrogens	Peroxidase
Chorionic gonadotropin	Peroxidase, acetylcholinesterase
Progesterone	β-Galactosidase
Digoxin	G6PD
Morphine	Lysozyme, malate dehydrogenase
Thyrotropin	Alkaline phosphatase
α_2-Globulins	Peroxidase
Cortisol	β-Galactosidase
Cholera toxin	Alkaline phosphatase
Streptolysin O	Glucose oxidase
Hepatitis B virus	Peroxidase
κ or λ L chains	Alkaline phosphatase
Hog cholera virus	Peroxidase
Rubella virus	Alkaline phosphatase
Malarial parasites	Alkaline phosphatase
Amphetamine	Lysozyme
Phenobarbital	G6PD
Methadone	Lysozyme

In the immunoenzymometric procedure an unknown quantity of antigen is reacted with an excess of labeled antibody, and then solid phase antigen is added. Centrifugation removes the unreacted enzyme-linked antibody molecules. Then enzyme actively associated with the soluble phase is measured, and this is an expression of the antigen concentration in the unknown sample.

The sandwich technique relies on the multivalence of antigen and its capacity to bind simultaneously with two molecules of antibody. The first antibody molecule is a solid phase reactant. It is used in excess to ensure binding of all the antigen molecules in the unknown sample. After this reaction is completed, an enzyme-labeled antibody is added and incubated with the complex resulting from the first phase. The labeled antibody now combines with the available determinants on the antigen. Excess antibody is removed by washing, and enzyme activity is determined (Fig. 14-3). As before, the amount of enzyme bound to the complex is an indirect expression of the amount of antigen in the sample. This procedure is also commonly described as an ELISA technique.

The homogeneous enzyme immunoassay system does not require a solid phase reactant. It relies on an inhibition of enzyme activity by combination of antibody with an enzyme-labeled antigen or hapten. This does not occur with all systems but is of regular enough occurrence to be a valuable serologic method for measuring haptens. Enzyme inhibition is presumed to occur because of steric effects. When the hapten is surrounded by the immunoglobulin, the enzyme is masked from its substrate.

The parallels between ELISA and RIA are apparent, and the simplicity and economy of the former indicate that ELISA may largely replace RIA in the future (Fig. 14-4).

FLUORESCENT ANTIBODY METHODS

Fluorescent antibodies (FAB), or, more accurately, the γ-globulin fraction of antisera, are antibody preparations that are chemically coupled to a fluorescent dye. The conjugation of the reactants is performed so that the serologic activity and specificity of the γ-globulin and the fluorescent character of the dyes are preserved in a single molecule. Efforts to label antibodies with visually detectable carriers are more than 50 years old. The first reagents were antibodies complexed with

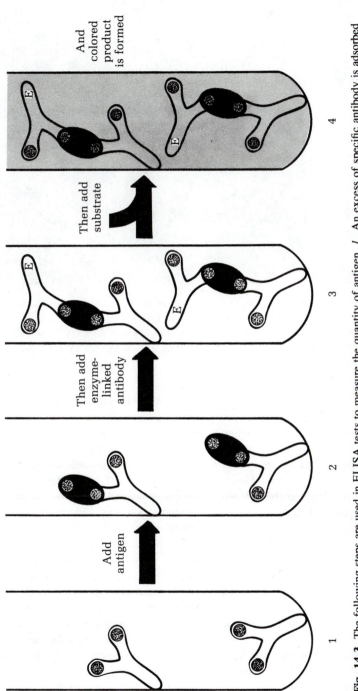

Fig. 14-3. The following steps are used in ELISA tests to measure the quantity of antigen. *1*, An excess of specific antibody is adsorbed to the vessel surface. *2*, The antigen is added and allowed to react with the antibody. *3*, Thereafter an enzyme-linked antibody is allowed to react with the antigen. *4*, When the enzyme substrate is added, the color of the enzyme product (*E*) is quantitated spectrophotometrically. The amount of color is proportional to the amount of antigen present.

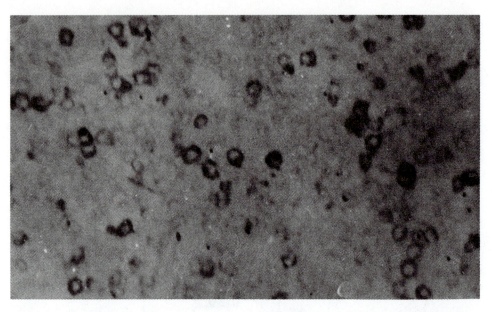

Fig. 14-4. The dark rings seen in this photograph represent the end product of an ELISA test in which a horseradish peroxidase–labeled antibody to human IgG was used to stain a preparation of lymphocytes. The enzyme substrate used was *o*-dianisidine, which forms an insoluble black product when oxidized. In the background the faint outline of cells that do not bear IgG on their surface is barely visible. (Courtesy Dr. E. Adelstein.)

azodyes, but little in the way of practical results came from their preparation and use. No true success was achieved until the early 1940s, when Coons developed the fluorescent antibody method.

The fluorescent technique makes use of special dyes referred to as fluors or fluorochromes. Fluors are chemical substances that are capable of absorbing a short wavelength of light and instantaneously emitting a longer wavelength light. The dyes used for fluorescent antibody absorb in the ultraviolet and short blue range (200 to 400 nm) and emit a visible light. The exact absorption spectrum of the fluor and that of its emitted light are characteristic for each fluor. The color of the emitted light is not a characteristic of the excitation light.

The fluorochromes usually chosen are fluorescein, a rhodamine such as lissamine rhodamine B, and 1-dimethylaminonaphthalene-5 sulfonic acid (DANSYL) (Fig. 14-5). One or another

of these is chosen because, although each fluoresces with high efficiency, a proper color is needed to avoid confusion with the blue-gray autofluorescence of tissues. Fluorescein and DANSYL give off a green or yellow-green light, and rhodamine gives off an orange-red hue. All three are easily bonded to the free amino groups of the antibody molecule. Fluorescein ordinarily is purchased in the form of fluorescein isothiocyanate, which forms a thiocarbamido linkage with amino groups of protein. Rhodamines and DANSYL more often are prepared as sulfonyl chlorides, which form sulfonamido bonds with proteins. Since free amino groups of lysine are not especially critical to the activity of the antibody, the covalent bonding of these ligands does not destroy the antibody activity unless carried to excess.

The antibody preparation to be labeled should be a purified γ-globulin preparation, since most fluors will label albumin and even α- and β-glob-

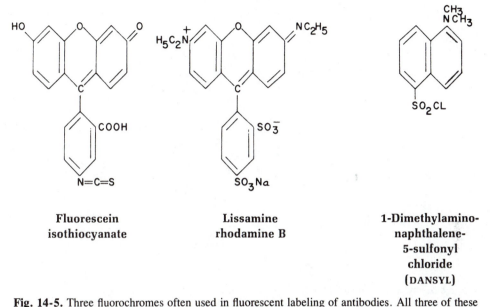

Fluorescein
isothiocyanate

Lissamine
rhodamine B

1-Dimethylamino-
naphthalene-
5-sulfonyl
chloride
(DANSYL)

Fig. 14-5. Three fluorochromes often used in fluorescent labeling of antibodies. All three of these compounds couple to the amino groups of proteins. Under ultraviolet illumination fluorescein and DANSYL emit a green or yellow-green light and rhodamine a red-orange light.

ulins much better than γ-globulins. Unless these serum proteins are excluded, the fluorescent antibody preparation will suffer from the dual handicap of low fluorescence and nonspecific staining by the other labeled serum proteins. The precipitation, agglutination, or some other serologic titer of the γ-globulin fraction of the antiserum should be determined before and after labeling. The immunofluorescent behavior of an antiserum is not dependent exclusively on its precipitation or other titer, since monovalent antibodies also function as fluorescent antibodies; but it is important to know if a great loss of antibody activity occurred during the labeling procedure. Specific labeling directions will differ slightly for different fluors and generally are based on specific dye/protein ratios. Careful adherence to the directions is necessary to avoid losses of antibody activity and nonspecific staining caused by overlabeling. Unreacted fluor can be removed by gel filtration or dialysis. Dilutions of the labeled antibody then should be tested on known preparations to determine its ac-

tivity and nonspecificity. Fluorescent antibody preparations with a high nonspecific background staining may be absorbed repeatedly with dried acetone powders of animal tissues to improve their quality. Background staining of tissue preparations with labeled albumin or simple dyes such as Evans blue or Congo red will quench nonspecific staining and improve contrast.

Fluorescence microscopy is more demanding than ordinary light microscopy, since objects are always much dimmer. A conventional microscope of good quality can be used. There is no need for quartz optics, even though an ultraviolet light source is used. The usual physical arrangement is depicted in Fig. 14-6. A high-pressure lamp emitting ultraviolet and short blue light is needed. The light is filtered by the primary filter to remove light longer than 450 to 500 nm. Heat filters usually are required because of the intensity of the mercury lamp. A front-surfaced mirror diverts the light into the condensor. A darkfield condensor is preferred, because it is easier to see a

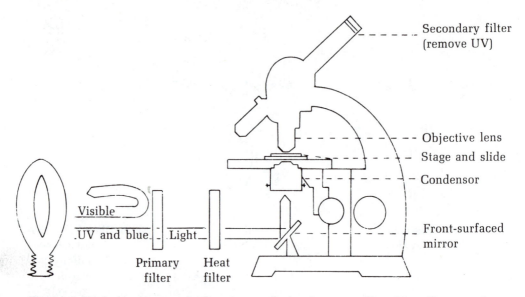

Visible
UV and blue . Light
Primary
filter
Heat
filter

Secondary filter
(remove UV)

Objective lens
Stage and slide
Condensor

Front-surfaced
mirror

Fig. 14-6. Physical arrangement for fluorescent antibody microscopy. The primary filter transmits only ultraviolet *(UV)* and blue light. Heat rays are removed by the heat filter, and the light is diverted into the darkfield condensor by a front-surfaced mirror. Visible light emitted by fluorescent-labeled materials passes through the tube of the microscope, where a secondary filter removes stray ultraviolet light rays. Quartz optics are not required.

point of colored light on a black field than against a bright white background. When the light coming through the condensor strikes the fluorescent antibody on the specimen slide, the fluor emits a visible light. This visible light, mixed with some ultraviolet light rays, progresses up the tube of the microscope to the observer. A secondary filter is used to remove the damaging ultraviolet light. Since the objects are often only faintly visible, this technique should be performed in a darkened room. For the same reason a monocular microscope may be preferred on some occasions.

Fluorescent antibodies are specific histochemical reagents capable of reacting with and identifying specific antigens. The antigen is fixed to an ordinary microscope slide. Impression smears, thin tissue sections, or alcohol-fixed bacterial smears may be used. In the direct fluorescent antibody procedure the labeled antibody is flooded onto the slide and allowed to react with the antigen. Gentle washing will remove the uncombined

antibody. The slide is dried and placed under the microscope. Wherever fluorescence is noted, one can be confident that the antigen is present, provided appropriate controls have been applied. The most suitable control is the blocking test. In the blocking test the antigen preparation first is reacted with an unlabeled portion of antiserum. Combination of this antiserum with the antigen will prevent the combination of the subsequently applied fluorescent antibody.

The blocking reaction is important from two aspects: it provides the most useful control for the direct test, and it provides a method of demonstrating antibody in a serum without the effort, time, and expense of attaching a fluor to each serum specimen. Thus the blocking test itself becomes a useful tool for identifying unknown sera.

The indirect fluorescent antibody method is based on the antiglobulin, or immunologic sandwich, procedure. Two steps are required; the first uses the antigen and an unlabeled antibody derived from some known species, possibly a rabbit, and is to this point the same as the first stage of the blocking test. After the uncombined antibody is washed away, the preparation is exposed to a fluorescent antirabbit globulin. This attaches to the rabbit globulin, which in turn is attached to the antigen (Fig. 14-7); thus the antigen is indirectly rendered fluorescent. A blocking control also can be applied to the indirect method.

The indirect method has certain advantages over the direct method: (1) it is more sensitive, since the unlabeled antibody, while serving as an antigen for the labeled antibody, provides many more combining sites than the original antigen itself; (2) it is more easily controlled, since more reagents are used and their concentrations are easily adjusted; and (3) it may conserve the number of fluorescent antibodies that must be prepared. In identification of a wide variety of antigens for which rabbit antisera are available, the only fluorescent reagent required is the labeled antirabbit globulin. Even this is not required if one prefers to use a fluoresceinated protein A as the second reagent. However, the indirect procedure does have the disadvantages of requiring more time and more reagents and being less specific.

A major drawback to microscopic fluorescent antibody procedures is the difficulty in quantitating the test. Most interpretations are simply expressed on a positive or negative basis. With expensive equipment the intensity of fluorescence can be evaluated in solid phase fluorescent antibody procedures conducted much like the corresponding RIA method.

The two procedures just described illustrate the two basic applications of the fluorescent antibody method: the identification of antigens with labeled antibody, as in the direct method, and the identification of antibody by either the blocking test or indirect method. Antibody also can be localized by using fluorescent antigens. These methods are adaptable to widely varying serologic problems.

The procedure used in the past for the diagnosis of animal rabies, when time is often of the essence, may require 3 weeks. With fluorescent antibody

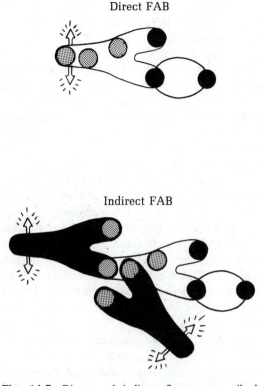

Fig. 14-7. Direct and indirect fluorescent antibody *(FAB)* procedures. In the direct procedure the antibody specific for the antigen is labeled. In the indirect procedure the antigen is reacted with its antibody, in this case of rabbit origin, and then with a fluorescent antibody versus rabbit γ-globulin. This diagram indicates why the indirect reaction produces a more brilliant fluorescence and a more sensitive test.

the time can be shortened to a few hours or a few days. Often when a person is bitten by a presumably rabid dog, the dog is killed. (This is absolutely the wrong thing to do, but in moments of panic the best judgment is seldom used.) The dog brain is then stained by Seller's method to identify the pathognomonic rabies inclusion bodies. If the brain has been severely damaged, or if the dog had only recently acquired rabies, these bodies may not be seen. If they are not, an emulsion of the brain is injected into mice. An incubation period of 3 weeks is allowed before the mice are examined to see if they have acquired rabies. In the meantime a decision has to be made as to the advisability of administering rabies vaccine to the bitten person. The Pasteur method of rabies vaccination has the inherent danger of initiating autoimmune encephalitis, so this vaccination procedure is not practiced recklessly. The application of fluorescent antibody to sections of the dog brain can obviate much of this problem. Such an antibody will specifically identify rabies virus in tissue, even in badly damaged tissue where the typical Negri inclusion bodies are absent by ordinary procedures. Within hours the decision becomes self-evident as to whether rabies immunization is needed.

A second major area of application of the fluorescent antibody method has been in the study of immunology itself—the site of antibody formation (Fig. 14-8), the nature of serum sickness, the autoimmune diseases, and other topics. Several approaches for locating the site of antibody formation have been employed. The first of these involves the direct fluorescent labeling of the antigen prior to injection. At appropriate time intervals the animals are sacrificed, and tissue sections are

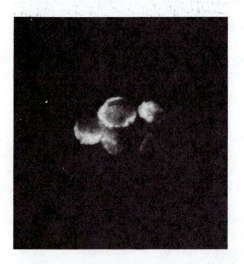

Fig. 14-8. A fluorescent antibody stain of a cluster of lymphocytes that are producing immunoglobulins. The antibody was specific for κ-chains. (Courtesy Dr. R. Lynch.)

prepared and examined for the fluorescing antigen. This method has a major drawback: the location of antigen is not necessarily the site of antibody formation. In fact good evidence already has been presented that the two are not the same. Certainly the location of many particulate antigens in phagocytic cells is one example. An alternative is to stain γ-globulins in tissues with a fluorescent antiglobulin. This has been justly criticized on the basis that all γ-globulins are not necessarily antibodies. Consequently the immunologic sandwich approach has been employed. Tissue sections of an immune animal are flooded with antigen first and then with fluorescent antibody. Only in this way is there an immunologically specific localization of tissue or cellular antibody. By using two differently labeled fluorescent antibodies in doubly immunized animals it has been found that each plasma cell makes antibody to only one antigen.

FERRITIN-LABELED ANTIBODIES AND ELECTRON MICROSCOPY

Ferritin is a protein of 465,000 mol wt whose biologic function is the transportation of iron. Nearly 23% of the molecule is iron, in the form of ferric hydroxide–phosphate salt. The complexed iron is situated in four discrete micelles about 55 Å in diameter. The iron micelles are electron opaque, and the electron microscopic location of antigens has been determined by using ferritin as the antigen.

Antibodies can be joined to ferritin (or other proteins) by divalent ligands. The compounds used for this purpose are difluorodinitro benzene, bisdiazobenzidine, toluene diisocyanate (or diisothiocyanate), m-xylene diisocyanate, carbodiimides, and others (Fig. 14-2). A complication arises from the use of these compounds with two proteins in that it is just as likely that two antibody molecules or two ferritin molecules will be joined as one antibody to one ferritin. Since two ferritins are much larger and two antibodies substantially smaller than one of each, the three forms of coupled protein molecules can be separated by gel filtration. The desired product can be used in the direct or indirect procedure to histochemically localize antigens or antibodies by electron microscopy (Fig. 14-9).

A recent labeling innovation, which is adaptable to both light and electron microscopy, is the use of enzymes. Two different enzymes, horseradish peroxidase and alkaline phosphatase, have been used. Horseradish peroxidase has a molecular weight of 40,000 and alkaline phosphatase a molecular weight of 80,000. Both these molecules are appreciably smaller than ferritin, so there is much less steric hindrance of immunoglobulin molecules bearing these enzymes than if they were labeled with ferritin. Because of this, several enzyme-labeled antibodies may attach to a single molecule of antigen that would have space for only one ferritin-labeled antibody. A second advantage of the enzyme-bound antibodies, as mentioned earlier in regard to ELISA tests, is that the enzymes are catalytic reagents which will convert many molecules of substrate to an electron-dense end product. These many molecules of product are much easier to detect than a single molecule of ferritin-labeled antibody. Thus the enzyme-labeled antibodies are more sensitive reagents.

IMMUNE COMPLEXES

The ability to detect free antibody or free antigen in serum, spinal fluid, or other specimens represents an ideal condition in which one of the

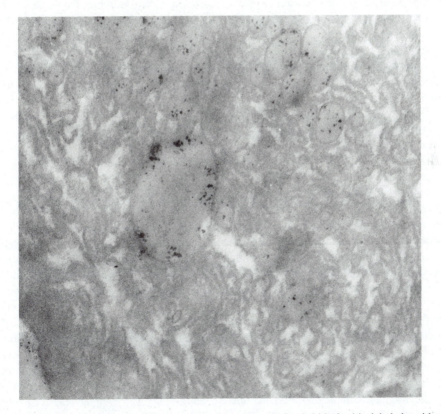

Fig. 14-9. Ferritin labeling of colloid vesicles of a thyroid gland with ferritin-labeled antithyroglobulin. The dark granules of ferritin are localized only in the homogeneously staining colloid. (Courtesy Drs. D. Senhauser and E. Adelstein.)

two reagents needed for a serologic reaction is present in excess. In the past few years it has been recognized that this is not always the case and that the antigen and antibody already have combined in vivo. This makes it difficult, if not impossible, to detect either of them by standard serologic reactions. These immune complexes may have incorporated complement into them, depending on the class of antibody involved. The complexes that contain an excess of antibody often are cleared rapidly by the phagocytic system. When the opposite is the case and antigen is in excess, the complex may circulate for 24 to 36 hours, during which time gradual deposition on target tissues occurs. Particularly when complement is bound into the matrix, the possibility of tissue damage and inflammation exists. For this reason it is important to recognize the presence of circulating immune complexes before tissue deposition creates tissue damage.

Immune complexes have been recognized in the blood of patients with malaria, leprosy, viral hepatitis, group A streptococcal infections, subacute bacterial endocarditis, dengue, schistosomiasis, and other infections. Indeed a transient "complexemia" can be anticipated in many infectious diseases. One whole subdivision of allergy is referred to as immune complex allergy. (See Chapter 19.) This includes conditions such as serum sickness, allergic pneumonitis, and the Arthus reaction. Several autoimmune diseases have an important component with the formation or deposition of immune complexes. Among these, rheumatoid arthritis, systemic lupus erythematosus (SLE), poststreptococcal glomerulonephritis, and rheumatic fever, pemphigus vulgaris, bullous pemphigoid, and myasthenia gravis (MG) are discussed in Chapter 21.

At present the techniques designed to detect immune complexes deposited in or on tissues are superior to the procedures used to recognize them in body fluids. Immune complexes in tissues are easily detected by fluorescent antibody methods using labeled antibodies specific for complement or a specific immunoglobulin. Fluorescein-labeled protein A will identify IgG in tissues. Among the currently employed techniques are those which rely on the presence of immunoglobulin in molecular aggregates larger than their expected size (150,000 to 900,000 mol wt). "Abnormal" sizes of antibody can be measured by ultrafiltration, gel filtration, gradient density centrifugation, etc., and when detected, they indicate the presence of antibody in association with other (antigen) molecules. Immune complexes frequently have different solubility properties than normal globulins, and this can be detected by precipitation in the cold (cryoglobulins are often antigen-complexed globulins) or with PEG. Antigen-complexed antibody can be recognized by antiglobulin methods either while held in the complex or after dissociation of the antibody from the complex and its separation from antigen. For example, an antibody to human γ-globulin, known as RF, can be adsorbed onto latex particles and used in passive agglutination tests to detect human IgG. If this reagent agglutinates in a fraction of human serum known to contain molecules greater than 150,000 mol wt, this indicates the presence of immune complexes in that fraction. Cryoglobulin precipitates formed in the cold can be dissolved at 37° C and tested with the reagent. Protein A has been adsorbed onto insoluble carriers and used as an immunosorbent for purifying IgG, and this technique is adaptable to measuring IgG in unusual size ranges typical of immune complexes.

The Fc region of the immunoglobulin in complexes usually remains exposed, even though the Fab portions are bound to the antigen. Many types of cells have receptors for the Fc region of immunoglobulins and respond differently on exposure to these complexes, depending on the nature of the cell. Platelets are aggregated by Fc domains in immunoglobulins, and it may be possible to capitalize on this so that only complexes and not free globulin will agglutinate platelets. Macrophages, neutrophils, B lymphocytes, Raji's cells, and K cells all have Fc receptors, and all but K cells have receptors for complement component C3b. When immune complexes are bound to Raji's cells, the globulin in the complex then is measured with radiolabeled antihuman globulin. Immune complexes that are not yet fully saturated with complement will bind additional complement in a modified form of the complement fixation test.

BIBLIOGRAPHY

Abraham, G.E., editor: Handbook of radioimmunoassay, New York, 1977, Marcel Dekker, Inc.

Albertini, A., editor: Radioimmunoassay of hormones, proteins, and enzymes, Amsterdam, 1980, Excerpta Medica.

Farr, A.G., and Nakane, P.K.: Immunochemistry with enzyme labeled antibodies: a brief review, J. Immunol. Meth. **47:** 129, 1981.

Hijmans, W., and Schaeffer, M., editors: Fifth international conference on immunofluorescence and related staining techniques, Ann. N.Y. Acad. Sci. **254:**1, 1975.

Ishikawa, E., Kawai, T., and Miyai, K.: Enzyme immunoassay, New York, 1981, Igaku-Shoin Medical Publishers, Inc.

Kawamura, A., editor: Fluorescent antibody techniques and their applications, Baltimore, 1977, University Park Press.

Luft, R., and Yalow, R.S., editors: Radioimmunoassay: methodology and applications in physiology and in clinical studies, Stuttgart, 1974, Georg Thieme Verlag.

Maggio, E.T., editor: Enzyme-immunoassay, Boca Raton, Fla., 1980, CRC Press, Inc.

Malvano, R., editor: Immunoenzymatic assay techniques, The Hague, 1980, Martinus Nijhoff.

Mayer, R.J., and Walker, J.H.: Immunochemical methods in the biological sciences: enzymes and proteins, New York, 1980, Academic Press, Inc.

Moss, A.J., Jr., Dalrymple, G.V., and Boyd, C.M.: Practical radioimmunoassay, St. Louis, 1976, The C.V. Mosby Co.

Mulé, S.J., and others, editors: Immunoassay for drugs subject to abuse, Boca Raton, Fla., 1974, CRC Press, Inc.

Nairn, R.C., editor: Fluorescent protein tracing, ed. 4, New York, 1976, Churchill Livingstone, Inc.

Newton, W.T., and Donati, R.M.: Radioassay in clinical medicine, Springfield, Ill., 1974, Charles C Thomas, Publisher.

O'Beirne, A.J., and Cooper, H.R.: Heterogeneous enzyme immunoassay, J. Histochem. Cytochem. **27:**1148, 1979.

Oellerich, M.J.: Enzyme immunoassays in clinical chemistry: present status and trends, J. Clin. Chem. Clin. Biochem. **18:** 197, 1980.

O'Sullivan, M.J., Bridges, J.W., and Marks, V.: Enzyme immunoassay: a review, Ann. Clin. Biochem. **16:**221, 1979.

Parker, C.W.: Radioimmunoassay of biologically active compounds, Englewood Cliffs, N.J., 1976, Prentice-Hall, Inc.

Parker, C.W.: Radioimmunoassay, Annu. Rev. Pharmacol. Toxicol. **21:**113, 1981.

Ransom, J.R.: Practical competitive binding assay methods, St. Louis, 1976, The C.V. Mosby Co.

Soini, E., and Hemmilä, I.: Fluoroimmunoassay: present status and key problems, Clin. Chem. **25:**353, 1979.

Sternberger, L.A.: Immunocytochemistry, ed. 2, Englewood Cliffs, N.J., 1978, Prentice-Hall, Inc.

Thorell, J.I., and Larson, S.M.: Radioimmunoassay and related techniques: methodology and clinical applications, St. Louis, 1978, The C.V. Mosby Co.

Weir, D.M., editor: Handbook of experimental immunology, ed. 3, Oxford, 1978, Blackwell Scientific Publications, Ltd.

Williams, R.C., Jr.: Immune complexes in clinical and experimental medicine, Cambridge, 1980, Harvard University Press.

Wisdom, G.B.: Enzyme-immunoassay, Clin. Chem. **22:**1243, 1976.

Yalow, R.S.: Radioimmunoassay, Annu. Rev. Biophys. Bioeng. **9:**327, 1980.

SITUATION: THE GRAD STUDENT MIXER

As the Graduate Student Association mixer was about to break up, a fellow you recognized as a student in the biochem. department approached you. He introduced himself and asked, "Can I pick your brain for the price of a beer?"

"Sure, as long as it's a mug!"

"Good, I need help from an immunologist. I've got a problem."

With that introduction he briefly outlined his doctoral research project. His advisor had been carrying a cell culture line for several years that was capable of producing nanogram quantities per milliliter of an exciting new hormone. All efforts to increase the yield of hormone by manipulating the composition of the growth medium had failed. This also was hampered by the fact that the biologic assay for the hormone, a molecule of only

17,500 mol wt, was expensive, time consuming, and subject to excessive variability. Now the possibility of selecting mutant cells with a greater hormone-synthesizing capacity was under consideration. Would it be possible to develop an immunoassay for tiny quantities of hormone that could be used to recognize the desired mutant cells and to more satisfactorily quantitate the hormone in culture fluids?

Questions

1. What are the antigen and immunization demands in problems such as the one just outlined?
2. What serologic procedures are sufficiently sensitive to quantitate nanogram amounts of an antigen or hapten?
3. Which serologic procedures are applicable to the recognition of specific antigens in or on cells?
4. Are the procedures meeting the demands of questions 1, 2, and 3 practical in terms of expense, time to develop (as for a Ph.D. dissertation), reproducibility, etc.?

Solution

To recognize and quantitate an antigen, it is necessary to produce a high-titer, specific antiserum. This is an aspect of research problems like the one being considered here which is often more troublesome than it first appears. The primary requirement, of course, is to have an adequate supply of a highly purified preparation of the antigen. "An adequate supply" was a deliberately chosen vaguely stated phrase. The immunologist would like to have several milligrams to enable the immunization of several rabbits or other species. Low molecular weight antigens are not as potent as those of larger size. Thus a large group of animals usually is selected for immunization with these antigens. This would make a larger demand on the ideal amount of antigen needed. When quantities of antigen are restricted, one should not ignore the possibility of using hybridoma technology. Clearly the use of adjuvants is important

in problems in which antigen supply is limited. Fortunately several good adjuvants are available. One method—an adjuvant-based method combined with antigen purification—might apply here. It is possible to identify an antigen in polyacrylamide gels where it has been electrophoretically separated from other antigens and use the antigen-gel mixture directly in the immunization. The matrix of the gel slows the release of antigen into the true physiologic milieu of the immunized animal and thus behaves as a depository adjuvant.

The most sensitive serologic procedures are the antigen- (or hapten-) binding reactions that economize on the amount of antigen used by eliminating the large amount of reactants needed to produce a second phase in the serologic reaction. The sensitivity of these tests almost always is related to the ability of a modified form of the antigen or antibody to display an easily detectable recognition signal. This may be done through the agency of fluorescent dyes, radioisotope or enzyme labels, or other alterations of the chemistry of the antigen or antibody.

The methods most adaptable to quantitating tiny amounts of antigen in solution would be RIA or enzyme-linked immunoassay. As described in this chapter, nanogram or picogram quantities per milliliter, or in some instances even per deciliter or liter, can be accurately determined by these techniques under ideal assay conditions. Preference for one or the other of these two methods would be based on criteria such as availability of radioisotope-counting equipment and general experience with radioisotopic or enzymatic techniques and related subjects, since the methods are very similar in sensitivity and in technical performance.

Immunohistochemical localization of antigens on cell surfaces is possible through techniques such as the horseradish peroxidase or ferritin antibody methods used in electron microscopy. Since there is no apparent need to involve electron microscopy in this problem, fluorescent or enzyme-linked methods would be preferred. Indirect methods are more sensitive than direct methods and would be recommended here. The limits of antigen detection by immunocytochemical methods are uncertain, but there is no reason to suspect other than success in their application here.

The practicality of the precedures outlined needs no further testimony than the abundance of such methods already available for problems with demands similar to those presented here. The development of RIAs, fluorescent antibody methods, etc. can be accomplished with expenditures ranging from only a few thousand dollars to tens of thousands of dollars and within periods of several months to several years. As with any research problem, a prediction as to time and cost must be tempered by the intangible: luck. Ordinarily the development of a completely satisfactory solution to the problems presented here would be more than an average Ph.D. candidate could accomplish in the time usually needed to complete degree requirements.

References

Clausen, J.: Immunochemical techniques for the identification and estimation of macromolecules, Amsterdam, 1971, North-Holland Publishing Co.

Skelley, D.S., Brown, L.P., and Besch, P.K.: Radioimmunoassay, Clin Chem. **19:**146, 1973.

Sternberger, L.A.: Immunocytochemistry, ed. 2, Englewood Cliffs, N.J., 1978, Prentice-Hall, Inc.

Weir, D.M., editor: Handbook of experimental immunology, ed. 3, Oxford, 1978, Blackwell Scientific Publications, Ltd.

CHAPTER
15

PRECIPITATION

GLOSSARY

CIEP Counterimmunoelectrophoresis.

counterimmunoelectrophoresis Electrophoresis of antigen and antibody toward each other through a gel.

crossed immunoelectrophoresis Electrophoresis of antigens through a neutral gel followed by electrophoresis at 90° C to the first axis and into an antibody-containing gel.

Elek's test A double immunodiffusion test similar to the Ouchterlony test.

Farr's test A test for soluble antigen-antibody complexes in which the radiolabeled complex is precipitated by reagents for γ-globulin.

flocculation 1. A specific type of precipitation that occurs over a narrow range of antigen concentration. 2. Aggregation of colloidal particles in a serologic reaction, as in syphilis serology.

immunodiffusion The diffusion of soluble antigens and/ or antibodies toward each other and their precipitation in gel.

immunoelectrophoresis An electrophoretic displacement of antigen(s) or antibodies followed by immunodiffusion.

incomplete antibody An antibody that does not continue into the aggregative phase of the reaction with antigen.

Mancini's test A radial immunodiffusion test, usually based on diffusion of antigen through a gel containing antibody.

monovalent antibody An incomplete antibody.

Ouchterlony's test An immunodiffusion test based on diffusion of both antigen and antibody through gels.

precipitation Formation of an insoluble complex of antibody with soluble antigen.

Quellung reaction Precipitation of specific antibody on the capsule of an organism, producing the appearance of capsular swelling.

radial immunodiffusion The Mancini test.

rocket immunoelectrophoresis The electrophoresis of an antigen into a gel containing antibody to form precipitates that are spear shaped.

The precipitation of antibodies by fluid antigens is one of the most useful of all serologic tests, partially because most antigens, if they are not already fluids, can be converted to fluid form by simple solubilization procedures. Fluid antigens are subject to rather easy purification, and immunologic study of highly purified materials is always a distinct advantage in explaining the mechanism of the reaction, in quantitating the reactants, and in other procedures. Another reason precipitation tests are so useful is that they can be varied in so many purposeful ways. Precipitation can be studied in either fluid or gelled media. Precipitation of antibody on cells, either as a histochemical reagent or as an aid to cell identification, has been of great value to immunologists, electron microscopists, pathologists, microbiologists, and a host of other biologic scientists. Precipitation tests can be converted to one of the most sensitive forms of the serologic reaction: the passive hemagglutination test.

Even when precipitation does not normally occur—as with the combinations of haptens and antibody—double antibody procedures can be used to develop the reaction as a precipitation test. This leads us to consider a number of variations of reactions with fluid but nonprecipitating antigens and haptens.

FLUID PRECIPITATION
Procedures

The phenomenon of serologic precipitation in a fluid medium was discovered in 1897 by Kraus, who found that culture filtrates of enteric bacteria would precipitate when mixed with homologous antisera but not with heterologous antisera. Kraus referred to the antigen as the precipitinogen (a precipitin generator) and to the antibody as the precipitin. This terminology gradually is falling into disuse but has had general application to other forms of antigens and antibodies, for example, hemagglutinins and agglutinogens.

In 1902 Ascoli modified the precipitation test to an interfacial, or ring type, test. In this form of precipitation small tubes partially filled with antiserum, which is usually the most dense of the reactants, are carefully overlaid with dilutions of the antigen. Mixing of the reagents must be avoided. As the reactants diffuse into each other, precipitation occurs at their interface. The plane of precipitate gives the illusion of a ring when seen from the side (Fig. 15-1).

Lancefield, when serologically typing the streptococci, adapted the Kraus method to a capillary precipitation technique. In this instance very small quantities of premixed antigen and antibody are drawn into capillary tubes that have an inside diameter of only 1.5 to 2 mm. Except for the quantity of reagents used, the capillary precipitation test is the same as that described by Kraus. In each of these methods incubation at room temperature

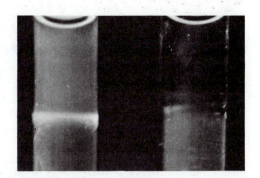

Fig. 15-1. Interfacial (ring precipitin) test. Antiserum to bovine serum albumin is seen in bottom of each tube. The left tube (positive) has been overlayered with bovine serum albumin and the right tube (negative) with human serum albumin. (Courtesy William Krass.)

for periods of a few minutes to 24 hours is allowed before the results of the test are recorded.

The exact physical form of the test is largely a matter of individual choice. Interfacial tests become positive rather quickly and tend to avoid prozone phenomena. The capillary test has two advantages: it conserves the serologic reagents, and it permits a rough quantitation of the reaction because the precipitate falls out of solution and accumulates at the bottom of the fluid column (Fig. 15-2). The height of this precipitate can be measured and used as an estimate of the amount of antibody present and the equivalence zone.

Since precipitation tests involve two reagents, both of which are in a fluid condition, two inherently different methods of procedure are possible. The method described by Ramon in 1922 specifies that dilutions of antibody should be mixed with a constant amount of antigen. The exact concentration of antigen used is the choice of the experimenter but is rarely greater than a 0.01% to 1% solution. Less concentrated antigen solutions will precipitate the antiserum at higher dilution and for this reason are usually preferred. In the second form of the test, advanced by Dean and Webb in 1926, the antibody concentration is held constant and is mixed with different dilutions of the antigen.

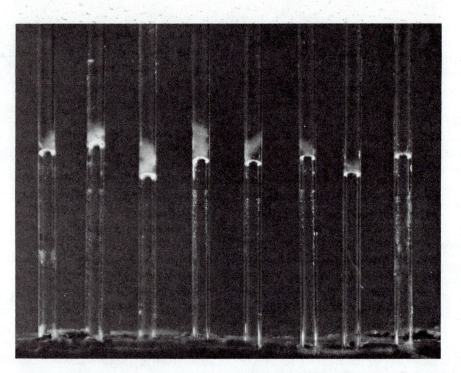

Fig. 15-2. A capillary precipitin test with dilutions of antigen (bovine serum albumin) premixed with the specific antiserum before being drawn into capillary tubes. Note the slight prozone because of antigen excess in the first two tubes and the postzone in the last tubes at right. The final tube contained no antigen and is a negative control. (Courtesy William Krass.)

The Dean and Webb method (the α procedure) is in reality a measure of the least amount of antigen that will coprecipitate with antibody, whereas the β procedure (Ramon's procedure) is a measure of the least amount of antibody that will react with a certain concentration of antigen. Despite the fact that, from a theoretic standpoint, the Ramon procedure is more satisfying (it is actually measuring antibody), the α procedure is more widely used. The reason for this is that the antigen can be diluted over a wide range, perhaps several hundredfold if one begins with a 1% antigen solution, and still yield a positive test with a high-titer antiserum. In this way antisera of different precipitating titers are distributed over a broad scale, and comparisons of sera with each other are easily made. In the Ramon method, with a 1% antigen solution, the antibody titers fall within a very narrow range. Use of a more dilute antigen solution will expand the titers over a wider range, but even so the comparative potency of different antisera is still difficult to establish. The comparison of antiserum potency by titer is not meaningful unless the exact conditions of the test are described. Antiserum potency is best determined by the quantitative precipitation method. Regardless of whether the α or β test is used, the results are still essentially the same, that is, the higher titers represent the more potent antisera.

The difference in the titers achieved in the α and β precipitation procedures is simply evidence that the procedures are fundamentally different. In the α, or antigen dilution, procedure the reactant being diluted is multivalent, whereas in the β, or antibody dilution, procedure a divalent reagent is being diluted. (IgM is not noted for its precipitating ability.) Moreover the antibody may be present at a level of only a fraction of a milligram per milliliter. Because of its usual low concentration and lower valence, antibody is more easily diluted beyond its functional concentration than is antigen.

In capillary precipitation tests the usual prozone and postzone are easily detected (Fig. 15-2). In this titration of bovine serum albumin versus its rabbit antiserum a partial prozone in the first two capillary tubes is evident. (Prozone in the case of the Dean and Webb procedure refers to the absence of precipitation in the presence of high quantities of antigen, just the opposite of the situation in other serologic tests in which the titer is determined by antibody dilution.) Following the region of prozone the tubes reveal a gradual increase in the amount of precipitate as the equivalence point is reached. Thereafter a gradual decrease in the amount of precipitate is evident as antigen dilution places the system gradually into the postzone area. Prozone phenomena rarely are observed in the interfacial test because the reactants diffuse into each other, diluting the reagents to a suitable concentration for precipitation. This may require a few minutes, but in general interfacial precipitation tests develop very rapidly.

Antigens and antibodies

The precipitation test places virtually no restriction on the type of antigen employed, except that it must be in a fluid condition. Proteins, polysaccharides, hapten-antigen conjugates, and contrived multivalent haptens all are usable as the antigen. The respective efficiency of IgG, IgM, and IgA in precipitation decreases in that order.

The maximum sensitivity of qualitative precipitation tests is in the range of 3 to 15 μg of antibody nitrogen per milliliter of serum. This is equivalent to approximately 25 μg of antibody protein. The qualitative and quantitative precipitation tests are of approximately equivalent sensitivity, depending to a considerable extent on the exact physical and chemical conditions employed in the two tests.

Applications

Precipitation tests have been adapted to a great variety of purposes, so only a few examples are illustrated here.

In forensic medicine it is sometimes necessary to determine if bloodstains are of human origin or lower animal origin, for example, in cases of suspected homicide. Cloth bearing the bloodstain is extracted with saline and is treated as antigen in precipitation tests. The antisera required are those against human and other species of serum proteins. A precipitation test is arranged with each antiserum and the stain extract. Precipitate formation with one of the antisera will identify the animal source of the bloodstain. Bloodstains can be identified not only as to their species origin but also as to their exact blood type by the use of specific antisera against the blood group antigens. Such information is obviously useful in criminal proceedings.

Fluid precipitation tests also are used to detect adulteration of beef with meat of a lower quality or with soybean protein. If hamburger is extracted with saline and is centrifuged, the supernatant can be considered as the antigen. Precipitation tests conducted with antisera to several domestic and wild animals and to soy protein will determine if the hamburger contains only beef or has been adulterated with "foreign" proteins.

The fact that mosquitoes feed on lower wild and domestic animals when there are no humans about was determined by grinding trapped mosquitoes in saline and using the clarified extract as an antigen. Precipitation tests were arranged with antihorse blood, antisheep blood, antirabbit blood, antisquirrel blood, and others. Whenever a positive test occurred, it meant that the mosquitoes contained that species of blood and had fed on that kind of animal.

One final application of quantitative fluid precipitation tests can be cited. C-reactive protein is an abnormal albumin-like protein found in the serum of persons experiencing an inflammatory condition. This is usually an infectious disease but also may include cancer or pregnancy. Under usual conditions C-reactive protein is absent from the blood of healthy persons. Fluid precipitation tests with anti–C-reactive protein sera and a person's serum as the antigen source are an inexpensive aid to the diagnosis of the conditions just stated.

QUANTITATIVE PRECIPITATION

Undoubtedly one of the most important advances in serologic technique occurred in 1932 when Heidelberger and Kendall developed the quantitative precipitation technique. This was soon followed by the application of quantitative chemical procedures to other serologic tests. Several kinds of information can be derived from quantitative serology; concerning precipitation this information includes the following points:

1. An exact expression of the amount of precipitating antibody in an antiserum (This is extremely important when comparing the potency of different lots of antisera.)
2. Proof of the antigen-antibody reaction in varying proportions
3. The functional valence of the antigen
4. An estimation of the relative heterogeneity of the antigen-antibody system
5. The distinction of precipitating and flocculating antisera
6. A measure of the contribution of serum complement to the serologic reaction
7. A quantitative expression of the amount of nonprecipitating antibody present

To perform the quantitative precipitation test, dilutions of antigen are mixed with a constant amount of heat-inactivated antiserum in a volume of 1 ml. (A smaller final volume may be used if microchemical techniques will be employed later.) Both the antigen and antibody solutions should be clarified by vigorous centrifugation if necessary. Controls containing the greatest concentration of antigen used and undiluted controls of antiserum adjusted to volume with buffer also are prepared. After proper mixing all tubes are stoppered and incubated, first for 30 minutes at 37° C and then for an additional 2 days at 4° C. The precipitates should be resuspended after the first

day in the refrigerator. After the second day the tubes should be centrifuged in the cold and the supernatant fluids used to determine the zones of equivalence, antigen excess, and antibody excess. The precipitates are washed with cold buffer three times and after the final wash are dissolved so that chemical analyses for protein content can be made. A plot of the amount of antigen added versus the amount of total precipitate is prepared.

The results of a hypothetical quantitative precipitin test are presented in Table 15-1 and Fig. 15-3.

Table 15-1 shows that the amount of precipitate formed in each tube increased as more antigen was added only until the sixth tube, after which the quantity of precipitate decreased. Tests of the supernatant fluids from each tube revealed that tube 6 is the only tube in which all the antigen and all the antibody were precipitated, and it is thus the equivalence point. For this tube the amount of antibody precipitated can be calculated by subtracting the amount of antigen added from the total amount of precipitate (0.734 − 0.043 = 0.691). This gives an exact expression of the amount of antibody in this antiserum.

Since all the antigen is precipitated in tubes 1 through 6, the amount of antibody contributing to the precipitate in each tube is easily determined by difference. When this is done, it is noted that the ratio of antibody to antigen in the precipitate varies. This is proof of the varying proportions of antigen and antibody in the serologic reaction. The proportions in tube 6 are useful in calculating the serologic valence of the antigen if its molecular weight is known and if it is assumed that IgG is the only species of antibody contributing significantly to the precipitate. The formula used is

$$\text{Valence} = \frac{\begin{array}{c}\text{Ratio of antibody to antigen} \times \\ \text{Molecular weight of antigen}\end{array}}{\begin{array}{c}\text{Molecular weight of antibody} \\ (150,000)\end{array}}$$

Since these data were derived from the use of bovine serum albumin as the antigen and it has a molecular weight of 36,000, the equation becomes

Table 15-1. Data from quantitative precipitation test

Tube	Antigen added (mg nitrogen)	Total precipitate (mg nitrogen)	Excess reagent*	Antigen precip-itated (mg nitrogen)	Antibody (mg nitrogen)	Antibody nitrogen/antigen nitrogen
1	0.003	0.093	ABY	0.003	0.090	30.0
2	0.005	0.145	ABY	0.005	0.140	28.0
3	0.011	0.249	ABY	0.011	0.238	21.7
4	0.021	0.422	ABY	0.021	0.401	19.1
5	0.032	0.571	ABY	0.032	0.539	16.8
6	0.043	0.734	—	0.043	0.691	16.1
7	0.064	0.720	Ag	—	—	—
8	0.085	0.601	Ag	—	—	—
9	0.171	0.464	Ag	—	—	—
10	0.341	0.386	Ag	—	—	—
11	0.525	0.314	Ag	—	—	—
12	0.683	0.241	Ag	—	—	—

*ABY, Antibody; Ag, antigen.

$$\text{Valence} = \frac{16.1 \times 36,000}{150,000} = \frac{579,600}{150,000} = 3.8$$

Naturally a whole integer should be the result, and the answer here would be rounded off to 4. This yields a functional valence of approximately 1 to 10,000 of molecular weight, which is in the expected range. Any great deviation from a whole number may be an indication of a large quantity of nonprecipitating antibody (that is, IgA, IgD, or IgE).

Fig. 15-3 shows a reasonably symmetric curve, plotted from the data of Table 15-1, typical of the results when a purified antigen is tested against its antiserum. The experimental curve is also typical of precipitating, or R type, antisera, as compared with H, or flocculating, antisera. R precipitation curves are typical of rabbit and human antisera. The H class, typified by horse antisera, precipitates only in a narrow range of antigen concentration, with soluble complex formation being the rule outside that zone. This is illustrated in Fig. 15-3 for comparative purposes. *Flocculation* is a term with a dual meaning in immunology. Its original use was for H precipitation tests, but it also has been used to describe aggregation of lipidlike particles that serve as the antigen in serologic tests for syphilis; flocculation in this sense is more akin to agglutination.

The contribution of serum complement to the system is determined by comparative trials using fresh and heat-inactivated sera. The increased amount of nitrogen precipitated in the former situation results from the contribution by complement.

Incomplete or monovalent antibody also can be detected by precipitation tests. This may seem startling to those who know that an incomplete or monovalent antibody is one which will combine with antigen but does not continue into the aggregative phase of the serologic reaction. It is rare that an antiserum is composed solely of monovalent antibody; usually it is present with complete antibody. A mixture of these two kinds of antibody in a single antiserum ordinarily would produce some precipitation with antigen because of its content of complete antibody. On seeing such a precipitate the experimenter may choose to ignore the possibility that monovalent antibody combined with the antigen may be present in the supernatant fluid or may attempt to measure this by the double antibody or antiglobulin technique or by the Farr procedure.

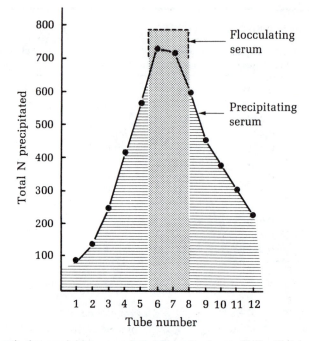

Fig. 15-3. A quantitative precipitin curve plotted from the data in Table 15-1 is seen in the solid line. Both the prozone and postzone effects (diminished amount of precipitate in the presence of excess antigen or antiserum) are apparent. A flocculating serum would precipitate over a narrow range of antigen concentration, as indicated by the broken line.

To perform the double antibody procedure for a nonprecipitating antibody, one must know the species origin of the incomplete antibody. For example, if rabbit antibody were used, the addition of goat, equine, or other antibody to rabbit γ-globulin would precipitate the monovalent antibody. The rabbit incomplete antibody serves as an antibody with the original antigen, a reaction that takes place exclusively via the Fab portions of the immunoglobulin molecule; but this leaves its Fc portions free to serve as antigen and to combine with the goat antirabbit γ-globulin. This precipitation produced by the antiglobulin can be quantitated exactly as in the usual precipitation test, and the amount of nonprecipitating antibody in a serum can be expressed in exact units of weight.

Although immunoglobulins that fail to illustrate the second phase of the serologic reaction are classified as incomplete or monovalent antibodies,

there is absolutely no evidence that they are structurally deficient in any way. For convenience in portraying serologic reactions these antibodies are shown as "one armed" models, devoid of an Fab unit; but all evidence indicates that they are structurally identical to complete antibodies. The reason they fail to complete the usual serologic reaction is not known.

The Farr test, an important modification of the precipitation test, is used to detect nonprecipitating antibody when the antigen is soluble in 50% ammonium sulfate solutions. The physical arrangement is the same as for the quantitative precipitation test, except that a ^{131}I or other appropriately marked antigen is needed. After precipitation the radioactivity in the precipitate is determined.

A second dilution series is prepared just as the first, but after the incubation ammonium sulfate is added to achieve a 50% saturated solution.

This will precipitate all the γ-globulin, and any labeled antigen attached to the γ-globulin (including that in unprecipitated antigen-antibody complexes) will be "salted out" of solution. As stated, the free antigen must remain soluble in 50% ammonium sulfate solutions. The greater amount of radioactivity precipitated in the second test is a measure of the amount of nonprecipitating antibody in the antiserum. A double antibody procedure must be used if the antigen precipitates in ammonium sulfate.

Laser beam technology has added a modern approach to quantitative serology by improving nephelometry. In nephelometry a light beam is passed through a solution or suspension, and the amount of light scattered from its original path is measured. The quantity of this scattered light is an index of the concentration of the suspension. Heretofore the measurement of immunoprecipitates or immune complexes by nephelometry was unsuitable because of its lack of sensitivity and inability to detect small differences in the amount of precipitate formed under different circumstances. This has been overcome by laser beams with a greater strength than the usual light sources and the ability to measure light that is deflected only slightly from its original path. Consequently immune complexes that produce only a slight haze in a solution can be quantitated, and nephelometric procedures are used in clinical immunology to quantitate several serum proteins. In performing these tests the antiserum and antigen solutions should be free of any contaminating particles.

IMMUNODIFFUSION

Between 1946 and 1948 three separate studies established that precipitation tests performed in gels could provide several advantages over fluid tests. One of the principal advantages of these tests is the ease by which multiple antigen-antibody systems can be identified. The report by Oudin (France) published in 1946 described a single diffusion system. Two years later Elek (England) and Ouchterlony (Sweden) both published

their data on a double gel diffusion technique. In 1953 a third technical variation of the gel immunodiffusion test was described, but this was also a double diffusion procedure and had no significant advantage over the Ouchterlony procedure. The three techniques are distinguishable on the basis of the number and dimension of the diffusion. Since only one reagent diffuses in the Oudin test, it is described as a single diffusion–single dimension system. Both the Elek and Ouchterlony procedures are double diffusion–two dimension systems, and the third procedure, devised by Oakley and Fulthrope, is a double diffusion–single dimension system. Obviously there can be at least one other class, a single diffusion–double dimension system. This often is called radial immunodiffusion and has been very useful in developing quantitative gel precipitation techniques. It was first devised by Feinberg in 1957 and was modified by Mancini in 1963.

Gel immunodiffusion tests are most commonly performed in purified agar gels. Ordinary bacteriologic grade agar is usually unsuitable; it has a slight yellowish gray tinge, it may contain finely dispersed particles that add a faint translucence to the gel, and it contains a large number of free carboxyl or sulfate groups that interfere with the simple diffusion of ionically charged reactants. Agar is a mixture of two principal linear polysaccharides: agaropectin, the portion containing the acid residues, and agarose, which is neutral. Agarose has replaced agar and is the most frequently used medium for immunodiffusion studies. Agar and agarose form gels that are essentially impermeable to molecules with a molecular weight greater than 200,000. Since most serologic precipitates exceed this molecular weight (one IgG plus two antigen molecules), the precipitates are held in the agarose while extraneous proteins are washed from the agar. Because of this, the immunoprecipitates can be stained for protein, lipid, or special enzyme activities, which adds to the information obtainable by gel diffusion analyses.

Agarose and agar are only two of the many gels

tested for immunodiffusion studies. Gelatin has been used but melts in warm rooms or incubators and has proved unsuitable. Cellulose acetate films are superb for many studies, but the film is very thin, a factor that makes it difficult to fill the wells and makes the precipitates difficult to see. This in turn makes staining a necessary additional step. Polyacrylamide gels are crystal clear, but the diffusion rate of most molecules is intolerably slow.

Single diffusion in one dimension

The Oudin procedure is a single diffusion–single dimension gel precipitation test. An antiserum or purified antibody is added to a 0.7% solution of agarose that has been melted and allowed to cool to about 50° C. Proteins in solution usually do not coagulate at temperatures below 60° to 65° C, and agarose congeals at about 45° C; so the temperature chosen will protect the antibody and allow adequate mixing of the reactants. This fluid agarose–antiserum mixture is placed in a tube of convenient size and is allowed to gel. Care should be taken to avoid depositing any of this mixture on the sides of the tube. The fluid antigen is layered over the gelled antiserum. The concentration of the antigen should be considerably greater than the equivalence concentration. If the tube is small enough in diameter to hold the fluid layer in place by surface tension, the tube is placed on its side. This eliminates any effect of hydrostatic pressure on the diffusion of the antigen into the antiserum layer.

As the fluid antigen diffuses into the agarose, it dilutes itself to the proper concentration to precipitate with the antiserum. A disc of precipitate will become visible in the tube when this occurs. The precipitin band that forms will move down the tube according to the time elapsed, the concentration of the antigen in solution, the concentration of antibody in the agarose, the temperature, and the pore space in the agar. Movement of the precipitin band is more apparent than real. As the increasing antigen concentration at the rear face forces the antigen concentration there into a zone of antigen excess, the precipitate dissolves. Simul-

taneous movement of the antigen at the front of the band forward into a new position for an equivalence concentration causes precipitation in front of the old precipitin band. Because of the dissolution and reformation of the precipitate, it appears to move down the precipitin tube. This process is repeated continuously until the position of the precipitate stabilizes. At this time the precipitate is observed as a sharp, distinct band with only a very faint fuzziness at its edges. This fuzziness is less likely to exist with "flocculating" sera, which form precipitates only within a restricted zone of antigen concentration, than with R antisera. A comparison of the behavior of R and H antisera is presented in Fig. 15-4. In the Oudin procedure only one of the reactants diffuses; this is in a straight line, so the procedure is aptly named a single diffusion–single dimension system.

In immunodiffusion tests a single antigen and its antibody will form only a single precipitin line. A mixture of antigen-antibody systems will present multiple bands, theoretically one band for each system. Exceptions occur when two antigens with equivalent diffusion rates diffuse into an antiserum that contains their respective antibodies in equal concentration. In such a case the equivalence concentrations in the two systems would occur in a single plane. The two precipitates thus would be superimposable and recorded as a single precipitate. Therefore in gel diffusion precipitation tests the number of precipitation bands observed will represent the minimal number of possible antigen-antibody systems functioning.

The exact identification of a single precipitation band in a mixture of antigen-antibody systems as being caused by certain antigen-antibody system is clumsy in the single dimension arrangements. The unknown precipitin band must be matched with that formed by the purified antigen in a replicate experiment. This is difficult, since the position of the band is partially dependent on the concentration of antigen used; also the concentration of one antigen in a mixture is not always easy to determine. Therefore the usual procedure is to add some of the purified antigen to the antigen mix-

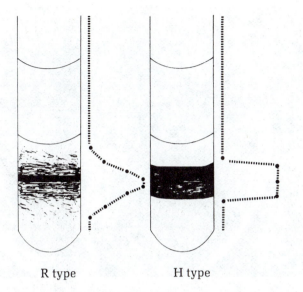

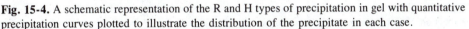

R type   H type

Fig. 15-4. A schematic representation of the R and H types of precipitation in gel with quantitative precipitation curves plotted to illustrate the distribution of the precipitate in each case.

ture, repeat the test, and determine which band is displaced further down the antiserum-gel column, but even this is sometimes difficult to determine. It is also possible to adsorb or precipitate one antibody out of the antiserum with the purified antigen, repeat the test, and observe which band has been deleted. These techniques do not have quite the precision that the two-dimension gel diffusion systems afford.

Double diffusion in one dimension

In the double diffusion–single dimension gel precipitation tests a zone of neutral agar is placed between the fluid antigen and fluid antiserum in a tube. The principles of the Oudin technique apply, the only variation being that both reagents are diffusable. Most of the advantages and disadvantages of the single diffusion test apply to the double diffusion method. The primary disadvantage of all single dimension tests is the difficulty in identifying an antigen-antibody precipitate as being caused by a known antigen and antibody; this is easier to do when double diffusion in two dimensions is used.

Double diffusion in two dimensions (Ouchterlony's technique)

To perform the double diffusion–double dimension test, better known as the Ouchterlony test, reservoirs are cut or molded into agarose on a flat surface. The exact number, position, and shape of the wells are mostly matters of choice, but square or rectangular reservoirs have the advantage of forming sharp angles of merging precipitin bands in comparative systems. The wells are filled with appropriate solutions of antigens and antiserum, covered to prevent evaporation, and observed periodically for several days. Precipitin bands may become visible in a few hours if concentrated reagents and/or a micromethod is used. The same general rules observed for the other gel diffusion tests concerning the number and position of the developing precipitin lines apply here as well.

If two wells for antigen are placed in opposition to a well containing antiserum, three principal types of reaction may be detected (Figs. 15-5 and 15-6). These differ physically in the way the two precipitation arcs from the separate antigen wells

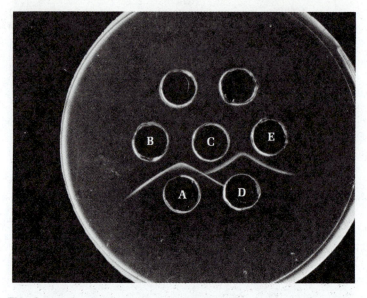

Fig. 15-5. This Ouchterlony immunodiffusion test shows two reactions of serologic identity and a reaction of nonidentity. Well A contains an antiserum to an *Escherichia coli* toxin. The toxin was placed in wells B and C. Well D contains antiserum to human lactoferrin. Lactoferrin was placed in wells C and E. (Courtesy Drs. R. Finkelstein and B. Marchlewicz.)

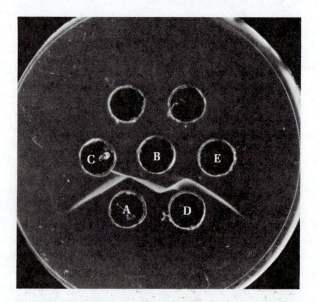

Fig. 15-6. In immunodiffusion reactions of partial identity spurred precipitation lines are seen. Well A contains an antiserum to a toxin from a human strain of *Escherichia coli*. This toxin was placed in well B. Toxin from a porcine strain of *E. coli* was placed in well C. Antiserum to the toxin of a porcine strain of *E. coli* was placed in well D and its corresponding antigen in well E. (Courtesy Drs. R. Finkelstein and B. Marchlewicz.)

merge. In a reaction of serologic identity the intercepts of the two precipitation lines merge into a single arc; this means that the antiserum cannot distinguish one antigen from the other. In reactions of nonidentity the lines cross completely; this is evidence that the two antigens are reacting with two entirely different antibodies. Both the second antigen and second antibody pass through the precipitate produced by the first antigen-antibody system. In reactions of partial identity, in which one antigen is cross-reactive with but not serologically identical to the other, a spurred intercept is noted. This is the result of precipitation of one antibody by determinants of the simplest antigen and the movement through that precipitate of antibody molecules with specificity only for determinants found in the more complex antigen. Viewed in another way, the simpler antigen adsorbs out its own antibody, but the antibody that is specific for the additional antigenic determinants of the second antigen passes

through that precipitate and reacts with the more complex antigen. Hence the spur points toward the simpler antigen. A fourth type of reaction (not illustrated) produces double spurs. Since this reaction is easily confused with reactions of nonidentity, it is fortunate that double partial identity reactions are rare. The ease with which two antigens can be established as serologically identical or different is the prime advantage of the Ouchterlony test over other immunodiffusion assays.

The morphology of the precipitin arc formed by diffusion from wells of equal size is concave around the well containing the lowest diffusion rate. The slowest diffusing molecule is usually the one with the highest molecular weight. A straight line indicates that the reactants are of nearly the same molecular weight. This is often useful in estimating the molecular weight of an antigen, since the precipitating antibody is IgG, with a molecular weight of approximately 150,000.

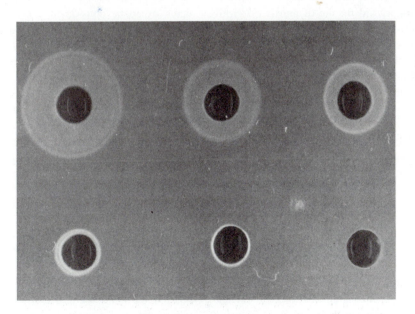

Fig. 15-7. The Mancini (radial immunodiffusion) test. Antigen in the upper wells was at a concentration of 10, 5, and 2.5 μg/ml, reading left to right. In the lower row only the left well received antigen (1.2 μg/ml). (From Barrett, J.T.: Basic immunology and its medical application, ed. 2, St. Louis, 1980, The C.V. Mosby Co.)

Radial quantitative immunodiffusion

A fourth form of immunodiffusion test first was described by Feinberg in 1957. It is now most widely known as the Mancini test or the radial immunodiffusion test. A major advantage of this technique is that it is a quantitative procedure. Microgram quantities of antigen can be accurately determined by the method. In terms of sensitivity, as little as 1.25 μg of antigen per milliliter can be quantitated in the Mancini test.

The Mancini technique is a single diffusion–double dimension system in which the antiserum is incorporated in the agarose gel, which is solidified on a flat surface. Small wells are cut in agarose and filled with antigen. Radial diffusion of the antigen produces a ring of precipitate, the diameter of which is proportional to the concentration of the antigen (Fig. 15-7).

The most intensive use of radial immunodiffusion is in clinical laboratories where it is necessary to determine the exact amount of various protein antigens in serum. Radial immunodiffusion is the best laboratory aid for the diagnosis of hypogammaglobulinemia of IgG, IgM, or IgA, the determination of myelomas of one of these immunoglobulin classes, and the quantitation of complement components C3 and C4, haptoglobin, lysozyme, α_1-antitrypsin, AFP, and of other serum proteins.

IMMUNOELECTROPHORESIS

There are two recognized handicaps to ordinary immunodiffusion tests. Incubations of several hours or even days are needed to ensure that equilibration of the system has occurred, and there is the possibility that two or more precipitation bands may form in the same plane and prevent an accurate enumeration of the antigen-antibody systems involved. Both these objections may be overcome in immunoelectrophoretic procedures. In immunoelectrophoresis a direct electric current is forced through a gel containing antigen and/or antibody. If the antigen is actually a mixture of antigens, the electrophoretic phase of the test generally will displace the antigens from one another.

The probability of two molecules having exactly the same electrophoretic mobility is unlikely. Because of this difference in the ionic properties of antigens, each will form a visibly distinct band of precipitate in the second immunodiffusion phase of the procedure.

In standard immunoelectrophoresis the electrophoretic portion of the method is followed by regular immunodiffusion. In a few variations of immunoelectrophoresis both antigen and antibody are set in motion by the electric field. In other instances the antigen is electrophoresed into a slab of antibody. In both cases the immunoprecipitates are formed quickly and are nearly complete during the electrophoretic phase of the test.

Counterimmunoelectrophoresis

The immunodiffusion technique in which both antigen and antibody are displaced electrophoretically (in opposite directions and toward each other) is the immunoelectrophoretic variant to the double diffusion–single dimension test. In some ways it can be considered a modification of the Ouchterlony test, even though this is a double dimension test, because the only dimension of interest in the Ouchterlony test is that between the antigen and antibody wells.

In counterimmunoelectrophoresis, countercurrent immunoelectrophoresis, or immunoosmophoresis, paired wells in an agarose film are charged with antigen and antiserum (or antibody). The agarose is buffered at pH 8.2 and is connected by paper wicks to buffer-filled reservoirs to complete an electric circuit. The electric potential is applied, and the reactants move toward each other if the test has been properly arranged. In the pH range below 8.2 the immunoglobulin molecules will carry a slight positive charge that will cause their movement toward the cathode. At pH 8.2 the immunoglobulins are essentially uncharged but are carried toward the antigen by the fluid through the gel, a process known as electroendosmosis. Antigens having an acidic isoelectric point will bear a negative ionic charge at alkaline pH and will be displaced toward the anode. Thus the serologic reactants will be driven toward each other by the electric potential, and this will accelerate their precipitation (Fig. 15-8).

Counterimmunoelectrophoresis is a time-saving procedure, qualitative rather than quantitative in nature, and most easily performed with electronegative antigens. Fortunately many antigens are negatively charged at an alkaline pH; these include the albumin, β- and α-globulins, many polysaccharides, nucleoproteins, and glycoproteins. This encompasses a wide range of antigens of practical interest: viruses, bacterial polysaccharides, serum proteins, etc. Moreover it is possible to improve the anodic migration of many proteins, including immunoglobulins, by acetylation or carbamylation reactions with their amino groups. When correctly performed, the addition reaction has no influence on the serologic reac-

tivity of the immunoglobulin, but these antibodies will move rapidly toward and precipitate more quickly with antigens that move little at pH 8.2. Contrariwise, acidic groups (COOH, SO_3H_2) can be added to neutral antigens to provide them the necessary mobility for standard counterimmunoelectrophoresis procedures.

Rocket immunoelectrophoresis

Rocket immunoelectrophoresis is the most used synonym for single crossed immunoelectrophoresis, spike immunoelectrophoresis, the Laurell technique, or electroimmunoassay. This is a quantitative method similar in concept and application to the Mancini test with the added dimension of electrophoresis.

To conduct this test, the antiserum is incorporated into an agarose film adjusted to pH 8.6,

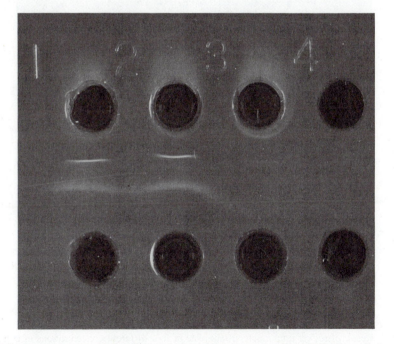

Fig. 15-8. Counterimmunoelectrophoresis of a heat-extracted antigen from *Bacteriodes fragilis* versus its antiserum produced the dual precipitation pattern seen in wells 1 and 2. A dilution of the antigen produced a trace precipitate in well 3. Well 4 was a control system in which normal rabbit serum was used. (Courtesy T. Ellis.) (From Barrett, J.T.: Basic immunology and its medical application, ed. 2, St. Louis, 1980, The C.V. Mosby Co.)

the isoelectric point of the immunoglobulins at which these proteins are electrophoretically immobile. The antigen specific for the antiserum is placed in small reservoirs along one edge of the antibody-containing slab or in a narrow film of neutral agarose placed against it. The electric potential is applied so that it will draw the antigen into the antibody-agarose layer, that is, with electronegative antigens at pH 8.6 the antigens would move toward the anode. As the antigen molecules contact the antibody molecules, precipitation begins. As the concentration gradient of the antigen changes, dissolution of the precipitate and reprecipitation take place at a steadily increasing distance from the antigen reservoir. At the end of the run the length of the cone-shaped precipitate is directly proportional to the concentration of the antigen (Fig. 15-9). When a series of antigen solutions of known concentration are examined, it is possible to construct a standard curve to determine the concentration of the antigen in an unknown preparation.

Crossed immunoelectrophoresis

This method initially was described by Ressler in 1960 but perfected by Laurell in the years following 1965. The method is also known as double crossed immunoelectrophoresis or two-dimensional immunoelectrophoresis.

This method requires, as its first stage, the simple electrophoresis of an antigen mixture in agarose. Thereafter this agarose strip is transferred to the edge of a second plate and positioned against an agarose slab containing an antiserum. Now

Fig. 15-9. Result of rocket immunoelectrophoresis of four different concentrations of complement component C3 against its monospecific antiserum. A twofold dilution series of the antigen was made beginning at the left and progressing to the right. Notice that the adjacent rocket heights do not differ by twofold, although the peak areas do. The left rocket did not form a perfect spear because of premature termination of the electrophoresis. (From Barrett, J.T.: Basic immunology and its medical application, ed. 2, St. Louis, 1980, The C.V. Mosby Co.)

the second electrophoretic step is applied, only this time the electric field is arranged at right angles to the original separation. This draws the antigens from their original positions in the neutral agarose slab into the antibody-containing film. As in counterimmunoelectrophoresis, the buffer system is adjusted to pH 8.6 to hold the antibody molecules immobile. As the antigens move into the antiserum layer, spears or rockets of precipitation develop (Fig. 15-10). Intercepts of these precipitation arcs will indicate their serologic unrelatedness or partial identity. Reactions of serologic identity are not observed.

Crossed immunoelectrophoresis is primarily a method for the enumeration of antigen-antibody systems in a mixture. It can become a quantitative

method if known standards are tested simultaneously with the unknowns and if their corresponding precipitation arcs are identifiable in the area of the plate containing the antigen mixture. This is often difficult; frequently a second property of the antigen, such as an enzymatic or hemolytic activity, is needed to identify it in a cluttered mixture of immunoprecipitation patterns.

Ordinary immunoelectrophoresis

The original immunoelectrophoretic modification of gel precipitation tests was the immunoelectrophoretic procedure of Grabar and Williams. The term *immunoelectrophoresis* was coined 2 years after they published the details of the method in 1953. The great advantage of immunoelectro-

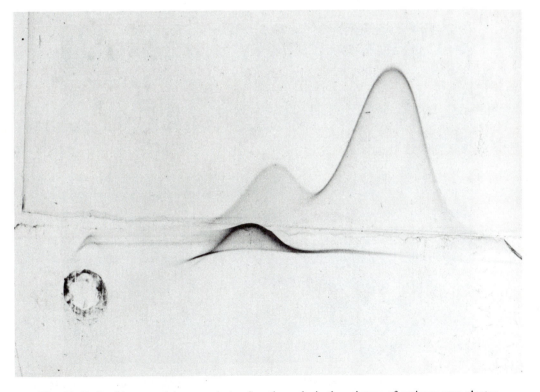

Fig. 15-10. In this crossed immunoelectrophoretic analysis the mixture of antigens was electrophoretically displaced from left to right followed by an immunoelectrophoretic development as the antigens moved to the top of the slide. Five antigen-antibody systems have produced precipitates. (Courtesy C. Helphingstine.)

phoresis, as pointed out earlier, is that the antigens in a mixture are separated from each other in two ways, first by electrophoresis through a gel and later by ordinary gel diffusion. According to this method (more so than with simple diffusion methods) the formation of a single precipitin line is more likely to be the result of a single antigen, since antigens of equal diffusion rate often differ electrophoretically.

The physical arrangement requires that an agarose film on a flat surface be placed in an electric field after the antigen mixture has been added to a small reservoir cut in the agar. Prior knowledge of the electrophoretic behavior of the antigens at the pH of the buffer used is desirable so that the electric force can be applied in sufficient strength and for a long enough period to permit an adequate separation of the antigens. After the electrophoresis a trough the length of the glass plate or slide is cut from the agarose and is filled with antiserum. Double diffusion in two dimensions begins, and after a suitable period of incubation areas of precipitate will develop just as in the usual Ouchterlony technique (Fig. 15-11).

Although immunoelectrophoresis is very useful in separating antigens and has a very high resolving power, it is somewhat difficult to identify a specific precipitin arc as originating from a known antigen. Parallel immunoelectrophoresis of a purified antigen preparation, even on the other half of the same slide, will not always present a perfect enough mirror image of the band in question to

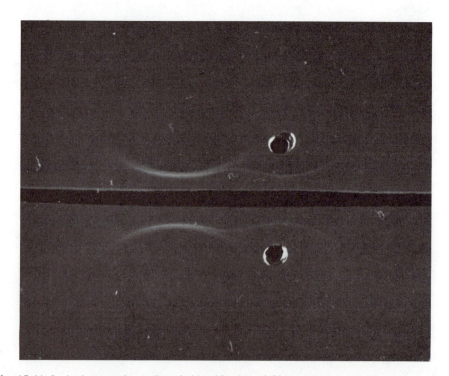

Fig. 15-11. In the immunoelectrophoretic identification of C3 proactivator and C3 activator a mixture of the two is placed in wells cut in an agarose film. The two proteins have dissimilar electrophoretic mobilities, with the proactivator moving further. When the plate is developed by adding antiproactivator serum to the trough, proactivator forms a heavy precipitation line and C3 activator a light precipitation line, with the latter nearer the starting point (the well). (From Barrett, J.T.: Basic immunology and its medical application, ed. 2, St. Louis, 1980, The C.V. Mosby Co.)

afford exact identification. This is especially difficult when several bands are situated closely together. To circumvent this handicap in antigen identification, the common antigen technique is employed. This involves the preparation of a second antigen trough, placed so that the electrophoretically separated antigens are between the antigen and serum troughs. This second trough is for the purified antigen, which diffuses toward the antiserum and precipitates with it in a straight line, except for that area where the antigen concentration was reinforced by the electrophoretically positioned antigen. In this region an arc is formed that fuses perfectly with the straight line, thus identifying the antigen involved. If prior immunoelectrophoretic analysis has located the position of an unknown band, the short trough technique is applicable to the identification of this band. In this instance the trough for antibody is cut only to the approximate center of the arc, and just beyond the end of this short antibody trough a well is made for the pure antigen. The antigen in this well should precipitate in a perfectly fused arc with the electrophoretically separated antigen.

CAPSULAR SWELLING (QUELLUNG REACTION)

One of the broader modifications of the precipitation test is the Quellung reaction. In 1902 Neufeld described the apparent swelling of the capsule of a bacterial organism when it was mixed with homologous antiserum. The German word *Quellung* means swelling, and the reaction has become known as the Quellung reaction. There is some disagreement as to whether capsular swelling actually occurs. The reaction may be viewed as the binding of antibody molecules to the periphery of the bacterial capsule, rendering its outline more visible. This fine precipitate actually may be at a point more distant than the apparent outer margin of the capsule because unstained capsules are very difficult to see under the ordinary light microscope. Thus swelling may be more apparent than real. It is rather doubtful that the volume of the cell and its capsule is increased enough by the addition of antibody molecules to create a visible increase in capsular size.

The capsular swelling technique, however inappropriate its name, has been extremely useful in the construction of an antigenic classification scheme for encapsulated bacteria. *Streptococcus pneumoniae* is a prime example. There are over 80 types of pneumococci, each with a capsule that is serologically (antigenically) distinct from all the others. The capsule, or specific soluble substance (SSS), is in fact a haptenic polysaccharide. The specific antiserum to each capsular type is clinically very useful in identifying pneumococci. Because of the rapidity of the Quellung reaction, the identification of presumed pneumococci in a sputum specimen may take no more than 20 to 30 minutes. It is not necessary to perform 80 separate Quellung reactions, since polyvalent or pooled antisera against the most commonly isolated types are available. Quellung typing and identification of other pathogenic bacteria—for example, *Neisseria meningitidis* and *Hemophilus influenzae*— also are practiced. In the Quellung test agglutination also occurs; this facilitates reading the test.

ARTHUS REACTION

The precipitin reaction can occur in vivo when sizable quantities of antigen are injected intradermally or subcutaneously into animals with a high antibody titer. The precipitate that develops blocks the local capillary bed and prevents the exchange of the nutrients and wastes from the injection site. This encourages the development of tissue necrosis, which is known as the Arthus reaction. (See Chapter 19.)

BIBLIOGRAPHY

Arquembourg, P.C.: Immunoelectrophoresis, ed. 2, Basel, 1975, S. Karger, AG, Medical and Scientific Publishers.

Axelson, N.H.: Quantitative immunoelectrophoresis, Baltimore, 1975, University Park Press.

Axelson, N.H., Krøll, J., and Weeke, B.: A manual of quantitative electrophoresis, Baltimore, 1975, University Park Press.

Crowle, A.J.: Immunodiffusion, ed. 2, New York, 1975, Academic Press, Inc.

Laurell, C.B., editor: Electrophoretic and electroimmuno-chemical analysis of proteins, Baltimore, 1977, University Park Press.

Løwenstein, H.: Quantitative immunoelectrophoretic methods as a tool for the analysis and isolation of allergens, Prog. Allergy **25**:1, 1978.

Verbruggen, R.: Quantitative immunoelectrophoretic methods: a literature survey, Clin. Chem. **21**:5, 1975.

SITUATION 1: A PIG IN A POKE

Dwight V., a 58-year-old businessman, left a meeting late at night in a city 25 miles from his home just as a heavy snowstorm struck. When he was still nearly 10 miles from home, a heavy flurry completely blinded him. Just then he felt his car strike a solid object. He pulled to the shoulder of the road as soon as he could see, stopped his car, got out, and with aid of a flashlight examined the roadway and car. Seeing nothing unusual, he proceeded homeward.

The next morning the newspaper lead story described a hit-and-run death in the snowstorm on the highway Dwight V. had taken and at about the distance from town where his own incident had occurred the night before. Clearly shaken, he went to the garage and looked at his car. Some blood and a small piece of flesh clung to the right front wheel suspension below the bumper.

Questions

1. What immunologic procedures could be used to determine if the blood and tissue are of human origin?
2. Are precipitin tests the only serologic means of identifying bloodstains?
3. If tests prove the human nature of the blood and tissue specimens, what tests could be conducted to further identify the individual source of these materials?

Solution

The time-proved method for identifying the origin of tissue is the precipitation test, customarily performed by the interfacial, or ring, technique. The test can be performed simply, inexpensively, and with known limits to its sensitivity. Basically the test depends on the extraction of protein and polysaccharide antigens from the unknown tissue, blood, or seminal stain with isotonic saline. In the case of solid tissue this will require grinding or homogenization of the sample in a small blender. The extract is clarified by centrifugation and layered over antisera of known specificity, such as antihuman albumin, antihuman serum, antidog serum, or antichicken serum. The development of positive tests identified the species origin of the sample.

The precipitation test has not been superceded by other methods, but other methods have been developed for identifying the species and blood group status of unknown samples and are proving satisfactory. In the realm of precipitation tests double immunodiffusion methods are useful substitutes for the interfacial test. In this method it is not always necessary to clarify the extract, since this is accomplished to some degree as the antigen-containing preparation diffuses through the agar. The test is more time consuming and less sensitive than interfacial precipitation tests. Counterimmunoelectrophoresis appears to combine the rapidity and sensitivity of the fluid precipitation test with the advantages of immunodiffusion. The principal antigens detected are albumin and the α-globulins, since they are the most electronegative.

For further identification of dried bloodstains the testing of extracts against anti-A, anti-B, and even anti-H(O) sera in precipitation tests remains the standard method. Other methods that may be used include mixed agglutination and absorption-elution. In the first method cotton or other cloth fibers bearing the stain are used directly, since the red cell debris is firmly adsorbed to the fibers. The fibers are incubated separately with anti-A and anti-B sera. Then A cells are added to the first mixture and B cells to the second. If A antigens are present on the fibers, the corresponding antibody will attach to the fibers and then to the indicator cells used in the second incubation. In negative tests the indicator cells are easily washed free from the fibers. The absorption-elution method is similar except the absorbed antibody is eluted from the fibers with heat and tested for its capacity to agglutinate indicator cells in a separate test.

Serologic methods are also available to identify proteins in which allotypic variations occur, such as the variants of hemoglobin, transferrin, double albumin, and haptoglobin. These markers are very helpful in the identification of specific individuals. For several enzymes in which electrophoretic variants are known, simple electrophoresis is useful in identifying the source of the bloodstain. Phosphoglucomutase and serum cholinesterase are examples. Methods to identify HLAs also are being developed but are not used frequently in forensic medicine. However, they definitely will be used in the future.

SITUATION 2: THE IMMUNOLOGY LABORATORY

Your advisor was called away from the university on Friday because of a death in his family. He expected to be absent until late Monday night. In a brief note he asked you to arrange for the Tuesday meeting of his immunology laboratory course. He informed you of the location of his stock antigens and antisera and specifically informed you his class should perform an experiment designed to display the multiplicity of antigens in a solution. He insisted that you pretest the experiment so that the proper concentrations of the reagents could be prepared by him Tuesday morning before his class.

Questions

1. What serologic tests are available to demonstrate that a solution contains more than one antigen?
2. How would you rank these tests according to their ability to reveal the multiple components in the antigen mixture?
3. Which of the tests would require the least amount of reagents?
4. In terms of reagent costs, equipment needs, and time of performance, which of these tests could you most conveniently pretest and then have a class perform in a 2-hour laboratory period?

Solution

There are, in fact, many serologic reactions which can be used to prove that a solution contains more than one antigen, including RIA, complement fixation, and quantitative fluid precipitation tests. With fluid antigen solutions it is possible to establish a dilution series of the antigen and test these dilutions with a constant amount of antiserum. When a bimodal response is observed, then one can be certain that two or more antigens are present in the antigen solution. The bimodal response is seen because the two antigens and their corresponding antibodies are rarely at equivalence at the same dilution. Thus, when one of the antigen-antibody systems is at equivalence, the other is in prozone or postzone. When the second system reaches equivalence, then the first is in antigen postzone. As more and more antigen-antibody systems participate, the response curve shifts from a simple bimodal to a trimodal form to a broad plateau, since one or more of the systems is in or near equivalence at every point in the antigen dilution series. For this reason quantitative fluid precipitation, RIA, complement fixation tests, etc. are not ideally suited for a situation such as that presented in this case.

Using antibodies, each bearing a different colored fluorochrome, radioisotope, enzyme, or other label, to different antigens in the mixture, it is possible to measure the simultaneous function of different antigen-antibody systems in a mixture. These methods usually are applied to particulate antigens and histochemical procedures but can be adapted to soluble antigens rendered insoluble or attached to particulate carriers.

The student in this situation should quickly

recognize the advantage of immunodiffusion techniques to solve the problem. The two major varieties of immunodiffusion are unaided, or simple, immunodiffusion and immunoelectrophoresis. In the first category are included the Ouchterlony, Preer, Oudin, and Mancini gel diffusion tests. Of these, the Mancini and Ouchterlony tests are easiest to arrange and to interpret and are consequently the most popular. The Mancini test is particularly suited to the quantitation of antigens but can be used for their enumeration as well, each antigen producing a separate ring of precipitate. The Ouchterlony test is more suited to the enumeration of antigens and can be used to identify an antigen in a mixture with a known antigen. Both tests suffer to some extent from delays in reading the results until diffusion is nearly halted, and the final results may not be available until several days after the tests were begun. This does not prevent recording data earlier as long as it is understood that the results may change slightly in the ensuing days. Depending on the physical circumstances of the test, as little as 3 μg of antigen per milliliter can be detected.

Because the diffusion rates of two antigens through a gel may be nearly identical, two antigen-antibody systems may precipitate at essentially the same location. This prospect is minimized if an electric potential is used to move the antigens, since the antigens will very likely have different isoelectric points. As a consequence, immunoelectrophoretic diffusion tests are more likely to display the multiplicity of antigen-antibody systems in a mixture of precipitating systems than is simple immunodiffusion. Of the available methods, ordinary immunoelectrophoresis and counter-immunoelectrophoresis are the simplest to arrange, although the restricted diffusion distance in the latter test may mask the true number of precipitating systems. Crossed immunoelectrophoresis, since it relies on antibody in an agarose slab, is unlike the previous two tests in that it is subject to prozone phenomena, which may prevent the formation of one or more precipitates. To prevent this, several pretitration runs may be necessary to establish the correct conditions.

Although immunoelectrophoretic diffusion tests are more sensitive in defining the number of antigens in a mixture, they are no more sensitive than simple immunodiffusion tests in measuring small quantities of an antigen, 1 to 3 μg/ml being the usual lower limit. This is true because the immunologic development in both types of tests usually takes place via simple diffusion.

Faced with the handicap of time and inexperience, it would probably be best for this student to prepare for the Ouchterlony immunodiffusion and either regular immunoelectrophoresis or counter-immunoelectrophoresis. If the student is fortunate, the Ouchterlony test might identify two serologic systems and the latter more than two.

All the simple immunodiffusion tests performed as microtechniques can be conducted with as little as 25 μl of antigen or antiserum, but larger volumes are needed if the tests are performed as macrotechniques. This is probably desired for a class exercise even though it may consume five to ten times more of the reagents. Students seldom are able to deposit 25 μl of solution in reservoirs of only 2 mm diameter in Ouchterlony plates without practice. Spilling the reagents on the agarose surface or deforming the reservoir will mar the results of the exercise. Since the Mancini and crossed immunoelectrophoretic procedures rely on antiserum incorporated into an agarose film, 0.1 to 0.5 ml of this reagent may be needed per test. Since the antiserum can be diluted fivefold to 500-fold, this does not stress the supply of antiserum. For immunodiffusion tests the amount of reagents used is seldom a limiting factor.

References

Crowle, A.J.: Immunodiffusion, ed. 2, New York, 1975, Academic Press, Inc.

Rose, N.R., and Bigazzi, P.E., editors: Methods in immunodiagnosis, ed. 2, New York, 1980, John Wiley & Sons, Inc.

Rose, N.R., and Friedman, H., editors: Manual of clinical immunology, ed. 2, Washington, D.C., 1980, American Society for Microbiology.

Williams, C.A., and Chase, M.W., editors: Methods in immunology and immunochemistry, vol. 3, New York, 1971, Academic Press, Inc.

AGGLUTINATION AND HEMAGGLUTINATION

GLOSSARY

ABO antigens Antigens on the major human blood group system.

agglutination Aggregation of a cellular or particulate antigen by an antiserum containing antibodies to one or more surface antigens.

agglutinin An antibody directed toward surface antigens and capable of causing agglutination.

agglutinin adsorption Removal of some of the antibodies in an antiserum by reacting them with the cellular antigen, which afterward is removed by physical procedures such as filtration or centrifugation.

blood group antigen Antigens that are genetically determined and which are present on the surface of red blood cells.

Boivin antigen A heat-stable antigen extractable from gram-negative bacteria; essentially synonymous with *endotoxin*.

Boyden's technique A procedure for attaching protein antigens to erythrocytes by first treating the cells with tannic acid.

Coombs' test A form of antiglobulin test in which the globulin antigen is a nonhemagglutinating antibody.

erythroblastosis fetalis A disease of the newborn in which maternal antibodies pass the placenta and contribute to destruction of fetal erythrocytes.

H antigen The flagellar antigen(s) of bacteria.

H substance An antigen on the human erythrocyte that is a precursor substance for the A and B antigens.

HDN Hemolytic disease of the newborn; *see* Erythroblastosis fetalis.

hemagglutination The agglutination of erythrocytes, especially by antiserum.

isohemagglutinin An antibody of an animal that will agglutinate erythrocytes from another animal of the same species.

lectin A PHA.

O antigen Surface somatic antigens of bacteria; not to be confused with ABO antigens of human erythrocytes.

passive hemagglutination Hemagglutination resulting from antibodies directed toward antigens adsorbed to the erythrocyte surface.

phytohemagglutinin (PHA) An extract of plant, usually legumes, that will agglutinate erythrocytes.

Rh antigens A system of human blood group antigens shared by the rhesus monkey.

tanned erythrocyte One treated with tannic acid in preparation for passive hemagglutination tests.

Widal's test A bacterial agglutination test.

Weil-Felix test An agglutination test used to diagnose certain rickettsial diseases.

The initial demonstration of immune hemagglutination was performed in 1900 by Ehrlich and Morgenroth, who immunized goats with the red blood cells of other goats (alloimmunization or isoimmunization). The resulting antisera were capable of distinguishing the red blood cells of different goats from each other, since some were hemagglutinated and some were not. This permitted the creation of the first blood cell groups. Human erythrocyte alloantibodies or isoantibodies (in human sera, of course) were described in the following year, 1901, by Landsteiner. This is the discovery which opened the way to successful blood transfusion, to a better understanding of erythroblastosis fetalis and other hemolytic diseases, to the potential prevention of these diseases, to the discovery and understanding of immune tolerance, and to the discovery of other tissue alloantigens or isoantigens so important in tissue transplantation. In 1930 Landsteiner received the Nobel Prize for his discovery of human blood groups.

ABO(H) BLOOD GROUP SYSTEM

Landsteiner made multiple crosses of erythrocytes and serum from himself and his associates and originally identified three types of persons, those currently designated A, B, and O. In a subsequent report the existence of a fourth group, AB, was noted. The relationship of these four groups to one another, recorded in Table 16-1, requires only a minimum of additional explanation. Every group A person has an antigen on the erythrocytes, which arbitrarily was designated as A, and has an antibody in serum that reacts with red blood cells bearing the B antigen. The reverse is true of the group B person, whose erythrocytes all contain the B antigen and whose serum contains an antibody to the A antigen. Persons in group O lack both the A and B antigens but have antibodies to both A and B antigens in their sera. The reverse situation is true for AB persons, who have both the A and B antigens on each erythrocyte but lack both A and B antibodies in their sera. It can be noted immediately that an antigen and its corresponding antibody do not coexist in one individual. This sometimes is referred to as Landsteiner's rule. Coexistence of a common antigen and antibody would be incompatible with life, since an in vivo hemagglutination reaction would result. This would block the circulation and destroy that person's red blood cells.

The blood group designations A, B, O, and AB are designations of phenotype, which in terms of genetic definition refers to the measured quality or characteristic that distinguishes one person or group from another. It has been postulated that the blood group antigens are inherited according to simple mendelian genetics involving three allelic genes, A, B, and O. These genes exist as pairs on the two sets of chromosomes present in the nucleus of all except the haploid germ cells (sperm and ovum). If the same characteristic is on both genes, then the person is homozygous. In the blood system this would be exemplified by the group O person, each gene lacking the A and B characteristic. The genotype of such a person would be OO. It is in fact artificial to refer to the O gene as a true gene, since it does not control the production of a specific product. The reference is made only for convenience at this point in the discussion. This is not the case with the A and B genes, which control the synthesis of definite antigens. An AB person, who produced both antigens, is heterozygous, that is, capable of producing germ cells of which half transmit the A gene and half the B gene to the zygote. In contrast to group O persons, who are restricted to the homozygous state, and to group AB persons, who are restricted to the heterozygous state, persons in groups A and B may be either homozygous (AA, BB) or heterozygous (AO, BO). This is important in solving cases of uncertain parentage or in identifying misplaced infants.

Group O persons are not absolutely devoid of antigens related to the A and B antigens, as was originally thought. Group O cells contain an H antigen, or H substance, which is a precursor to the A and B antigens; this is why the ABO blood group system now is usually referred to as the

Table 16-1. ABO(H) blood group system

Blood group phenotype	Antigen on red blood cells*	Antibody in serum	Genotype	Distribution in United States (percent)
A	A	Anti-B	AA, AO	42
B	B	Anti-A	BB, BO	10
O(H)	Neither A nor B	Both anti-A and anti-B	OO	45
AB	Both A and B	Neither anti-A nor anti-B	AB	3

*Cells of all blood groups contain the H substance.

ABO(H) system. The H gene regulates the production of the H substance, some of which is converted to the A and B antigens by products of the A and B genes. Some of the H substance remains unconverted and can be detected on A and B cells.

The distribution of the ABO(H) blood groups in the United States is approximately 45% O, 42% A, 10% B, and 3% AB. These values will differ slightly in separate racial or ethnic groups, which represent "isolated" genetic populations because of the tendency to marry within the group. For example, the distribution in blacks is 49% O, 28% A, 20% B, and 3% AB.

About 80% of A and AB blood cells are easily agglutinated by anti-A serum, but the remaining 20% are difficult to clump because of the presence of A_1 and A_2 subgroups within the A group. The A_1 cells have both the A_1 and A_2 antigens, and the A_2 cells have only the A_2 antigen. Since the usual anti-A serum contains both anti-A_1 and anti-A_2, it is a more potent reagent for the A_1 cells than it is for A_2 cells. Extracts from the plant *Dolichos biflorus* have a 500-fold greater hemagglutinating activity on A_1 than on A_2 cells and also have been used to distinguish these two cell types. Incubation of anti-A serum with A_2 cells will remove the A_2 antibody (agglutinin adsorption) and leave an antiserum that is specific for the A_1 antigen. Of the 42% of the population referred to as group A, actually about 34% (42 × 0.8) are A_1, and 8% are A_2. Likewise, the AB persons are divisible into those who are A_1B (2.5%) and those who are A_2B (0.5%).

Less important subgroups of the A antigen include A_3, A_x, and A_m. Variants of the O and B groups also are known but are quite rare.

ABO(H) antigens

Antigens of the ABO(H) system are present on erythrocytes from fetal life onward and can be found on most other cells as well. In each instance the antigen exists as an integral part of the cell wall. Estimates of the number of A sites on a single erythrocyte have varied widely, from as low as 120,000 to as high as 1,170,000. The number of B sites has been estimated to be from 310,000 to 830,000 per cell. A figure of 500,000 for each is probably a satisfactory compromise of these estimates at present.

Information concerning the chemistry of the A, B, and H antigens has come from three major sources: (1) the agglutination of erythrocytes by lectins (PHAs), (2) the enzymatic and chemical degradation and analysis of the blood group substances from human and lower animal sources, and (3) inhibition of the serologic reaction between red blood cells and antibodies by monosaccharides and oligosaccharides of known structure. The results of these independent approaches have been mutually supportive, and now the structure of the immunodominant portion of these molecules generally is agreed on.

Hemagglutination by extracts of plants has been known since 1888. The active substance (PHA, phytoagglutinin, plant agglutinin, or lectin) is seldom specific for a single blood type, probably because it combines with additional or different chemical sites than the blood group determinant, but a few are blood type specific. Those lectins with blood group specificity have replaced animal sera in the identification of blood for clinical blood banking purposes and in the characterization of the blood group antigens.

The common lima bean, *Phaseolus limensis,* is the source of a highly specific lectin for the blood group A antigen. *Vicia crassa* (vetch) extracts are also A specific. The specificity of *Dolichos biflorus* lectin and A_1 has been mentioned already. Few anti-B lectins are available, and none has been adopted for routine clinical use. Several lectins are specific for the H substance, including those from *Ulex europaeus* (common gorse), other *Ulex* species, and *Lotus* and *Laburnum* species. Since the H substance is present on cells of all four blood types, H-specific lectins have not been useful in blood grouping, but they have been useful in chemical studies of the ABO(H) antigens.

Preincubation of an anti-A lectin with enzymatically or chemically produced fragments of the soluble blood group A substance seriously impairs its hemagglutinating capacity. Chemically these fragments are largely polysaccharide; when various monosaccharides were tested for their ability to inhibit anti-A lectins, it was found that N-acetyl-D-galactosamine was the most efficient. This saccharide is also a potent inhibitor of the microbial enzymes that hydrolyze the A substance, presumably by an end product inhibition. Perhaps most important is that all human anti-A alloantibodies are inhibited by N-acetyl-D-galactosamine. The disaccharide N-acetyl-D-galactosaminyl-β-1,3-D-galactose is an even better inhibitor. An extension of the saccharide inhibition studies has revealed that the immunodominant portion of the A antigen consists of the hexasaccharide N-acetyl-D-galactosaminyl-α-1,3-(L-fucosyl-α-1,2)-D-galactosyl-β-1,3 or β-1,4-N-acetyl-D-glucosyl-β-1,3-D-galactosyl-β-1,3-N-acetyl-D-galactosamine. This structure is illustrated in Fig. 16-1. This oligosaccharide is only the terminal portion of a large glycoprotein, which may have a molecular weight of several hundred thousand. The remainder of this molecule is relatively unimportant, since it is toward this hexasaccharide that blood group–specific antibodies are directed.

End group analysis of the B and H substances by the techniques just described indicate that they have structures very similar to that of the A substance (Fig. 16-1). The B antigen has an unsubstituted D-galactose as its terminal unit but is otherwise like the A antigen. The H substance has the same pentasaccharide core as the A and B substances but is devoid of their terminal D-galactose and N-acetyl-D-galactosamine, leaving L-fucose as the final monosaccharide. Because of the similarity of these structures, it was assumed that their biosynthetic pathways were closely interrelated; this has proved to be the case and is described after a brief consideration of secretors and the Lewis blood group system.

Secretors and the Lewis blood group system

In roughly 78% of the population the ABO(H) blood group antigens can be found in a soluble form in the body secretions: saliva, serum, urine, gastric juice, seminal fluid, ovarian cyst fluids, etc. These persons are referred to as secretors and have an inherited characteristic regulated by the Se gene. Both homozygous SeSe and heterozygous Sese persons are secretors, since the se gene is recessive. Nonsecretors (sese) represent 22% of the population. The soluble forms of the major blood group antigens have been a useful source of the antigens free of unwanted cellular debris, a factor that has facilitated the immunochemical study of these antigens. Moreover geneticists have found the secretors to be an interesting subject of study because of their relationships with the Lewis blood group.

Originally it was believed that the Lewis antigens were an integral part of the erythrocyte cell wall just like the other blood group antigens. This later was proved fallacious. The Le[a] and Le[b] substances are complex glycoproteins or glycolipids that are found free in the serum and which, like

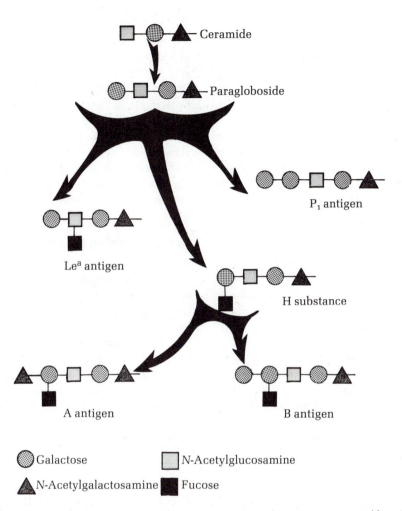

Fig. 16-1. The common origin of several blood group antigens from precursor ceramide and globiside molecules. Addition of a terminal galactose to the globiside produces the P_1 antigen, addition of a fucose to the *N*-acetylglucosamine produces the Le^a antigen, and addition of fucose to the terminal galactose produces the H substance. The A and B antigens are synthesized by the addition of *N*-acetylgalactosamine or galactose, respectively, to the terminal, fucose-bearing galactose of the H substance.

many polysaccharide-containing compounds, have a natural ability to adsorb to red blood cell surfaces. In fact the chemistry of the Lewis substances is very similar to that of the antigens of the ABO(H) system. It now is generally agreed that the Le^a and Le^b antigens arise from the same precursor as the ABO(H) antigens. This precursor

substance consists of a protein core to which four saccharides are attached (Fig. 16-1). The final two saccharides are D-galactose and *N*-acetyl-D-glucose. These two sugars are joined by β-1-3 glycosidic bond. The Le^a gene regulates a fucosyl transferase, which adds L-fucose to the substituted glucose moiety of the precursor via an α-1-4 linkage to create the Le^a antigen. Alternatively the precursor substance is operated on by the H gene, which also controls a fucosyl transferase. In this case L-fucose is added through an α-1-2 linkage to the terminal galactose to form the H substance. The Le^a and H genes are structural genes for enzymes that have slightly different functions. The H substance is a key intermediate in the pathway to the A, B, and Le^b antigens. To reach the A antigen, an *N*-acetyl-D-galactosamine transferase adds that sugar to the final galactose of the H substance via a β-1-3 bond. To reach the B antigen, D-galactose is added to the previously terminal galactose of the H substance by a D-galactose transferase. Finally, to reach the Le^b antigen, a third type of L-fucosyl transferase adds a fucose molecule via an α-1-4 bond to the *N*-acetyl-D-glucose. Thus the structures of the A, B, O(H), and Lewis antigens are closely related to each other.

ABO(H) antibodies

One of the great mysteries of the ABO(H) blood group system is that the alloantibodies are naturally present in the sera of all but group AB persons. The antibodies are barely detectable in the sera of newborn infants, but in the first few months after birth these agglutinins gradually increase in titer. This fact has been used to determine if infants are undergoing a normal maturation of their "bursal dependent," or immunoglobulin-producing, system. The uniform upward progression of ABO agglutinin titers in infancy and early childhood has been cited as evidence that an immunizing experience, occurring during these early months of life, is responsible for their production. It is known that during this same period enteric bacteria of several types begin to colonize in the intestinal tract. Some of these bacteria are noted for their polysaccharide antigens, which are described in chemical terms later in this chapter. Exposure of this sort to an organism with an antigen that is structurally related and cross-reactive with the ABO antigens may be the source of the alloantibodies.

This hypothesis for human A and B isohemag-glutinin formation has been supported by experiments in germ-free chickens. Chickens reared in the usual fashion have anti-human B in their sera, but germ-free chickens do not. If these germ-free chickens are deliberately contaminated with *Escherichia coli,* which synthesizes a B-like antigen, anti-B appears in the chicken sera. A- and B-like antigens are also present in *Shigella, Salmonella,* and other coliform bacteria. The reason that group A persons produce only anti-B is that their own A antigens produced early in fetal life have rendered them immunotolerant to the A antigen.

Hemagglutination testing

Hemagglutination relies on the bridging of red blood cells with antibody molecules. Since several thousand copies of each antigen are present on each erythrocyte, there is ample opportunity for the lattice formation needed to create easily visible clumps of erythrocytes. Most of the naturally occurring allohemagglutinins are antibodies of the IgM class. Partially because of their high serologic valence, these immunoglobulins are very efficient hemagglutinins. They function well in the ordinary hemagglutination tests in physiologic saline diluent and are by definition "complete" antibodies. Many of these IgM hemagglutinins are known as cold agglutinins because of their unique thermal amplitude, functioning much better at 25° or even 4° C than at 37° C, at which they are essentially inactive. When hemagglutination tests that are positive at 4° C are warmed to 37° C, the clumped cells redisperse, and the test becomes negative. These qualities differ from those frequently associated with the immune hemagglutinins of human or other animal origin which are more commonly of the IgG class. Antibodies that function best at 37° C such as the IgG agglutinins are known as warm agglutinins.

Possibly because of their smaller size or lower serologic valence, the IgG antibodies are less efficient hemagglutinins than the IgM antibodies, and some, but not all, may fail to clump erythrocytes in standard physiologic saline. By definition, then, these are "incomplete" antibodies. There is as yet no evidence that incomplete antibodies are structurally different from complete IgG antibodies, but traditionally they have been portrayed as "one-armed," or monovalent, molecules; this convenience is continued here. Cells coated with incomplete antibody can be induced to aggregate, provided their normal electronegative repulsive charge, known as the zeta potential, is reduced. This can be accomplished by several methods. Exposing the unreacted cells to proteolytic enzymes such as bromelin, papain, ficin, or trypsin will release electronegative groups from the cell surface, lowering the zeta potential from the normal value of 18 or 20 mV to about 8 mV. A second method involves the modification of the dielectric constant of the diluting fluid by adding albumin (hence the false term *albumin antibodies*). Increasing the salinity of the diluent to 1.85% saline rather than the standard 0.85% is a third satisfactory method. Cells coated with incomplete antibodies also can be agglutinated with Coombs' reagent (antihuman globulin), as explained in the discussion on Rh antigens in this chapter.

Hemagglutination tests are interpreted by two different methods. In the standard tube test dilutions of the antiserum are incubated with a volume of red blood cells, usually 1 or 2 ml at a concentration of about 2%, and then observed macroscopically for clumping. In the case of weak agglutination, or when time is important and the incubation period must be abbreviated, light centrifugation of the tubes is helpful. After centrifugation the tubes are tapped gently with the finger to resuspend the cells. Cells that do not disperse evenly are agglutinated; agglutinated cells usually are graded as to heavy, moderate, or weak agglutination. Vigorous resuspension of centrifuged cells must be avoided, or cells that are feebly clumped may be separated from each other. In cases of questionable agglutination microscopic examinations are recommended. Rouleaux formation, a nonimmune aggregation of cells in which the cells seem stacked on each other, can be distinguished from true agglutination, in which the cells are bonded haphazardly to each other.

The cell sedimentation pattern also can be used to interpret hemagglutination, either in tubes or in wells molded in plastic blocks (Fig. 16-2). The latter have become very popular in microtitrations performed in a final volume of 0.25 or 0.5 ml. For this test more dilute erythrocyte suspensions are used and are mixed with antiserum and incubated as usual. Centrifugation may be employed if needed. The settling pattern in the bottom of

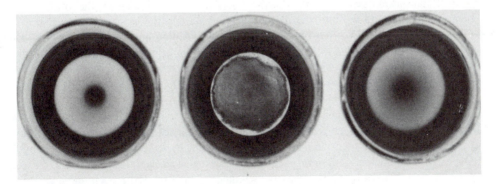

Fig. 16-2. Hemagglutination as seen by the settling patterns of the erythrocytes. A dark center indicates no hemagglutination, whereas a uniform distribution of erythrocytes across the bottom of the tubes is evidence of positive hemagglutination. These tubes would be read as negative, very strongly positive, and questionable or very weakly positive (*left* to *right*).

the wells is examined; when the cells form a dark red central button, the test is recorded as negative. Agglutinated cells are spread evenly over the bottom of the well, except in instances of very heavy agglutination, when ragged or "torn" edges of the cell pattern are typical.

Certain erythrocytes are agglutinable by all samples of normal serum. This phenomenon is known as panagglutination or polyagglutination and is caused in nearly every instance by the in vitro contamination of erythrocyte preparations with bacteria. Enzymes released by these bacteria hydrolyze surface components of the erythrocytes to expose the T antigen. Since antibody to the T antigen exists in all human sera, mixture of such cells and normal sera will result in hemagglutination. Panagglutination from this cause is referred to as the Thomsen-Friedenreich phenomenon, after two of the earliest investigators to study this phenomenon.

Hemagglutination tests usually require antisera with an antibody content of only 0.001 to 0.01 μg/ml. As will be seen in the discussion of passive hemagglutination, less sensitive serologic tests may be converted to hemagglutination tests for improved sensitivity in detecting antibodies.

Rh BLOOD GROUP SYSTEM

The Rh factor was described by Landsteiner and Wiener in 1940 as an antigen common to 85% of all human erythrocytes and those of the rhesus monkey. (The symbol for the Rh system has been taken from the first two letters of the word *rhesus*.) This shared antigen was discovered by hemagglutination testing of human red blood cells with antisera prepared in rabbits against rhesus monkey erythrocytes. Natural alloagglutinins against the Rh antigen do not occur; this fact probably accounts for the 40-year gap between the discovery of the ABO and the Rh blood group systems. Since the discovery of the initial Rh antigen it has become clear that more than 30 antigens must be considered as Rh antigens (Table 16-2). For practical reasons only the major Rh antigens are included in this discussion.

Nomenclature

Three independent nomenclature systems have arisen for the Rh antigens, two of which are in widespread use. In the Fisher-Race system capital and lower case letters (C, D, E, c, d, e,) are used to designate the six most commonly detected antigens. Actually only five of these may exist, since it has been impossible to produce antisera to the d antigen. Consequently d may represent only the absence of D. The D antigen is the most potent of these antigens and is synonymous with Rh antigen, as used in the original sense of Landsteiner and Wiener, or the Rh_0 antigen in the Wiener nomenclature system. Thus the 85% of the population who are Rh positive have the D antigen (Rh_0 antigen) on their red blood cells, and the 15% lacking this antigen are referred to as Rh-negative.

According to the interpretation by Fisher and Race the genes that regulate the synthesis of the Rh antigens exist as the allelic pairs Cc, Dd, and Ee, which reside at three separate but neighboring loci. Currently this interpretation is less favored than that of Wiener, but because of its simplicity, the Fisher-Race nomenclature remains a popular system in many laboratories.

The Wiener nomenclature system is more complex than the Fisher-Race system, since the letters *Rh* are varied between capital and lower case and are modified with subscripts (Rh_0, rh_1) or superscripts (Rh^A) to identify the different antigens. Consequently there is a greater chance for error in bookkeeping and in written records. However, this system appears to be gaining popularity. In the Wiener system rh', Rh_0, and rh'' represent C, D, and E of the Fisher-Race system, and hr' and hr'' are c and e (Table 16-2). Wiener's proposal for the inheritance of these antigens is that multiple alleles may exist at a single locus. At the time this hypothesis was forwarded by Wiener, it was viewed skeptically, since such a mode of inheritance had never been suggested previously for blood group antigens. Now, however, the HLAs are believed to be inherited in this fashion. This belief has strengthened the acceptance of this method for naming the Rh antigens.

Table 16-2. Partial list of human blood group systems

System	Number of antigens	Antigens			
ABO(H)	4	A_1, A_2, B, H plus four interactions with the I system			
Rh	33	Rh1	Rh_0, D	Rh18	Hr
		Rh2	rh', C	Rh19	hr^s
		Rh3	rh'', E	Rh20	VS, e^s
		Rh4	hr', c	Rh21	C^G
		Rh5	hr'', e	Rh22	CE
		Rh6	hr, f, ce	Rh23	D^w (Wiel)
		Rh7	rh_i, Ce	Rh24	E^T
		Rh8	rh^{w1}, C^w	Rh25	LW
		Rh9	rh^x, C^x, ce^s	Rh26	c-like (Deal)
		Rh10	hr^v, V	Rh27	cE
		Rh11	rh^{w2}, E^w	Rh28	hr^H
		Rh12	rh^G, G	Rh29	RH
		Rh13	Rh^A	Rh30	Go^a, C^{Cor}
		Rh14	Rh^B	Rh31	hr^B
		Rh15	Rh^C	Rh32	Troll (Reynolds)
		Rh16	Rh^D	Rh33	Ro^{Har}
		Rh17	Hro		
MN	28	M, N, S, s, U, U^B, M_1, M^A, M^C, M^g, M^V, Tm, Sj, Mi^a, Vu, Mur, Hill, Hu, He, M^e, Vr, St^a, Mt^a, Ri^a, Cl^a, Vr^a, Ny^a, Sul			
P	4	P_1, P_2, p, Tja, plus one interaction each with ABO (Luke) and with I (IP)			
I	5	I, i, i_2, I^t, I^D			
Lutheran	3	Lu^a, Lu^b, Lu^{ab}			
Kell	10	K, k, Kp^a, Kp^b, Js^a, Js^b, Kp^o, K^w, KL, $U1^a$			
Lewis	6	Le^a, Le^b, Le^c, Le^x, Le^{ab}, Mag			
Duffy	3	Fy^a, Fy^b, Fy^3			
Kidd	2	Jk^a, Jk^b			
DBG	4	Ho, Ho-like, Ot, DBG			

Low-frequency antigens, not grouped: Be^a, By, Evans, Good, Box, Job, Kam, Lev, Mag, Nij, Or, Rd, Rm, Sf, Spl, Ta^a, Tr^a, Ven, Wb, Zd, and many others

High-frequency antigens not grouped: AT^a, Bra, Co^a, Ge, Kelly, Lan, Sd^a, Yus, and many others

The third nomenclature system is a simple numeric system proposed by Rosenfield in 1962 in which $Rh1 = Rh_0 = D$, etc. (Table 16-2). The numeric system has not yet been widely accepted as a neutral solution for those debating the merits of the Wiener and Fisher-Race systems.

Regardless of the system of nomenclature or the exact modes of inheritance, it is agreed that an allelic system is followed. Thus an Rh-positive person may be either homozygous or heterozygous, but an Rh-negative person is necessarily homozygous. This is an important consideration when discussing HDN caused by maternal-fetal Rh incompatibility.

Rh antigens and antibodies

The number of Rh_0 (D) antigen sites on human erythrocytes has been variably estimated to be between 2,000 and 33,000 per cell. If we accept 10,000 to 15,000 as an average value, then the number of A or B sites per cell exceeds the number of Rh_0 sites by about fortyfold. The Rh antigens can be detected on fetal erythrocytes by 6 weeks of age. Efforts to arrive at chemical formulas for the immunodominant portions of these antigens have been handicapped by several factors; lectins with a specificity for the Rh antigen are still unknown, and highly purified soluble Rh antigens are difficult to prepare. Chemical hydrolysis of partially purified preparations and inhibition of antibodies by saccharides suggest that Rh_0 contains neuraminic acid as part of its structure, but the chemistry of the Rh antigens is largely unknown.

Human immunoglobulins to the Rh antigens differ from the hemagglutinins to the ABO(H) antigens in that the former arise from genuine alloimmunization and do not exist as ''natural'' antibodies. Thus an Rh-negative person does not axiomatically have antibodies to the Rh_0 antigen. As described earlier, Rh-negative means the absence of Rh_0, or D; so an Rh-positive person cannot make antibodies to an antigen that does not exist. (Notice that this applies only to D and d; a person who is genetically CDE [and Rh-positive] can make antibodies to antigens c and e.) Alloantibodies directed toward the Rh antigens may be of the IgM or IgG class. The route of immunization is from improper transfusion of Rh-positive blood into an Rh-negative recipient or maternal immunization by Rh-positive fetal erythrocytes. Mild or recent antigen exposure will favor IgM, and more intensive immunization will favor IgG. Both classes of immunoglobulin usually can be detected by hemagglutination tests, although the IgM antibodies are considered the more efficient hemagglutinins, as discussed earlier.

HDN

Erythroblastosis fetalis, one of the more severe forms of HDN, is frequently the result of a so-called Rh incompatibility. The conditions for development of HDN exist when an Rh-negative mother carries an Rh-positive child and through alloimmunization produces antibodies to the Rh antigen. This antibody, if of the IgG class, can pass the placental barrier and react with the fetal erythrocytes (Fig. 16-3). These erythrocytes are removed from the circulation and lysed, causing a hemolytic condition in the fetus. An attempt by the erythropoietic tissue of the fetus to compensate for this loss of mature red blood cells results in an outpouring of immature erythrocytes (erythroblasts) into the blood. From this the name of the condition is derived. Depending on the severity of the disease, the fetus may be aborted, may be stillborn, or may be born alive with evidence of a hemolytic disease.

Until recently there has been little agreement on the origin of maternal Rh alloimmunization. Earlier it had been noted that the first Rh-incompatible pregnancy rarely resulted in HDN but that the risk for erythroblastosis fetalis steadily increased with each succeeding pregnancy. From this it was deduced that the greatest opportunity for maternal immunization was associated with the trauma of childbirth, and there are methods by which fetal contamination of maternal blood can be detected. For example, the hemoglobin of fetal erythrocytes is quickly leached from red blood cells by dilute acid, whereas adult hemoglobin is not. Periodic examination of a mother's blood during pregnancy and especially after delivery has proved that the child's red blood cells can be present in the maternal circulation in the last trimester of pregnancy and after childbirth. Radiolabeled erythrocytes placed in the uterine cavity immediately after delivery were detected in the maternal circulation in 10 of 30 instances. Fluorescent antibody to human γ-globulin that is attached to Rh-positive cells can detect one antibody-coated cell in a population of 1 million Rh-negative cells. This means that as little as 0.01 ml of fetal blood can be detected as foreign in the maternal circulation. By such methods, used in different patient study groups, it has been revealed that 20% to 50% of the mothers are exposed to the blood of their children at delivery.

First Rh-positive pregnancy   Second Rh pregnancy

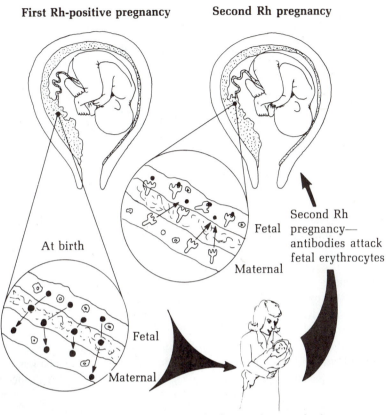

Second Rh
pregnancy—
antibodies attack
fetal erythrocytes

At birth

Fetal

Maternal

Fetal

Maternal

Mother makes antibodies

Fig. 16-3. Erythroblastosis fetalis is the result of maternal immunization to fetal erythrocytes in a first pregnancy, usually at birth, followed by the transplacental migration of these antibodies to attack fetal red blood cells in a subsequent pregnancy.

Rh immunoprophylaxis. To the knowledge that immunization occurred most often at delivery, additional pieces of information have been added to produce an immunologic method for the control of erythroblastosis. One of the added bits of information is that blood group O, Rh-negative mothers have fewer infants with hemolytic disease than statistics would predict. It was suggested that the maternal anti-A and anti-B combined with any A, Rh-positive or B, Rh-positive fetal cells at the moment they entered the maternal circulation and contributed to their speedy removal without antibody formation. It also was shown that Rh-

negative men given Rh_0-positive cells precoated in vitro with anti-Rh_0 were protected from making anti-Rh_0. This led to experiments in which pregnant women were given anti-Rh_0 γ-globulin if immunization from an Rh-positive child was anticipated. In one of the studies conducted in the United States 0.2% of mothers passively immunized with anti-Rh_0 globulins developed anti-Rh_0, whereas nearly 7% of untreated mothers produced the antibody. In a study in England 21% of non-passively immunized controls produced anti-Rh_0, compared with only 0.6% of immunized mothers. The studies have been so convincing that passively administered anti-Rh$_0$ now is given at every delivery or induced abortion for an Rh-negative woman and is considered routine perinatal care for the mother. A typical recommendation is that 100 to 200 μg of anti-Rh$_0$ be given within 72 hours of delivery unless there is a heavy load of fetal erythrocytes entering the maternal circulation, in which case 1,000 μg of antiserum is given. Interestingly it is believed that incomplete Rh$_0$ antibodies are largely responsible for the protection and that complete, hemagglutinating antibodies are ineffective. The only serious risk to the procedure that has been noted so far is that recipients who are unable to synthesize IgA may become sensitized to this immunoglobulin and be subject to anaphylactic shock on reexposure as a result of later pregnancy. It is believed that Rh immunoprophylaxis may reduce Rh-mediated HDN to 1 in every 20,000 opportunities.

Coombs' tests. However, feedback control of Rh immunization by the passive administration of anti-Rh$_0$ globulins at the time of delivery only controls future Rh disease and can do little to regulate erythroblastosis when the mother already has been immunized by a previous Rh-positive pregnancy or improper blood transfusion. In these instances the attending physician must in some way measure the potential for HDN. He could assume that maternal anti-Rh could be detected by merely incubating the mother's serum with Rh-positive erythrocytes and determining if they are agglutinated. Such would be the case if the mother had produced the usual complete antibody. Experience has shown, however, that incomplete antibody is as likely as complete antibody to cause erythroblastosis, even though incomplete antibodies do not function in the ordinary hemagglutination test. Fortunately Coombs and his associates have devised a test to demonstrate incomplete antibodies in maternal sera or on fetal or newborn erythrocytes. The Coombs tests, for actually there are two, are known as antiglobulin tests or double antibody tests. In immunologic jargon such tests sometimes are described as immunologic sandwich procedures.

The direct Coombs test is used to detect monovalent maternal antibody already present on the infant's erythrocytes (Fig. 16-4). These antibodies are often anti-Rh in character but could be directed as well toward other erythrocyte antigens. For positive tests it is necessary for the maternal antibody to pass the placenta, enter into the circulation of the unborn child, and attach to his or her red blood cells. If the mother has a low titer of these antibodies, caused either by the decay of hemagglutinin titers developed from an early exposure to antigen or by recent immunization in this pregnancy, insufficient antibody may be present in the fetus to cause death or even serious hemolytic disease prior to birth. However, it is not unusual in such instances for gradual jaundice of the baby to develop within the first few days after birth as a result of red blood cell destruction. This may require total blood exchange transfusion. Therefore it is important to test the baby's red blood cells for antibodies that might cause hemolysis. This is accomplished by the direct Coombs test, which requires only one incubation, that is, newborn red blood cells (coated with incomplete antibody) with an antibody to human γ-globulin. The latter product is available commercially and is prepared by immunizing rabbits, goats, or other animals with human γ-globulin. The Coombs antiglobulin reagent must be a divalent antiglobulin that will combine with the human γ-globulin on the red blood cells and produce hemagglutination. The incomplete anti-Rh serves as both an antibody and an antigen and is the filling in the immunologic sandwich. A negative direct Coombs test is interpreted as an absence of maternal antibody on the child's erythrocytes.

The indirect test is designed to detect the presence of incomplete anti-Rh globulins in maternal sera (Fig. 16-5). Two incubations are needed, as compared with the single incubation in the direct test. Maternal serum is incubated with known Rh-positive cells, after which the cells are washed to remove extraneous serum proteins. This is followed by incubation of the coated cells (in the case of tests that will be positive) with Coombs'

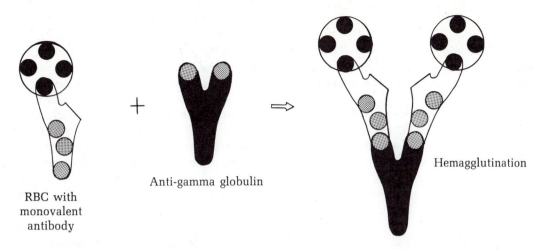

Fig. 16-4. Direct Coombs' test. Erythrocytes coated with a monovalent antibody that is incapable of hemagglutination become agglutinated by an antibody versus the antierythrocyte globulin. Although the monovalent antibody, as illustrated, lacks one Fab fragment, the evidence is that the monovalent and divalent antibodies differ only in function and not in structure.

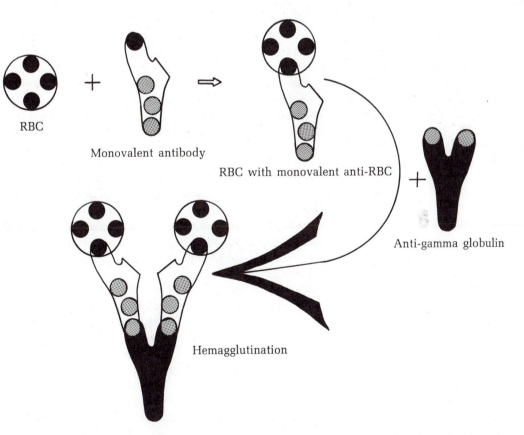

Fig. 16-5. Indirect Coombs' test. This test is the same as the direct test except that the monovalent antierythrocyte globulin must be combined with the red blood cell prior to addition of the antiglobulin in the second stage of the reaction.

reagent, which then agglutinates the cells. Naturally there is no need to perform the indirect Coombs test on maternal sera that contain complete hemagglutinins.

As mentioned briefly, the Coombs test is applicable to the detection of any incomplete immunoglobulin. HDN may arise from incompatibilities between antigens other than the Rh antigen; when monovalent antibodies are incriminated, they can be measured by the Coombs antiglobulin test.

MISCELLANEOUS HUMAN BLOOD GROUP SYSTEMS

The second blood group system to be discovered, the MN system, was reported by Landsteiner and Levine in 1927, more than a decade prior to the discovery of the Rh system. These antigens were detected by the use of specific sera produced in rabbits, and the letters *M* and *N* were chosen arbitrarily. The two original antigens of this system are inherited in the same way as the A and B antigens so that three blood groups are possible: MM, MN, and NN. There is no group corresponding to O. The frequency of the M, MN, and N groups in the white population is 29%, 50%, and 21%, respectively. Human anti-M is fairly frequent; anti-N is more rare. Detection of M and N antigens now is accomplished with a lectin of *Iberis amara* for the M antigen and of *Vicia graminea* or *Bauhinia purpura* for the N antigen.

The MN system now has been expanded to include at least 28 different antigens. The best known of these additional antigens are S, s, and U. Nearly 100% of whites and 95% of blacks have the U antigen. The S and s antigens are inherited in a four-gene complex with M and N, permitting the combinations MS, Ms, NS, and Ns. Much is yet to be learned about the chemistry of these antigens, but the evidence currently available indicates that M and N are dependent on a complex polysaccharide core modified by *N*-acetylneuraminic acid groups. These antigens are rarely involved in HDN.

Antigens and antibodies of the I blood group system have some interesting relationships to several disease conditions and to human development. The discovery of the I blood group was made in 1956 by Wiener and his associates, who suggested that the cold agglutinin found in patients with hemolytic anemia was directed against a specific antigen. This antigen, the I antigen, is present on virtually 100% of human adult red blood cells and is one of the two major antigens in this group, the other antigen being i. Agglutinins with anti-I activity are thus autoantibodies, and, as indicated, most of these antibodies have a unique thermal amplitude, reacting at 4° C but hardly at all at 37° C. Anti-i exists with a high frequency in patients with infectious mononucleosis, but the basis for this relationship is uncertain.

Fetal erythrocytes and those taken from cord blood or newborn infants do not react with anti-I. During the first months of life these i cells tend to disappear and by the second year of life are replaced by I cells of the adult type. Adult type cells still contain traces of the i antigen; so this i → I transition probably is related to an enzymatic "maturation" that converts the i substance to the I antigen. Red blood cells of persons with chronic hemolytic anemia or hypoplastic anemia react strongly with anti-i. Thus immature erythrocytes originating from natural or disease conditions are deficient in I but have the precursor i substance.

The first antibody in the Kell blood group system was described in 1946 by Coombs, Mourant, and Race as a result of the first clinical uses of the Coombs antiglobulin test. It was realized that the fetal erythrocytes were coated in this instance with a non-Rh, incomplete antibody that was termed "anti-Kell," after the family name. The antigens originally identified were labeled K and k, which are inherited in the expected manner, but with K being present in only 9% of the population, KK in 2%, and Kk in 7%. The predominant group is thus kk, at an incidence of about 82%. Since 1957 several new antigens have been added to the Kell system; currently it is composed of at least 10 antigens (Table 16-2). Of these, the K and k antigens still appear to be the most potent. The Kell system is often involved in HDN, more often than one would expect from the low frequency of the K antigen.

One sex-linked human blood group antigen, Xg^a, has been discovered. It should be recalled that females are genetically XX and males XY in reference to the sex chromosomes. Thus daughters must receive an X chromosome from each parent, whereas sons receive the X chromosome only from their mother and the Y from their father. Inheritance of the Xg^a antigen follows this genetic principle. An Xg(a+)Y father and Xg(a−a−) mother can produce Xg(a−)Y sons and Xg(a+a−) daughters. An Xg(a+)Y father and Xg(a+a−) mother will produce Xg(a+a−) daughters and half Xg(a+) and half Xg(a−) sons.

The Duffy blood group system is of considerable interest to anthropologists. Of the two major antigens in the system, Fy^a and Fy^b, the Fy^a antigen is present on approximately 65% of white erythrocytes and lacking on a similar percentage of Negroid cells. Likewise, the Fy^b antigen is infrequent on Negroid cells; so nearly 70% of blacks can be classified as Fy(a−b−). No other erythrocyte system so clearly distinguishes whites and blacks. The Fy^a antigen incidence is even higher in Mongolians than in whites, exceeding 99.5%.

New blood cell antigens continuously are being discovered. When it can be shown that the inheritance of two or more antigens is interrelated, then the antigens are placed in a blood group. If the inheritance of these antigens is unrelated to the inheritance of a preexistent group, the creation of a new blood group system is justified. The time required to make these decisions is often considerable, perhaps several years. During this time the presumed new antigen or blood group has to be named in some way so that it is not confused with existing blood group systems. The first red cell antigens to be discovered were assigned capital letters A and B, and then later M and N, and still later C and D of the Rh system. When the suggestion of an alphabetic order was broken in the formation of the MN group, then one or more

letters from the name of the first individual known to have the antigen or antibody was used, as in Rh (rhesus), K (Kell), and Le (Lewis). The letters need not come from the first part of the name; the name ending also can be used, as in Fy (Duffy). As additional antigens were discovered within a group, subscripts, superscripts, changes in case, and combinations of these were used to name the new antigens. In this way A_1, rh', rh'', Rh_0, Le^a, and others were created. Currently there is a tendency to use the first three or more letters of the person's last name for new blood group antigens. The result of this mixture of nomenclature systems is that there is no simple method for learning blood group antigens.

Blood cell antigens often are described as public or private antigens, depending on their incidence. ''Public'' antigens are those which are unusually common but not a part of a known group; At^a, Co^a, Ge, and Lan are examples. In many instances these antigens later are placed in new or existing groups. ''Private,'' or ''family,'' antigens generally have an incidence of less than 0.25%. Such antigens are especially useful in identifying specific individuals or groups and are valuable genetic tools.

Blood group systems depending on antigenic variations of white blood cells and platelets also have been constructed. Those based on leukocyte antigens are discussed in Chapter 11, where their importance as histocompatibility antigens is explained.

APPLICATIONS OF HEMAGGLUTINATION
Blood transfusions

The practical importance of blood groups and blood grouping in modern medicine is immeasurable. The increasing use of blood transfusions has made hemagglutination the most frequent serologic test performed. In blood transfusions it is essential that the recipient be given exactly his or her own type of blood insofar as possible. For example, a group A person should not receive group B blood, since the blood would be destroyed by the B alloagglutinins of the group A person. A group A person might be given group O blood, despite the known content of anti-A in the latter. This is often a safe procedure, since in the transfusion the anti-A globulins will be diluted extensively in the recipient, possibily beyond the titer of their activity. It is on this basis that the group O person has been described as the "universal donor" and the group AB person as the "universal recipient." In emergencies this may be an acceptable operating procedure, but in everyday blood banking an exact matching of donor and recipient blood is the goal.

All laboratories perform two tests to determine the suitability of a transfusion. These are called the major and minor cross matches. The major cross match, called major because it is of greater importance, is performed by mixing the serum of the recipient with the blood cells of the donor. If agglutination occurs, this blood cannot be given to the recipient for the obvious reason that the recipient has antibodies which will destroy the donor cells. In the minor cross match the recipient's cells are mixed with the donor's serum. If agglutination occurs, the blood should not be given because the donor's serum contains antibodies capable of attacking the recipient's cells. It is only during a true emergency that such blood can be given. A positive minor cross match destroys the concept of O blood being the universal donor, since it contains both anti-A and anti-B globulins and only can match with O blood. Similarly, since AB blood is agglutinated by all except group AB sera, an AB person is not a universal recipient.

To these considerations of the ABO system must be added identical considerations with the other major blood group antigens, the Rh system, MN, P, S, and others. Because of the vast and expanding number of these systems, coupled with the increased frequency of blood transfusion, the importance of the major and minor cross match cannot be overemphasized.

In actual practice the minor cross match is not used extensively, and the major cross match, now called the compatibility test, is the only test being used. Compatibility testing has the major limitation that it does not detect antigens. For example, the Rh antigen would not be detected in a donor's blood by cross matching with a nonimmune Rh-negative person. Transfusion of such blood would actively immunize the recipient and set the stage for a subsequent transfusion reaction if similar Rh-positive blood were given again. Incomplete antibodies can be identified in the compatibility test by performing the Coombs test after the incubation of donor cells and recipient serum.

Blood transfusion reactions historically have been thought of as resulting only from mismatched red blood cells interacting with immunoglobulins. This is still the major cause of hemolytic transfusion reactions, but reactions caused by foreign white blood cells or platelets are a common cause of transient fever after transfusion. An awareness of previous immunization to plasma proteins such as IgA is also necessary to ensure safe transfusions.

Because of the many problems associated with whole blood transfusion—the immunologic problems just discussed plus problems relating to the collection and storage of large quantities of blood, not to omit the expense of whole blood—the search for a total blood substitute has been a constant research endeavor. Heretofore limited success has met the search for blood volume expanders, in the form of dextran or albumin, to replace the fluid portion of blood. Now it appears that an oxygen-transporting substitute may exist in the form of perfluorochemicals which can replace red blood cells. Perfluorochemicals, such as perfluorobutyltetrahydrofuran or perfluorotributylamine, are chemical compounds in which all H atoms have been replaced by F. Many of these compounds will carry sufficient dissolved oxygen so that animals totally immersed in solutions of the perfluor continue to live. When the animals are removed from the solution and the perfluorochemical is drained from their lungs, they appear perfectly normal and respire in the usual way. These fluorocompounds are prepared in the form of emulsions for intravenous use and have successfully replaced red blood cells. More data, especially on the toxicity of these compounds in long-term use, are needed, but the future is promising. Although these compounds may replace the erythrocyte portion of the blood, it is not expected that suitable replacements for the leukocytes, the clotting or the buffering systems, or the macromolecular components of blood will be easily located. Thus, future hematologists may escape laborious erythrocyte-typing tests and still be plagued by transfusion difficulties associated with the other elements of blood; but even this would be a remarkable feat.

Personal identification

Because of the large number of blood group antigens that are now known, it is almost possible to identify a specific individual by his or her own special combination of antigens. This fact, coupled with an understanding of genetic principles, has led to a number of forensic applications based on erythrocyte antigens. In paternity suits certain combinations of blood types in the mother and child will exclude the possibility of certain men being the father. For example, an AB man cannot father a group OO child; an A woman and an A man cannot produce a B child; an A_1 woman and an A_1 man cannot produce an A_2 child; and an O, Rh-negative woman and an O, Rh-negative man cannot produce an O, Rh-positive child. Blood group testing can only exclude a putative father from fatherhood; this is now generally accepted in courts of law. By means of similar tests "mixed babies" in the newborn nursery often can be identified as belonging to a specific mother-father combination.

Another forensic application of blood grouping occurs in cases of violent deaths with loss of blood. As described in the previous chapter, serologic testing with specific antisera can identify the species and blood type of stains that are days, weeks, or even years old. Proof of the origin of bloodstains is often very useful in cases of suspected homicide, suicide, or severe bodily injury.

Passive hemagglutination and passive agglutination

The type of hemagglutination described in the previous paragraphs may be categorized as immune, direct hemagglutination. This implies two other forms of hemagglutination: nonimmune and indirect. Actually a few examples of the former already have been presented. The agglutination of erythrocytes by phytoagglutinins or lectins is accomplished via a nonimmune mechanism. To this could be added hemagglutination by viruses, especially the myxoviruses such as influenza virus and Newcastle's disease virus. A few bacteria also are capable of effecting direct hemagglutination. Antibodies to these direct agglutinating viruses or bacteria will inhibit hemagglutination; this is the basis for hemagglutination inhibition tests, which have been useful in quantitating sera against certain pathogens.

Indirect, or passive, hemagglutination is based on the red blood cell as an inert carrier (Schlepper) of antigens (Fig. 16-6). Erythrocytes often are preferred to other particles as the carrier because hemagglutination is a familiar serologic test and the results are easily interpreted. Hemagglutination tests are easily converted to hemolytic tests by the addition of complement, and hemolytic tests are adaptable to exact quantitation by colorimetry or spectrophotometry. This permits an exact measurement of the amount of antibody in an antiserum. Of course spontaneous lysis of erythrocytes is one complaint about passive hemagglutination testing. This interferes with the reading of the test and precludes long-term storage of antigen-coated cells. This handicap has been overcome in two ways: by the use of glutaraldehyde- or formaldehyde-treated erythrocytes as the antigen carrier and by the use of carrier particles that are less fragile or totally resistant to osmotic lysis. Aldehyde-treated cells take on a brown color and resist lysis. They even can be frozen and thawed

RBC with attached antigen   Antibody

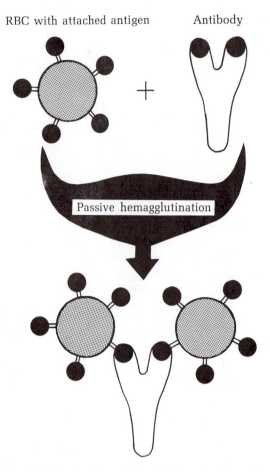

Passive hemagglutination

Fig. 16-6. Passive hemagglutination by using the erythrocyte as an inert carrier of an antigen.

or lyophilized so that an antigen-coated red blood cell can be preserved almost indefinitely. Other types of cells, yeast, or bacteria or other materials such as polystyrene spheres, polyacrylamide, and particles of latex or of charcoal, which are more osmotically resistant and in some cases easier to prepare, are replacing erythrocytes as the carrier. For example, polystyrene latex particles of various sizes can be purchased in a concentrated stock preparation dyed a light blue to make them more visible. These can be diluted, coated with antigen, and used very simply in passive agglutination tests.

There are many variations of the passive hemagglutination test. In the simplest form the antigen is incubated with the erythrocytes, and antigen adsorption takes place spontaneously. The antigen-coated erythrocytes are washed to remove excess free antigen and then are incubated with antiserum to the adsorbed antigen to produce hemagglutination. The biochemical class of molecule most easily adsorbed on erythrocytes is polysaccharide or polysaccharides that are conjugated with lipids or proteins. LPS is a typical example. Pure protein antigens cannot be used in this type of test because they do not attach to the red blood cells. Only tiny amounts of the polysaccharide antigens are required—about $100 \ \mu g/10^{10}$ cells. This is equivalent to about 2,000 molecules per erythrocyte.

The erythrocyte receptors for polysaccharides have never been identified. The red blood cells are still agglutinable by anti-A, anti-B, or anti-Rh sera; so these antigens still are available in an unmasked form. Receptor-destroying enzyme, which removes the attachment receptor for viral hemagglutination, does not remove the polysaccharide receptors. Several types of receptors may be present, or at least several antigens can be coated onto the cells simultaneously. These receptors apparently are present on other blood and tissue cells, since they can be used also in passive agglutination tests.

One handicap of simple adsorptive coating of erythrocytes by antigen is that the antigen-erythrocyte bond is strictly a physical bond, and the antigen can dissociate easily from the cell. This is of special concern because any antigen released into solution will ''tie up'' antibody and prevent its combination with the antigen present on the red cells. The consequence of this is that the free antigen behaves as a blocking antigen and seriously reduces the hemagglutinating titer of the antiserum.

Protein antigens can be complexed with erythrocytes that have been pretreated with tannic acid according to the technique of Boyden. These tanned erythrocytes do not lose their polysaccharide receptors, so they still will bond to these antigens as well. Tannic acid, in a final concentration of 1:20,000 to 1:40,000, is used to alter the cell and reveal new protein receptors. Spontaneous agglutination of the red cells occurs if they are overexposed to tannic acid. Buffers containing colloids prevent this. Tanned cells are especially liable to lysis, so formalinized cells are recommended. Certain metals (for example, chromium salts) will complex proteins to erythrocytes and provide a more stable antigen preparation than is afforded by the usual adsorption process.

The principal disadvantage of the aforementioned tests, from an immunologic point of view, is that the antigens are only loosely bound to the erythrocyte carrier. Dissociation of the antigen from the ordinary or the tanned erythrocyte can occur without notice and can invalidate the red blood cells as the "antigen." To overcome this deficit, methods designed for covalent bonding of antigens to erythrocytes have been developed. Dinitrodifluorobenzene, bisdiazotized benzidine, toluene diisocyanate, and other dually reactive compounds, such as those applied to ferritin labeling of antibodies, have been used. The antigen, erythrocyte, and coupling reagent, when mixed in the correct proportions, will yield a covalently linked red cell–antigen conjugate of almost interminable life expectancy. Such a preparation can be lyophilized in small portions and rehydrated for use, which obviates the repeated preparation and standardization of smaller, individual batches of antigen.

One useful modification of the passive hemagglutination technique is the reversed passive hemagglutination test, whereby the antibody is united covalently with the carrier and is used to detect antigen. Inhibition tests also can be devised wherein free antigen reacts with antibody to prevent its agglutination of antigen-coated erythrocytes.

The principal purpose of all passive hemagglutination tests is to convert precipitation reactions to hemagglutination reactions and to increase the sensitivity of the test. Passive hemagglutination tests are among the most sensitive serologic procedures available; under ideal conditions as little as 0.003 μg of antibody nitrogen will yield a positive test. Consequently passive hemagglutination titers of 1:1,000,000 and higher are not unusual.

Both IgG and IgM function in passive hemagglutination tests because of the good IgG response to protein antigens and IgM response to polysaccharide antigens.

Several passive agglutination or reversed passive agglutination tests now are used in clinical laboratories. These include tests for antibodies to nucleoproteins diagnostic for LE, antibodies to thyroglobulin and RF important in detecting Hashimoto's thyroiditis and rheumatoid arthritis, and antibodies formed in specific diseases, including histoplasmosis and trichinosis. Reversed passive agglutination is used to determine the presence of C-reactive protein in human serum and the blood level of fibrinogen or of γ-globulin. Passive agglutination inhibition tests are used to measure the presence of antigens or low molecular weight substances. The most common of these is the test for human chorionic gonadotropic hormone in pregnancy testing. One of each of these three types is discussed in the following paragraphs.

The C-reactive protein is an unusual protein produced in the liver and excreted into the bloodstream only on certain occasions; at other times the blood is free of this protein. The protein is found in the blood in instances of inflammatory or infectious diseases or cancer and during pregnancy. C-reactive protein was so named because it precipitates with the C substance, a somatic polysaccharide of pneumococci. C-reactive protein is not an antibody; it is not even a γ-globulin. It is merely a unique protein produced during conditions of poor health that attaches to phosphorylcholine residues in complex oligosaccharides. Of interest is the fact that it is antigenic. Antibodies from experimental animals will precipitate C-reactive protein; if these antibodies are attached to latex particles, the particles passively agglutinate in sera containing the C-reactive protein. The test is a reversed passive agglutination test used as an index of an inflammatory disease.

To diagnose Hashimoto's thyroiditis, a passive hemagglutination test has been developed based on the attachment of human thyroglobulin to inert carrier particles. A positive slide agglutination test with these particles and a patient's serum indicates the presence of anti–human thyroglobulin in the serum. This autoantibody is not an absolute index of autoimmune thyroiditis, but it often is used as a screening test for patients potentially suffering from this disease.

The passive agglutination inhibition test for human chorionic gonadotropin has become the most rapid, least expensive, and most popular test for this hormone, replacing the earlier rabbit and frog tests for pregnancy. Several forms of the test are available commercially; in one kit two main reagents are provided. The first is an antiserum to the hormone, which has a molecular weight of 30,000 and is an acceptable antigen. The other reagent is a formalinized erythrocyte preparation to which the hormone is attached. A mixture of the two reagents will produce a passive hemagglutination. Preincubation of fluids containing the hormone (urine or serum of pregnant women) with the antiserum will cause a serologic reaction (invisible because of the concentration of antiserum used) which will bind the antiserum so that it cannot agglutinate the hormone-bearing cells. This test is so simply performed that self-test kits now have been marketed. With obvious modifications it is adaptable to the measurement of other antigens and haptens.

BACTERIAL AGGLUTINATION
H and O bacterial agglutination

The discovery of bacterial agglutination by Grüber and Durham in 1896 and the popularization by Widal of the agglutination test as a diagnostic aid for bacterial infections are described in Chapter 1. It now is recognized that practically all cells—bacteria, yeasts, erythrocytes, leukocytes, sperm, and others—can be agglutinated by specific antiserum. The agglutination of bacteria has been one of the key methods used to identify and classify these microorganisms which lack the gross identifying features present in higher life forms.

Bacterial agglutination tests may be performed in tubes or on slides (Fig. 16-7). In the tube agglutination test a dilution series of antiserum is prepared, and, to each tube, a suspension of bacteria is added so that the final concentration of the organisms is approximately 900×10^6 per milliliter. Bacteria at this concentration will give a light opalescence to the suspension. The dilution of the antiserum is determined on the basis of the total volume in the tube after all reagents have been added. The tubes are incubated, removed, and examined. Agglutination frequently is difficult to detect at this time, and so refrigeration of the test overnight often is practiced to allow further aggregation. At this time the titer can be determined by merely examining the tubes to see which still contain a cloudy suspension and which are clear; agglutinated cells do not remain in a uniform suspension and will settle to the bottom of the tube. This can be confirmed by tapping the tubes and looking for aggregates of bacteria, which rise from the sediment in the tubes exhibiting agglutination.

In the slide agglutination test small volumes of the antiserum are dispensed onto a slide and mixed with a dense suspension of organisms. The slide is tilted gently to and fro or rotated for 3 to 5 minutes. Agglutinated cells are seen as large clumps of bacteria. The slide test is more rapid and economic but is less precise than the tube test.

In either the tube or the slide test a difference in the physical size of the clumped bacteria may be noted, depending on the nature of the organism and the antiserum used. If the antiserum is prepared against a whole, intact, motile organism, such as *Salmonella typhi*, and if the same organism is used in the agglutination test, the clumps will be rather large and light or snowflake in appearance. This is referred to as the H type of bacterial agglutination; H is taken from the German word *Hauch*, which means a film, breath, or haze, much as one might see on a steamed glass. Motile

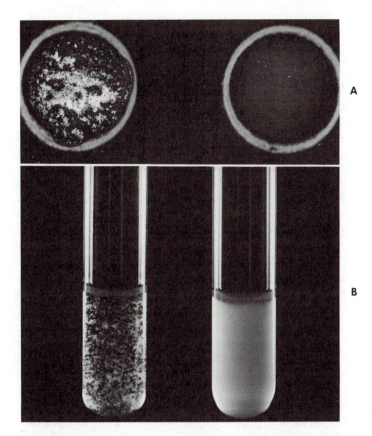

Fig. 16-7. A, Slide agglutination of bacteria is a rapid method of identifying unknown bacteria with known antisera or the reverse. **B,** Tube agglutination can be used for the same purpose and to quantitate the antibody content in an antiserum. In each case the positive test is seen at left and the negative control at right.

bacteria will produce a thin, nearly transparent type of growth on a moist agar plate. This loose flocculant type of agglutination is indicative of the operation of flagellar antigens (H antigens) and their respective antibodies in the test. The flagella, extending as they do some distance from the bacteria, are "glued" to each other by antibody molecules. This unites the bacteria into an agglutinate even though the bacterial cells proper are still some distance from each other. The result is a loosely woven lacework of clumped cells, which produces a light, snowflake type of agglutination.

Quite the opposite occurs in the O type of ag-glutination (O from the German *ohne Hauch,* meaning without a film, hence aflagellate). In this instance agglutination is the result of antibodies to somatic (cellular) antigens, which hold the cell walls of the bacteria very closely together (Fig. 16-7). The consequence of this is the formation of a very compact, granular or hailstonelike mass of agglutinated bacteria.

Bacterial agglutination results largely from antibodies of the IgM class. In describing H and O agglutination or H and O antigens it is necessary to distinguish between human blood cell antigens and bacterial agglutination systems.

Bacterial antigens

It is obvious that the chemical nature of the agglutinogens will vary as widely as the bacteria that produce them. For this reason only the O antigens on the genus *Salmonella* are considered in detail, with a more general discussion of those of gram-positive bacteria.

Antigens of gram-positive bacteria. The chemistry of the cell walls and plasma membranes of gram-positive bacteria is dominated by the teichoic acids, which are absent from gram-negative bacteria. Teichoic acids are polymeric phosphate esters of glycerol and ribitol substituted with alanyl and glycosyl groups. The teichoic acids found in the cell membrane are always of the glycerol type and covalently joined to a glycolipid. For this reason they are designated as lipoteichoic acids. Teichoic acids of the cell wall may be based on either a glycerol or ribitol structure covalently linked to a peptidoglycan. Cell wall teichoic acids and some lipoteichoic acids are sufficiently surface oriented to combine with antibodies. For example, the group D antigen of streptococci is a lipoteichoic acid that is not found in cells walls, only the plasma membrane, yet it participates in agglutination reactions.

Lipoteichoic acids are responsible for many of the cross-reactions of gram-positive bacteria, but this does not mean that the teichoic acids are identical among all cross-reacting bacteria. These acids contain several antigenic determinants, including the glycerol phosphate backbone of the polymer, the alanyl and glycosyl side groups, and the glycolipid, although antibodies directed against the latter are rare. Those determinants need not be all identical in cross-reacting species. In some instances, as in the group D and also the group A, F, and N streptococci, lipoteichoic acids common to members of the group form the basis for the serologic grouping. Other streptococci possess other teichoic acids, and this is expressed by the failure of them to cross-react with the antilipoteichoic sera used to establish the separate antigenic groups.

Antigenic classification of *Salmonella* organ-ism. The antigenic complexities of the enteric bacilli have been most thoroughly studied of all bacteria, both on a serologic and on a chemical basis. As a result of systematic serologic experiments, largely by Kauffmann and White, approximately 1,100 serotypes within the genus *Salmonella* alone have been distinguished. These are determined on the basis of somatic, or O, antigens, flagellar, or H, antigens, and virulence, or Vi (somatic), antigens. A unique combination of these in an organism creates a unique serotype. In the classification of the salmonellae each new serotype has been treated and named as a new species. The fallaciousness of this practice, as it might be extended to higher life forms, now has been recognized, and species names in the genus *Salmonella* have been revised.

On the basis of common somatic O antigens the individual serotypes (species) of the genus *Salmonella* are placed in groups designated by the latters A to I. All group B species, for example, contain somatic antigen 4, and all group C_1 members contain antigens 6 and 7. There are actually some 60 different O antigens used to define the 40 groups. These serogroups are divided into serotypes on the basis of their H antigens. The virulence antigen is not used in the construction of either serogroups or serotypes. The Vi antigen is a somatic antigen situated external to the O antigens and may prevent bacterial agglutination by anti-O sera. The Vi antigen is destroyed easily by mild heating, by dilute acid, or by repeated transfer of the organism on artificial media. The H antigens are destroyed by alcohol or by extensive heating. To prepare an antiserum that contains anti-Vi globulins, a fresh isolate of the organism must be used. Of course the antiserum also will contain antibodies to the H and O antigens. An antiserum that contains only anti-H and anti-O immunoglobulins can be prepared by using midly heated, acid-exposed, or repeatedly transferred cells as the vaccine. Such cells are referred to as H cells. O cells can be prepared by alcohol treatment of H cells.

Agglutinin adsorption and cross agglutina-

tion. By proper adsorption experiments pure antisera against the Vi or H antigens can be prepared. It is not necessary to resort to agglutinin adsorption to prepare O antisera, since O cells contain only O antigens.

If an antiserum against the Vi cell is incubated with the H organism, the H and O antibodies will attach to the bacteria. If the bacteria are removed by centrifugation, these H and O antibodies also are removed. This leaves only pure Vi antibody in the solution. This process is called agglutinin adsorption. Pure H antibody can be prepared by agglutinin adsorption with O cells and antiserum to the H cells. Note that one cannot prepare pure flagella by mixing H cells with anti-O sera, since all parts of the cell are removed when the cells are agglutinated and removed.

As discussed earlier, all the species of the genus *Salmonella* in one group share at least one somatic antigen. Consequently an O antiserum against the antigen will agglutinate all the bacteria in that group. Several unshared antigens also may exist between any two organisms. These shared and unshared O antigens have been identified and arbitrarily assigned numbers on the basis of cross agglutination tests and agglutinin adsorption experiments with anti-O sera. From these sources it has been possible to assign an antigenic formula to the somatic (and by the use of specific anti-H sera, to the flagella) antigens of each organism. *Salmonella typhi* is designated as 9, 12, Vi, and d; 9 and 12 represent the two ordinary somatic antigens, Vi the virulence antigen, and d a certain flagellar antigen. Antigenic formulas are exactly known for all the *Salmonella* species, since it is on the basis of an individual combination of antigens that new species were created in the past.

Salmonella O antigen chemistry. The first chemical studies of the Salmonella O antigens by French workers revealed that trichloroacetic acid extraction of salmonellae would liberate a phospholipopolysaccharide-protein complex. This material behaves predominantly as a polysaccharide; for example, it is not denatured by boiling. It is antigenic and is a potent endotoxin with marked pyrogenic activity for rabbits. This preparation, known as the Boivin antigen, also has an adjuvant effect. Phenol-water extractions of the salmonellae liberate an LPS antigen that contains only traces of the peptide (Fig. 16-8). The Boivin antigen, when saponified with alkali, is reduced to a structure of about 200,000 mol wt with the simultaneous liberation of fatty acids. Further alkali treatment produces a polysaccharide with a molecular weight of 20,000 to 30,000. This polysaccharide is free of lipid, which is released during the hydrolysis. The endotoxic activity of the parent complex is associated closely with the lipid, whereas the O-specific antigen property is retained entirely by the polysaccharide fraction.

Polysaccharides from all salmonellae, regardless of their O antigenic grouping, contain five common monosaccharides. These are D-glucose, D-galactose, D-glucosamine, L-glycero-D-manno-heptose, and 2-keto-3-deoxyoctonic acid. This suggests that a unit polysaccharide core is present in all *Salmonella* species. This core may be modified by the addition of other monosaccharides to create the specific O antigens for that organism. Proteins and lipids are not involved in O antigen specificity, since all O activity is present in the pure polysaccharides. Studies of R (rough) mutants, which lack the O antigen, support this hypothesis. Several R chemotypes have been identified that lack one or more of the five core constituents, but the complete core has been identified in several mutants.

Attached to each core are the unique and specific monosaccharides for the individual O antigens. These may consist of additional hexoses or substituted hexoses (D-mannose, D-galactosamine), methyl pentoses (L-fucose, L-rhamnose), and ribose in unique combinations with or without a 3,6-dideoxyhexose. The 3,6-dideoxyhexoses originally were isolated from *Salmonella* species; four of these novel sugars are related to specific O antigens. The four sugars are abequose (3,6-dideoxy-D-galactose), colitose (3,6-dideoxy-L-galactose), paratose (3,6-dideoxy-D-glucose), and tyvelose (3,6-dideoxy-D-mannose); their structures

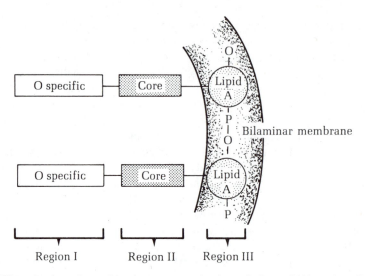

Fig. 16-8. The somatic antigen of many gram-negative bacteria has a lipid portion (lipid A) attached to a polysaccharide core common to all the antigens. The antigen specificity resides in region I.

are presented in Fig. 16-9. Serologic analysis reveals that these dideoquose sugars are part of the immundominant group of O antigens. This indicates their terminal, external location in the oligosaccharide chain. Hapten inhibition studies with specific O antisera have shown that abequose contributes strongly to antigens 4 and 8, paratose to antigen 2, tyvelose to antigen 9, and colitose to antigens 35 and 40. Additional sugars contribute to these antigenic determinants. Other somatic antigens contain more common sugars in their immunodominant center: for example, glucose in antigens 1, 12, 19, and 37.

The flagellar antigens (flagellins) are usually pure proteins of 20,000 mol wt *(Proteus vulgaris);* 20,000 to 30,000 molecules may be associated into the flagellar structure itself. Tryptophan often is missing, and unusual amino acids, for example, ϵ-N-methyl lysine, may be present.

The availability of antisera that are specific for certain species of pathogenic bacteria or specific for certain antigens of pathogenic bacteria has provided a valuable time-saving method for the identification of microorganisms isolated from patients with infectious diseases. In many instances the bacteriologic identification of these isolates requires several days after they are available in pure culture. A bacterial loop full of such an organism is sufficient for several slide agglutination tests, which might establish the identity of the organism in only a few minutes and surely in less than a half hour. Moreover, when pathogenic bacteria cannot be isolated from patients, it is possible to make a serologic diagnosis of the disease. This is done by drawing two samples of blood from the patient, the first during the acute phase of the illness, usually when the patient first seeks medical assistance, and the second, or convalescent, sample 1 or 2 weeks later. Sera from the acute and convalescent samples are tested for their agglutinating capacity with known bacteria. The species of bacteria selected are those which produce an illness similar to that the patient has or had. A difference in agglutination titer of fourfold between the acute and convalescent serum samples with a specific bacterium is accepted as evidence of an antigenic exposure to that organism. This in turn is taken as proof of the cause of the disease.

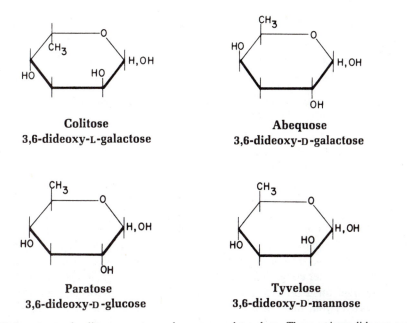

Colitose
3,6-dideoxy-L-galactose

Abequose
3,6-dideoxy-D-galactose

Paratose
3,6-dideoxy-D-glucose

Tyvelose
3,6-dideoxy-D-mannose

Fig. 16-9. Structures of colitose, paratose, abequose, and tyvelose. These unique dideoxy sugars are part of the immunodominant portion of several *Salmonella* species somatic antigens.

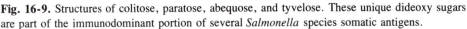

This evidence is only usable when both the acute and convalescent serum samples are analyzed. Patients may have a high agglutinating titer against a certain organism as the result of a cross-reaction, prior disease, or immunization with that organism; so single, high values are not easily interpreted. Among the pathogenic bacteria analyzed in this way are *Escherichia, Hemophilus, Brucella, Listeria, Corynebacterium, Leptospira, Bordetella, Shigella, Staphylococcus, Streptococcus, Proteus,* and *Salmonella* organisms and many more outside the realm of human medical microbiology.

Special terms are used in clinical serologic laboratories to describe these agglutination tests. A test for febrile agglutinins usually means for agglutinins against *Salmonella typhi, Salmonella paratyphi* A (and possibly *Salmonella paratyphi* B), and *Brucella* and *Francisella* organisms. The Widal test refers to agglutination of *Salmonella* species. A Weil-Felix test refers to agglutinins for *Proteus* species and is used to investigate the possibility of rickettsial disease.

BIBLIOGRAPHY

Boorman, K.E., Dodd, B.E., and Lincoln, P.J.: Blood group serology, ed. 5, Edinburgh, 1977, Churchill Livingstone.

Bryant, N.: Disputed paternity, New York, 1980, Thieme-Stratton, Inc.

Davey, M.: The prevention of rhesus isoimmunization, Clin. Obstet. Gynaecol. **6:**509, 1979.

Erskine, A.G., and Socha, W.W.: The principles and practice of blood grouping, ed. 2, St. Louis, 1978, The C.V. Mosby Co.

Fudenberg, H.H., and others: Basic immunogenetics, ed. 2, New York, 1978, Oxford University Press.

Giles, C.M.: The LW blood group: a review, Immunol. Commun. **9:**225, 1980.

Gopelrud, C.P.: Remaining problems in the prevention of Rh_0 isoimmunization, Semin. Perinatol. **1:**177, 1977.

Jann, K., and Westphal, O.: Microbial polysaccharides. In Sela, M., editor: The antigens, vol. 3, New York, 1975, Academic Press, Inc.

Lis, H., and Sharon, N.: Lectins: their chemistry and application to immunology. In Sela, M., editor: The antigens, vol. 4, New York, 1977, Academic Press, Inc.

Mollison, P.L.: Blood transfusion in clinical medicine, ed. 6, Oxford, 1979, Blackwell Scientific Publications, Ltd.

Ørskov, I., and others: Serology, chemistry and genetics of O and K antigens of *Escherichia coli,* Bacteriol. Rev. **41:**667, 1977.

Sandler, S.G., Nusbacher, J., and Schanfield, M.S., editors: Immunobiology of the erythrocyte, New York, 1980, Alan R. Liss, Inc.

Watkins, W.M.: Genetics and biochemistry of some human blood groups, Proc. R. Soc. London (Biol.) **201:**31, 1978.

Watkins, W.M.: Biochemistry and genetics of the ABO, Lewis, and P blood group systems, Adv. Hum. Genet. **10:**1, 1980.

Wicken, A.J., and Knox, K.W.: Lipoteichoic acids: a new class of bacterial antigens, Science **187:**1161, 1975.

Zmijewski, C.M.: Immunohematology, ed. 3, New York, 1978, Appleton-Century-Crofts.

SITUATION 1: THE WORRIED BRIDEGROOM

Your roommate has just returned to the dormitory and announced that he and Louise, his steady since they were sophomores, are pinned. It looks like a summer marriage. After congratulations and a quick trip to The Pub for a brief celebration a sudden cloud passes over your mind, and you ask, "What's Louise's blood type?" Your roommate doesn't know, but then it hits him: "That's right—when we took Immunology 420 I checked out group A,M,Rh+(D). What if she's Rh negative?"

Questions

1. What is an "Rh-incompatible" marriage?
2. Is an Rh-negative mother doomed to produce children with hemolytic disease?
3. Can hemolytic disease result from conditions other than Rh incompatibilities?
4. How is HDN caused by Rh antigens prevented?

Solution

When an Rh(D)-negative woman takes an Rh(D)-positive man as her husband, the possibility exists that their children will inherit the Rh(D) antigen. If the father is genetically Rh+/Rh−, then mathematically only half the children would be Rh positive. Naturally 100% of the children would be Rh positive if the father were homozygous. A marriage between an Rh-positive man and an Rh-negative woman may be described as Rh incompatible, but when the father is heterozygously Rh positive, then only half the children are "incompatible" with the mother. The incompatibility exists because the Rh(D) antigen inherited by the child is considered a foreign antigen by the immune system of the mother. Any fetal cells reaching the maternal lymphoid system will stimulate an anti-Rh(D) response.

The time of almost unavoidable immunization of the mother occurs during childbirth with an Rh-positive child. The rupture of placental membranes releases fetal Rh-positive cells into the womb and activates the immune response. Rh immunization also may result from transfusion of Rh-positive blood into an Rh-negative woman. The first Rh-positive child is unaffected by the incompatibility if his or her birth is the immunizing experience. In a second Rh-positive pregnancy the antibody titer may rise because of exposure to Rh antigens during the gestation period. There is also the possibility of a shift to IgG from IgM antibodies as a result of the booster immunization. The former class of antibodies is more dangerous, since they can migrate freely across the placental barrier. The maternal anti-D globulins move into the fetal circulation and attach to and accelerate the destruction of fetal erythrocytes. The fetus becomes jaundiced and anemic and is delivered with HDN.

Anti-D is the most common cause of HDN. In 99% of all cases of HDN anti-D immunization was known to occur. Even so only about 4% of mothers who have delivered two Rh-positive babies become immunized. Women with Rh-positive children who are compatible with their mother in the ABO or MN groups are more likely to develop anti-D than when their children are ABO incompatible. The maternal anti-A or anti-B tends to minimize immunization with the fetal erythrocytes.

These facts applied to this situation indicate a risk for HDN because of the Rh(D) antigen. If Louise is group O or B, her natural anti-A may reduce somewhat her risk for an affected child, presumably by speeding their elimination and reducing the risk for immunization.

The administration of anti-D to every Rh-negative mother within 72 hours of childbirth has proved fantastically successful in preventing HDN. In one study of 1,662 women so treated only two formed anti-D, whereas in 1,168 untreated control subjects 111 developed anti-D. The mother must be tested to ensure that she is D negative, or a serious reaction could develop when she is passively immunized with anti-D.

References

Erskine, A.G., and Socha, W.W.: The principles and practice of blood grouping, ed. 2, St. Louis, 1978, The C.V. Mosby Co.

Issitt, P.D.: Applied blood group serology, Oxnard, Calif., 1970, Becton, Dickinson & Co.

SITUATION 2: A PEACH OF A PEAR

It was Bob G. from the horticulture department. "Dave, I thought I'd give you a call about this discovery we've made. You dummies kept telling me my pear trees couldn't make antibodies, right? Even if they were resistant to the bacterial infections that killed the other pear trees, right? Well, we just did an agglutination test, and my resistant trees were positive, and the sensitive trees were negative. Now tell me again about plants not making antibodies."

Further discussion with Bob revealed that he had made an extract of pear leaves from his resistant line and from his sensitive line a few hours after infecting each with the bacterial pathogen. The extract from the resistant tree agglutinated the bacterium, a gram-negative bacillus, but the other extract did not. Extracts from the resistant tree line made prior to infection failed to clump the organisms.

I asked him a few questions about controls and gave him my advice.

Questions

1. What is nonimmune agglutination of bacteria, and how does it differ from immune?
2. What substances are capable of nonimmune bacterial agglutination?
3. What types of experiments or controls are used to distinguish nonimmune and immune agglutination?
4. What are lectins? Will they agglutinate bacteria?

Solution

Spontaneous agglutination of bacteria is a common finding in the study of certain species or genera and is separated easily from nonimmune agglutination. Spontaneous agglutination describes the clumping of bacteria, such as that seen with several corynebacteria and mycobacteria, which takes place in ordinary buffers or saline. This phenomenon makes it almost impossible to use these organisms in agglutination tests, since they already are clumped.

Nonimmune agglutination is defined as the agglutination of cells by nonantibody forces. This has been most extensively studied in the form of hemagglutination, but many of the same principles apply to nonimmune bacterial agglutination. Unsuitable pH, metal ions, and other forces that influence the ionic condition of the bacterial cell may cause agglutination. Thus clumping of red blood cells and bacteria often can be induced by mixing them with electropositive proteins—histones, lysozyme, protamines, etc. These materials bind firmly to the electronegative bacteria and neutralize their repellant electric charge. The bacteria are enabled to contact each other and remain attached, particularly if there is an adhesive structure such as a polysaccharide capsule on their surface.

Since immune agglutination is a property of immunoglobulins, it is possible to identify this type of agglutination by identifying the proteins responsible for it. If one removes all the proteins or only the globulins from a serum, it should no longer agglutinate. Sera that have agglutinated will leave a coat of γ-globulin on the bacteria. These antibodies can be recognized by various antiglobulin tests such as enhanced agglutination by the antiglobulin, fluorescent antiglobulin, and enzyme-labeled antiglobulin. This aspect of the present problem was investigated, but it was not possible to identify any adsorption of globulins by the bacteria.

The adaptive nature of the agglutinating response developed by the pear trees in this problem is characteristic of the immune response. Since no new globulins could be detected on the surface of the agglutinated bacteria, the cells were examined for their adsorption of other substances. This resulted in the finding that a protein high in polysaccharide content, a glycoprotein, seen in the extract as small structures almost viral in dimension, had attached to the bacteria. This substance in the pear leaf extracts was assumed to be lectin. When the extract was tested for its ability to agglutinate close relatives to the bacterial pear tree pathogen, they all were agglutinated. Other, more distantly placed taxonomic bacteria occasionally were agglutinated.

Further studies indicated that this agglutination was caused by a pear lectin that was normally present in the plant but which accumulated in leaves and twigs heavily parasitized by bacteria because of fluid imbalances created in these tissues during the infection. Lectins (phytoagglutinins, PHAs) are known to be normal constituents of plants that have an affinity for polysaccharides found on the surface of erythrocytes, tissue culture cells, bacteria, and other sources. Some of the lectins are multivalent and can bridge to cells (or two sites on the same cell) to hold them together. Agglutination of *Escherichia coli* by Con A and the agglutination of other bacteria by lectins have been reported. The genetics of this has been studied by using bacterial mutants.

References

Maruyama, H.B., Arisawa, M., and Ono-onitsuka, M.: Simplified assay for concanavalin A–dependent bacterial agglutination by using cell surface mutants, Infect. Immun. **11**: 1320, 1975.

Sharon, N., and Lis, H.: Lectins: cell-agglutinating and sugar-specific proteins, Science **177**:949, 1972.

Toms, G.C., and Western, A.: In Harborne, J., Boulter, D., and Turner, B.L., editors: Chemotaxonomy of the leguminosae, New York, 1971, Academic Press, Inc.

SECTION FOUR

IMMUNOPATHOLOGY

CHAPTER

17

INTRODUCTION TO ALLERGY

GLOSSARY

allergen A substance (antigen or hapten) that causes an allergy, that is, stimulates IgE synthesis or causes a delayed hypersensitivity.

allergy An altered state of reactivity to an antigen or hapten; used synonymously with *hypersensitivity*.

anaphylactic allergy An allergy caused by IgE.

anergy The inability to respond to an antigen, especially in the allergic sense.

cytotoxic allergy An allergy dependent on an antibody- and complement-mediated cell toxicity.

delayed hypersensitivity Synonym of *cell-mediated hypersensitivity;* a form of allergy expressed by T lymphocytes, not involving immunoglobulins, and developing slowly when provoked dermally.

hypersensitivity An unexpected, exaggerated reaction to an antigen.

immediate hypersensitivities Allergies relatable to IgE, or similar immunoglobulins in lower species, such as hay fever, food allergies, certain drug allergies, and other allergies of the immediate type.

immune complex disease A disease caused by or associated with the formation of antigen-antibody complexes, for example, glomerulonephritis and serum sickness.

T cell–mediated allergy An allergy expressed by antigen-sensitized T cells.

IMMUNOLOGIC BASIS OF THE HYPERSENSITIVITIES

Immunization and the formation of antibodies does not uniformly lead to a state of resistance or immunity. This is most obvious when the antigen employed in the immunization has nothing at all to do with infectious organisms or their toxins: for example, immunizations with bovine γ-globulin, sheep red blood cells, or ragweed pollen. Many times the synthesis of specific immunoglobulins and the later reaction of these antibodies with the antigen can be detrimental to the host's well-being. In such cases the immunization may be referred to as a sensitization, which more accurately describes the result of the antigenic exposure than does immunization. Whether the term *immunization* or *sensitization* is used is largely dependent on the response of the treated animal to a subsequent exposure to antigen and not to any substantial difference in the cellular and chemical events that follow the injection of the antigen. Certain manipulative procedures such as the administration of rather small quantities of an antigen may favor sensitization by restricting the quantity of antibody formed, but this only emphasizes that the difference between immunization and sensitization is more quantitative than qualitative.

The untoward or unusual reaction that is seen following the second exposure of the animal to the antigen reveals the existence of the sensitiza-

343

tion. This is the allergic or hypersensitive response. *Allergy* is defined as an altered ability to react; in immunology this means an altered reactivity to an antigen or a hapten. Strictly interpreted, *hypersensitivity* means a heightened reactivity and is not synonymous with *allergy,* but on the basis of common usage the terms are interchangeable. Hyposensitivity is defined as a condition of diminished reactivity, and anergy refers to an absolute failure to react when a reaction otherwise would be expected.

Allergic or hypersensitive responses are unquestionably immunologic in origin. The initial stage in their development is an exposure to an antigen or an autocomplexing hapten. This is the sensitizing exposure. The sensitized animal is not immediately capable of displaying its sensitivity. An immunologic waiting period of 5 to 10 days must elapse before the sensitization is expressible. This is the interlude customarily associated with the production of antibodies. After this the animal is sensitive; this sensitivity can be demonstrated by the injection of a second, or shocking, dose of antigen. The manifestation of shock will vary according to the condition used to elicit it, including the kind of sensitivity the animal has developed, the route, form, and dosage of antigen, plus other variables. Provided the shock has been of sufficient yet sublethal intensity, the animal will progress into a temporary state of hyposensitivity. This condition can be induced deliberately, without serious harm to the animal; it is described as desensitization.

In all these events (sensitization, shocking, and desensitization) the ground rules of immunologic specificity apply. Antigenic and haptenic materials are required for sensitization. The shocking dose is ineffectual until an immunologic waiting period has expired. The shocking antigen must be the one initially used in the sensitization or one that is serologically cross-reactive with that antigen. Specific desensitization is possible only with the sensitizing antigen or known cross-reacting antigens. These factors all point to an immunologic origin of the hypersensitivities.

CLASSIFICATION OF THE HYPERSENSITIVITIES
Immunoglobulin relationships

The immunoglobulins that are associated with allergic diseases fall into two classes: the heat-stable and the heat-labile immunoglobulins (Table 17-1). The heat-stable antibodies are the ordinary immunoglobulins considered in detail earlier (Chapter 6) and represented by IgG, IgA, and IgM. It is uncertain what role IgD may take in the hypersensitivities. The "classic" immunoglobulins resist destruction when held at 56° to 60° C for periods of 30 minutes to 4 hours. Since these immunoglobulins will produce visible serologic reactions in vitro when incubated with specific antigen, hypersensitivities involving these globulins sometimes are referred to in the older literature as the precipitin allergies.

Allergies caused by the classic antibodies can be passively transferred through the placenta to the fetus if IgG is involved. When passive transfer is made with serum from the allergic individual to the skin of a normal individual, it is found that these antibodies remain fixed to the skin for only a few hours. During this time a local skin reaction can be produced in the recipient by the injection of the offending antigen into the skin site, but thereafter the dermis returns to its usual nonreactive state typical of the nonallergic individual.

Until the last few years the exact immunologic basis of the allergies related to heat-labile antibodies was uncertain. The term *reagin* was used to describe a heat-labile (56° to 60° C for up to 3 hours) serum reagent, immunoglobulin-like in nature, that was correlated with a second type of hypersensitivity. Now reagin has been positively identified as a fifth immunoglobulin, IgE. IgE combines in vitro with its specific antigen, but the serologic reaction cannot progress to the second, or aggregative, stage. For this reason in vitro serologic tests with IgE cannot be performed, and reagin is described as a nonprecipitating antibody. The type of immediate hypersensitivity caused by IgE also is described as an atopic illness or an atopic allergy. The word *atopy* means for-

Table 17-1. Comparison of the properties of classic immunoglobulins and IgE

	Classic immunoglobulins	IgE
Immunoglobulins included	IgG, IgA, IgM, IgD (?)	IgE (reagin)
Stability at 56° to 60° for 30 minutes to 4 hours	Stable	Labile
In vitro reactions with antigens	Yes: precipitation, agglutination, complement fixation, etc.	Combination but no directly observable reaction
Associated class of allergy	Cytotoxic and immune complex	Immediate, nonprecipitating or atopic
Types of antigens involved	Ordinary, including hapten-antigen conjugates, cellular for cytotoxic reactions, soluble for immune complex reactions	Chemistry poorly understood but probably not unusual, often in a cellular form (spores, pollens, etc.)
Origin of immunoglobulin	Usually associated with heteroimmunization and autoimmunization	Associated with natural (oral and respiratory) and artificial immunizations
Placental passage	IgG	No; does not pass to fetus from mother
Fixation to skin on passive transfer	Relatively short time	Relatively long time (several days)
Desensitization	Difficult, seldom attempted	Yes, by hyperimmunization to form blocking antibody; temporary

eign, unusual, or out of place and indicates that the allergy has arisen from a rare or even unknown antigenic stimulus. Now it is generally agreed that most reaginic allergies result from natural oral or respiratory immunizations from food- or air-borne antigens, but even these may result in anaphylactic death.

Since IgE does not pass the placental barrier, an allergic mother will not give birth to a passively sensitized child. The child may have a hereditary disposition to form IgE against naturally occurring antigens in the environment because of his or her inheritance of specific Ir genes. Passive transfer of serum from sensitized individuals to the skin of normal persons will allow the provocation of the hypersensitivity reaction in the recipient for several days after the transfer. This is considered proof that IgE fixes for relatively long periods to the skin on transfer. Desensitization of the atopic allergies is dependent on the production of high levels of circulating immunoglobulins of the usual type. In this instance these antibodies which minimize or prevent the allergy are referred to as blocking antibodies. Further details of desensitization of the IgE allergies are discussed later, but it should be recognized that the sensitivity would return if the titer of the blocking, classic antibodies became significantly lowered.

The hypersensitivities traditionally have been separated on the basis of the time they appear after exposure to the shocking dose of antigen. On this basis there are two types of hypersensitivities: immediate and delayed. The immediate hypersensitivities are IgE mediated, whereas the delayed, or cell-mediated, allergies depend on the activities of sensitized T cells. Decades of study have revealed that immediate and delayed hypersensitivities differ in more fundamental respects than the times of their appearance (Table 17-2). Hypersensitivities also are classified on an immunopathologic basis (Table 17-3).

Immediate hypersensitivity

The immediate response appears within a few seconds or a few minutes after the administration of the shocking dose of antigen. This reaction

Table 17-2. Comparison of IgE- and T cell–mediated hypersensitivities

	IgE mediated	T cell mediated
Timing of response after shocking exposure	Appears within a few minutes, fades within a few hours; immediate	Develops and fades gradually; maximum at 24 to 72 hours; delayed
Special target tissue	Usually smooth muscle, but organ varies with species	Generalized tissue involvement
Tissue death	May occur; variable	Occurs but not typical of ordinary reaction
Humoral factor involvement	Yes; IgE	None yet identified
Cellular factor involvement	Only in that immunoglobulins are produced by B lymphocytes and plasma cells; mast cells	T lymphocytes, directly, not via immunoglobulin
Passive transfer	With immunoglobulins	With T lymphocytes
Type of tissue involved	Vascular	Vascular, but relatively avascular suitable also
Histology of skin reactions	Predominantly neutrophils and eosinophils; edema obvious, with wheal and erythema	Tendency toward mononuclears, with some neutrophils; species variation; less edema and wheal; erythema and induration
Mediators	Histamine, serotonin, kinins; species variation	Lymphokines
Moderators	Antihistamines and smooth muscle relaxants (adrenergic compounds)	Steroids (antiinflammatory compounds)
Immunotherapy (desensitization)	Yes; relatively easy, temporary; via neutralizing antibodies or formation of blocking antibodies	Yes; with difficulty, temporary; usually not attempted

fades or disappears rapidly so that in a few hours there may be no obvious external indication that the reaction even occurred. If a systemic response is evoked by the shocking dose of antigen, the symptoms of the immediate hypersensitivity will be noted to affect special target tissues. The exact tissue involved will vary but usually will include smooth muscle.

The immediate allergic reaction results from the presence of specific IgE in the sensitized individual. For this reason cells are involved in creating the sensitivity only in the requirement of plasma cells to produce the antibody. This means that the sensitivity can be passively transferred by serum. It also means that, to demonstrate an immediate hypersensitivity on a local or an isolated tissue basis, a vascularized tissue must be chosen. If this tissue is skin, and if the change in histology of the reaction site is observed over a period, it will be noted that neutrophils migrate quickly into the affected tissue. Eosinophils also aggregate in large numbers. Mononuclear cells are relatively rare early but increase in number later in the reaction sequence. This skin reaction in its outward physical appearance is very similar to that which follows the intradermal injection of small amounts of histamine. The triple response of erythema accompanied by edema and wheal formation is typical in both cases. Other vasoactive amines also may produce the triple response; in some animal species these amines (serotonin, kinins) may be more responsible for the hypersensitive response than is histamine itself. These amines usually arise from mast cells, basophils, or platelets; therefore a cellular participation at this level is required.

Chemotherapy and chemoprophylaxis of the immediate hypersensitivities thus are logically based on these classes of drugs: those which oppose the action of histamine as competitive metabolites (antihistamines), those which physiologically oppose the physiopharmacologic action of histamine (smooth muscle relaxants such as adrenaline and other adrenergic compounds), and those which stabilize mast cells. Desensitization is relatively easy as far as the immediate hypersensitivities are concerned; it depends on the cautious neutralization of antibody and the formation of blocking antibody. The desensitized state is only temporary.

T lymphocyte–mediated hypersensitivity

The behavior of the delayed hypersensitivities is almost always the opposite of the immediate hypersensitivities for each of the criteria listed in Table 17-2. To begin with, the shock response in delayed hypersensitivities is slow in developing and does not reach its maximum until sometime between 24 and 72 hours after the exposure to antigen. On the whole animal basis no special target organs seem to be involved; rather vague, generalized symptoms are observed, such as headache, fever, backache, and malaise. In this reaction cell death is uncommon.

The delayed hypersensitive reaction does not depend on circulating immunoglobulins. Instead the delayed reaction is dependent on specifically sensitized T lymphocytes; therefore the passive transfer of this kind of allergy to a normal recipient requires the transfer of lymphocytes. It is possible to effect this transfer in some species with soluble products from the T cells. Since delayed hypersensitivity does not depend on free proteins of the circulatory system, theoretically the reaction could be evoked equally as well in relatively avascular tissue, such as the external layers of the dermis or the cornea, as it is in vascular tissue. The major requirement is simply that the tissue be situated close enough to the vascular system that lymphocytes can emigrate from it to the point of antigen deposition.

The ordinary locus for detecting delayed hypersensitivity is the skin. Compared with the immediate skin reaction there is less edema and virtually no wheal, only erythema and induration. In delayed hypersensitivity the cellular infiltrate is dominated by mononuclear cells and less by granulocytes than in the immediate skin reactions. Variation in the cellular response from species to species has been noted. No chemical basis for the delayed allergic state has been definitely established. The lymphokines described earlier are chemical associates of the reaction, but the biochemical basis for the activity of these compounds has only recently come under investigation. Since the chemical mechanism is unknown, it has been impossible to devise a logical chemoprophylactic or chemotherapeutic suppression of the delayed hypersensitive state. Steroids and other antiinflammatory drugs will minimize the shock reaction but cannot totally prevent it. Desensitized individuals will display no shock reaction; this condition is relatively difficult to create, and since the delayed hypersensitivities are seldom life threatening, this is not often practiced.

When sensitization to an antigen develops, it does not develop solely in the form of an immediate hypersensitivity with the exclusion of any delayed or cell-mediated component; neither does an exclusive delayed type of hypersensitivity develop. One or the other form may very well dominate the allergic state, but the two forms are usually mutually present. It is often the method of testing that causes one of the forms of hypersensitivity to be detected in the absence of the other.

Immunopathologic classification of the hypersensitivities

A second system of classification for hypersensitive responses was forwarded by Gell and Coombs in England over a decade ago (Table 17-3). Although four types of hypersensitive reactions are included in this system, the first three are but subdivisions of the immunoglobulin-dependent hypersensitivities, and the fourth is the cell-mediated, or delayed, hypersensitivity.

The anaphylactic type of reaction is that in which homocytotropic or heterocytotropic immunoglobulins of the IgE type, synthesized by plasma cells, become attached to mast cells and basophils via their Fc portion. The two Fab regions protrude from the cell surface and, when combined with antigen, alter the permeability of these cells. Phar-

Table 17-3. Classification of hypersensitive reactions

	Anaphylactic	Cytotoxic	Immune complex	T cell dependent
Immunoglobulin	IgE	IgG, possibly other	IgG, IgM, etc.	None
Antigens involved	Heterologous	Autologous or hapten modified	Autologous or heterologous	Autologous or heterologous
Complement involved	No	Yes	Yes	No
Cellular involvement	Mast cells and basophils	Red and white blood cells, platelets, etc. as targets	Host tissue cells	Host tissue cells
Chemical mechanism	Mast cell products and others	Complement-dependent cytolysis	Complement-dependent reactions	Lymphokines
Examples	Anaphylaxis, hay fever, food allergy	Transfusion reactions, Rh disease, thrombocytopenia	Arthus reaction, serum sickness, pneumonitis	Allergy of infection, contact dermatitis

macologically active substances, such as histamine and serotonin, released by the cells affect the shock tissues, primarily smooth muscles. Serum complement is not required in this reaction. The immunoglobulins are described as cytotropic or homocytotropic antibodies because of their affinity for tissue cells.

In the cytotoxic allergy reaction antibodies of the IgG and possibly IgM classes react directly with antigens or hapten-antigen complexes on the surface of the tissue cell. Complement participates in this reaction and promotes cytolysis or cytotoxic reactions such as those seen in hemolytic reactions and thrombocytopenic purpura. Elements of this type of reaction may be present in several autoimmune diseases, drug allergies, and allograft rejection.

In the immune complex reaction antigen-antibody complexes form in the soluble or fluid phase of tissues or in blood and then deposit on vessel walls, glomerular membranes, and elsewhere to interrupt normal physiologic processes. These immunoglobulins may be of the IgG, IgM, or possibly other classes. Complement becomes activated in many of these reactions and releases chemotactic factors. The attracted leukocytes release enzymes and possibly other agents that in-

jure local tissues. Immune complex reactions are typified by the Arthus reaction, portions of serum sickness, and aspects of autoimmune disease such as SLE and glomerulonephritis.

The delayed type reaction is the cell-mediated hypersensitive reaction involving antigen-sensitized T cells, which respond directly or by the release of lymphokines to exhibit contact dermatitis and allergies of infection.

BIBLIOGRAPHY

Barber, H.R.K.: Immunobiology for the clinician, New York, 1977, John Wiley & Sons, Inc.

Cohen, S., Ward, P.A., and McCluskey, R.T., editors: Mechanisms of immunopathology, New York, 1979, John Wiley & Sons, Inc.

Criep, L.H.: Clinical immunology and allergy, ed. 3, New York, 1976, Grune & Stratton, Inc.

Freedman, S.O., and Gold, P., editors: Clinical immunology, ed. 2, New York, 1976, Harper & Row Publishers, Inc.

Gell, P.G.H., Coombs, R.R.A., and Lachmann, P., editors: Clinical aspects of immunology, ed. 3, Oxford, 1974, Blackwell Scientific Publications, Ltd.

Miescher, P.A., and Müller-Eberhard, H.J., editors: Textbook of immunopathology, ed. 2, New York, 1976, Grune & Stratton, Inc.

Movat, H.Z., editor: Inflammation, immunity and hypersensitivity: cellular and molecular mechanisms, ed. 2, New York, 1979, Harper & Row Publishers, Inc.

IMMUNOGLOBULIN E–MEDIATED ALLERGY

GLOSSARY

adrenergic drugs Drugs such as adrenalin that constrict blood vessels, relax smooth muscles, and in general function in the opposite way as histamine; synonym of β-adrenergic drug.

anaphylactoid reaction A pseudoanaphylactic reaction and similar to it in all respects except that it is not created by antigen-antibody reactions.

anaphylaxis An unexpected, detrimental reaction to a second exposure to antigen in which histamine, serotonin, etc. are released by reaction of the antigen with IgE on the surface of mast cells (*ana*, without; *phylaxis*, protection).

antihistamine A drug that is an inhibitor, usually a competitive inhibitor, of histamine.

atopy An IgE-dependent allergy often arising from unknown exposure to an antigen or autocoupling hapten.

blocking antibody An antibody that prevents the action of another antibody, as exemplified by antibodies formed during desensitization against atopic allergies.

bradykinin A specific peptide of nine amino acids formed during anaphylaxis that produces pain.

catecholamine An adrenergic drug such as adrenalin.

cromolyn A mast cell stabilizing drug.

cytotoxic allergy An allergy dependent on an antibody- and complement-mediated cell toxicity.

cytotropic antibody An antibody that attaches nonspecifically to mast cells and basophils.

desensitization Elimination or reduction of allergic sensitivity, usually through a programmed course of antigen treatment.

ECF-A Eosinophilic chemotactic factor of anaphylaxis.

heterocytotropic antibody An antibody from one species that will attach to mast cells of another species.

histamine A specific chemical compound released from mast cells and producing vasodilation, smooth muscle contraction, and edema during anaphylaxis.

homocytotropic antibody An antibody that will attach to the mast cells of the species producing it.

kallidin Lysylbradykinin or kinin 10.

kallikrein Protease(s) that releases kinins from kininogen; synonymous with *kininogenase*.

kininogenase *see* Kallikrein.

kininogens α-Globulin proteins of serum that are precursors to kinins.

kinins Peptides or polyamines released during anaphylaxis that possess vasodilating and muscle-contracting activity.

leukotriene *see* Slow-reacting substance of anaphylaxis.

mast cell A cell found in connective tissue in which heparin and histamine are stored in numerous intracytoplasmic granules.

PAF Platelet-activating factor from basophils.

PG Prostaglandin.

P-K test The Prausnitz-Küstner test.

Prausnitz-Küstner test A test for immediate hypersensitivity performed in a normal subject who has been passively sensitized by immunoglobulin from the allergic individual.

prekallikrein Prokininogenase.

prokininogenase The proenzyme precursor to kininogenase.

prostaglandin A derivative of arachidonic acid.

reagin 1. IgE, with specificity for allergens. 2. Syphilitic reagin, with specificity for cardiolipin antigens.

Schultz-Dale reaction An in vitro anaphylactic response of sensitized uterus or gut when exposed to antigen.

serotonin A chemical mediator of anaphylaxis (5-hydroxytryptamine).

slow-reacting substance of anaphylaxis A material that causes a slow or prolonged contraction of smooth muscle released during anaphylaxis; leukotrienes C, D, and E.

SRS-A Slow-reacting substance of anaphylaxis.

vasoactive amine An amine or peptide that produces vasodilation.

Hypersensitivities caused by IgE may assume any of several forms from the life-threatening anaphylactic reactions to the milder discomforts associated with food allergies. Regardless of their severity, these depend on the presence of an IgE with a serologic specificity for the offending allergen. The combination of the allergen with IgE on the surface of mast cells and basophils releases pharmacologic agents that trigger an immediate physiologic response. These immediate hypersensitivities or anaphylactic hypersensitivities are compared with other forms of allergy in Chapter 17, which should be consulted for review.

The IgE-dependent allergies are known by several synonyms; reaginic allergy and atopic allergy are two. *Reagin* was the early term used to denote that there was an antibody-like substance in the serum of many allergic persons. Now it is recognized that reagin and IgE are identical substances.

The word *atopy* means foreign, unusual, or out of place and indicates that the allergy has arisen from a rare or even unknown antigenic stimulus. Many reaginic allergies result from natural oral or respiratory immunizations from food- or air-borne antigens, but IgE allergies also may arise from known, artificial exposures to antigens or haptens, as exemplified by penicillin allergy.

ANAPHYLAXIS
Systemic anaphylaxis

Total body or systemic anaphylaxis is the most devastating form of the IgE-mediated hypersensitivities. The first complete description of this phenomenon was given by Portier and Richet in 1902 following their anaphylactic shock of dogs. These investigators attempted to immunize dogs against the toxins of the sea anemone by administering spaced injections of small, nonlethal quantities of the toxin. When the animals received secondary injections of sublethal quantities of the toxin, at a time when it might be expected that they would be immune, the dogs entered the shock syndrome that Richet designated as anaphylaxis. This word indicates that the prior injections of the antigen had produced the converse of the expected situation, prophylaxis.

The initial injection of the toxin must be considered as the sensitizing exposure, which was followed by an immunologic waiting period necessary for immunoglobulin synthesis. Anaphylaxis was demonstrated when the dogs were exposed to a later shocking dose of antigen. For the easiest provocation of systemic anaphylaxis the shocking dose of antigen should be given in fluid form directly into the circulation so that it can be rapidly distributed throughout the body. For this reason the intramuscular injection of bacterial vaccines or precipitated toxoids rarely causes anaphylaxis.

The symptoms of anaphylaxis vary from species to species because of the central involvement of different shock organs. In virtually every instance smooth muscle contraction, dilation of the vascular system, and edema are among the major changes.

Richet stated that nonfatal systemic anaphylaxis

in the dog results in restlessness, an increased respiratory rate, an increased pulse rate, pruritus, diarrhea, and urination. In fatal anaphylaxis immediate and frequent vomiting follows the shocking exposure to antigen. This increases in severity until the vomit is bilious or fecal in character. The diarrhea is more extreme than in nonfatal shock and may become bloody. The respirations are short and frequent, the blood pressure drops, the heartbeat is accelerated, and the animal soon collapses. Although death appears imminent, dogs usually survive for 2 or more hours. At autopsy extensive edema is seen in the intestinal mucosa and lungs, and hemorrhage and congestion in the liver, gastrointestinal tract, and heart are noted. The liver may contain as much as 60% of the animal's total blood volume because of constriction of hepatic blood vessels. The result of this is that the dog essentially bleeds to death.

The symptoms of anaphylaxis in the guinea pig first appear as ruffling of the hair on the back of the neck, restlessness, sneezing, and pawing at the nose. These quickly progress to coughing and retching, combined with gasping for air. Tremors may course through the animal's body. Cyanosis is evident by the pallor or bluish cast assumed by the mucous membranes. Defecation, urination, and collapse of the animal followed by convulsive kicks and continued respiratory failure lead to death, frequently within 5 to 10 minutes after the injection of the antigen. The most obvious finding at autopsy is the marked inflation of the lungs from constriction of the bronchial musculature. Hemorrhages may be noted in the viscera and on the diaphragm, but the animal dies of asphyxiation.

Anaphylaxis is established less predictably in the rabbit than in the guinea pig. Successful anaphylactic shock first is manifested by a flush and then a pallor of the ears. Defecation and urination precede a few convulsive kicks, collapse, and death, which usually is not as sudden as in the guinea pig. The major finding at autopsy is a dilation of the right side of the heart and inferior vena cava as a result of the constriction of the pulmonary arterioles. Heart failure probably is responsible for death.

The symptoms of anaphylactic shock in humans are more similar to those in guinea pigs than in any other animal. Shortness of breath, increased heart rate, and a tingling in the throat precede collapse. Death may follow within a few minutes. Edema of the throat, brain, and lungs and inflation of the lungs are observed at autopsy.

Some species, such as the rat, mouse, and hamster, are quite refractory to lethal anaphylaxis, but anaphylactic sensitivity can be induced by repeated exposures to antigen. Anaphylaxis has been demonstrated in virtually all species tested, provided the species is capable of immunoglobulin synthesis.

Active sensitization to anaphylactic shock can be induced by any antigen; proteins, polysaccharides, conjugated antigens, and autocoupling haptens have been used. The amount of antigen needed for sensitization depends on the species of animal, the antigen, and the manner of sensitization. Large amounts of antigen or intensive immunization (sensitization) schedules usually should be avoided, except in markedly resistant animals. A single injection of 0.001 to 1 mg of soluble proteins given intraperitoneally will provide uniform sensitivity in guinea pigs, which usually are not susceptible to shock until the eighth day after antigen exposure and display maximal sensitivity at 21 days. The immunologic waiting period for most species is 1 to 2 weeks, which matches closely the known latent period for immunoglobulin synthesis.

Rapid and immediate saturation of the animal with antigen by the shocking dose of antigen favors lethal anaphylaxis. For this reason it is important that the antigen be fluid and that it be given by the intravenous or intracardial route. A total amount of 0.1 to 1 mg of antigen is adequate, but since a prozone phenomenon with excess antigen is not observed, larger quantities of antigen can be sued.

Animals that escape death after the administration of the shocking dose of antigen are specifically desensitized for a period of several days to several weeks, after which their sensitivity returns.

Variants of anaphylaxis

Cutaneous anaphylaxis or local cutaneous anaphylaxis is merely the provocation of the immediate type of skin reaction in a sensitized individual by injecting the allergen responsible for the sensitivity into the skin. This can be accomplished by intracutaneous injection, prick, or scratch testing. A skin test of this sort should be conducted if it is necessary to administer an antigen systemically to a person, because it will reveal if the person is susceptible to anaphylactic shock.

Active systemic or cutaneous anaphylaxis has variants that have provided considerable insight into the immunologic basis for the phenomenon. The ability to passively transfer anaphylactic sensitivity from the actively sensitized to an untreated animal has proved that a serum substance, now recognized as IgE, is responsible for anaphylaxis. The observation that the passively sensitized animal may not be shockable for several hours after being passively sensitized indicates that some second event must occur before IgE can complete its sensitization.

Passive cutaneous anaphylaxis (PCA) experiments and the Schultz-Dale reaction indicate that this event is the attachment of IgE to tissues. In PCA serum from an anaphylactically sensitized animal is injected into the skin of a normal animal. When antigen is injected systemically several hours later, an edematous and erythematous reaction develops at the skin site. In fact one may delay the antigen injection for several days and still elicit the immediate skin reaction. This long period of skin fixation is not typical of other immunoglobulins such as IgG and IgM and suggests that a novel type of immunoglobulin is responsible for the PCA reaction.

When the PCA reaction is conducted in man, it is known as the Prausnitz-Küstner (P-K) reaction, named for the German physicians who first performed this test. Küstner was allergic to cooked fish. If Küstner's serum was injected into the skin

of the nonallergic Prausnitz, and this was followed the next day by the injection of an extract of cooked fish into the same site, an immediate skin reaction developed. It is interesting that extracts of raw fish did not elicit the reaction, which indicates that Küstner was allergic to a heat-denatured antigen.

In the Schultz-Dale reaction, or in vitro anaphylaxis, evidence for a fixed antibody is revealed by the fact that tissues from a sensitized animal can be washed free of serum proteins and still undergo anaphylactic shock, as described more fully later.

Pathway to anaphylactic shock

Immunoglobulin formation and fixation. The immunologic basis for anaphylaxis is antibody of the reaginic type, that is, IgE. Three conditions offer strong evidence against a dependence of anaphylaxis on circulating antibody. One of these is that an actively sensitized animal can be placed in shock even though it has no detectable antibody in its blood. Indeed sensitization is usually optimal when a single dose of a small quantity of antigen is used, that is, when the antigenic stimulus has been quite modest. This might be interpreted only as evidence that anaphylaxis is a more sensitive detector of circulating antibody than standard in vitro serologic tests, but it could mean as well that a second form of antibody, a form that is not free in the circulation, is the source of anaphylactic shock. A second line of evidence is that animals with a high titer of circulating antibodies are quite refractory to shock. That circulating immunoglobulins are involved at all is demonstrable by passive sensitization experiments. When antiserum with a good reaginic titer is taken from an actively sensitized animal and injected into a normal animal, the recipient becomes sensitized to anaphylaxis. The recipient is not immediately susceptible to anaphylactic shock, however; a waiting period of a few hours to a day is essential to permit full sensitivity to develop. It is now well accepted that this latent period is necessary to allow the fixation of serum antibody to tissue cells.

The IgE that is free in the circulation of allergic persons thus is not the cause of their allergic condition; it is the IgE that has become bound to cells. IgE is a cytophilic, or cytotropic, antibody. Although the latter term is used more commonly than the former, there is no difference, except by use, in their meaning. Cytotropic antibody has come to mean that type of antibody which binds to mast cells. A homocytotropic antibody is one that binds to cells of its own species. This distinguishes it from a heterocytotropic antibody, which will bind to cells of other species.

The original experiment that illustrated the necessity of cell-bound (cytotropic) antibody for anaphylaxis is the Schultz-Dale reaction. Schultz and Dale found that the uterus or a segment of ileum removed from a sensitized guinea pig, if heavily perfused, can be washed free of circulating immunoglobulins. When suspended between a fixed and a movable pole in an isotonic bath solution, muscles in these tissues will contract when the sensitizing antigen is added to the bath. This contraction is recordable by contact of a pen on the movable pole against a turning drum (kymograph). The Schultz-Dale reaction is thus an in vitro anaphylactic reaction that is dependent on cell-bound antibody. In vitro anaphylaxis has been very useful in establishing the antigenic specificity of anaphylaxis, in studying specific immunologic desensitization and the effect of certain drugs in mimicking, and in preventing anaphylaxis.

Mast cells and basophils. The next problem obviously is to determine what cells bind IgE. One would immediately suspect the muscle cell, since it is affected so profoundly during anaphylactic shock. Unfortunately no evidence has yet been presented that muscle cells bind antibodies. It was suggested in 1909 that in vivo serologic reactions liberated a special anaphylatoxin, possibly from the antigen involved in the reaction. This idea was abandoned when it was found that many different kinds of antigens were capable of inciting anaphylactic sensitivity and when it became statistically unlikely that they were all producing the same or a similar kind of anaphylatoxin.

Examination of the blood of animals undergoing anaphylactic shock reveals that the blood has an extended clotting time and is toxic to the skin of normal animals given intradermal injections of serum or blood. It also has been noted that anaphylactic shock in the guinea pig has many points in common with histamine shock. In the late 1920s the triple response of skin to histamine injections was observed to parallel very closely the immediate hypersensitive skin response of sensitized guinea pigs to intradermal injections of the offending antigen. This response consists of immediate erythema and edema at the injection site followed by wheal and flare, or pseudopodial spread, of the reaction. Subsequent inquiries now have defined histamine as a primary pharmacologic mediator of anaphylaxis in guinea pigs. Other compounds with profound physiopharmacologic activity also are released during anaphylaxis. Tissue mast cells and basophils are two important cell sources of these molecules.

Mast cells were discovered and named by Ehrlich. These cells are widely distributed throughout the body but are especially populous in connective tissues, in lung and uterus, and around blood vessels. They are abundant in liver, kidney, spleen, heart, and other organs. The individual mast cell is ovoid and about 10 to 15 μm in diameter (Fig. 18-1). It has a poorly developed endoplasmic reticulum, contains only a few mitochondria, and has a heavily granulated cytoplasm (Fig. 18-2). The granules are about 0.5 to 2 μm in diameter, stain unevenly, and are surrounded by a limiting membrane. These granules may be so numerous as to totally obscure the cell nucleus in stained preparations, and it is not unusual for a single cell to contain 200 to 500 of these granules. The tissue mast cell is similar in appearance to the basophilic leukocyte. The granules in both cells consist of a complex of heparin, histamine, and zinc ions, with the heparin existing in an approximate ratio of 6:1 with histamine. The actual heparin content is about 70 to 90 μg/10^6 cells, and the histamine content is about 10 to 15 μg/10^6 cells.

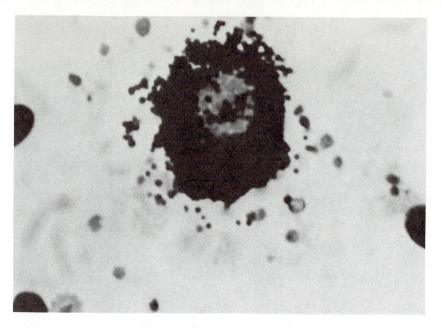

Fig. 18-1. A mast cell that has begun to discharge its granules. The light area in the center of the cell, partially shielded by granules, is the nucleus.

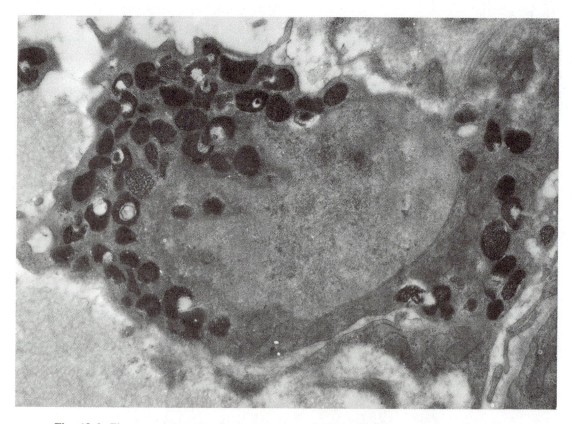

Fig. 18-2. Electron micrograph of a human mast cell. Note the fine granular structure of the numerous cytoplasmic granules, which store histamine and heparin. (Courtesy Dr. E. Adelstein.)

The basophil is the least common of the blood granulocytes. There are only about 40 such cells per cubic millimeter of human blood, in which the basophils constitute up to about 2% of the cells. Basophils are the smallest of the granulocytes with a range in diameter from 8 to 18 μm. The nucleus is not as well segmented as in the neutrophils and eosinophils. The cytoplasm of basophils contains a few mitochondria and other structures but is most noted for its numerous round or ovoid granules, which are basophilic in their staining properties. These granules average 0.5 μm in diameter and under electron microscopy are observed to have an internal subgranular structure composed of particles of only 100 to 150 Å in diameter. The morphologic resemblance of basophils and mast cells is very striking and accounts for the description of the mast cell as the tissue basophil and of the basophil as the circulating mast cell (Fig. 18-3). This is an oversimplification, since these cells arise from separate stem cells.

The morphologic unity of mast cells and basophils is repeated in their chemical composition. Basophils contain several enzymes, but as with mast cells, the most important is histidine decarboxylase. This enzyme is the catalyst for the formation of the biogenic amine found in the basophil, just as it is in the mast cell. The histamine content of basophils is some 20 to 50 times less than in mast cells, seldom exceeding 2.5×10^6 μg/cell.

Mast cell degranulation

General immunology. The histamine and heparin held within the granules of mast cells and baso-

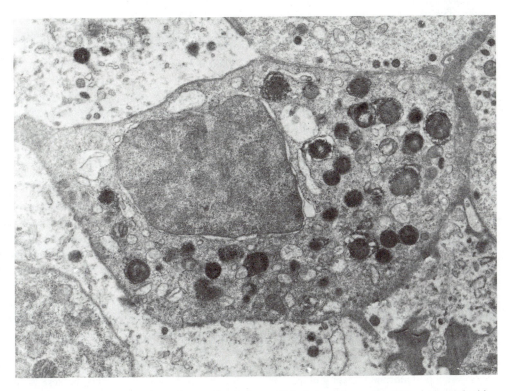

Fig. 18-3. This electron photomicrograph of a basophil in bone marrow should be compared with that of a mast cell in Fig. 18-2. The granules in basophils contain histamine. (Courtesy Dr. E. Adelstein.)

phils are released when these cells are exposed to specific immunologic or chemical agents.

Mast cell degranulation can be accomplished in any of three immunologic ways. The first of these is to use mast cells as the antigen for immunization of a heterologous species of animal. Passive administration of the anti–mast cell serum to the species that was the source of the mast cells used in the immunization will initiate a complement-dependent immunolytic reaction that will destroy the mast cell and release histamine and heparin.

The second serologic method of mast cell degranulation is by the passive administration of antibody to the animal's IgG, IgA, or IgE. The reaction of these antiglobulins with these classes of antibody bound to the mast cell surface activates the complement cascade and results in a typical complement-dependent immunocytolytic anaphylactic reaction. Presumably the same type of cell destructive reaction would occur if the specific antigen for the homologous cell-bound antibody were injected.

The third method of mast cell degranulation depends on the fixation of IgE to the cell surface and the reaction of these cell-bound antibodies with antigen. The subsequent release and dissolution of granules does not depend on the fixation of complement or on mast cell lysis.

Mast cell lysis need not result solely from the combination of antibody and antigen on its surface. Rabbit, rat, and guinea pig neutrophils that have engulfed antigen-antibody complexes release polyamino compounds which are mastocytolytic. In the case of rabbit mastocytolytic factor (MCF) partial purification has identified the compound as having a molecular weight of 1,200 to 2,400. This polycationic protein is composed of nearly 25% arginine. Many synthetic histamine releasers are polycationic compounds. MCF is heat stable, dialyzable, and inactive on smooth muscle and does not release histamine from either basophils or platelets. The polymorphonuclear cell is not affected by MCF and retains its structural integrity for a considerable period under the in vitro conditions designed to study MCF release.

IgE. The existence of a heat-labile antibody, originally termed *reagin,* in the sera of persons displaying various allergies was first recognized by Prausnitz and Küstner in 1921. It was noted that reagin was specific for the allergen or antigen which evoked its production. It would not pass the placenta to passively hypersensitize the newborn child; it would not give the usual in vitro serologic tests such as precipitation, agglutination, complement fixation, or others associated with the heat-stable immunoglobulins; and on passive transfer to a normal individual it would "fix" in the skin for several days or weeks. It is this latter characteristic which is the basis for the P-K test.

Reagin has long been known to migrate in the γ_1 fraction of allergic sera, and many efforts were made to identify reagin with other immunoglobulins migrating in this region of the electrophoretic profile. DEAE cellulose ion exchange chromatography and Sephadex gel filtration resulted in the isolation of a reagin-rich serum fraction that was devoid of IgG, IgA, IgM, and IgD. Immunization of rabbits with this reagin-rich fraction resulted in an antiserum that would remove the reaginic activity of sera by serologic precipitation. Adsorption of this rabbit antiserum with the four well-known immunoglobulins did not delete the antibody that precipitated reagin. By the extensive use of radio-immunodiffusion experiments it was shown that reagin was a new, distinct immunoglobulin; it was named IgE. The letter *E* was assigned because the reagin most studied was specific for antigen E of ragweed. Now IgE refers to reagin in the general sense, and its specificity for an antigen must be designated in the same way as for any other immunoglobulin.

Since IgE occurs in only minute quantities in normal sera (16 to 97 ng/ml of serum), critical biochemical studies were hampered for several years after its discovery. Even though serum levels of IgE in allergic individuals may be elevated to 50 times the normal serum levels, sera from these allergic persons simply are not available in quantity. This dilemma was circumvented by the discovery in Sweden of a patient with a unique myeloma protein, originally designated as the ND myeloma protein. This paraprotein was not antigenically related to any previously known myeloma protein or immunoglobulin H chain, although it was related to immunoglobulins by virtue of its λ L chain determinants. This ND protein soon was proved to be serologically identical to IgE. This discovery and the attendant availability of large quantities of IgE opened the way to a precise biophysical characterization of this new immunoglobulin, and the following data cited for IgE actually are taken from studies of the ND (γE) myeloma protein (Table 18-1).

IgE migrates electrophoretically as a fast γ- or $γ_1$-globulin with a molecular weight of 188,000 to 190,000. It has a half-life of 2.3 days. It is synthesized at a rate of 2.3 μg/kg body weight/day. Carbohydrate represents about 10.7% to 11.7% of the total weight of the molecule. Based on the assumption that IgE is a globular protein, its $S_{20,w}$ value has been reported as 7.92 to 8.2. Reductive mercaptan cleavage followed by alkylation with iodoacetamide revealed the presence of λ L chains with a molecular weight estimated as 22,600. Typical κ-chains also have been identified in IgE. This means that the H chain—the ε-chain—must have a molecular weight of 75,000. It now is accepted that this extra size of the ε-chain is a result of its content of a fourth C_H domain. A single disulfide bond unites the ε- with the λ-chain. Carbohydrate, previously believed to be shared between the λ- and ε-chain, is exclusively restricted to the latter, indicating that the molecular weight of the ε-peptide is 61,000. Papain digestion of IgE produces several fragments, including the two Fab units and an Fc unit, but also an L chain fragment, λ C, Fc″, and a $7S_{20,w}$ fragment. Fc has a molecular weight of 98,000 and an $S_{20,w}$ of 5.1S. This Fc fragment is the only papain fragment that inhibits the P-K reaction. This is proof that is contains the cytotropic region of intact IgE. Fc″ is an amino terminal portion of the Fc unit that seems to bear the carbohydrate associated with the ε-chain. Two Fab fragments have been identified, one of which has a detectable component of car-

Table 18-1. Chemical and physical properties of immunoglobulin E

Current designation	IgE
Older name	Reagin
Molecular weight	190,000
$S_{20,w}$ value	8.2
Electrophoretic mobility	$γ_1$
Carbohydrate content (percent)	11.7
Resistance to — SH reagents	Low
Concentration (mg/dl serum)	0.1 to 1.0
Amount of serum immunoglobulins	<1%
Half-life (days)	2.3
Rate of synthesis (μg/kg body weight/day)	2.3
Light chain types	κ or λ
Heavy chain class	ε
General formula	$ε_2κ_2$ or $ε_2λ_2$
Light chain allotypes	Km
Heavy chain subclasses	None
Heavy chain constant domain	4
Stable at 56° to 60° C	No

bohydrate. Tryptic and peptic proteolysis of IgE also have been performed, the latter producing F(ab′)₂ units of 140,000 mol wt and an $S_{20,w}$ of 6.7. The Fd′ unit has a molecular weight of 45,000.

Because of the paucity of IgE in normal human serum, sensitive serologic procedures must be used for its quantitation. These include the radioimmunosorbent test (RIST), the radioallergosorgent test (RAST), and enzyme immunoassays. The Mancini radial diffusion test also may be used, since potent antisera now have been prepared against IgE myeloma proteins.

The RIST procedure is dependent on the availability of an ^{125}I-labeled ND protein and its specific antibody, the latter used in the solid phase of this RIA procedure. Competition of IgE in an unknown serum sample with radiolabeled ND in the binding reaction with the immobilized antibody is measured as a decrease in bound label and is a direct measure of the IgE in the sample. This test measures total serum IgE and is a typical competitive inhibition RIA test.

The RAST test uses a specific allergen bound to a solid phase carrier, which then is incubated with a serum sample containing an unknown amount of IgE specific for the allergen. When radiolabeled anti-IgE is added, the amount of label bound is a measure only of the allergen-specific IgE in the serum. IgG or other antibodies to the allergen could be detected by specifically labeled antibodies for IgG, etc.

By these procedures it has been determined that the healthy adult usually will have 61 to 100 ng of IgE per milliliter of serum. IgE in cord sera of newborn infants averages 37 ng/ml, or about 15% of the adult average. There is no correlation between the maternal and newborn serum IgE levels, which indicates that fetal IgE synthesis can occur. From infancy to puberty the IgE levels progress gradually toward the adult norm. Levels of IgE in colostrum are 20% higher than in serum, and urinary IgE values are also often high, suggesting the local production and secretory nature of this immunoglobulin. In various atopic allergic diseases, especially hay fever and asthma, IgE levels may rise to nearly 6,000 ng/ml of serum, with a mean value of 1,191. Consequently values over 1,000 are considered pathologic. Very high levels have been noted in children with roundworm infection. Hyposensitization therapy for hay fever also increases the serum levels, which seem to remain high for several months. The effectiveness of hyposensitization obviously is not through its effect on IgE levels.

The chemistry of the rat mast cell receptor for IgE has been partially characterized. There are nearly 10^6 such receptors distributed over the surface of the cell, each of which binds a single IgE molecule. The receptor molecule has two protein subunits: the α-chain and the β-chain. The α-chain (about 50,000 mol wt) contains about two thirds of its weight in protein and one third in polysaccharide. A region identified as the α_1-domain bears the carbohydrate. The β-chain has a molecular weight of approximately 30,000 and contains no polysaccharide. It too can be divided into two domains: β_1, which anchors the receptor in the cytoplasmic membrane of the mast cell, and the exposed β_2-domain. The α- and β-chains are noncovalently joined, with the α-chain located more exterior in relationship to the cell surface.

Cellular biochemistry. A mechanism by which secretory cells in different organs, such as the endocrine glands, are stimulated to release storage materials from intracellular granules has been carefully described and documented over the past decade. For these cells an extracellular stimulus or first messenger is "read" at the cell surface to stimulate an increase in membrane-bound adenylate (adenyl) cyclase. This enzyme generates cyclic 3,5-AMP from ATP inside the cell. Whenever the intracellular concentration of cAMP reaches a certain level, the cell is stimulated to secrete its intracellular store of hormone, lipid, water, or other substance. It has been noted that the adenylate cyclase system works in reverse for mast cells; that is, when the intracellular level of cAMP is lowered, mast cell degranulation follows (Fig. 18-4). Exactly why this system should function in the reverse fashion in mast cells and basophils is unclear at the moment. For example, epinephrine and some other catecholamines stimulate adenylate cyclase and the formation of cAMP, yet they inhibit the allergic reaction. Theophylline blocks the enzyme phosphodiesterase, which hydrolyzes cAMP to linear AMP; this is turn maintains a high intracellular pool of cAMP. Theophylline also protects mast cells against degranulation. Thus, if high levels of cAMP depress mast cell degranulation, then the surface reaction of IgE with antigen must decrease the cellular level of cAMP, since this reaction causes mast cell degranulation. Statistical analyses indicate that it may be necessary for antigen to bridge two IgE molecules on the mast cell surface before degranulation will occur.

Anaphylactic shock, then, is the summation of immunoglobulin formation, the fixation of these immunoglobulins to mast cells and basophils, an in vivo antigen-antibody reaction, the degranu-

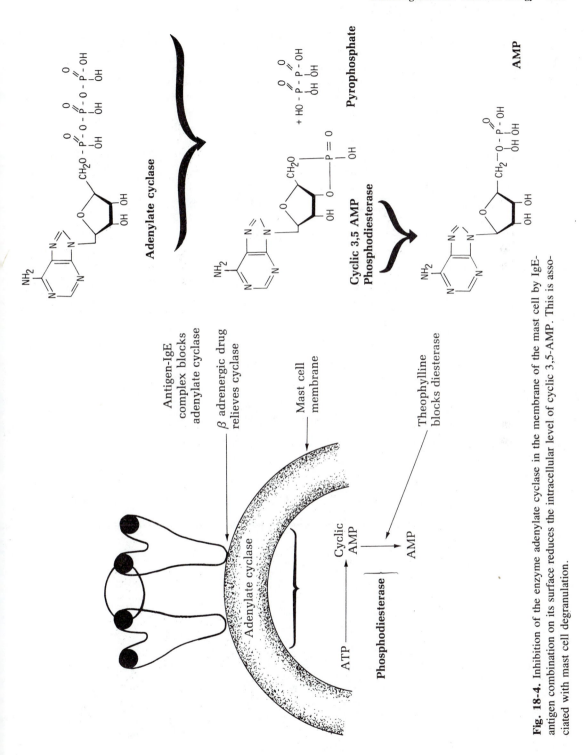

Fig. 18-4. Inhibition of the enzyme adenylate cyclase in the membrane of the mast cell by IgE-antigen combination on its surface reduces the intracellular level of cyclic 3,5-AMP. This is associated with mast cell degranulation.

lative release of histamine and other vasoactive compounds, and the pharmacologic activity of these drugs primarily on smooth muscle (Fig. 18-5). In this light, additional details of the anaphylactic reaction can be considered.

Mediators of anaphylaxis. Several important

pharmacologically active compounds are discharged from mast cells and basophils during anaphylaxis (Table 18-2). These include histamine, heparin, serotonin, ECF-A, and slow-reacting substance of anaphylaxis (SRS-A). Additional substances also are known to participate. The

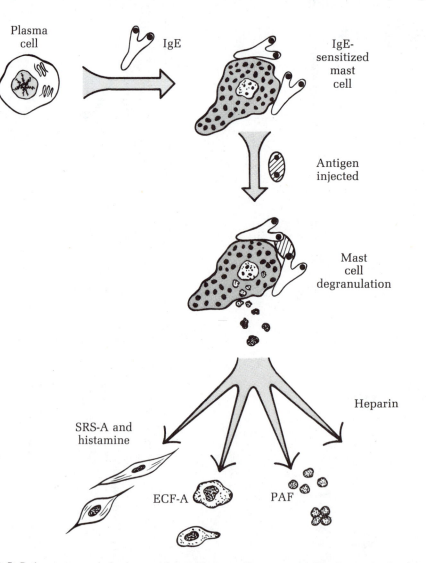

Fig. 18-5. Pathway to anaphylactic sensitivity. Plasma cells are responsible for synthesis of the immunoglobulins that are released and circulate through the blood. The homocytotropic immunoglobulins attach to mast cells. On injection of antigen a cell-fixed antibody-antigen reaction releases histamine and SRS-A to contract smooth muscle, ECF-A to attract eosinophils (eosinophil chemotaxis), PAF to aggregate platelets, and heparin to affect blood clotting.

importance of each of these is directly correlated to its relative proportion (in a physiopharmacologic sense) in the mixture of substances liberated during anaphylaxis, to the sensitivity of smooth muscle and vascular tissue of the animal species involved to the specific action of the compound, and to the rate and mechanism of its detoxification or degradation.

Histamine. Histamine is a simple chemical with a molecular weight of 111. It is formed by the action of the enzyme histidine decarboxylase and its cofactor, pyridoxal phosphate, on histidine (Fig. 18-6). The required enzyme is abundant in tissue mast cells and basophils. The human lung is well supplied with mast cells and contains 25 μg of histamine per gram of wet weight. In the mast cell histamine is held in an ionic complex with heparin in the mast cell granules. Heparin is a substituted polysaccharide consisting primarily of alternating units of α-D-glucuronic acid-2-sulfate and α-D-glucosamine-3,6-disulfate united by

a 1,4-glycosidic bond. Heparin has a molecular weight of approximately 17,000. The ionized sulfate and carboxylate groups in heparin hold histamine in an ionic complex through its protonated nitrogen atoms. Degranulation of mast cells dissociates this complex and releases heparin and histamine. As a consequence, the anticoagulant activity of heparin and the vasodilating and smooth muscle contracting properties of histamine are identified easily in the individual suffering from anaphylactic shock.

Histamine constricts smooth muscle (Fig. 18-5), and in humans the musculature of the respiratory system and the smooth muscle of the venules are highly sensitive to histamine. Serious allergic reactions are accompanied by respiratory distress in which the individual takes rapid, short inhalations without an equal exhalation phase. The blood pressure may drop as the capillaries expand, a compensatory action for venule constriction. This forces fluids into the tissue bed (edema), and the

Table 18-2. Mediators of immediate hypersensitivities

Mediator	Description	Primary activity	Antagonist
Histamine	From histidine in mast cell, 111 mol wt, a heterocyclic amine	Contracts smooth muscle	Antihistamines
Serotonin	From tryptophan in mast cells, 171 mol wt, an aromatic amine	Contracts smooth muscle	Methysergide
ECF-A	From mast cells, about 380 mol wt, a peptide	Attracts eosinophils	None known
SRS-A	Leukotrienes	Prolonged contraction of smooth muscle	Arylsulfatases
Bradykinin and related kinins	From plasma kininogens, near 1,000 mol wt	Contracts smooth muscle slowly	None known
Anaphylatoxins	C3a, 8,900 mol wt C4a, 9,000 mol wt C5a, 11,000 mol wt (not involved in IgE-regulated activities)	Release histamines	Ana INH
PG	Twenty-carbon unsaturated fatty acids, connection to allergy uncertain	Increase cAMP, dose-dependent effect on histamine release, contract smooth muscle	Indomethacin, aspirin
Platelet-activating factor	Substituted phosphorylcholine	Causes platelet degranulation	Phospholipases

accompanying capillary engorgement is observed as erythema.

These activities eventually subside as histamine is detoxified by methylation and oxidation to methylhistamine and imidazoleacetic acid, which do not have the pharmacologic activity of their precursor amine (Fig. 18-6).

A role for histamine as a mediator of the inflammatory reaction received its first significant support from the studies of Lewis, who described the triple response of the skin to the intradermal injection of histamine. This response included an immediate edema, erythema, and wheal or spread

of these effects into the surrounding tissues. It was recognized that these were the exact characteristics of the immediate hypersensitivity reaction which could be provoked in allergic individuals by the intradermal administration of the offending antigen. It also was known that during anaphylaxis a substance appeared in blood which could be injected into the skin of a normal animal and elicit the triple response. Not until 1953 was it possible to associate this activity with histamine. Even at that time it was recognized that histamine probably was not the sole mediator of the immediate allergic response.

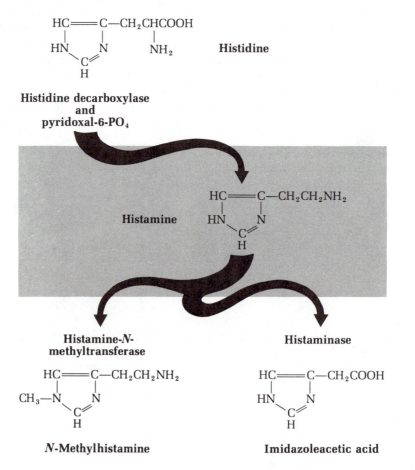

Fig. 18-6. Histamine is formed in the mast cell, as indicated in upper portion of diagram. Two methods of detoxifying histamine are indicated in lower portion.

Serotonin. Serotonin (5-hydroxytryptamine) is derived from the amino acid tryptophan after two enzymatic reactions, the first being a hydroxylation at the 5 position in the ring and the second being the decarboxylation of 5-hydroxytryptophan (Fig. 18-7). Species variation in the distribution and content of serotonin is marked. Most mammals have appreciable serotonin in the gastrointestinal tract and brain. Serotonin is present in the mast cells of many species but not those of the human, mouse, dog, or cat. Platelets are a source of serotonin in several species.

Serotonin has basically the same pharmacologic action as histamine; it causes a rapid contraction of smooth muscles and increases vascular permeability. Rodents seem especially sensitive to its action; in both rats and mice there are data that definitely implicate serotonin as a primary mediator of anaphylactic shock. This is not true for humans, guinea pigs, or dogs. The participation of serotonin in anaphylaxis in rodents is defended by several independent lines of evidence: (1) rodent tissues are very susceptible to serotonin, the injection of which produces a reaction that closely mimics anaphylactic shock; (2) serotonin release into the blood during shock has been proved; (3) antihistamines provide poor protection of rodents against anaphylaxis; and (4) protection is provided by small amounts of lysergic acid, a known serotonin antagonist.

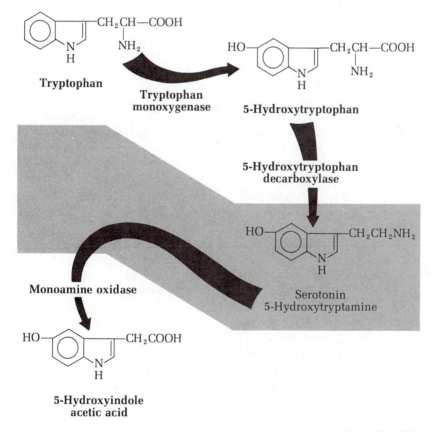

Fig. 18-7. Biochemical pathway for formation of serotonin in the mast cell is indicated in upper half of diagram. Lower half illustrates how detoxification of serotonin occurs.

ECF-A. A third product of mast cells that contributes to the immediate hypersensitive response is ECF-A. Human lung sensitized with IgE and then exposed in vitro to the specific antigen releases an attractant for eosinophils that, although of low molecular weight, could be easily distinguished from histamine and serotonin (Fig. 18-8). ECF-A has a molecular weight near 380, and it is preformed and present in mast cell granules. It is resistant to proteolysis by trypsin and chymotrypsin. Despite the resistance of ECF-A to destruction by pancreatic proteases, its susceptibility to pronase and subtilisin indicates that it has a peptide nature.

ECF-A activity has been attributed to two tetrapeptides from mast cells: Val-Gly-Ser-Glu and Ala-Gly-Ser-Glu. Both molecules are very active on eosinophils, and less chemoattractant to neutrophils, and have no influence on monocyte motility.

Several other chemotaxins have been described as mast cell products in addition to the low molecular weight ECF-A. An intermediate sized ECF-A with a molecular weight between 1,500 and 3,000 is attractive to eosinophils. Neutrophils respond to a molecule of greater than 75,000 mol wt, described as a high molecular weight neutrophil chemotactic factor (HMW-NCF, or NCF). The chemistry of these molecules is under further study.

SRS-A. The treatment of guinea pig lung with cobra venom will release a substance that produces a slow contraction of guinea pig ileum. This material was designated as SRS (for slow-reacting substance) by Feldberg and Kellaway, its discoverers, in 1938. Since that time similar substances elaborated during anaphylaxis also have been noted, and it was suggested that these be designated SRS-A to denote their anaphylactic origin. SRS-A is a family of compounds that have in common their ability to cause the prolonged contraction of certain smooth muscles, to produce increases in vascular permeability as measured in skin, and to be synthesized and released on immunologic order. These molecules do not exist preformed in mast cells.

The initial attempts to purify and characterize SRS-A molecules were handicapped by the heat lability of SRS-A activity; however, this activity was identified as residing in lipid or lipid-soluble substances that contained sulfur atoms. During this same period a great interest developed in PG chemistry and metabolism. Recently SRS-A activity has been identified in three products of the leukotriene pathway of PG and arachidonic acid metabolism: leukotrienes C, D, and E, abbreviated LTC_4, LTD_4, and LTE_4.

Arachidonic acid is found in the cytoplasmic membrane of cells where it is esterified into the structure of sphingomyelin. When liberated from sphingomyelin, arachidonic acid is subject to alteration by two principal pathways: the cyclooxygenase or lipoxygenase pathway. The PGs and several chemotactic molecules (thromboxanes) are produced in the former pathway. In the lipoxygenase pathway additional chemotaxins (HETE) and the leukotrienes are synthesized. Although changes may be made in theories about this pathway in the future, the current concept is as presented in Fig. 18-9. Arachidonic acid is oxidized to 5-hydroperoxyeicosatetraenoic acid, which decomposes spontaneously to form LTA. LTA itself is unstable but becomes stabilized by the addition of glutathione to form LTC. This is accomplished by the enzyme glutathione S transferase. The loss of glutamic acid forms LTD, and the further loss of glycine from the remainder forms LTE, which has only cysteine as its amino acid substituent.

These SRS-A molecules are liberated from mast cells, basophils, neutrophils, and even macrophages when these cells are stimulated by either IgE- or IgG-mediated serologic reactions on their cell surface. The muscle-contracting property of LTC, LTD, and LTE is inactivated by arylsulfatase A and B, found in eosinophils to regenerate the inactive LTA, which is degraded further by other enzymes.

PGs. The confirmation that SRS-A activity was resident in the leukotriene derivatives of arachidonic acid stemmed from earlier suggestions that PGs were involved in IgE-mediated reactions. The prostaglandins (PG), so named because they

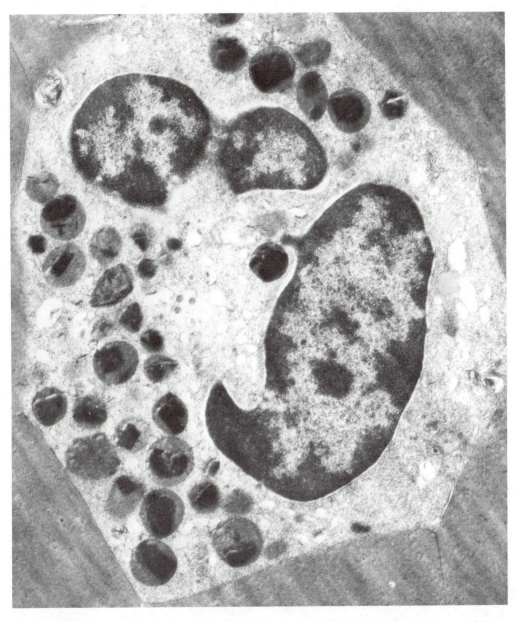

Fig. 18-8. Angular structure of the eosinophil in this electromicrograph is an artifact created by the dense red cell population surrounding it. Notice that the eosinophil is polymorphonuclear, and its cytoplasm contains many granules. These granules contain a crystalloid bar, which allows them to be distinguished from basophilic or neutrophilic granules. Other than their response to ECF-A, the role of eosinophils in IgE-mediated reactions is uncertain. (Courtesy Dr. E. Adelstein.)

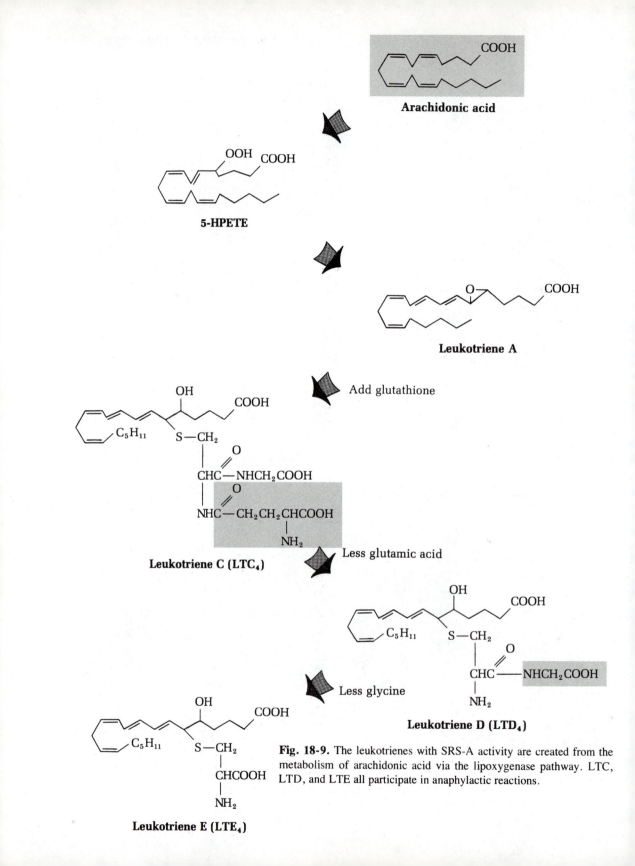

Arachidonic acid

5-HPETE

Leukotriene A

Add glutathione

Leukotriene C (LTC₄)

Less glutamic acid

Leukotriene D (LTD₄)

Less glycine

Leukotriene E (LTE₄)

Fig. 18-9. The leukotrienes with SRS-A activity are created from the metabolism of arachidonic acid via the lipoxygenase pathway. LTC, LTD, and LTE all participate in anaphylactic reactions.

were first identified in the prostate gland, are 20-carbon unsaturated fatty acids that have a cyclopentane ring embodying positions C8 through C12. The PGs are identified as prostaglandins A, B, E, and F, according to the position of keto or hydroxyl substitutions and unsaturated bonds in the cyclic pentane ring. Subscripts, as in PGE_1, denote the position of additional double bonds in the aliphatic portion of the molecule, but the number does not refer to the carbon number of the bond; PGE_1 is unsaturated between carbons 13 and 14, PGE_2 between carbons 6 and 7, and PGE_3 between carbons 17 and 18. PGE and PGF compounds are the two best known series in terms of their biologic activity.

Histamine will initiate PG release, notably PGE and $PGF_{2\alpha}$, from lung tissue. $PGF_{2\alpha}$ causes bronchospasm, bronchodilation, and changes in vascular permeability. PGE stimulates vasodilation and increased vascular permeability and lowers the concentration of intracellular cAMP. This would release histamine and cause lung muscle generation of more PGE and $PGF_{2\alpha}$. The intricacies of these interrelationships undoubtedly will be very interesting when resolved, as will further details of PG inactivation by dehydrogenases.

Platelet-activating-factor (PAF). Basophils have been identified as a source of 1-0-alkyl-2-acetyl-glyceryl-3-phosphorylcholine (Fig. 18-10), better known as platelet-activating-factor (PAF) because of its profound activity on platelets. PAF is generated during anaphylaxis (it does not exist preformed) in rabbits, the species most studied in regard to PAF. The involvement of platelets in the anaphylactic reaction is of interest because platelets contain granules that are released when they are aggregated by PAF (Fig. 18-11). Platelet granules store serotonin, thus further contributing to the anaphylactic reaction. Phospholipases A, C, and D, which cleave substituted glycerides, will inactivate PAF.

Bradykinin and other kinins. The term *kinin* was applied to a number of vasoactive substances on the basis of their similar activity long before their chemical structures were known. This ac-

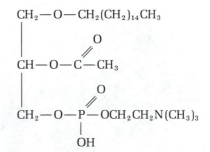

Fig. 18-10. PAF is substituted phosphorylcholine whose alkyl group has a carbon length of 16 to 18 carbons.

tivity includes the slow contraction of smooth muscle (*brady,* slow; *kinin,* to move), an extremely potent vasodilating effect, and an enhancement of capillary permeability. The first of these compounds to be characterized chemically was bradykinin itself (Fig. 18-12). It is a peptide composed of only nine amino acids. Closely related to bradykinin in structure are two other compounds, lysyl-bradykinin (kallidin) and methionyl-lysylbradykinin, also known as kinin 10 and kinin 11, respectively. They all are formed from the same parent compound(s) by what is proving to be a complex biochemical pathway. Not only is the pathway intrinsically complex, involving several compounds in an interrelated sequence of enzyme activation steps (Fig. 18-13), but it also involves a confusing set of nomenclature.

The generation of these kinins begins with the Hageman factor. Hageman's factor, known as factor XII in the blood clotting cascade, is a globulin with a molecular weight reported to be between 80,000 and 100,000. Hageman's factor is enzymatically inert until it is activated by contact with soft glass, colloidal silica, carbon particles, proteases, or antigen-antibody aggregates to become a proteolytic enzyme. In this activation step, fragments that resemble albumin in molecular weight and isoelectric point are liberated, and these albumin fragments are also proteolytic. Both activated Hageman's factor and the Hageman factor albumin fragments can catalyze the activation of plas-

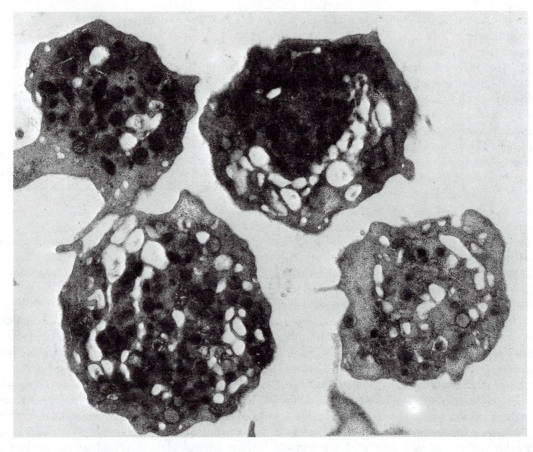

Fig. 18-11. Platelets have numerous granules and vacuoles, as is apparent in this electron micrograph. (Courtesy Dr. E. Adelstein.)

minogen proactivator to form the plasminogen activator. This enzyme and its proenzyme are both γ-globulins with molecular weights near 100,000. Plasminogen activator converts plasminogen, a β-globulin with a molecular weight of 80,000, into plasmin, an active proteolytic enzyme. Plasmin converts a proenzyme, prokininogenase, also known as prekallikrein, into its enzymically active form kininogenase, or kallikrein. This involves a peptide bond cleavage in the 108,000 mol wt proenzyme (also cited to exist in two forms with molecular weights nearer 90,000) to produce its enzyme. Hageman's factor and its albumin fragments also are able to effect this hydrolysis to form kininogenase.

The substrates for kininogenase are the kininogens. These are naturally occurring serum proteins separated into high molecular weight and low molecular weight subclasses. These differ in size from species to species and from report to report, but the high molecular weight molecules range between 80,000 and 125,000 mol wt, and the low molecular weight forms are near 50,000 mol wt. Both types of kininogen contain the sequence of bradykinin within their structure; bradykinin is situated centrally in high molecular weight and terminally in low molecular weight kininogens (Fig. 18-14). Thus the activation of four proenzymes, all found in plasma, culminates in the generation of the kinins.

Human kininogen I

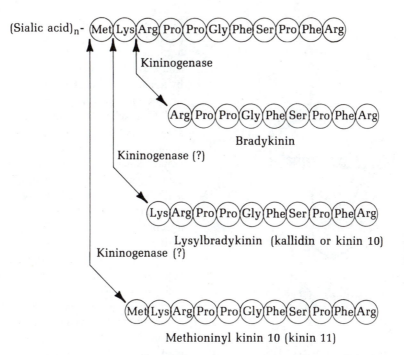

Kininogenase

Bradykinin

Kininogenase (?)

Lysylbradykinin (kallidin or kinin 10)

Kininogenase (?)

Methioninyl kinin 10 (kinin 11)

Fig. 18-12. Several kininogens and kininogenases in human tissues are known. This diagram suggests how bradykinin and its related kinins may be formed from kininogen I.

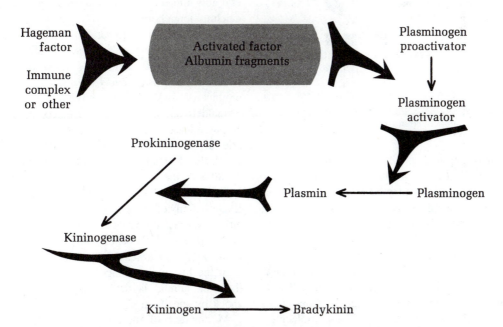

Fig. 18-13. Multistage proenzyme-enzyme reactions through which bradykinin and other kinins are released begin with the activation of Hageman's factor by immune complexes or enzymes, starch, agar, drugs, and other substances that produce anaphylactoid reactions. (From Barrett, J.T.: Basic immunology and its medical application, ed. 2, St. Louis, 1980, The C.V. Mosby Co.)

High molecular weight kininogen

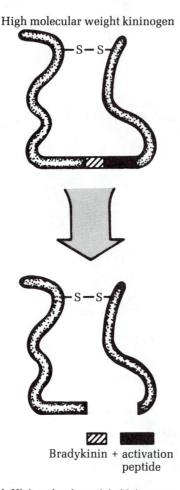

Bradykinin + activation
peptide

Fig. 18-14. High molecular weight kininogen contains a centrally located bradykinin *(striped bar),* which is liberated with an activation peptide by kininogenase.

Various peptidases, which can use kinins as substrates, destroy their biologic activity. Kininases in certain tissues may be highly specific; for example, a specific oligoendopeptidase in brain hydrolyzes only bradykinin and not other substrates.

Anaphylatoxins. Anaphylatoxins are, by definition, molecules of biologic origin that can induce the release of histamine from mast cells. Three anaphylatoxins are known to originate from complement: C3a, C4a, and C5a. These molecules produce edema and erythema in human skin. Their vasoactive property is dependent on a terminal arginine and is lost when this arginine is removed. The knowledge that the activation of complement by nonantibody mechanisms through the properdin or alternate pathway would release C3a, C4a, and C5a suggests these anaphylatoxins may be very important in nonantibody-mediated immediate allergic reactions (anaphylactoid reactions). Since IgE does not activate the complement system, the anaphylatoxins are of importance here only for comparative purposes.

Anaphylactoid reactions can be produced by the injection of agar, starch, india ink, colloidal iron, barium sulfate, and several other nonantigenic materials. These immunologically inert materials activate serum and tissue proteases and the alternate pathway of the complement system. This is the basis of anaphylactoid reactions.

Anaphylactoid reactions. Direct chemical degranulation of mast cells may be the cause of anaphylactoid reactions resulting from the injection of complex macromolecules, or these may function by first causing anaphylatoxin formation. Several low molecular weight agents, including the calcium ionophore A 23187, guanidine, strychnine, aromatic and aliphatic monoamines or diamines, and quaternary amines, will liberate histamine from mast cells. The most thoroughly studied of these is probably 48/80, a condensation product of *p*-methoxyphenethylmethylamine and formaldehyde, which is an extremely potent histamine releaser. The administration of large quantities of 48/80 will throw an animal into a synthetic duplicate of anaphylactic shock. The injection of 48/80 into the skin produces the triple response typical of immediate hypersensitive skin reactions. Examination of biopsy tissue specimens after either experience reveals that mast cells indeed are degranulated. If the chemically initiated release of histamine in a sensitized animal is continued until the histamine storage depots are exhausted, then the animal is desensitized to anaphylactic shock by specific antigen.

Moderators of anaphylaxis. It is clear that the

biochemical regulation of anaphylaxis is possible at several stages in the pathway to anaphylactic shock. Regulation of immunoglobulin synthesis by the use of immunosuppressants is one theoretic mechanism. The use of fragments of the Fc portion of ε-chains from the hinge region will block ε-chain binding to mast cells and may become a practical approach to the prevention of IgE-mediated allergies. A third possibility is the controlled chemical degranulation of mast cells, but other chemical approaches currently are preferred.

Chemical methods. Since such a variety of chemical substances are involved in the immediate allergic reaction, and since smooth muscle is an important target organ, it is clear that antagonists of those chemicals and smooth muscle relaxants would be superior combatants of these reactions. The body's natural moderators of anaphylaxis are the enzymes that decompose the mediators of anaphylaxis.

Antihistamines. Histamine acts on mammalian cells by combining with histamine receptors on their cell surface, of which there are two distinct types, H1 and H2. Molecules other than histamine which combine with these receptors may behave then as histamine antagonists. The H1 receptor is more important to immunology than the H2 receptor, since it is associated with smooth muscle contraction, venule dilation, and pruritus. The classic antihistamines competitively inhibit this receptor. The H2 receptor is associated with non-immunologic events such as histamine-induced gastric secretion and mucous secretion, but it also may be important in suppressing T cell activities.

Antihistamines frequently are substituted amines or ethanolamines that have only a vague resemblance to the structure of histamine (Fig. 18-15). Nevertheless these compounds plus certain substituted piperazines, phenothiazines, and hydroxyzines are considered competitive inhibitors of histamine because they block histamine receptors on nerve endings. Antihistamines have no effect on histamine release from mast cells or basophils. In humans antihistamines are effective antagonists of edema and pruritus, which probably

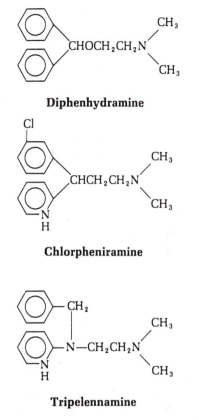

Diphenhydramine

Chlorpheniramine

Tripelennamine

Fig. 18-15. Structures of three antihistamines. These compounds all are substituted diamines. Literally dozens of compounds with antihistaminic activity are known.

are related to their blockage of histamine-induced increases in capillary permeability. Antihistamines are relatively less effective in humans in preventing bronchoconstriction.

The competitive function of histamine analogs is best displayed when they are administered prior to the release of histamine. Since this is rarely the case in human allergies, these drugs have been thought less effective than experimental situations indicate. Drug effectiveness always must be evaluated in terms of side effects, and sedation is a major undesired effect of many antihistamines.

Catecholamines. The terms *adrenergic* drug, *sympathomimetic drug,* and *catecholamines* are used interchangeably to described a series of sub-

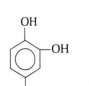

**Adrenaline
(epinephrine)**

Norepinephrine

Isoproterenol

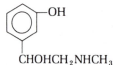

Phenylephrine

Ephedrine

Fig. 18-16. Adrenaline and several related adrenergic drugs.

stituted amines that have a potent bronchodilating and smooth muscle relaxant activity. The physiologic response to these compounds is best explained on the basis of the concept of α- and β-receptors on the effector cells with which the catecholamines react. Attachment and blockage of the β-adrenergic receptor on mast cells allows adenylate cyclase to accumulate cAMP, which in turn stabilizes mast cells. The β-receptors on smooth muscle of the bronchi influence muscle relaxation, and the α-receptors regulate constriction.

The various adrenergic drugs differ in their ability to block the α- and β-receptors, but since they act directly on mast cells, they inhibit histamine release, which then reduces the amount of muscle constriction and edema, and have a second direct action on muscle cells to relax them. These compounds have both a prophylactic and therapeutic application. The best known of these compounds are adrenaline, ephedrine, propranolol, and isoproterenol (Fig. 18-16), but there are many adrenergic drugs available to treat and reverse IgE-mediated allergic reactions.

Cromolyn. Extracts of the seeds of the plant *Ammi visnaga* contain a complex heterocyclic compound—cromolyn sodium—that just recently has been tested for its effect in modifying allergic reactions. The compound is absorbed poorly from the intestinal tract (Fig. 18-17); therefore it is administered by inhalation. The field trial successes of its use can be attributed to its prevention of histamine and SRS-A release from mast cells, which cannot degranulate in the presence of cromolyn. Cromolyn is a prophylactic drug and is not antagonistic to SRS-A or histamine.

Methyl xanthines. Relaxation of smooth muscle by the methyl xanthines caffeine, theophylline, and theobromine has encouraged their use as bronchodilators. These compounds also function at the level of the mast cell by increasing the concentration of cAMP and reducing mast cell degranulation. An undesirable effect of the methyl xanthines is their diuretic function.

Antiserotonins. Inhibition of 5-hydroxytryptophan-induced constriction of smooth muscle is possible with lysergic acid derivatives, but be-

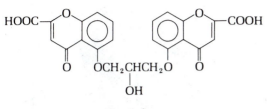

Cromolyn

Fig. 18-17. Structure of cromolyn.

cause of the hallucinogenic activity of these compounds, they are not used extensively.

Immunologic methods

Neutralization. When skin tests reveal that an intended recipient is allergic to an antigenic injectable or inhalant allergen, the existing cell-bound IgE can be neutralized. This can be accomplished and yet avoid the life-threatening hazard of a massive release of histamine if minute and increasing dosages of the antigen are injected over a few hours. The first small amounts of antigen provoke only a minimal amount of histamine release, and this is rapidly converted to the inert imidazoleacetic acid. When symptoms of histamine shock have disappeared, another of antigen is given, and this is continued until the individual can tolerate the therapeutic dose of the injectable or further desensitizing doses of the allergen.

Before IgE neutralization is attempted, it is prudent to administer antihistamines and to have adrenaline ready to reverse any accidental severe shock. This desensitization is temporary and in fact consists of booster exposures to the antigen. A week or so after neutralization has been completed, the production of IgE may place the individual in a state of heightened hypersensitivity.

Blocking antibody. It does not necessarily follow that repeated exposure to an allergen will accentuate the hypersensitivity. Specific desensitization procedures are based on booster injections of antigen spaced over periods of weeks rather than hours to prompt the formation of blocking antibodies. These blocking antibodies are circulating IgG antibodies which combine with the antigen

in the vascular system and prevent antigen diffusion into the tissues where IgE-coated mast cells reside. This mechanism of action for blocking antibodies was first proved in desensitization to insect stings, in which case the level of IgG blocking antibodies is well correlated with the degree of protection against the allergic reaction. Blocking antibodies now have been proved to be the protective antibodies formed by desensitization to several allergens. It does not matter that the desensitization increases IgE levels; there was previously sufficient IgE present to render the individual seriously allergic. What is important is that cell-bound IgE has less chance to react with allergen in the face of high levels of circulating IgG.

ATOPY

Approximately 10% to 20% of the population in the United States has some type of allergy. Of these, it has been estimated that 8,000,000 persons have hay fever, 3,000,000 have asthma, and 9,000,000 have atopic allergies to other agents—certain foods, animal dandruff or feathers, dust, antibiotics, wool, insect stings, and a countless variety of other substances. These atopic allergies (*atopy,* a strange disease) are for the most part naturally occurring conditions for which the antigenic exposure is not always known. Until the past decade it was not known what type of immunoglobulin was associated with these diseases, but now it is agreed that IgE is the responsible molecule.

Atopic illnesses were among the first antibody-associated diseases noted to have a strong familial or hereditary tendency. More than 50 years ago hay fever, bronchial asthma, and food allergies were observed to be family-associated in almost half the reported instances. About 58% of all allergic children had parents who were both allergic, and only 12.5% of such children had allergy-free parents. Knowledge of the genetic basis for allergies thus has a long history, and a genetic basis for the synthesis of all immunoglobulins is now well accepted.

Genetic studies in humans first suggested specific haplotypes were associated with atopic allergy to ragweed, but this was not supported by subsequent analyses. Nevertheless genetic studies in mice have determined that poor IgE responders are under Ir gene control via Ts cells. The failure to demonstrate this in humans may mean the human IgE response is under multigene regulation.

Respiratory allergy

Probably the most commonly offending inhalant antigens are pollens or spores of higher plants and molds. Animal danders, vegetable and cereal dusts, and house dust should not be excluded from this list of excellent natural sensitizers. The pollens of higher plants such as the several species of ragweed (genus *Ambrosia*), many different trees, and grasses are responsible for the condition known as hay fever. It has been estimated that a single ragweed plant produces as many as 1,000,000 pollen grains annually. A square mile of ragweed would liberate about 16 tons of pollen into the air in one season (Fig. 18-18). The pollen grains are very light and can be carried for miles by a gentle summer breeze. Contact of the pollen with the mucous membranes of the eye, nose, and throat is the normal manner of sensitization. Reexposure of these surfaces, perhaps in a subsequent pollen season, causes the local allergic reaction known as hay fever. Sneezing, watery reddened eyes, an itching and running nose, and respiratory distress are all part of the usual episode. Although this might be described as a mild form of anaphylaxis, local in nature because of the mode of contact and insoluble state of the pollen, hay fever sufferers certainly would not refer to their condition as a mild illness.

It would be impossible to consider the chemistry of the many pollen antigens, even if they were known. The principal antigens of the low ragweed plant, *Ambrosia elatior,* are two proteins designated as antigens E and K. These have been purified by a combination of ammonium sulfate precipitation, Sephadex filtration, and ion exchange chromatography. Both antigens have molecular weights of about 38,000, and both are pure proteins containing less than 1% carbohydrate. Anti-

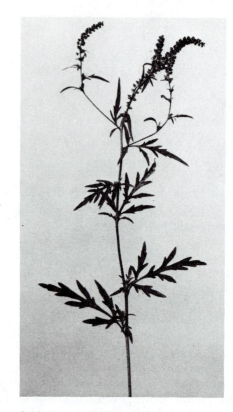

Fig. 18-18. Ragweed plant with pollen-bearing stems at the top.

gen E represents 6% of the total protein in the pollen and antigen K about 3%. These two antigens, which are not cross-reactive, represent the two most important allergenic proteins in low ragweed. Although other antigens are present in the pollen, they have a much weaker sensitizing ability.

Other offending pollens include those of *Ambrosia trifida* (giant ragweed), those of most trees, including elm, oak, and pines, and those of grasses such as rye, timothy, and bluegrass. Many flower pollens are allergy inducers.

Allergy to house dust is surprisingly constant over widely dispersed geographic areas from which the dust has clear differences in composition because of the nature of the soil itself and the plants which grow in these areas. A common feature of house dust is its population of dust mites, which live in carpets and soil. Many persons allergic to house dust react to extracts of the mites *Dermatophagoides farinae* and *D. pteronyssinus*.

Food allergy

Food allergies represent another major class of atopic allergies. An allergy to food may arise at any age; it may be expressed locally by oral inflammation, canker sores, and cramping and by nausea, gaseous distention, and diarrhea of the intestinal tract. The symptoms may erupt in the skin as splotches of urticaria known as hives. Respiratory symptoms also may develop, especially with dry foods to which respiratory exposure is almost guaranteed. Based on skin sensitivity testing of 200 allergic children below the age of 8 years, the following percentages of allergy were determined for these foods: chocolate 19%, cow's milk 15%, wheat or wheat products 26%, orange 25%, strawberries 33%, and codfish 45%. Other "good" allergens include tomatoes, peanuts, egg, and rye and other cereals. Food avoidance rather than desensitization is recommended to prevent recurrence of food allergies.

Miscellaneous allergies

Anaphylactic allergy arising from the injection of antigens also can exist as an atopic allergy. In the United States about 40 deaths are reported each year as the result of insect stings. The principal insects involved are represented by the common honey bee, yellow jacket, yellow hornet, paper wasp, and others in the order *Hymenoptera*. Only the females of these insects sting, and when they do so, several different proteins, including the enzymes phospholipase, hyaluronidase, and phosphatase, may sensitize the individual by stimulating an IgE response. A repeated sting may incite a serious, even lethal anaphylactic response to these enzymes contained within the venom. Bee keepers who are insensitive to bee stings have high levels of IgG, in the company or absence of high circulating levels of IgE.

Physical allergies to heat, cold, sunlight, and pressure are not as life threatening as those related to injectables. Heat, cold, and ultraviolet light are believed to cause a physicochemical derangement of proteins or polysaccharides of the skin and transform them into autoantigens that are responsible for the allergic reaction. Prevention of these allergies is based on avoidance of the incitant. Dermographism (dermatographism, or skin writing) is seen as edematous and mildly erythematous eruption in the track of mild pressure applied to the skin.

PENICILLIN ALLERGY

With the demise of antiserum therapy as a major hypersensitizing treatment of persons suffering from acute infectious or toxic disease has arisen an equally dangerous hypersensitizing treatment: the injection of low molecular weight antibiotic drugs. Although penicillin is undoubtedly one of the least toxic of all drugs used in the therapeusis of human and animal diseases, it has been responsible for an increasing number of allergic reactions and anaphylactic deaths since its introduction on the pharmaceutical market approximately 40 years ago. It now is estimated that over 300 anaphylactic deaths occur each year from treatment with penicillin.

Penicillin is a complex, although relatively low molecular weight, compound that is subject to decomposition by several different routes to a diverse array of products. Most intermediates and end products have been isolated or synthesized and used as haptenic sensitizers of humans and experimental animals. Immunization with hapten-antigen conjugates also has been practiced. Studies of the dermal sensitivity or antiserum reactivity with specific degradation products have indicated that penicilloic acid derivatives, and to a lesser extent derivatives of penicillamine and penicillenic acid, are the key sensitizing agents (Fig. 18-19). All these are capable of covalent bonding with proteins, the latter two through sulfhydryl exchange reactions. Penicilloyl conjugates are formed by amidination reactions, which open the oxazole ring of penicillenic acid. Thus in one sense penicilloic acid derivatives are in actuality penicillenic acid derivatives.

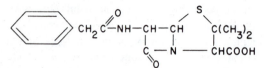

Penicillin G

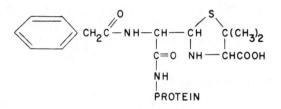

Penicilloic acid–protein complex

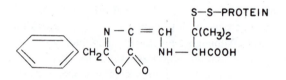

Penicillenic acid–protein complex

Penicillamine–protein complex

Fig. 18-19. Three hypersensitizing derivatives of benzyl penicillin (penicillin G). The penicilloic acid compound is formed by opening of the oxazolone ring of penicillenic acid during conjugation.

Detection of anaphylactic sensitivity to one or another of the haptenic metabolites of penicillin is complicated by several problems associated with skin tests with haptens. One of these is that the hapten alone apparently is incapable of releasing the pharmacologic mediators of immediate hypersensitivities because haptens cannot bridge two IgE molecules. Second, on combination with the antibody the free hapten may block the binding of any in vivo–formed hapten-protein conjugate and thus mask the hypersensitivity that is present. A

third problem is that in vivo formation of the hapten-protein conjugate may be so rapid and extensive that systemic anaphylactic shock rather than a mild skin reaction may be elicited. A fourth factor is that the skin test with the hapten may serve as a hypersensitizing experience and produce sensitivity in a previous nonsensitive individual.

It is clear that the use of hapten-protein conjugates would eliminate some of the faults of testing with pure haptens alone, since it could be made multivalent with respect to penicillin determinants and used in a standardized fashion. Testing with hapten alone always leads to some confusion, since the amount of autocoupling from person to person varies considerably. One major fault inherent in the use of conjugates is that one can become sensitized to the protein carrier. Egg albumin, milk casein, and certain other proteins that humans regularly contact in their diet should not be used as carriers. A clever solution to this dilemma was realized when penicilloyl poly-D-lysine became available. After testing it was found that this reagent is a very sensitive detector of penicillin hypersensitivity in the human when other tests are negative. Furthermore it does not induce penicillin allergy or allergy to poly-D-lysine, since this carrier is nonimmunogenic. The use of this reagent has greatly reduced the incidence of allergic reactions to penicillin, since individuals whose skin test results are positive now can be selectively excluded from the anaphylactic risk group by being given an alternative therapeutic.

DETECTION OF THE IgE-DEPENDENT HYPERSENSITIVITIES

Diagnosis of atopic allergies is dependent on the specificity of the immediate skin reaction observed after the intradermal exposure to the allergen. This may be done by scratch, prick, or intracutaneous testing. A droplet of the allergen extract is placed in a superficial scratch on the skin and observed for local edema. Literally a score of such tests can be applied to the back and forearms of a patient at one sitting. In prick testing a series of small skin punctures is made with a needle, and a droplet of allergen is placed on the skin. Scratch and prick testing are about a hundred times less sensitive than intracutaneous testing. Ophthalmic testing, with observation for conjunctival irritation, is little better than intracutaneous testing, although it may involve slightly less risk. Diagnosis is also possible on the basis of the P-K test. The P-K test now is used only when it is necessary to avoid multiple skin testing of a child or of a seriously ill individual.

With the knowledge that IgE is the allergic antibody, in vitro testing procedures for total IgE content of sera (RIST) or IgE specific for specially selected antigens (RAST) soon may replace much of the skin testing currently used in diagnosing atopic allergies. The IgE testing procedures certainly will be more quantitative and may even prove superior to skin testing. The radial quantitative immunodiffusion test now can be used as a less expensive substitute for the RIST test.

BIBLIOGRAPHY

Austen, K.F.: Biologic implications of the structural and functional characteristics of the chemical mediators of immediate-type hypersensitivity, Harvey Lect. **73**:93, 1979.

Bahna, S.L., and Heiner, D.C.: Allergies to milk, New York, 1980, Grune & Stratton, Inc.

deWeck, A.L., and Blumenthal, M.N.: HLA and allergy, Basel, 1977, S. Karger, AG, Medical and Scientific Publishers.

Dorrington, K.J., and Bennich, H.H.: Structure-function relationships in human immunoglobulin E, Immunol. Rev. **41**:3, 1978.

Foreman, J.C.: The pharmacologic control of immediate hypersensitivity, Annu. Rev. Pharmacol. Toxicol. **21**:63, 1981.

Galant, S.P., Bronsky, E.A., and Gillman, S.A.: Pediatric allergy case studies, Garden City, N.Y., 1980, Medical Examination Publishing Co., Inc.

Gell, P.G.H., Coombs, R.R.A., and Lachmann, P., editors: Clinical aspects of immunology, ed. 3, Oxford, 1974, Blackwell Scientific Publications, Ltd.

Gerrard, J.W.: Food allergy, Springfield, Ill., 1980, Charles C Thomas, Publisher.

Gupta, S., and Good, R.A., editors: Cellular, molecular, and clinical aspects of allergic disorders, New York, 1979, Plenum Publishing Corp.

Hugli, T.E.: Chemical aspects of the serum anaphylatoxins, Contemp. Top. Mol. Immunol. **7**:181, 1978.

Ishizaka, K.: Cellular events in the IgE antibody response, Adv. Immunol. **23**:1, 1976.

Johnson, F., and Spencer, J.T., Jr., editors: Allergy: immunology and medical treatment, Chicago, 1980, Year Book Medical Publishers, Inc.

Katz, D.H.: Prospects for the clinical control of IgE synthesis, Prog. Clin. Immunol. **4**:127, 1980.

Kazimierczak, W., and Diamant, B.: Mechanisms of histamine release in anaphylactic and anaphylactoid reactions, Prog. Allergy **24**:295, 1978.

King, T.P.: Chemical and biological properties of some atopic allergens, Adv. Immunol. **23**:77, 1976.

Lessof, M.H., editor: Immunological and clinical aspects of allergy, Philadelphia, 1981, J.B. Lippincott Co.

Middleton, E., Jr., Reed, C.E., and Ellis, E.F., editors: Allergy: principles and practice, St. Louis, 1978, The C.V. Mosby Co.

Movat, H.Z., editor: Inflammation, immunity and hypersensitivity: cellular and molecular mechanisms, ed. 2, New York, 1979, Harper & Row Publishers, Inc.

Mygind, N.: Nasal allergy, ed. 2, Oxford, 1979, Blackwell Scientific Publications, Ltd.

Norman, P.S.: A review of immunotherapy, Allergy **32**:62, 1978.

O'Connell, E.J.: Pediatric allergy, Garden City, N.Y., 1980, Medical Examination Publishing Co., Inc.

Oppenheim, J.J., Rosenstreich, D.L., and Potter, M., editors: Cellular functions in immunity and inflammation, New York, 1981, Elsevier/North-Holland, Inc.

Parwaresch, M.R.: The human blood basophil, Berlin, 1976, Springer-Verlag.

Piper, P.J.: SRS-A and leukotrienes, New York, 1981, John Wiley & Sons, Inc.

Schachter, M.: Kallikreins (kininogenases)—a group of serum proteases with bioregulatory actions, Pharmacol. Rev. **31**:1, 1979.

Sobotka, A.K., and others: IgE-mediated basophil phenomena: quantitation, control, inflammatory interactions, Immunol. Rev. **41**:171, 1978.

Turk, J.L.: Immunology in clinical medicine, ed. 3, New York, 1978, Appleton-Century-Crofts.

Vane, J.R., and Ferreira, S.H., editors: Inflammation, New York, 1978, Springer-Verlag New York, Inc.

Weller, P.F., and Goetzl, E.J.: The regulatory and effector roles of eosinophils, Adv. Immunol. **27**:339, 1979.

SITUATION: ANAPHYLACTIC OR ANAPHYLACTOID?

The elevator for employees stopped on the fifth floor, and I expected to see one of my friends from the physiology department get on. Sure enough, John S., pushing a cart ahead of him, stepped on and pushed the ground floor button. As we started down, I asked him how his research was going.

"You've got the answer right in front of you. On that cart is the sixth animal in a row that died before we could complete the experiment. Every one of them lately has died of anaphylaxis."

"How do you know it's anaphylaxis? What's your experimental set up?"

"Well, we've been wanting to check the effect of a new drug used for parasite infections on kidney function. We've set up a series of intravenous injections of the compound, increasing the dose stepwise. At various times we give them tests for kidney function and take kidney biopsies. Now that we have increased the dose to 5 mg the animals all roll over dead in about 10 minutes."

"I don't know, John. It might be anaphylaxis, and it might not. Let me check you out on a few things. You know what an anaphylactoid reaction is, don't you?"

Questions

1. What is an anaphylactoid reaction?
2. What types of agents cause anaphylactoid reactions?
3. What are the major characteristics that distinguish anaphylactoid and anaphylactic reactions?
4. How can anaphylactoid reactions be prevented or treated?

Solution

An anaphylactoid reaction may be defined as any reaction having the characteristics of anaphylaxis but not based on immunologic phenomena.

Anaphylactoid reactions are acute, life-threatening reactions that follow the intravascular administration of nonantigenic materials. Substances that provoke anaphylactoid reactions also lack the qualities of autocoupling haptens. Nevertheless in sufficient doses these agents through direct actions on the kinin system of the blood, or on basophils and mast cells, cause the release of histamine, serotonin, kinins, and other mediators that are responsible for the anaphylaxis-like reaction. Small quantities may produce symptoms so mild as to go unnoticed by inexperienced observers, and larger doses may produce pronounced symptoms or death. A direct-dose response relationship is not a constant observation in anaphylactoid reactions, however. A dose of a given magnitude may produce an anaphylactoid reaction on one occasion and fail to do so at another time.

Anaphylactic reactions are dose dependent, but this is difficult to demonstrate, since such tiny amounts of antigen can elicit the full response. An important feature which distinguishes these two reactions is the failure to observe antibodies in individuals who demonstrate anaphylactoid reactions.

Among the substances causing anaphylactoid reactions, starch, organic iodine, agar, bromphenol blue, and contrast media used in urographic analysis can be mentioned. The latter are important human causes of anaphylactoid reactions. These reactions are so unpredictable and rare (only 0.05% of all patients subjected to intravenous pyelography had acute reactions) that little is done to prevent them. Treatment is also uncertain, but corticosteroids, fluid replacement, and adrenergic drugs have been used.

In this situation the death of the animals almost certainly was caused by anaphylactoid reaction to the large doses of the drug used in the later injections.

References

Obeid, A.I., and others: Fluid therapy in severe systemic reaction to radiopaque dye, Ann. Intern. Med. **83:**317, 1975.

Witten, D.M., Hirsch, F.D., and Hartman, G.W.: Acute reactions to urographic contrast medium: incidence, clinical characteristics and relationship to history of hypersensitivity states, Am. J. Roentgenol. Radium Ther. Nucl. Med. **119:**832, 1973.

Zwieman, B., Mishkin, M.M., and Hildreth, E.A.: An approach to the performance of contrast studies in contrast material reactive persons, Ann. Intern. Med. **83:**159, 1975.

CHAPTER 19

IMMUNOGLOBULIN G–MEDIATED ALLERGY

According to the Gell and Coombs classification of hypersensitivity the cytotoxic and immune complex reactions depend on heat-stable antibodies, in contrast to the anaphylactic allergies associated with the heat-labile IgE described in the preceding chapter. The cytotoxic allergies of alloimmune origin include conditions such as transfusion reactions and HDN. Autoimmune cytotoxicity, described in Chapter 21, also is seen in several blood-vascular conditions, including autoimmune hemolytic disease, autoimmune thrombocytopenia, and autoimmune granulocytopenia. The immune complex reactions also can develop from alloimmune or autoimmune phenomena. This chapter includes only immune complex phenomena related to xenoantigens.

Historically the cytotoxic and immune complex allergies have been categorized as precipitin allergies because the antibodies involved normally precipitate with or on the antigen. Moreover the antigens involved (foreign serum or injectable solutions) were often fluids that were simply identified as antigens by precipitation reactions. The term *precipitin allergy* seldom is used today but is still an appropriate term to separate these allergies from those which rely on IgE or T cell activities.

SERUM SICKNESS

Serum sickness develops in approximately 50% of normal human beings who receive a single injection of bovine or horse antitoxin against tetanus, gas gangrene, or other toxins for prophylactic or therapeutic purposes. Since antitoxin therapy is less frequently practiced today because of the superiority of immunity developed on active immunization with toxoids, the allergic response to serum per se as the cause of serum sickness is diminishing. An exception to this can be noted in persons receiving ALS for immunosuppression of graft rejection reactions. The majority of these patients develop serum sickness within a few weeks of therapy even though given chemical immunosuppressives simultaneously. Penicillin is now one of the most common causative agents of serum sickness, especially penicillin injected in long-acting repository form.

Primary serum sickness

Ordinary serum sickness, an allergic reaction to a foreign serum or autocoupling hapten, is marked by hives, extensive edema (especially about the face, neck, and joints), joint pain, malaise, and fever. These symptoms usually are first seen about 7 to 10 days after the injection and persist for several days, after which they gradually subside. Transitory eosinophilia, complementemia, and albuminuria occur. von Pirquet and Schick presented the first full description of the disease, although it had been described previously by several investigators. von Pirquet's interest in serum sickness stemmed from his conviction that the onset of many diseases with an inflammatory quality resulted from the formation and reaction of antibodies with an antigen. The current indications that inflammation is the result of anaphylatoxic components arising from complement activation during antigen-antibody reactions are the most modern reaffirmation of the genius and forethought of von Pirquet.

Primary serum sickness is caused by the mutual presence of antigen and antibody in the blood following the primary immunization. By about the fifth to eighth day after an initial immunization with a substantial quantity of fluid antigen a portion of the antigen still will be circulating. By this time the initial traces of antibody are detectable in the blood. IgG and possibly other immunoglobulins combine with the antigen in the circulation and are deposited at various locations throughout the body. These immune complexes can be seen in the blood vessel walls and in the kidney, where they can be stained with fluorescent anti-C3

or anti-IgG. Immune complex nephritis is a regular finding in serum sickness. These immune complexes of antigen, antibody, and complement activate the complement cascade. C5a draws neutrophils to the complex, which then is phagocytosed. The neutrophils may release lysosomal enzymes and contribute to local tissue damage. The C3a, C4a, and C5a anaphylatoxins cause degranulation of mast cells, which results in the appearance of histamine, ECF-A, and SRS-A in the blood. This pathway accounts for the hypocomplementemia, edema, joint pain, and eosinophilia seen in patients with serum sickness.

The role of cell-bound antibody (IgE) in serum sickness is uncertain. Presumably there is some contribution. When cell-fixed antibodies combine with the antigen, the serologic reaction on the cell surface, just as in systemic anaphylaxis, triggers the release of histamine, eosinophilic chemotactic factor, etc. Since each molecule of antibody is able to combine with antigen and release histamine at the moment the antibody molecule fixes to cells, there is never the sudden release of lethal quantities of pharmacologic amines and peptides. Likewise, IgG-antigen complexes, through C3a, C4a, and C5a, would release histamine and other kinins gradually, a molecule at a time. Moreover histamine detoxification mechanisms continually reduce the quantity of histamine in the circulation as it is formed. Thus the symptoms of serum sickness are more chronic and less life threatening than those of anaphylaxis, even though IgE may add to the mast cell effects of the anaphylatoxins.

Since the symptoms of serum sickness do not appear until several days after the injection of the antigen, the disease has been called protracted anaphylaxis. This is a poorly chosen term. Anaphylaxis is clearly an IgE-mediated condition. Serum sickness is largely an IgG-mediated disease, although other immunoglobulin classes, including IgE, may contribute to the symptomatology. Protracted anaphylaxis also has been used to describe the delayed lethal effect produced by injecting antigen into anaphylactically sensitive animals by routes that ensure slow antigen absorption.

Accelerated serum sickness

An accelerated form of serum sickness can be provoked in persons who were sensitized several years previously to an antigen that they now are given a second time. The appearance of the symptoms within 2 to 5 days is typical in these cases. The hastened onset of accelerated serum sickness compared with primary serum sickness is due to the anamnestic response which follows this second exposure to antigen. Even though the individual may have been sensitized to the antigen years previously, the anamnestic response will result in a rapid outpouring of IgG and other immunoglobulins into the blood. Within a brief time a sufficient quantity of immune complexes will be available for the patient to express the symptoms of serum sickness.

Experimental serum sickness can be produced in experimental animals by a single large injection of a fluid antigen. The edematous response is not as striking in lower animals as in humans, but otherwise the disease is very similar to that in the human, both in its symptomatology and in its immunologic aspects.

THE ARTHUS REACTION

Local anaphylaxis was the term used by Arthus in 1903 to describe the development of dermal necrosis in antigen injection sites in rabbits that have a high level of circulating antibody. In the Arthus reactions the first indication of an allergic reaction is the development of an extensive zone of erythema and edema surrounding the bleb created by the intradermal injection of antigen. Within a few hours a cyanotic center develops within an erythematous ring. Later this assumes a deep purplish black cast indicative of cellular necrosis. Over the succeeding day or two this necrotic zone may enlarge to 2 to 3 cm in diameter. The size of the edematous area may be three times the size of the central necrotic zone. The dead tissue dries, and over a period of a week or more healing becomes complete (Fig. 19-1).

This local reaction is the result of intravascular precipitate formation and thrombosis. Diffusion of the antigen into the vascular bed surrounding the injection site creates a local area of mutually high concentration of antigen and circulating antibody, resulting in antigen-antibody complexing and precipitation. Precipitate formation becomes so extensive as to physically blockade the small venules. Deprivation of gas exchange, coupled with the inability to adequately eliminate tissue waste products or supply nutrients, results in local tissue destruction. Tissue destruction is further favored by the participation of serum complement in the reaction and the release of chemotactic factors. Massive infiltration of PMNs follows. Within a few hours, after the shocking dermal dose of antigen, the leukocytes begin to disintegrate and release their lysosomal enzymes, which contribute to the damage. Within 1 or 2 days most of the damage has been done, and healing begins.

The pivotal role of neutrophils in the Arthus reaction is demonstrated by the effect of certain alkylating agents on the reaction. In particular the nitrogen mustards have a powerful depressing effect on the level of circulating neutrophilic leukocytes and almost totally eliminate the Arthus reaction. Since these leukocytes are attracted to the site by the action of complement-derived leukotaxins, the complement-fixing antibodies, that is, IgG and IgM, not IgE, are responsible for the Arthus reaction. A good appraisal of the circulating IgG titer of an animal can be determined by measuring its Arthus response to antigen.

Variants of the Arthus reaction include the passive Arthus and the reversed passive Arthus (RPA) reactions. The first of these is simply the provocation of the Arthus reaction in an animal that has been passively immunized. In the RPA reaction the antiserum is injected into the skin (rather than systemically), and the antigen then is given systemically (rather than intradermally). Both injections are made at about the same time so that a sufficient amount of antibody will remain near the injection site to precipitate with the antigen and cause local necrosis.

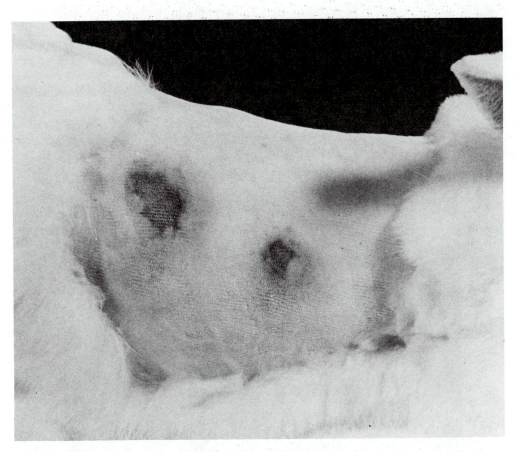

Fig. 19-1. Two Arthus reactions in rabbit skin. The larger reaction has an extensive zone of erythema and edema surrounding its necrotic center.

Table 19-1. Distinctions between PCA and RPA reactions

	PCA	RPA
Quantity of antibody required	Very little	Large amount
Cytotropic antibody required	Yes; homocytotropic or heterocytotropic	No
Latent period after transfer	Yes	No
Histamine release	Yes	No
Antihistamines effective	Yes	No
Complement required	No	Yes

Technically the RPA and PCA reactions are performed in the same way, that is, antibody is placed in the skin, and antigen is administered intravascularly, but the RPA and PCA reactions are distinct immunologic phenomena (Table 19-1).

PCA AND RPA REACTIONS

Sensitization to systemic passive anaphylaxis results from the transfer of serum containing homocytotropic or heterocytotropic (IgE or IgE-like) antibodies into the vascular system of a nor-

mal recipient. When a latent period of 4 to 18 hours is allowed for fixation of the antibody to mast cells and basophils, the animal is sensitized. At that time a shocking dose of antigen given intravascularly will evoke total body anaphylaxis. If the antiserum is injected intradermally, however, only the PCA reaction follows (Fig. 19-2). This is expressed as the triple response of edema, wheal, and erythema, which is difficult to observe on the skin of some animal species. The reaction area is stained a light blue if Evans blue dye is

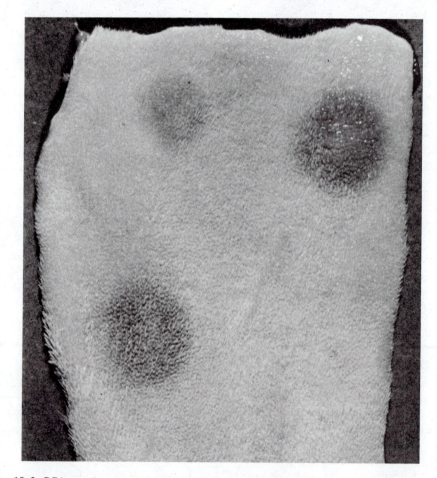

Fig. 19-2. PCA reactions in guinea pig skin. Antiserum dilutions were placed intradermally 18 hours before an intravenous injection of Evans blue dye and antigen. The skin was excised 45 minutes later. The saline control site is on lower right, where no reaction is shown. The positive sites are dark and correlate directly with the dilution of the antiserum injected.

included in the antigen solution. Since the anaphylactic reaction increases the permeability of the vascular bed around the reaction site, blood proteins and the dye leak into and stain the surrounding tissue. The area of this reaction site is useful in evaluating the quantity of IgE-like antibody in the serum.

The PCA reaction is one of the most sensitive serologic tests available. With protein antigens the injection of 0.1 ml of antiserum containing as little as 0.003 μg of antibody nitrogen per milliliter will produce a positive test. The Arthus reaction is positive only when a large quantity of antibody is given. Since the Arthus reaction is independent of cell-fixed antibody, no latent period is required. For the PCA reaction a period of 4 to 18 hours is necessary to allow antibody to fix to cells before a positive test can be elicited by the shocking dose of antigen. Since the Arthus reaction does not depend on mast cell degranulation and histamine release, antihistamines are ineffective in preventing the RPA reaction, but they will moderate the PCA reaction. Any species of antibody will function in the RPA test, but certain species of heterocytotropic antibodies—for example, antibody from ungulates—do not fix to guinea pig tissue, and these cannot be used in the PCA test.

IMMUNE COMPLEX PNEUMONITIS

The human ailments referred to by the terms *hypersensitivity pneumonitis, allergic pneumonitis,* and *immune complex pneumonitis* are natural expressions of the Arthus reaction. This condition has a plethora of synonyms, most of which are derived from some occupation or avocation associated with the disease. Thus we have farmer's lung, laundry worker's lung, pigeon breeder's disease, etc. as names for a kind of pneumonitis that is immunologically the same in all affected persons (Table 19-2).

A cardinal feature shared by all persons afflicted by immune complex pneumonitis is a regular exposure to an atmosphere heavily laden with antigen. This exposure need not be constant and in fact is more often intermittent. Such an atmosphere is created, for example, by farmers working with hay or silage, by mushroom workers preparing mushroom beds, by pigeon breeders and bird fanciers as they clean the bird roosts, or by the birds as they fly in and around their coops. Such air is heavily charged with antigens that vary to some extent according to the source of the dust but usually include spores of a fungus or an excretory product from an involved animal. Media such as moist hay, silage, wood bark, cotton, and fertilized soil favor mold growth, which terminates

Table 19-2. Various forms of immune complex pneumonitis and their cause

Disease	Source of antigen	Antigen
Farmer's lung	Moldy hay	*Micropolyspora faeni* spores
Mushroom worker's lung	Moldy compost	*Thermoactinomyces sacchariii* spores
Bird fancier's lung	Dry bird droppings	Bird proteins
Pigeon breeder's disease	Pigeon droppings and dander	Pigeon proteins
Bagassosis	Moldy sugar cane (bagasse)	*Thermoactinomyces vulgaris* spores
Maple bark pneumonitis	Moldy maple bark	*Cryptostroma corticale* spores
Malt worker's lung	Moldy barley	*Aspergillus clavatus* spores
Miller's lung	Contaminated flour	*Sitophilus granarius* (wheat weevil)
Cheese washer's disease	Cheese casings	*Penicillium caseii* spores
Humidifier lung	Home humidifiers	*Thermoactinomyces candidus* spores
Sequoiosis	Moldy redwood or other sawdust	Spores of *Graphium* and *Pullularia* species

in sporulation. Fungal spores, most of which are less than 10 μm in diameter, are inhaled deeply into the lung. Fungal spores may be present in bird manure, but it is more likely that antigens of these materials or in animal dander are the offending substances.

The respiratory route is a very satisfactory avenue of immunization. Patients with hypersensitivity pneumonitis develop high levels of IgG and may have elevated levels of IgE as well. If both antibodies are present, a reexposure to the antigen will produce a biphasic response. The earliest is the IgE-dependent response characterized by sneezing, edema of the respiratory tract, increased nasal discharge, and the symptoms of an atopic respiratory condition. These symptoms typically disappear within a few hours.

The distinguishing feature of allergic pneumonitis, however, is delayed for several hours after the exposure to antigen. This reaction embodies a dry cough, shortness of breath, fever, and general malaise, all appearing within 6 to 8 hours. Within a few days the person feels perfectly healthy again. Another exposure to the antigen source will trigger another episode of disease.

The immunohistology of lung tissue from patients with allergic pneumonitis is very revealing. A neutrophilic infiltration of the alveolar capillaries, a deposition of fibrin and platelets, and the accumulation of IgG precipitates are completely harmonious with those seen in the Arthus reactions. The present opinion is that all these conditions are examples of the Arthus reaction produced in the lung because of a respiratory exposure of sufficient magnitude and frequency to stimulate high levels of IgG, which precipitate with the antigen in capillaries of the lung. In every instance removing the source of the antigen terminates the disease.

THE SHWARTZMAN REACTION

The Shwartzman reaction is a dermal reaction characterized by intense hemorrhage and necrosis. To provoke this reaction, the skin first is sensitized by the intradermal injection of a culture filtrate of a gram-negative bacterium. Almost any such organism can be chosen, including the typhoid, cholera, or common colon bacillus. This initial injection produces only a local erythema, which can be directly correlated with the LPS or endotoxin content of the injected material. Twenty-four hours later, when an intravenous injection of the same filtrate or one from a dissimilar organism is given, the hemorrhagic necrosis at the initial skin site develops. The Shwartzman lesion can be detected within 2 hours and is usually maximal by the sixth hour.

For years the Shwartzman reaction (or its systemic equivalent, the Shwartzman-Sanarelli reaction) has been considered a nonimmunologic mimic of immediate skin hypersensitivity. Part of the evidence that this is a toxic rather than an immunologic reaction was based on the rather restricted time interlude after sensitization within which the shocking dose must be administered to produce the reaction. Thirty-six hours after sensitization the sensitivity has vanished. The ability to sensitize with one material and shock with a second, unrelated (or even nonantigenic) material such as starch or agar argues strongly against a dependence on immunologic mechanisms. Currently the most favored theory of the mechanism for the Shwartzman reaction is that the endotoxin contained in the first material injected causes local intravascular coagulation and gradual deposition of fibrin on the blood vessel walls. At first the cells of the RES are stimulated by the LPS and attempt to remove this debris by phagocytosis. Later the LPS depresses the RES, and this permits the accumulation of fibrin in the blood vessels. The second injection again stimulates fibrin deposition on the original fibrin matrix, creating a blockade of the small blood vessels and causing tissue necrosis. When agents other than endotoxin are used in the second injection, fibrin accumulation is also the result but by uncertain pathways, possibly by the activation of Hageman's factor and the blood-clotting sequence.

BIBLIOGRAPHY

Gell, P.G.H., Coombs, R.R.A., and Lachmann, P.J., editors: Clinical aspects of immunology, ed. 3, Oxford, 1974, Blackwell Scientific Publications, Ltd.

Gupta, S., and Good, R.A., editors: Cellular, molecular, and clinical aspects of allergic disorders, New York, 1979, Plenum Publishing Corp.

Kirkpatrick, C.H., and Reynolds, H.Y., editors: Immunologic and infectious reactions in the lung, New York, 1976, Marcel Dekker, Inc.

McCluskey, R.T., Hall, C.L., and Coloin, R.B.: Immune complex mediated diseases, Hum. Pathol. **9:**71, 1978.

Middleton, E., Jr., Reed, C.E., and Ellis, E.F., editors: Allergy principles and practice, St. Louis, 1978, The C.V. Mosby Co.

Miescher, P.A., and Müller-Eberhard, H.J., editors: Textbook of immunopathology, ed. 2, New York, 1976, Grune & Stratton, Inc.

Oppenheim, J.J., Rosenstreich, D.L., and Potter, M., editors: Cellular functions in immunity and inflammation, New York, 1981, Elsevier/North-Holland, Inc.

Parker, C.W., editor: Clinical immunology, vols. 1 and 2, Philadelphia, 1980, W.B. Saunders, Co.

Pepys, J.: Hypersensitivity diseases of the lungs due to fungi and organic dusts, Basel, 1969, S. Karger, AG, Medical & Scientific Publishers.

Ward, P.A.: The immunopathologic basis of hypersensitivity pneumonitis, Monogr. Pathol. **19:**88, 1978.

SITUATION: THE CHRISTMAS BREAK

It was good to be home. The semester had been rough, but three As and a B weren't bad. Dad would need the help during the holiday season, always the busiest of the year. And Mom said the old man hadn't been feeling all that well lately. A few good hard days at the bakery would be tiring, but to the body, not to the mind. I was looking forward to it this Christmas break.

It was only 2 PM, but for the early shift bakers it was quitting time. Dad and I headed for the shower. This time I was sure of it. He was having trouble breathing, not wheezing exactly, but trouble anyway. Seemed like he'd been OK after that little episode at the early coffee break. As we walked along, things began to fit into place. I didn't get that A in immunology for nothing, so I said to him, "Dad, you better check with Doc. I think you've got allergic pneumonitis."

Questions

1. What is allergic pneumonitis?
2. How does allergic pneumonitis differ from asthma and other allergic respiratory complaints?
3. What antigens are involved in allergic pneumonitis in bakers and those with other occupations?
4. Can allergic pneumonitis be treated? If so, how?

Solution

Allergic pneumonitis is only one of several synonyms for an IgG-mediated respiratory disease characterized by an Arthus-like necrosis in the alveoli. Allergic alveolitis, extrinsic allergic pneumonitis, and hypersensitivity pneumonitis are generic equivalents for specific names such as farmer's lung, pigeon breeder's disease, bird fancier's lung, and mushroom worker's disease. These conditions all were named to reflect a specific hobby or vocation associated with the disease. The common thread to all these conditions is a sporadic exposure to an atmosphere heavily contaminated with some form of dust. For the farmer it is dusty hay, straw, or silage; for the pigeon breeder and bird fancier it is the dusty atmosphere of the bird loft or coop, heavy with bird dander and pigeon droppings; and for the baker it is the flour-filled air of the bake shop. Proteins in the flour are absorbed from the inhaled particles and stimulate the production of IgG. Subsequent inhalation of the flour and absorption of the antigens into the capillary bed of the alveoli results in intravascular precipitation and the development of numerous, small Arthus lesions.

The respiratory distress associated with the necrotic Arthus lesions develops several hours after inhalation of the antigens. It is very common for an early episode of respiratory distress to precede this. The early reaction is dominated by a local IgE reaction with the antigen. This biphasic condition is characteristic of allergic pneumonitis and eases differentiation from asthma, which is more chronic and constant once symptoms are evident. Asthma is not related to IgG, as is the case here. Baker's asthma has been described as an IgE-dependent condition characterized by immediate skin tests to flour, histamine release of leukocytes incubated with flour, and positive P-K tests. Bakers are often allergic to insects found in grain or flour and may express a contact dermatitis of the delayed type to proteins from wheat, rye, or other grains.

Allergic pneumonitis cannot be treated with chemotherapeutics such as the antihistamines or adrenergic drugs. Mast cell products have little to do with the severest portions, the second necrotizing phase of the illness, so treatment with these drugs is doomed to failure. These drugs will moderate the earlier, less serious phase of the disease. The only successful treatment is avoidance of antigen exposure.

References

Pepys, J.: Hypersensitivity diseases of the lungs due to fungi and organic dusts, Basel, 1969, S. Karger, AG, Medical and Scientific Publishers.

Popa, A., George, S.A., and Gavanescu, O.: Occupational and non-occupational respiratory allergy in bakers, Acta Allerg. **25:**159, 1970.

Wilbur, R.D., and Ward, G.W., Jr.: Immunologic studies in a case of baker's asthma, J. Allergy Clin. Immunol. **58:**366, 1976.

T CELL–MEDIATED ALLERGY

GLOSSARY

allergy of infection An allergy, often of the delayed type, resulting from an infection.

CBH Cutaneous basophilic hypersensitivity.

cell-mediated hypersensitivity A T cell hypersensitivity of the delayed type.

contact dermatitis A delayed or cell-mediated hypersensitivity response to cutaneously applied allergens.

cutaneous basophilic hypersensitivity A T cell hypersensitivity characterized by a basophilic infiltration.

delayed hypersensitivity Synonym of *cell-mediated hypersensitivity;* a form of allergy expressed by T lymphocytes, not involving immunoglobulins, and developing slowly when provoked dermally.

DH Delayed hypersensitivity.

Jones-Mote reaction An older synonym of cutaneous basophilic hypersensitivity.

Koch's phenomenon Rejection of subcutaneously placed tubercle bacilli by tuberculous animals as an expression of CMI.

OT Old tuberculin.

PPD Purified protein derivative of tuberculin.

Tdh cell The T cell responsible for delayed hypersensitivities.

TF Transfer factor.

transfer factor A ribonucleotide (700 to 4,000 mol wt) that can transfer (in some species) the cell-mediated hypersensitivities of the lymphocytes from which it is extracted.

tuberculin A concentrate of the growth medium of *Mycobacterium tuberculosis* used to test skin for delayed hypersensitivity to this organism.

urushiols Catechols found on poisonous plants responsible for contact dermatitis.

In the introductory pages of Chapter 17 the characteristics of the cell-mediated, or T cell–dependent, hypersensitivities are described and compared with the characteristics of the immediate, immunoglobulin-related hypersensitivities. The hallmarks of the delayed hypersensitivities, as listed in Table 17-2, include their slow development following the shocking exposure to the antigen, lack of tissue specificity, requirement for T lymphocytes and their products, collectively described as lymphokines, lack of any known dependence on humoral antibodies, tendency toward mononuclear cell infiltrates in affected tissues that can be combated by steroids, and the difficulty in achieving relief from these allergies by specific antigen desensitization. These same features characterize and identify hypersensitivities (Table 17-3) expressed by antigen-sensitized T lymphocytes. Of course lymphocytes are involved in the immediate and other immunoglobulin-mediated allergies, but these lymphocytes are of the B type. Lymphocytes involved in the cell-mediated hypersensitivities consist of the Lyt-1 or Tdh subset of T cells of the mouse. The T cell subset essential to delayed hypersensitivity in humans has not been identified yet.

A brief reminder about terminology is appropriate. The term *T cell–mediated allergy* or *hypersensitivity* has been equated with two closely related terms: *cell-mediated immunity* (CMI) and *cell-mediated hypersensitivity*. Although these three phrases customarily are interchangeable, their meanings are not exactly the same. CMI in sensu stricto should refer to protection acquired from cellular activities. This can and does include the bactericidal and other protective actions of blood and tissue phagocytes as well as certain activities of T lymphocytes. Activities of the phagocytes are not antigen specific, but those of the lymphocytes are; their activities are best expressed on reexposure to antigen. Cell-mediated hypersensitivity refers to antigen-specific properties expressed by T lymphocytes that contribute to the delayed inflammatory allergic reaction, as seen in contact dermatitis to certain chemicals and allergies of infection. These may have no relationship at all to body protection and are in fact allergies or hypersensitivities.

There is good evidence that these older terms prefixed by cell mediated should be dropped. In these hypersensitivities the lymphocytes are operating mainly through extracellular products: the lymphokines. These lymphokines differ immensely from immunoglobulins, but their existence indicates that cell-mediated hypersensitivities are really no more cell mediated than the IgE- or other immunoglobulin-mediated hypersensitivities. They merely are dependent on a different class of lymphocyte.

ALLERGY OF INFECTION

The discovery of the delayed hypersensitivities is credited to Koch; he described the Koch phenomenon and the unique skin reactions to tuberculin exhibited by persons who have or who previously had tuberculosis. The tuberculin reaction is considered the prototype of the delayed hypersensitive skin reaction.

Two separate materials may be used in the tuberculin skin test: OT or PPD prepared from OT. OT is prepared by first growing *Mycobacterium tuberculosis* in a special broth for several weeks (Fig. 20-1). Thereafter the broth is concentrated on a steam bath to one tenth its previous volume. The mycobacteria are removed by filtration, and the product is OT. Other tuberculin preparations,

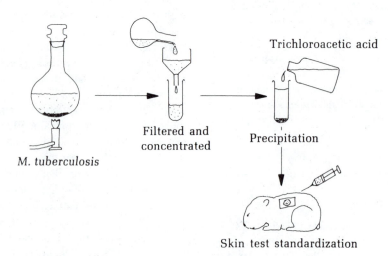

Trichloroacetic acid

Filtered and concentrated

Precipitation

M. tuberculosis

Skin test standardization

Fig. 20-1. Important stages in the preparation of PPD.

similar in nature and including extracts of the organism, have not been proved superior to the original tuberculin.

The active principal in OT can be precipitated from it by trichloroacetic acid or ammonium sulfate. One of the small proteins of about 2,000 mol wt in this precipitate contains virtually all the tuberculin activity. This fraction, PPD, is remarkably stable when dried and has a constant activity; therefore it is gradually replacing OT as the skin-testing reagent of choice.

Several different techniques are used in cutaneous tuberculin testing. In the von Pirquet test, one of the first forms of the test to be critically evaluated, tuberculin is rubbed into scarified skin. Variations of this test include the tine test, or multiple puncture method. In this procedure a drop of OT or PPD is placed on a bed of needles, which is used to puncture the skin. Two other procedures are in greater use. In the Mantoux test the allergen is injected intradermally. The Vollmer patch test is used widely for tuberculin testing of children, since no injection is necessary. The patch is simply a square of paper impregnated with OT and held

to the skin with a piece of tape. The commercially available tape strip incorporates a normal broth control. A positive test develops slowly and reaches its maximum at about 48 to 72 hours after application or injection of the reagent. The skin is erythematous and indurated (hardened), and in the Mantoux test the reaction site must be at least 10 mm in diameter to be considered positive (Fig. 20-2). In highly sensitized individuals a small vesicle develops in the center of the inflamed zone. Central necrosis may develop but usually does not do so.

The skin of many animals is not adaptable to intradermal skin testing for hypersensitivities. The mouse is a prime example, having a very thin skin that is almost laminated in structure. Intradermal injections are unsatisfactory because the skin appears to split, and the fluid injected does not remain localized. Solutions injected into the footpad or into the ear remain localized and in this vascular tissue can be approached by lymphoid cells and immunoglobulins. Footpad and ear swelling, if determined after any immediate hypersensitive response has subsided, can be measured

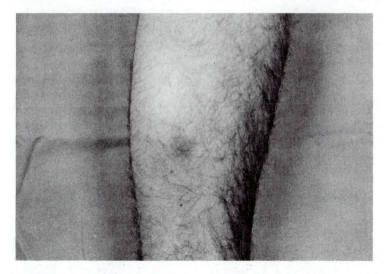

Fig. 20-2. A delayed skin reaction exhibiting an erythematous but nonedematous zone 15 mm in diameter at 48 hours. A control site, inoculated higher on the forearm, shows no reaction at this time.

exactly with calipers for a precise quantitation of the reaction. This method serves as a useful substitute for typical delayed skin reaction in other small animals, including hamsters, rats, guinea pigs, and gerbils.

Systemic reactions to tuberculin follow intravenous injections in experimental animals, and constitutional reactions have been noted in humans. A sharp rise in body temperature, malaise, and pain in the extremities are the major symptoms; these usually subside within 24 hours. Fatal tuberculin shock can be produced in laboratory animals.

The tuberculin reaction has been described as an allergy of infection. Not all allergies to infectious organisms are of the delayed type, but the tendency toward delayed reactions has been so prominent that the term *allergy of infection* is used synonymously with *delayed hypersensitivity*. Other examples are the delayed skin reactions associated with leprosy, histoplasmosis, coccidioi-domycosis, blastomycosis, brucellosis, mumps, lymphogranuloma venereum, and smallpox virus (Table 20-1).

It must be remembered that positive skin reactions with PPD, lepromin, histoplasmin, etc., are not diagnostic tests for a current illness. Allergies of infection generally are persistent throughout life and remain positive long after the infection itself has disappeared. This is because of the longevity of the Tdh cells responsible for the delayed hypersensitive reactions.

Another interesting aspect of these skin tests is that some of the eliciting products—histoplasmin, for example—are themselves antigenic. The consequence of this is that repeated skin testing of a nonreactor may convert him or her to a positive state and also induce the formation of antibodies. These events could confuse the diagnosis of disease on the basis of both a false positive skin test and a false positive serologic test. Since the active ingredient in OT and PPD has a molecular weight

Table 20-1. Delayed hypersensitive skin tests for allergies of infection

Disease	Skin test	Reagent
Bacterial diseases		
Tuberculosis	Mantoux, Vollmer, etc., according to method	OT or PPD
Leprosy	Lepromin (Mitsuda)	Extract of lepromatous tissue (lepromin)
Diphtheria	Moloney	Diphtheria toxoid
Brucellosis	Brucellergin	Heat-killed organism
Tularemia	Foshay	Bacterial protein antigen
Streptococcal infection	—	Streptokinase-streptodornase
Viral diseases		
Lymphogranuloma venereum	Frei	Inactive virus
Smallpox	—	Vaccinia virus
Mumps	—	Mumps virus vaccine
Fungal diseases		
Histoplasmosis	Histoplasmin	Concentrate of culture filtrate (histoplasmin)
Coccidioidomycosis	Coccidioidin	Concentrate of culture filtrate (coccidioidin)
Blastomycosis	Blastomycin	Concentrate of culture filtrate (blastomycin)
Candidiasis	Candidin	Concentrate of yeast culture

of only 2,000, these events are unlikely with the use of these reagents.

CONTACT DERMATITIS

Dermal sensitivity of the delayed type may follow contact with chemicals from many sources, including cosmetics, insecticides, topically applied disinfectants and ointments, metals, hair and clothing dyes, photographic chemicals, rubber goods, leather goods, and many others (Table 20-2). In many of these instances specific chemicals in the product are known to be the incitant: for example, formaldehyde, mercury, and other heavy metals in insecticides; nickel and copper in coins, metal buckles, watchbands, and jewelry; potassium dichromate in leather goods and yellow dyes; paraphenylenediamine in black, brown, and blue dyes for human and animal hair or cloth; and phenyl-β-naphthylamine in rubber goods. Allergies to "poisonous" plants such as poison ivy, poison oak, and poison sumac or primrose are caused by specific compounds, often substituted urushiols on the surface of their leaves.

Poison ivy and poison oak represent interesting examples of contact dermatitis common in the rural United States. *Rhus radicans* (poison ivy), *Rhus toxicodendron* (poison sumac), and *Rhus diversiloba* (poison oak) cause contact dermatitis because of the common catechols present in the plant sap and on the surface of bruised leaves. Urushiol is the name given to the mixture of four catechols found in the poison ivy plant. These catechols differ from each other only in the degree of saturation of their pentadecyl side chain. The fully saturated compound is 3n-pentadecylcatechol; the compound that is singly unsaturated has a double bond at position 8 to 9; the doubly unsaturated compound has a double bond at positions 8 to 9 and 11 to 12; and the trienyl compound has a double bond at positions 8 to 9, 11 to 12, and 14 to 15 (Fig. 20-3). These compounds exist in urushiol in the ratio of 3, 15, 60, and 22, respectively; thus it is not surprising that patients show more strongly positive reactions to the latter two than to the former two compounds.

Catechols are haptenic and can couple to tissue proteins by virtue of their ready oxidation to quinones, the sensitizing form of these compounds. Blocking quinone formation by substituting the hydroxyl groups renders the catechols inert. When it is applied to skin, only 44% of pentadecylcatechol remains at the site of application; the remainder is recoverable from feces, urine, lymph nodes, and internal organs. The exact form of the catechol-protein conjugate and the identity of specifically involved proteins are not known. (Dinitrochlorobenzene, a potent skin sensitizer, binds to 15 different proteins in skin.) Many of these

Table 20-2. Sources of contact dermatitis and the allergens involved

Object	Sources	Compounds involved
Metal	Jewelry, belt buckles, watches, watchbands, scissors, thimbles, cosmetics	Nickel, chromium, iron, cobalt, copper, mercury
Clothing		Animal and plant fibers, anthraquinone and other dyes, vinyl, acrylate, glycol, and other permanent press agents, formaldehyde
Rubber	Swim wear, garters, shoes, condoms	Hydroquinone and other antioxidants, benzothiazole and other accelerators
Cosmetics	Rouge, lipstick, eye shadow, hair dye, depilatories, perfumes, lotions, sprays	Iron and cobalt dyes, sulfide depilatories, phenylenediamine and other dyes, balsam
Leather	Belts, shoes, leather watchbands	Potassium dichromate, dyes
Plants	Poison ivy, oak, sumac, etc.	Catechols

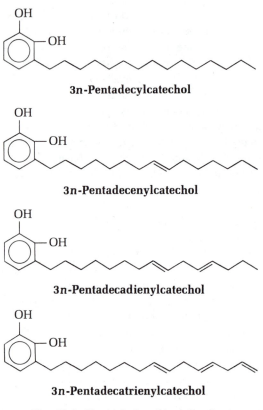

3n-Pentadecylcatechol

3n-Pentadecenylcatechol

3n-Pentadecadienylcatechol

3n-Pentadecatrienylcatechol

Fig. 20-3. Urushiols found in poison ivy.

low molecular weight chemicals such as the substituted nitrophenols and oxazolones are classifiable as autocoupling haptens. When these compounds contact the skin, they combine with skin or tissue antigens to form neoantigens against which the hypersensitivity develops. Cutaneous reapplication of the compound will produce the allergic reaction at that site. The application of complete antigens to healthy skin rarely produces a contact dermatitis, yet intracutaneous injection of these antigens or hapten-antigen conjugates is effective in inducing a delayed hypersensitivity.

INDUCTION OF T CELL HYPERSENSITIVITY
Antigens and haptens

Delayed hypersensitivity, as it occurs naturally in allergies of infection and contact dermatitis,

has been proved to result from sensitization to protein antigens and autocoupling haptens. Polysaccharide antigens have never been incriminated in delayed hypersensitivities apparently because T cells do not respond to them. Synthetic polyamino acids that are antigenic also will induce delayed hypersensitivity. There are many examples of low molecular weight allergens, including the aforementioned halogenated nitrobenzenes, catechols, oxazolones, sulfonyl and sulfenyl chlorides, and anhydrides, most of which are known to possess autocoupling potentiality.

The exact size of the antigenic determinant required to induce and detect delayed hypersensitivity may vary from one situation to another. Sensitivity to picrylated antigens (proteins conjugated with picryl chloride) extends beyond the hapten and includes portions of the carrier protein. Skin tests with the carrier antigen often produce stronger delayed tests than when the complete antigen is used, which is reflective of the sensitivity of T cells to the carrier and B cells to the hapten in hapten-antigen complexes. It probably is safe to assume that the size requirements of T cells are not too different from those of B cells for immunoglobulin synthesis.

Adjuvant

Sensitization for delayed hypersensitivities is encouraged by (1) incorporating the material in Freund's adjuvant, (2) using microgram quantities of the allergen and testing early, or (3) sensitizing by percutaneous application of the allergen. How Freund's adjuvant stimulates delayed hypersensitivity is not known; it does not result entirely from the waxes associated with the dead mycobacteria, since incomplete Freund's adjuvant is active. Freund's adjuvant also promotes good immunoglobulin formation. Quantities of antigen in the range of 1 to 3 μg in Freund's complete or incomplete adjuvant will sensitize for delayed skin reactivity. Antigen-antibody complexes have been used for sensitization, but it is doubtful that the presence of antibody serves any great advantage. Skin tests should be applied between the fifth and tenth day so that the delayed reaction is not overcome by Arthus-type sensitivity. The application of allergenic drugs to the skin tends to encourage the delayed hypersensitive response. One suggested mechanism for the high-sensitizing activity of dermal applications is that the oils of the skin function as adjuvants; this does not appear to be an especially strong argument.

Antigens on cell surfaces function as the best incitants, an observation attributed to the ''dual signal'' activation of T cells.

Macrophage requirement

The dual signal activation of T cells involves both antigen determinants and MHC markers on macrophages. (See Chapter 3.) The need for macrophages in delayed hypersensitivity has been demonstrated by experiments that simultaneously diminish the macrophage population and render an animal resistant to sensitization. Langerhans' cells, the most populous macrophages found in skin (over 900 per mm^3 in guinea pig epidermis), are depleted by exposure to ultraviolet light. Haptens painted on the skin normally home in the neighboring Langerhans cells, and their absence virtually precludes sensitization. Hapten that escapes the Langerhans cells may be carried to macrophages in the neighboring lymphatic system and still induce a low-grade sensitivity.

T cell requirement

The proof that viable T cells were responsible for the delayed hypersensitivities stemmed from the success of transfer experiments from a sensitive donor to a naive recipient with lymphoid cells but not with serum. The first successful transfer experiment, described by Landsteiner and Chase in 1942, used live peritoneal exudate cells from a guinea pig sensitized with picryl chloride. Twenty-four hours after the transfer the recipient developed a typical delayed skin reaction to the dermally applied drug. Heat-killed cells were ineffective. Three years later the transfer of tuberculin hypersensitivity in guinea pigs was accomplished by a similar method. Living lymph node cells, peripheral white blood cells, peritoneal exudate cells, and other sources rich in small lymphocytes (the T lymphocytes) all are capable of transferring sensitivity from an actively sensitized donor to a normal recipient. More recent experiments have defined the Lyt-1 T cell subset as the responsible T cell (the Tdh cell) in the mouse. Lyt-1 cells of the mouse also are described as Th cells, but the Th and Tdh cells probably represent different compartments of the Lyt-1 cells. That Tdh cells are under MHC control is demonstrated by the success of cell transfer experiments with syngeneic animals and their failure in most allogeneic transfers. Successful transfers now have been related to the Ir region of the MHC.

Transfer factor

Delayed hypersensitivities of humans, higher primates, cattle, dogs, rats, and mice, but not guinea pigs, can be transferred by lysates of sensitized white blood cells prepared by repeated cycles of cell freezing and thawing. Sensitivity to streptococcal M substance, diphtheria toxoid, tuberculin, coccidioidin, and histoplasmin has been successfully transferred in humans and to tuberculin and *Schistosoma mansoni* in *Macaca mulatta* (rhesus monkeys). The newly acquired sensitivity persists for a few weeks to several months (Fig. 20-4). It also has been found that antigen-sensitive lymphocytes incubated with specific antigen elaborate into the fluid phase, a substance that will transfer the delayed sensitivity. Under these circumstances the cells become deficient in transfer activity. An examination of transfer-competent extracts, prepared as just described or by distilled water lysis or ultrasonication of lymphocytes, was inaugurated by Lawrence and his associates in an attempt to characterize transfer factor. Human transfer factor is a molecule of less than 10,000 mol wt and is not antigenic to rabbits or humans. Based on the assumption that transfer factor might be a protein, lymphocyte extracts were treated with trypsin, but transfer factor activity was not destroyed. Since the passively acquired delayed hypersensitivities are so persistent, it was thought that transfer factor might be a DNA and function much like the transforming DNA of bacteria, which can transmit genetic in-

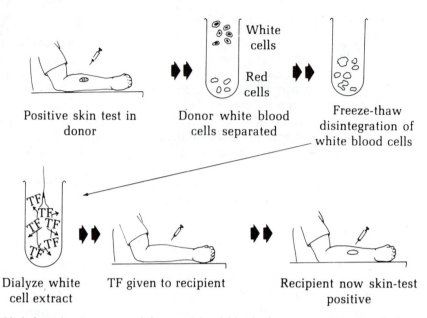

Fig. 20-4. Lymphocytes separated from peripheral blood of a person with a T cell–dependent (delayed) skin reaction to a specific antigen can be used as the source of transfer factor *(TF)*. This molecule will diffuse through the pores of a dialysis bag and can be used to convert a normal individual to the same reactive status as that of the transfer factor donor.

formation from one cell to another. However, neither DNAase nor RNAase treatments inactivate transfer factor.

Subsequent examination of human transfer factor partially purified by Sephadex G-200 and G-25 filtration has identified several transfer-competent fractions. The higher molecular weight fraction contains γ-globulins and α_1-lipoprotein, neither of which is believed to be the active agent. The lower molecular weight fraction, estimated to contain molecules between 700 and 4,000 mol wt, has an absorption spectrum compatible with a high nucleic acid content. The chemical structure of transfer factor has escaped exact identification. Transfer factor is sensitive to heat at 56° C or higher. This may be related to a heat-labile protein moiety or to a dsRNA. The latter, as opposed to ssRNA, is heat sensitive and RNAase resistant. It is sensitive to pronase, indicating some protein component. Both hypoxanthine and uracil in a 2:1 ratio are present in transfer factor. Further chem-

ical studies obviously are needed to clarify the nature of this ribonucleoprotein factor, although putative structures have been forwarded.

The ability of transfer factor to convert a nonsensitive recipient to the status of delayed hypersensitivity of the transfer factor donor is antigen specific, and on this basis transfer factor is not justifiably listed as a lymphokine, which are all antigen nonspecific. The antigen specificity of transfer factor has not gone unnoticed by the medical profession. Resistance to many fungal and viral diseases is associated with the development of CMI. Resistance to tumors is provided by the same mechanism. Of 11 patients with chronic mucocutaneous candidiasis included in one study, seven have been clinically improved by injections of transfer factor from donors with a cutaneous sensitivity to monilial antigens. The skin clears, heals, and reassumes its normal appearance. Restored good health of these patients has persisted for at least a year. Three of three instances of generalized vaccinia virus infections have been halted by specific transfer factor from sensitive donors. The claim also has been made that 30 of 33 patients with carcinoma, 8 of 10 with leukemia, and 11 of 13 with sarcoid disease have had their cell-mediated hypersensitivity reconstituted by transfer factor injections. All these persons have not been cured of their illness, but on strictly immunologic grounds one should expect them to have an improved survival benefit from the transfer factor injections.

IMMUNOSUPPRESSION OF T CELL–MEDIATED ALLERGIES

Most of the treatments that have been used to suppress immunoglobulin synthesis also have been tested for their ability to impede the development of delayed hypersensitivity. This includes all three of the major categories of immune suppression: physical, chemical, and biologic.

Physical methods

Irradiation. The development of delayed hypersensitivity in guinea pigs is considerably more resistant to the effects of x rays than is immunoglobulin formation. Heavy irradiation, even doses that will prove lethal, given just before or just after sensitization has little or no effect on the development or the expression of delayed hypersensitivity in this animal. Rabbits, however, are more sensitive to x rays. Doses of 400 to 800 R suppress the development of tuberculin sensitivity in rabbits; this condition persists for at least 1 month.

Thymectomy. It will be recalled from the discussion in Chapter 5 that surgical removal of the bursa of Fabricius from birds severely handicaps their antibody response to antigenic stimuli. The division of the immune mechanism into two central lymphoid tissues in birds has revealed the dominant role of the thymus in the regulation of delayed hypersensitivity. Interestingly the initial experiments in chickens did not reveal the thymic role in the development of delayed hypersensitivity. This is because at the time of hatching the delayed hypersensitive mechanisms in chicks already are dispersed to peripheral tissues and have partially matured. Combined surgical thymectomy and irradiation, the latter for the purpose of inactivating peripheral lymphoid tissue, have placed the role of thymectomy in the regulation of delayed hypersensitivity in sharper perspective.

Thymectomy of mammals also affects cell-mediated hypersensitivities. Neonatal thymectomy of mice will allow them to retain allogenic grafts longer than is customary. Rats thymectomized at birth fail to develop delayed hypersensitivity to tuberculin or bovine serum albumin. Surgical removal of the thymus from newborn guinea pigs or rabbits has little effect on their ability to develop delayed hypersensitivity, since this arm of their immune responsiveness is nearly mature at birth.

Chemical methods

Unfortunately many of the studies with immunosuppressant chemicals have ignored the widely known antiinflammatory action of these drugs. When drug therapy is continued up to the time of skin testing, the results do not differentiate the effect of the drug on the development of the hypersensitivity and the expression of the hypersensitivity. To determine only the former, the administration of the drug must be terminated several days before skin testing.

Steroids. The powerful antiinflammatory effect of corticosteroids at times has confused an interpretation of their effect on the development of delayed hypersensitivity. All these compounds are excellent suppressors of the expression of delayed allergies and are used to ameliorate drug hypersensitivities and to ensure longer survival of homografts. Steroidal derivatives significantly reduce the number of immunoblasts associated with homograft rejection and prevent the development as well as the expression of delayed hypersensitivity.

Alkylating agents. Nucleophilic chemicals, represented here by the nitrogen and sulfur mustards, reduce the expression of delayed allergies.

Cyclophosphamide prolongs graft survival; in studies with tuberculin and picryl chloride sensitivity this drug has been demonstrated to have a central and an antiinflammatory role.

Purine and pyrimidine analogs. Treatment of guinea pigs with 6-mercaptopurine in an effort to prevent delayed hypersensitivities has presented conflicting results. Tuberculin sensitivity was inhibited, but in two separate studies dinitrochlorobenzene and picryl chloride sensitivities developed normally. Since protein synthesis is an integral part of the development and expression of delayed hypersensitivity, one should expect these compounds to have a depressant effect.

Folic acid analogs. Methotrexate, which has no antiinflammatory activity, inhibits the development of delayed hypersensitivity to picryl chloride, oxazolone, diphtheria toxoid, and ovalbumin. Skin graft survival also is prolonged by this drug.

Biologic methods

Essentially the same biologic procedures used to block the formation of circulating antibodies have been used in efforts to halt the development of delayed hypersensitivity. The methods include specific immunologic tolerance, competition of antigens, ATS, and the identification of genetic or acquired incapacity to develop delayed hypersensitivities. Feedback control experiments in delayed hypersensitivity are difficult to construct because of the persistent nature of the sensitivity.

ATS. ATS or its γ-globulin fraction (ATG) is quite effective in prolonging allograft survival in the human, mouse, monkey, rat, and pig. An effect of ATG on T cell–dependent humoral responses advanced its use in depressing delayed hypersensitivities, because T cells are responsible for these allergies.

One must realize from the outset that all ATS or ATG preparations are far from equivalent. There are decisions to be made as to what tissue will be the lymphocyte antigen source, what animal will be immunized and by what type of dosage and schedule, how the antilymphocyte titer and immunosuppressive activity of the product will be determined, and how its clinical appraisal will be determined. The following lymphocyte sources have been used as the antigen: blood lymphocytes, thymocytes, cells from patients with chronic lymphocytic leukemia, thoracic duct lymphocytes, spleen, and fractions of many of these cells. These preparations differ tremendously in their proportions of T and B lymphocytes; so it is no wonder that the ATS had remarkably divergent activities from one study to another. Thymocytes and thoracic duct lymphocytes contain the greatest preponderance of T cells. Since much ATG is being used in human treatment of graft recipients, there is an advantage in selecting the horse over the rabbit as the animal source. Variations in immunization schedule and testing procedures, however, have made it impossible to claim one animal as being superior to another.

ATG has been prepared from ATS by the usual antiserum purification procedures of DEAE cellulose chromatography and cold ethanol or ammonium sulfate precipitation. Purification concentrates the antibody activity and eliminates extraneous serum proteins that may be involved in toxic reactions. Adsorption with erythrocytes and lymphocyte-poor tissues will remove undesired antibodies to other host cells. Testing of the effectiveness of the remaining ATG is fraught with many problems. ATG is species specific, which means that antihuman ATG must be standardized in humans or closely related primates. This is virtually impossible to do in terms of graft survival, so in vitro tests have been substituted. But which in vitro test is best? Sensitization of lymphocytes to phagocytosis by ATG has proved a rather poor parallel with in vivo activity, and in general, phagocytic tests are difficult to standardize. Lymphocyte agglutination and lymphocyte cytotoxicity tests agree rather poorly with actual immunosuppressive results of ATG. Inhibition of lymphocyte activities in culture—MIF production, inhibition of target cell destruction, and other in vitro correlates of cell-mediated hypersensitivities—has not proved satisfactory. Probably the most acceptable is the inhibition of rosette formation by normal lymphocytes, incubated in vitro with sheep red blood cells. Note that this is not the same as the rosette test used to detect immunoglobulin-synthesizing cells, but rather it involves normal lymphocytes. The basis for this type of rosette formation is uncertain, but its inhibition is probably the best correlate of ATG activity. In any event the research worker or clinician does the best he or she can to find some measure for the genuine antilymphocytic activity of the ATG and uses what is available.

The use of ATG is not without hazard. Since ATG is necessarily prepared in heterologous species, its administration may induce serum sickness or even anaphylactic shock. Admittedly this danger is less with purified ATG than with ATS, but it is still a problem. Many, if not most, human recipients of ATG demonstrate a hypersensitive response to the foreign proteins in about 2 weeks, even with the simultaneous use of chemical immunosuppressives. Persons receiving ATG should be monitored closely for the development of viral diseases and tumors, since body defenses against these are mediated by T lymphocytes, which are being suppressed by ATG.

Desensitization and tolerance. Specific desensitization of delayed hypersensitivities can be accomplished by the intravenous injection of the allergen in sublethal quantities. Experiments in which large doses of the allergen are inoculated within a few minutes or hours after a smaller sensitizing dose of the allergen are interpreted more fairly as experiments in immunologic unresponsiveness than in desensitization. Even discounting these reports, it is possible to desensitize guinea pigs without much trouble. Desensitization of the human appears to be more difficult. The mechanism of desensitization is not entirely known but possibly is based on the same mechanisms that produce tolerance rather than sensitization.

The phenomenon of tolerance was discovered during Sulzberger's studies of delayed hypersensitivity to neoarsphenamine in which he found that no sensitization occurred if the usual sensitizing dose was followed by a large dose (6 mg) of the drug. Later it was observed that feeding picryl chloride or dinitrochlorobenzene to guinea pigs prior to dermal contact with these haptens prevented the development of contact sensitivity. Whereas skin painting with haptens customarily elicits contact sensitivity, intravenous or intralymphatic injections, like feedings, render the animal resistant to sensitization. Adult guinea pigs can be made tolerant with as little as 10 μg of bovine γ-globulin injected into the mesenteric vein in divided doses 1 week apart. Fetal and neonatal animals can be rendered tolerant prior to the time their T cell system matures. The most recent technique for inducing tolerance to contact sensitivity is to inject the hapten coupled to lymphoid cells. This is considered superior to other "tolerizing" procedures.

Tolerance can be transferred from the tolerant to an untreated animal with T cells. Although this transfer is successful only during a 2- to 3-week period beginning about 5 days after exposure to the tolerogen, the duration of the tolerant state in the recipient is nearly 2 months. The time difference of transferability and duration of tolerance has suggested that Ts cells in the transferred cell population may not be responsible for maintaining tolerance.

On the other hand, there is good evidence that Ts cells are present in actively tolerized animals and can transfer tolerance between syngeneic animals. Transfer of tolerance is MHC restricted, again in concordance with the dual signal hypothesis for the activation of T cells. In vitro cultivation of lymph node cells from tolerant mice causes the appearance of a soluble suppressor factor (SSF) in the culture medium. SSF is a cell-free, tolerogen-specific molecule with a molecular weight between 35,000 and 60,000. Immunoglobulin markers and hapten have not been found in SSF. SSF may prove to be identical to SIRS from Ts cells, which impedes the immunoglobulin response.

Both SSF and SIRS contain determinants coded for by genes of the MHC, probably the I-J region.

Although Ts cells are induced by tolerogenic exposure to haptens, tolerogens also may suppress Tdh precursor cells. If the proliferative and differentiating steps that lead to functional Tdh cells are prevented, then immune tolerance would develop.

CUTANEOUS BASOPHILIC HYPERSENSITIVITY

A form of skin reaction described as the Jones-Mote reaction and previously described as an evanescent delayed hypersensitive response now is generally known as cutaneous basophilic hypersensitivity (CBH). In experimental laboratory animals intradermal reexposure to antigen 5 to 7 days after the initial exposure initiates the CBH reaction. Within the first 24 hours a nonedematous area of erythema develops, which persists for only another 24 to 48 hours. Eosinophils are identified as the first cells to infiltrate the reaction site, and these are supplanted by basophils by the forty-eighth hour.

Earlier evidence that suggested the CBH reaction was under T cell control included (1) the ability to develop the reaction in hypogammaglobulinemics, (2) the ability to evoke the reaction before circulating antibodies appear, (3) the sparse amount of edema associated with the reaction and its resemblance to the tuberculin reaction, and most critically (4) the failure to transfer the reaction with serum but the ability to do so with viable T cells.

CBH is a transitory reaction that precedes by several days the expression of the classic delayed dermal reaction and is no longer demonstrable when the classic delayed reaction can be elicited.

BIBLIOGRAPHY

Caplin, M.: The tuberculin test in clinical practice, London, 1980, Ballière Tindall.

Claman, H.N., and others: Control of experimental contact sensitivity, Adv. Immunol. **30:**121, 1980.

Cronin, E.: Contact dermatitis, Edinburgh, 1980, Churchill Livingstone.

Crowle, A.J.: Delayed hypersensitivity in the mouse, Adv. Immunol. **20:**197, 1975.

Dahl, M.V.: Clinical immunodermatology, Chicago, 1981, Year Book Medical Publishers, Inc.

Dvorak, H.F., Galli, S.J., and Dvorak, A.M.: Expression of cell-mediated hypersensitivity in vivo—recent advances, Intern. Rev. Exp. Pathol. **21:**119, 1980.

Fregert, S.: Manual of contact dermatitis, ed. 2, Copenhagen, 1981, Munksgaard, International Bookseller & Publishers, Ltd.

Gell, P.G.H., Coombs, R.R.A., and Lachmann, P.J., editors: Clinical aspects of immunology, ed. 3, Oxford, 1974, Blackwell Scientific Publications, Ltd.

Gupta, S., and Good, R.A., editors: Cellular, molecular, and clinical aspects of allergic disorders, New York, 1979, Plenum Publishing Corp.

Khan, A., Kirkpatrick, C.H., and Hill, N.O., editors: Immune regulators in transfer factor, New York, 1979, Academic Press, Inc.

Lockey, R.F., editor: Allergy and clinical immunology, Garden City, N.Y., 1979, Medical Examination Publishing Co., Inc.

Middleton, E., Jr., Reed, C.E., and Ellis, E.F., editors: Allergy principles and practice, St. Louis, 1978, The C.V. Mosby Co.

Miescher, P.A., and Müller-Eberhard, H.J., editors: Textbook of immunopathology, ed. 2, New York, 1976, Grune & Stratton, Inc.

Parker, C.W.: Drug allergy, N. Engl. J. Med. **292:**511, 732, 957, 1975.

Parker, C.W., editor: Clinical immunology, vols. 1 and 2, Philadelphia, 1980, W.B. Saunders Co.

Patterson, R., editor: Allergic diseases; diagnosis and management, ed. 2, Philadelphia, 1980, J.B. Lippincott Co.

Polak, L.: Immunological aspects of contact sensitivity, Basel, 1980, S. Karger, AG, Medical and Scientific Publishers.

Polak, L., Turk, J.L., and Frey, J.R.: Studies on contact hypersensitivity to chromium compounds, Prog. Allergy **17:**146, 1973.

Turk, J.L.: Delayed hypersensitivity, ed. 3, Amsterdam, 1980, Elsevier/North Holland Biomedical Press.

SITUATION: ANTIPERSPIRANT ALLERGY

Kevin, a 45-year-old business executive, contacted his physician about an itch under both axillae on his return from an extended vacation in Europe. On examination an eczematous rash was apparent. The history was revealing. The rash began approximately 10 days after arrival in southern Spain and was more bothersome in that warm climate than at home, although it had continued on his return. Kevin feared that he had some kind of "crabs." A pubic rash was not seen. On further questioning it was revealed that he had failed to pack his usual toilet articles and had been forced to buy new supplies while on vacation.

Questions

1. What "underarm" applications are likely to lead to dermatitis?
2. What treatment is suggested for contact dermatitis?

Solution

In the absence of any convincing sign of arthropod infestation of other hairy parts of the body, axillary rashes are most likely to be caused by depilatory preparations in women or by antiperspirants in either sex. The efficacy of most antiperspirants on the market in the United States is based on the activity of aluminum salts—aluminum chloride, most commonly—which are not considered effective sensitizers. Formaldehyde, which is in widespread use in European antiperspirants, and glutaraldehyde are active sensitizers. Formaldehyde may not appear as such on the label of the product, since it may be incorporated in a condensed form with other compounds, as in methenamine. Formaldehyde products sometimes are used as accelerators in rubber products and may be released from the valves of pressurized atomizer dispensers, thereby causing the sensitization.

Most patients with axillary dermatitis recognize the source of their sensitivity as an antiperspirant and discontinue use of the product. In this instance the patient was inclined to think of other causes of his condition. When he returned to the use of a formaldehyde-free product, his symptoms disappeared.

References

Dahl, M.V.: Clinical immunodermatology, Chicago, 1981, Year Book Medical Publishers, Inc.

Patterson, R., editor: Allergic diseases; diagnosis and management, ed. 2, Philadelphia, 1980, J.B. Lippincott Co.

AUTOIMMUNITY

GLOSSARY

cold agglutinin An agglutinin or hemagglutinin that is active at 4° C but not at 37° C.

cross-reactive antigen An antigen that will react with an antibody induced by some other antigen.

EAE Experimental allergic encephalomyelitis.

horror autotoxicus Fear of self-poisoning, as related to the usual inability of an antigen to serve as an autoantigen.

LATS Long-acting thyroid stimulator.

LE Lupus erythematosus.

LE cell A polymorphonuclear cell that has engulfed the enlarged nucleus of another white blood cell which was distorted by antinuclear antibody.

Masugi's nephritis A form of glomerulonephritis produced by passive immunization with antikidney serum.

MBP Myelin basic protein.

MG Myasthenia gravis.

MS Multiple sclerosis.

neoantigen A "new" antigen, formed by modification of an "old" antigen by haptenic addition or other means.

relative risk A calculation that relates HLA antigens with susceptibility to an autoimmune disease.

RF Rheumatoid factor.

rheumatoid factor An IgM with specificity toward IgG associated with arthritis.

sequestered antigen An antigen not found in the circulatory system.

shared antigen A cross-reactive antigen.

SLE Systemic lupus erythematosus.

Witebsky's postulates A set of conditions that must be met before a disease can be accepted as an autoimmune illness.

warm agglutinin An agglutinin or hemagglutinin that is active at 37° C but not at 4° C.

The autoimmune diseases represent a group of conditions in which immunoglobulins or T cells display a specificity for self-antigens, or autoantigens. In certain situations this "forbidden" immune response can be defended as the etiologic basis of the disease, but more often this is not the case. Then one can only describe these autoimmune phenomena as correlates of the disease. This is quite unlike the alloimmune diseases (blood transfusion reactions, HDN, graft rejection) or the heteroimmune diseases (serum sickness, anaphylaxis, hay fever) where the immune response is clearly the cause of the disease.

AUTOIMMUNIZATION AND HORROR AUTOTOXICUS

Autoimmunization is the use of self-antigens or autoantigens to produce circulating immunoglobulins or sensitized lymphocytes, which react with the autoantigen. According to the concept of horror autotoxicus forwarded by Ehrlich, one does not develop an immune response to the normal circulating antigens. A combination of these two definitions reveals that autoantigens must be noncirculating or abnormal. Only under those conditions can the two definitions remain intact.

Etiology of autoimmune disease

Actually there are five major avenues through which an individual may develop an autoimmune response:

1. A response to antigens that do not normally circulate in the blood (the hidden or sequestered antigen theory)
2. A response to an altered antigen (The alteration could arise through chemical, physical, or biologic means, such as hapten complexing, physical denaturation, and mutation, respectively.)
3. A response to a foreign antigen that is shared or cross-reactive with self-antigens
4. A mutation in immunocompetent cells to acquire a responsiveness to self-antigens
5. A loss of immunoregulatory power by Th or Ts cells

Sequestered antigen. An unfortunate attraction of the sequestered, hidden, or noncirculating antigen notion is that it is based on a negative concept, the inability to identify these "normally hidden" antigens in the circulation under conditions of normal health. Even very sensitive detectors require that nanogram quantities of an antigen be present before a positive test can be observed. Consequently any antigen not found in the blood at that concentration is described as a noncirculating or sequestered antigen. This can easily be a fallacious assumption.

Antigens often grouped as noncirculating antigens are lens proteins of the eye, milk casein, antigens of the reproductive system (especially of the male), thyroglobulin, etc. Although some antigens (lens proteins may be an example) are unusually stable and have very little metabolic turnover, others such as those of the thyroid gland or male reproductive tract might be expected to undergo degradation and elimination just like antigens of the kidney, liver, and other tissues. Then they very easily could be present in the circulatory system at levels too low to detect and be erroneously classified as hidden antigens. Until more knowledge of the elimination pathway of effete antigens is available, the possibility of hidden antigens being autoantigens must be considered, but it is difficult to determine exactly what criteria should be used to determine if an antigen is hidden or not.

Altered antigen or neoantigen. Altered antigens or neoantigens may be created by chemical, physical, or biologic means. Convincing proof that new antigens are formed by autocoupling haptens already has been advanced as a mechanism for contact dermatitis and anaphylactic sensitivity to low molecular weight compounds. When a portion of the immune response is directed against the carrier antigen, then an autoimmune disease may result. Physical autoallergies to visible light, ultraviolet light, physical pressure, and cold arise through a similar mechanism. In these instances the physical forces reform the molecule to expose or create a new antigenic determinant or determinants against which the response might be developed. Photosensitization—the labilization of a compound by a photoreactive dye—would combine the chemical and physical means of antigen alteration. By mutation in an antigen-producing cell a new and structurally different antigen might be produced that would no longer be recognized as self by one's immune machinery and thus would stimulate an immune response.

Shared or cross-reactive antigen. A third potential for autoimmunization is that exogenous antigens exist which are cross-reactive with self-antigens. Because of the size of antigenic determinants, the possibility exists that complex structures which are recognized as foreign could include simpler parts that are identical or similar to self-structures. This would result in immunologic cross-reactivity. If this is viewed in the sense of Ehrlich's lock and key hypothesis of antigen-antibody combination, it is not inconsistent with immunologic specificity. A fit of the key (autoantigen) into only a small part of the lock (auto-

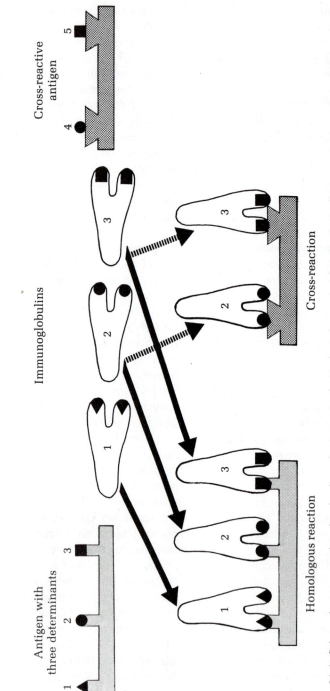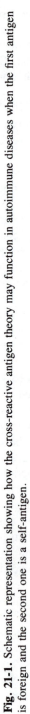

Fig. 21-1. Schematic representation showing how the cross-reactive antigen theory may function in autoimmune diseases when the first antigen is foreign and the second one is a self-antigen.

antibody or T cell receptor) might be perfectly adequate to initiate an autoimmune disease (Fig. 21-1).

Mutation. The mutation of an immunocompetent cell to acquire an unnatural responsiveness to self-antigens would be a de facto abrogation of the concept of horror autotoxicus. The inclusion of hypermutable cells in one form of the clonal selection theory to account for the apparent pluripotentiality of the antibody response from a limited number of cells almost ensures an expanded antigenic responsiveness to self-antigens in later life. Such an age relationship with autoantibodies is described earlier. The mutations responsible could occur at the level of the macrophage, T or B lymphocytes, or their progenitor cells.

The synthesis of new antigens as a result of mutation is mentioned previously under the section on altered antigen.

Loss of immunoregulation. The recognition that Th and Ts cells have pronounced effects on B cells and certain T cell subsets suggests that diminished suppressor cell activities, resulting from a total functional loss of these cells or only a relative loss compared with helper cells, would be reflected in heightened immunoglobulin levels or T cell responses. Evidence that this is the basis for both experimental and natural autoimmune disease already has been provided.

This loss of immunoregulation is synonymous with a loss of self-tolerance. Tolerance to self-antigens exists as the natural result of embryonic development. Most potential antigens are present in the fetus prior to the time of immunologic maturation and, as illustrated experimentally, induce a tolerogenic state in the immunocompetent cells or their progenitors as they develop. The continued presence of the antigen ensures a continuation of the tolerance until such time that mutation or loss of immunoregulatory powers permits an escape from that condition and self-antigens behave as foreign antigens. This forbidden response results in autoimmune disease.

Witebsky's postulates

There are many diseases associated with autoimmune phenomena (Table 21-1). Whether these autoantibodies merely are associated with the dis-

Table 21-1. Human diseases expressing autoimmune phenomena

Disease	Antigen	Immunoglobulin and/or T cell response
Postvaccinal and postinfectious encephalomyelitis	Myelin, cross-reactive	T cell
Aspermatogenesis	Sperm	T cell
Sympathetic ophthalmia	Uvea	T cell
Hashimoto's disease	Thyroglobulin	IgG and T cell
Graves' disease	—	Long-acting thyroid stimulator (LATS)
Autoimmune hemolytic disease	I, Rh, and others on surface of red blood cells	IgM and IgG
Thrombocytopenic purpura	Hapten-platelet or hapten-adsorbed antigen complex	IgG
MG	Acetylcholine receptor	IgG
Rheumatic fever	Streptococcal cross-reactive with heart	IgG and IgM
Glomerulonephritis	Streptococcal cross-reactive with kidney	IgG and IgM
Rheumatoid arthritis	IgG	IgM to Fc(γ)
SLE	DNA, nucleoprotein, RNA, etc.	IgG

ease or play a central role in the cause of the illness is not always easy to determine. Much the same problem confronted microbiologists in their initial efforts to identify which organisms isolated from patients actually were responsible for disease. Koch created four criteria to be used by microbiologists interested in the accurate assignation of microbes as the agents of infectious disease. These standards have become known as Koch's postulates. Witebsky has erected the following very similar criteria for immunologists who wish to determine the relationship of immunologic phenomena to disease etiology.

1. The autoimmune response must be regularly associated with the disease.
2. A replica of the disease must be inducible in laboratory animals.
3. Immunopathologic changes in the natural and experimental diseases should parallel each other.
4. Transfer of the autoimmune illness should be possible by the transfer of serum or lymphoid cells from the diseased individual to a normal recipient.

Among the most obvious immunologic findings associated with autoimmune diseases are one or more of the following: general hypergammaglobulinemia, specific self-directed immunoglobulins, decrease in total serum complement levels (hypocomplementemia) or in specific complement components, increase in activities attendant to activation of complement, especially chemotactic attraction to sites where γ-globulin and complement are bound to tissues involved in the disease, and the appearance of T lymphocytes with self-directed activities. Serologic tests directed toward identification of these unusual immunologic manifestations are useful screening procedures for the diagnosis of autoimmune disease.

Replicas of most of the human autoimmune conditions described in this chapter have been developed in experimental animals. In most instances these mimics have been created by removing a portion of some tissue, treating it as an antigen, emulsifying it with adjuvant, and injecting this into the same animal which donated the tissue. This procedure is very convenient when the tissue source exists as a paired organ (such as thyroid or gonad). Half the organ then serves as the antigen and its remainder as an indicator tissue for any evidence of autoimmune phenomena resulting from the autoimmunization. Injections of haptenic materials also have been used to generate autoimmune replicas.

Alloimmunization and even xenoimmunization with exogenous antigens also can produce replicas of autoimmune diseases. This is not unexpected when the alloantigens or xenoantigens involved share antigenic determinants with the autoantigen. Since this has been proved in only a few instances, acceptance of these alloimmune or xenoimmune copies as embodying the precise phenomena of the autoimmune condition should be guarded.

Other models of human autoimmune diseases may be found in a natural autoimmune counterpart in experimental animals. Mice, rats, dogs, chickens, and other species sometimes are affected by diseases which closely parallel those observed in humans. Particularly in mice, where our depth of knowledge about the immune response often exceeds what we know about the human system, these spontaneous autoimmune diseases have been very informative. In chickens the separation of the central lymphoid tissues into the bursal and thymic compartments has been especially important in evaluating the role of immunoglobulins against T cells in the cause of autoimmune disease.

The reaction of self-antigens with autoantibodies or autosensitized T lymphocytes is the natural result of their simultaneous existence in an individual. In certain instances it is believed that this reaction is the final immunologic event in the development of the disease. The autoimmune hemolytic diseases and thrombocytopenic purpura can be cited as examples. In a greater number of cases in which immunologic reactions are occurring, it is uncertain or even doubtful whether they cause the disease with which they are associated. In many instances these immunologic events appear to be only secondary aspects of the disease which, although they may contribute to the perpetuation of it, have little or nothing to do with the origins of the illness. In still other instances immunologic phenomena appear to have little, if anything, to do with the continuation of the disease.

One indirect line of evidence that an immunologic event is critical to the continuation of an autoimmune disease stems from the types of treatment that are most effective for the disease. In the past decade the availability of a large number of cytotoxic agents with immunosuppressive action has resulted in their therapeutic application to several autoimmune diseases. Corticosteroids, purine and pyrimidine analogs, and alkylating agents have been used in diseases such as autoimmune thyroiditis, LE, rheumatoid arthritis, and autoimmune hemolytic disease. Most of these compounds have a potent antiinflammatory effect, and both T and B lymphocytes are highly sensitive to their cytotoxic action. The prolonged use of these drugs is not without hazard, since the total immune capabilities of the subject are depressed, and constant supervision of patients for the development of infectious diseases is a necessity. Temporary or intermittent treatment with the more potent drugs is necessary to avoid undesirable side effects, but, as logic would indicate, autoimmune diseases do respond favorably to these compounds. Healing of tissue damage or other pathologic lesions that already have developed is not promoted by these compounds, which halt the progress of but do nothing to repair prior damage caused by the illness.

THE MHC AND AUTOIMMUNE DISEASE

Although the major source of our knowledge about the MHC and its relationship with the immune response evolved from the study of the murine H-2 system, our knowledge about the relationship of the MHC to autoimmune disease is largely, if not entirely, the result of studying the human animal. These investigations quickly followed those in mice which correlated the susceptibility of the mouse to leukemia with its H-2 antigens and have been a steadily expanding field of study.

To determine if an autoimmune disease is a genetic trait, two approaches are possible: family studies and population studies. When family members with a presumed autoimmune disease can be identified as sharing common HLA haplotypes, then a link between the disease and HLA clearly is suggested. Because large families displaying autoimmune disease are not always available because of death from the disease or awareness of the disease as a family characteristic and a consequent restriction of family size, population studies must be used. In this approach antigen frequencies among large groups of patients with a specific illness are compared with those of a group of healthy control subjects. Since the frequency of most HLA antigens is 0.20 or less, statistically significant associations are frequently impossible, even when large groups are studied. Instead a calculation of relative risk is used to indicate the HLA-disease relationship. Relative risk is calculated as follows:

$$\text{Relative risk} = \frac{\begin{array}{c}\text{Frequency of}\\\text{patients with}\\\text{the HLA}\\\text{antigen}\end{array} \times \begin{array}{c}\text{Frequency of}\\\text{control subjects}\\\text{lacking the}\\\text{HLA antigen}\end{array}}{\begin{array}{c}\text{Frequency of}\\\text{patients lack-}\\\text{ing the HLA}\\\text{antigen}\end{array} \times \begin{array}{c}\text{Frequency of}\\\text{control subjects}\\\text{with the HLA}\\\text{antigen}\end{array}}$$

The autoimmune disease with the highest relative risk is ankylosing spondylitis, where the HLA-B27 antigen yields a relative risk of approximately 90% (Table 21-2).

Currently the autoimmune diseases expressing HLA associations have identified antigens in the B series as those most related to the disease. In one sense this is an artifact of the available technology. The D/DR region of the human MHC is the Ia region, and hence immune responses should be associated with D/DR antigens. Unfortunately antisera to identify these

Table 21-2. Relationship of HLA and autoimmune human diseases

Disease	HLA	Antigen frequency (percent)		Relative risk
		Patients	Control subjects	
Ankylosing spondylitis	B27	79 to 100	4 to 13	90
Addison's disease	B8	20 to 69	18 to 24	1 to 7
Reiter's syndrome	B27	65 to 100	4 to 14	36
Graves' disease	B8	25 to 47	16 to 27	1.8 to 2.4
Yersinia arthritis	B27	58 to 78	9 to 14	18
Salmonella arthritis	B27	60 to 69	8 to 10	18
Sjögren's syndrome	Dw3	68 to 69	10 to 24	8 to 16
Adult rheumatoid arthritis	Dw4	38 to 65	18 to 31	4.4
Autoimmune thyroiditis	Bw35	63 to 73	9 to 14	16.8
Anterior uveitis	B27	37 to 58	7 to 10	9.4
MG	B8	38 to 65	18 to 13	4.4
Multiple sclerosis (MS)	B7	12 to 46	14 to 30	1.7

human Ir products are available for only a few of the proteins. Until such antisera are available, relative risks must be calculated for antigens of the A, B, and C series, for which antisera exist. The higher relative risk values associated with the B antigens are a result of the closer proximity of the B locus to the D/DR locus compared with the position of the A and C genes.

Table 21-2 presents a list of the relative risk calculations for several human diseases. Although some of these conditions appear to be infectious diseases, this actually is not the case. For example, arthritides associated with bacterial infections are not the direct result of the bacterial infection but are sequelae that stem from the infection.

ANIMAL MODELS FOR AUTOIMMUNE DISEASES

The obvious handicaps in experimentation with human subjects have emphasized the importance of the search for and the value of experimental animal models for human diseases. Such animals have proved especially valuable as mimics of diseases such as LE, autoimmune hemolytic disease, immune complex glomerulo-nephritis, autoimmune thyroiditis, arthritis, and a few others such as the slow virus infections.

T CELL–ASSOCIATED AUTOIMMUNE DISEASES

In this section the human autoimmune diseases and some of their experimental counterparts that have well-documented associations with T cell phenomena are considered. It bears repeating that unexpected immunoglobulin activities often are associated with these diseases, and it may be difficult to determine whether the undesired T cell activities actually dominate these conditions. This is best determined by successful transfer of the disease with T cells.

Allergic encephalomyelitis

Postvaccinal and postinfectious encephalomyelitis. Postvaccinal encephalomyelitis following immunization against rabies is an undesired sequela to the use of the Pasteur rabies vaccine. The earlier vaccines customarily were prepared by phenolizing extracts of spinal cord of rabbits that had experimental rabies. In both a chemical and an immunologic sense the antigen is extremely crude and contains, in addition to the inactivated rabies virus, many different antigens from the central nerve tissue of the rabbit. For rabies immunization daily inoculations of this vaccine over a 2-week period are prescribed. In rare instances (1 in 4,000) symptoms of encephalomyelitis appear about 2 weeks after the immunization. Backache, headache, muscle weakness, and changes in reflex response are noted. Persons who survive the acute stages invariably recover without permanent neurologic disorders. Rabies vaccines free of neural tissue have replaced the Pasteur vaccine and largely eliminated this problem.

Rabies vaccine encephalomyelitis has been recognized since the 1930s as an immunologic disorder. Circulating immunoglobulins have been detected in the sera of these patients, but anti–brain tissue globulins are found in many vaccinated persons who do not develop the encephalitis. On the basis of comparative studies in experimental allergic encephalitis the cause is more likely to derive from a cell-mediated allergic response.

A second form of postvaccinal encephalomyelitis is known to accompany vaccination with attenuated viruses. These vaccines for smallpox, measles, rubella, mumps, and chickenpox do not contain nerve tissue antigens; however, the viruses in these attenuated vaccines are able to initiate an abbreviated, normally mild disease. These viruses may invade cells of the central nervous system during the course of their modified disease. This usually occurs early in the disease, and later, when active viral particles are no longer detectable, the symptoms of encephalomyelitis appear. These include an elevated temperature, drowsiness perhaps proceeding to a comatose state, convulsions, and paralysis of the legs. Following the use of attenuated measles vaccines the encephalitis rate is about 1 in 1,000. The fatality rate is about 10% of the affected individuals. The survivors may demonstrate mental retardation, epileptic seizures, or other neurologic symptoms, although many survivors remain free of secondary effects. Incidents of postvaccinal encephalomyelitis have been the dominating force in efforts to improve these vaccines.

These examples of postvaccinal encephalomyelitis are artificially induced instances of post-

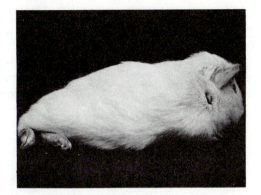

Fig. 21-2. Hind quarter paralysis in a guinea pig with EAE. (Courtesy Dr. C.W. Purdy.)

infectious encephalomyelitis, which may develop after natural infections with viruses. In 1968 it was reported that 22% of all cases of encephalitis were associated with childhood diseases, practically all of which had a viral origin. Among the RNA viruses involved are those of measles, mumps, rubella, and influenza; viruses of the DNA group that have been incriminated include chickenpox (varicella), herpes zoster, herpes simplex, and vaccinia. The association of these childhood viral diseases with encephalomyelitis is what prompted the development of the attenuated vaccines for their prevention. This reduced the incidence of viral associated encephalomyelitis but did not eliminate it as a risk of exposure to viruses.

The best model for both postvaccinal encephalomyelitis and postinfectious encephalomyelitis is experimental allergic encephalomyelitis.

Experimental allergic encephalomyelitis. The postvaccinal and postinfectious encephalomyelitides have heteroimmune-alloimmune counterparts that serve as excellent models. The best model, experimental allergic encephalomyelitis, or EAE (Fig. 21-2), customarily is produced by the inoculation of brain extracts in Freund's adjuvant into the animal to be studied. There is virtually no species barrier to this disease; extracts of the brain of most common domesticated mammals are equally effective in inducing EAE in rats. The symptoms of EAE in the rat begin at about the tenth to fourteenth postsensitization day. Grossly these include an ascending, flaccid paralysis that may disappear after 2 weeks accompanied by complete recovery. Histologic lesions in the brain are variable, but focal perivascular areas of inflammation containing lymphocytes, mononuclear cells, and plasma cells are common in most species. Complement-fixing anti–brain tissue globulins usually are produced in response to the immunization, but these are unable to transfer the disease. However, it is possible to passively transfer EAE with sensitized lymphocytes.

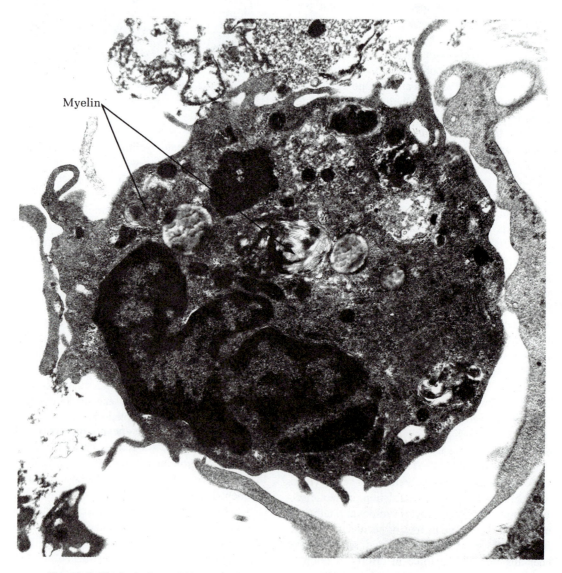

Fig. 21-3. The inclusions within this granulocyte are not all identifiable, but the ones identified by the arrows are myelin. (Courtesy Dr. E. Adelstein.)

Chemical fractionation of brain extracts that successfully produce EAE in rats, guinea pigs, mice, rabbits, and other animals has incriminated the myelin basic protein (MBP) as the key encephalitogen (Fig. 21-3). This protein alone represents about 30% of the protein in the central nervous system myelin. It has a molecular weight of 18,500 and is composed of 169 amino acid residues. Its isoelectric point is 10.2 because of the presence of 31 residues of lysine and arginine. The amino acid sequence of the MBP from several species has been completely determined. MBPs from the species studied are virtually identical with very few amino acid substitutions, and this permits the equally effective routes of xenoimmunization or alloimmunization to induce the disease.

Although MBPs from diverse species are nearly identical, the encephalitogenic sequences differ for the different species. For the rabbit the encephalitogenic determinant encompasses amino acids 44 to 89 and specifically the region 66 to 74; for the rat the determinant includes amino acids 75 to 84, for the guinea pig amino acids 114 to 122, and for the monkey amino acids 154 to 167. Thus, when describing EAE, one need not refer to the species source of the MBP but only to the species tested, since the encephalitogenic peptide varies with the test species, as follows:

1. For rabbit, 66 to 74: Thr-His-Tyr-Gly-Ser-Leu-Pro-Gln-Lys
2. For rat, 75 to 84: Ala-Gln-Gly-His-Arg-Pro-Gln-Asp-Glu-Asn
3. For guinea pig, 114 to 122: Phe-Ser-Trp-Gly-Ala-Glu-Gly-Gln-Lys
4. For monkey, 154 to 167: Phe-Lys-Leu-Gly-Gly-Arg-Asp-Ser-Arg-Ser-Gly-Ser-Pro

Among separate guinea pig strains, strain 2 is very resistant to EAE, whereas strain 13 is very sensitive. Strain 2 and 13 guinea pigs are well known to differ in their immune response to several antigens, and this is taken as further evidence that multiple sclerosis (MS) and the postvaccinal and postinfectious encephalitides are in fact autoimmune diseases.

A recent discovery may help clarify why some strains of rats or other species are more refractory to the development of EAE. This also may be taken as prime evidence for immune tolerance in a more general sense as the reason autoimmune diseases are relatively uncommon. The experiment was simply an investigation of the blood of young animals, which are characteristically resistant to EAE, for some factor which could contribute to this resistance. It was found that these animals, and adults of EAE-resistant strains, had an antigen in their vascular system that appears to be nearly identical to the myelin peptide. The hypothesis is that the continued presence of this peptide in the blood maintains self-tolerance to neural tissue. Failure to secrete this material permits a response to the peptide with the undesired consequence of EAE in experimental animals or postvaccinal or postinfectious encephalomyelitis in humans.

Aspermatogenesis

Autoimmunization of guinea pigs with sperm was one of the first experimental autoimmunizations ever conducted and dates back to the work of Metalnikoff in 1900. Since spermatic and testicular antigens develop after the immunologic apparatus has matured, and since they are sequestered antigens, the ability of these tissues to serve as autoantigens is not considered unusual. More recently demographers (population and birth control experts) have looked on experimental human aspermatogenesis as a potential method of limiting the world increase in population, even in the face of effective drug control of female fertility.

Spermagglutinins are found in a small number (2% to 3%) of male partners of infertile marriages. These agglutinins are present in the seminal fluid, where they produce agglutination and immobilization of sperm, which logically could impair the opportunity of sperm to contact and fertilize the ovum. Since these antibodies are found in such a low proportion of infertile males, it seems unlikely that they are a major cause of infertility.

Immunization of guinea pigs or rats with autologous testis extracts in Freund's complete adjuvant has been very successful in producing an experimental aspermatogenesis. As in hypothyroiditis, half the tissue system is used for immunization and the remainder for assaying the disease. Aspermatogenesis is almost the only result of testis immunization; there is very little generalized tissue damage to the gland. About 3 weeks after the immunization the seminiferous tubules are almost devoid of cells. Interstitial cell infiltration is evident, but it is localized rather than generalized. This condition persists, with some testicular atrophy, for 3 to 6 months, after which regeneration of the spermatogenic capacity occurs; after 1 year normal sperm production is regained. Since these changes can be produced by the injection of sperm just as easily as by the use of homologous or autologous testis extracts, the potential for birth control vaccines in humans exists. One advantage of such vaccines is that the interruption of sperm production is temporary.

The aspermatic condition is accompanied by circulating antibody formation and anaphylactic sensitivity, but the experimental disease is not transferrable with serum. However, aspermatogenesis can be passively transferred with viable cells, although not all such experiments have been successful. Experimental aspermatogenesis thus is dependent on the cell-mediated hypersensitive response.

The potentiality of birth control of the female by immunization with sperm antigens is a second, perhaps even more promising, possibility. It was noted over a generation ago, before efficient chemical and mechanical control of fertilization was possible, that the incidence of pregnancy in prostitutes, was not totally compatible with their exposure. Among the suggested explanations for this was that such women produced sperm agglutinating and immobilizing antibodies as a result of immunization through the vaginal mucosa. Sperm-immobilizing antibodies have been identified in human vaginal washings; these very well could protect against impregnation. Experiments with lower animals generally, but not always, have demonstrated protection of the female by immunization with homologous sperm.

Sympathetic ophthalmia

Sympathetic ophthalmia is a chronic inflammatory reaction in a healthy eye within a few days to a few weeks following surgical or traumatic injury to the other eye. At the cellular level this is characterized by an infiltration of mononuclear cells that engulf the uveal pigment. Clusters of lymphocytes and occasional eosinophils are seen. Attempts to demonstrate circulating antibodies in persons with sympathetic ophthalmia usually have met with failure.

Sympathetic ophthalmia appears to be representative of an autoimmune disease that is dependent of the response of antigen-exposed T cells rather than on immunoglobulin synthesis. Skin reactions of the delayed type are present in patients with the disease. The skin test intensity often parallels that of the disease, whereas antibody titers, when detected, show little correlation with the symptomatology. The ability of steroids to control the disease also is suggestive of a delayed hypersensitive mechanism. The critical passive transfer experiments in experimentally produced ophthalmia have not been performed. Reproducible animal models for sympathetic ophthalmia that might clarify its immunopathology have not been developed.

Cataract removal sometimes is followed by a postoperative intraocular complication known as phacoanaphylaxis. Histologic examination reveals that the lens is invaded by leukocytes and macrophages. It is believed that lens antigens, which escape during the surgical procedure, hypersensitize the individual. These patients exhibit immediate skin reactions when tested with lens proteins. The exact immunologic cause of this disease is uncertain, but it appears that circulating antibodies are involved.

Hashimoto's thyroiditis

A form of thyroiditis unique and readily distinguished from other types of thyroiditis on a histologic basis was the first disease that satisfied Witebsky's criteria for an autoimmune disease. Hashimoto's disease (hypothyroiditis) is characterized physiologically by a deficiency in thyroid

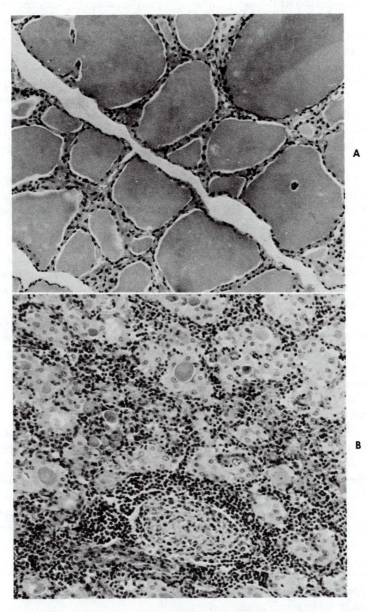

Fig. 21-4. A, Normal thyroid. **B,** Thyroid of Hashimoto's disease. In the normal thyroid the colloid fills the vesicles, whereas in the diseased gland only isolated deposits of colloid are seen. The cell infiltrate is lymphoid in nature. In the lower center is a germinal center. (From Anderson, J.R., Buchanan, W.W., and Goudie, R.B.: Autoimmunity, Springfield, Ill., 1967, Charles C Thomas, Publisher.)

hormone and anatomically by an enlarged thyroid gland infiltrated with plasma cells and lymphocytes (Fig. 21-4). In the sera of a certain proportion of patients with Hashimoto's disease a single gel precipitin line between the serum and an extract of human thyroid gland is produced. This same precipitin band is produced when purified thyroglobulin is the antigen. Because of the relative insensitivity of the gel precipitin test, recourse to passive hemagglutination was made to identify antithyroid globulins. Both IgG and IgM may have antithyroid activity.

Thyroglobulin is stored as a distinct colloid that fills the vesicles in a normal thyroid gland and is the reservoir of thyroxin, the thyroid hormone. In Hashimoto's disease little colloid can be detected in the gland. Many plasma cells and lymphocytes are present. Formation of antithyroglobulin and the mononuclear cell population of the thyroid gland are compatible with an autoimmune origin of this disease. This supposition is supported by the identification of other antibodies in patients' sera that are reactive with specific portions of thyroid epithelial cells and colloid and with cell nuclei. The fluorescent antibody method has been very useful in distinguishing these antibodies from each other.

Experimental thyroiditis can be produced in rabbits by autoimmunization with thyroid gland extracts emulsified in Freund's complete adjuvant. One lobe of the gland is used as the immunizing antigen, and the disease is assayed in the intact, remaining lobe. The formation of circulating antibody and the histologic changes in the rabbit thyroid parallel very closely the condition in the human. The disease now has been created in other common laboratory mammals.

It has not been possible, either in the human patient or in the experimental animal, to establish an exact correlation between serum antithyroglobulin titers and the severity of the thyroiditis. Transmission of the disease by passive immunization with serum is very difficult, and infants of mothers with Hashimoto's disease are unaffected by the maternal antithyroglobulin antibodies. Delayed hypersensitive skin reactions to thyroglobulin correlate in intensity with the severity of the disease; the transfer of the disease by lymphocytes strongly indicates a cell-mediated origin of the disease. However, the initial insult which permits the development of this autoallergic illness has not been identified yet, nor can one state unequivocally that this is a T cell–related disease.

Spontaneous autoimmune thyroid disease develops in the Buffalo strain rat and the Obese strain (OS) chicken. In the rat model the presence of high titers of antithyroid globulins parallels the development of thyroiditis. Mononuclear cell infiltration of the thyroid gland is similar to that observed in Hashimoto's disease. All animals' skin tested with rat thyroid gland extract failed to exhibit a delayed skin reaction, and no MIF could be detected in their sera. Thymus cell transfers failed to increase the incidence of disease. These features of the disease tend to negate any direct role of T cells and suggest an immunoglobulin dependence of the disease.

The avian model for autoimmune thyroiditis (Hashimoto's disease) is especially interesting because of the clear division of the immunologic functions into bursal and thymus-dependent compartments in birds. The conclusion that B cell activities dominate this disease is supported by microscopic evidence that the mononuclear cell invasion of the thyroid gland heavily favors B cells, that antithyroglobulin titers parallel the severity of the disease, that bursectomy reduces the severity of the disease, and that denser populations of B cells are present in OS chickens compared with normal chickens. The possibility of T cell control of these B cell–mediated functions is indicated by the experiments in which thymectomy resulted in a greater frequency and intensity of thyroiditis in the affected chickens.

IMMUNOGLOBULIN-ASSOCIATED AUTOIMMUNE DISEASES
Autoimmune hemolytic disease

Autoimmune hemolytic diseases represent a complex assortment of disorders that share the major feature of anemia and accelerated blood cell loss associated with the simultaneous presence of immunoglobulins specific for the person's own erythrocytes. In a surprisingly large percentage of instances the anemia may be almost nonexistent, but in others, such as paroxysmal cold hemoglobinuria, red blood cell lysis is a striking feature of the illness. In 50% to 75% of the cases the cause is unknown; these are the so-called idiopathic acquired hemolytic anemias. In the remainder the condition develops secondary to disease of the RES, other lymphoid illnesses, or drug therapy.

The immunoglobulins associated with hemolytic diseases may be of the cold agglutinin type or the warm type (Table 21-3). The former function well at 4° C or other low temperatures but are feebly active at room temperature and almost, if not totally, inactive at 37° C. These may or may not be hemolytically active with complement. The warm agglutinins are usually poor complement fixers, which is compatible with the rarity of severe hemolytic episodes in patients with this type of antibody. These warm agglutinins are also feeble agglutinators, and their presence usually is detected by antiglobulin tests for human IgG on the affected red cells. The cold agglutinins are most commonly of the IgM class, and they, too, are easily detected by antiglobulin tests of erythrocytes. Complement components also may be detected on the erythrocytes. It is not definitely known if these antibodies develop from a break in

tolerance to normal antigens or if neoantigens are formed by infectious agents. Hemolytic anemias following primary atypical pneumonia or infectious mononucleosis are so common as to support the neoantigen concept.

Autoimmune hemolytic disease caused by warm antibodies rarely occurs in childhood. The antibody is invariably an IgG and most often directed against an Rh antigen. About one third of the cases involve other than Rh antigens. The antibodies are not highly active; in vivo little anemia develops, although there are exceptions. Autoagglutination of erythrocytes from these patients is uncommon except in high-protein media (plasma).

Autoimmune hemolytic diseases caused by cold antibodies of the IgM class are often anti-I. The I antigen is formed after birth during "maturation" of red cell development. Agglutination of erythrocytes by cold agglutinins is reversed by warming the cells to 37° C. Necrosis of the fingertips, earlobes, tip of the nose, or other chilled parts of the patient's body may result from vascular plugging by the agglutinated cells. The simplest protection against these episodes is to keep warm.

Cold autoantibodies of the IgG class also are known to participate in hemolytic disease. These antibodies bind to erythrocytes at low temperature and at body temperature fix complement and function as hemolysins. This temperature dependence clearly is related to the disease with which these antibodies are most regularly associated: parox-

Table 21-3. Autoantibodies found in autoimmune hemolytic disease

	Warm antibody	Cold antibody
Immunoglobulin class	IgG	IgM
Temperature optimum	37° C	4° C
Antigen involved	Rh and other	I and other
Hemolysis	Less hemolytic	More hemolytic
Complement fixation	Less fixation	More fixation
Age attack range	Any age	Tendency toward older persons
Anemia	Variable	Variable
Associated diseases	SLE	*Mycoplasma* infection

ysmal cold hemoglobinuria. After cold shock these patients experience a severe hemolytic episode. This can be duplicated by immersing the hand and forearm in ice water. The low temperature promotes antibody–red cell combination, and the warmer temperature promotes lysis. This form of hemolytic anemia is a complication of tertiary syphilis, although it may have other origins as well. The autoantibody is to the P antigen of the human red blood cell.

Drug-induced autoimmune hemolytic anemia has been associated with many different chemotherapeutics, such as quinine, quinidine, the sulfonamides, penicillin, cephalosporin, tetracycline, aspirin, antihistamines, and cytotoxic drugs used in cancer therapy. These drugs stimulate antibody formation by complexing with the erythrocyte surface to create new antigenic determinants, by forming new determinants with serum proteins, which then adsorb to the red cell surface, or by modifying the erythrocyte surface so that its new determinants are expressed. Only the latter does not contain the drug-hapten complex as an integral part. Antibodies formed against any of these would react with the antigen on the erythrocyte surface and cause anemia.

Thrombocytopenic purpura

Thrombocytopenic purpura is an illness characterized by lowered platelet count (thrombocytopenia) in the circulation and the appearance of purpuric or petechial hemorrhages in the skin and tissues. The known contribution of thrombocytes to blood clotting is fully compatible with a close association of these two expressions of the disease.

Thrombocytopenic purpura in infants can arise through alloimmunization in much the same way that erythroblastosis fetalis develops, that is, the transplacental migration of maternal antifetal thrombocyte globulins. An autoimmune form of thrombocytopenic purpura is seen in adults. Invariably the afflicted persons are on a continued drug regimen of some sort. The offending drug may be aspirin, a sulfonamide, an antihistamine,

quinine, digitoxin, or a tranquilizer. During the time the drug therapy is maintained, the purpura and thrombocytopenia are evident, but when the drug is withdrawn, the disease abates. Reinitiation of the therapy causes an exacerbation of the illness. The disease is truly iatrogenic in origin. An in vitro mixture of the patient's serum with human platelets of any origin plus the offending drug results in complement fixation and lysis of the platelets. If complement is absent, platelet agglutination may occur, but lysis cannot. If the offending drug is absent, the patient's serum has no effect on the platelets. These features indicate that a hapten-antigen complex in which the hapten dominates the determinant site is the incitant of the disease.

Two immunologic hypotheses have been formulated for this disease. One assumes that the hapten (inciting drug) complexes naturally with platelets to create a neoantigen and that the antibody is formed against this complex. Therefore normal platelets are not agglutinated or lysed by the antibody in the absence or presence of complement; these reactions require the drug (Fig. 21-5). The other proposal suggests that the drug binds to a serum protein to form the hapten-antigen complex. This complex adsorbs to the platelet surface and causes agglutination or lysis in the presence of the specific antibody and/or complement. Whatever the exact mechanism, there can be no question that this is a hapten-mediated condition which is directly associated with circulating antibody. Passive transfer of the patient's serum will convey the disease to a normal person, provided the latter receives the drug also.

MG

MG is a disease in which a gradual progressive weakness of striated muscle is a prominent external sign and which becomes so severe that even eating is laborious. MG affects 1 in every 10,000 to 40,000 persons. About 10% to 20% of its victims have a thymoma of mixed epithelial and thymocytic nature. A number of immunologic aberrations are seen in MG patients. Germinal

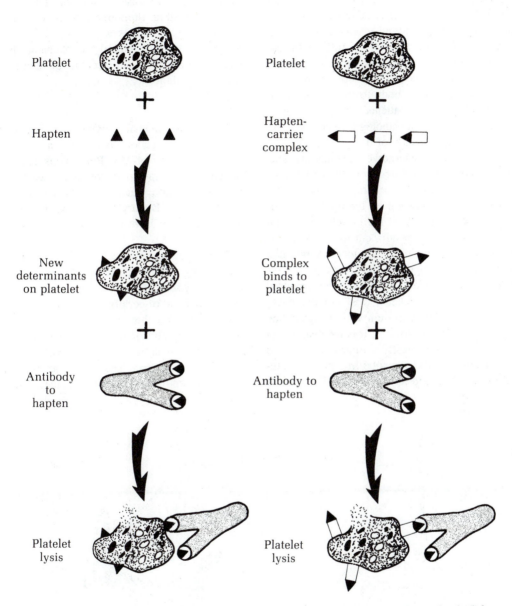

Fig. 21-5. Two hypotheses for the autoimmune origin for thrombocytopenia purpura. On the left, a hapten combines with the surface of a platelet to create new antigenic determinants. The resulting antibody reacts with the platelet and complement to cause cell lysis. On the right, the hapten combines spontaneously with a carrier molecule, which adsorbs to the surface of the platelet. The new antigenic determinant involves the hapten and carrier but not the platelet.

centers are detectable in the thymus gland, which normally is devoid of these structures. Antinuclear antibodies (ANA) are found in about 20% of the patients. RF is present in 5% to 10% of the patients, and antibodies that react with striated muscle are quite common (30% to 40% frequency). The presence of an antibody to the acetylcholine receptor in 80% of the patients is the most important of these immunopathologic features. This autoantibody is frequently of the IgG3 isotype.

At the normal muscle-nerve (myoneural) junction acetylcholine is released from the nerve when it stimulates the muscle to contract. The acetylcholine binds to a receptor on the muscle surface and initiates contraction of the muscle. When antibody is adsorbed to or adjacent to this receptor, this event is inhibited. Consequently muscular contraction and strength are impaired (Fig. 21-6).

Experimental models of MG can be produced in species such as chickens, rats, rabbits, mice, and monkeys by immunization with acetylcholine receptors from the electric eel. It is interesting that this receptor is antigenically similar in the eel and several mammals. Experimental MG in mice is related to the MHC and an increase in Th cells. In humans there is an association with HLA-B8.

An interesting alloimmune form of MG exists in neonates of mothers who have MG. This is a temporary disease entirely explainable by the placental transfer of antireceptor IgG and its half-life in the infant.

MS

Partial loss of vision, nystygmus, facial palsy, and muscular incoordination are a few of the varied symptoms of MS. Remissions and exacerbations are characteristic of this disease, which may affect more than 250,000 persons in the United States. Dietary, infectious, and immunologic causes all have been proposed for the disease.

The major pathologic feature of MS is an inflammatory lesion of the myelin in the central nervous system. Myelin of the central nervous system and that of peripheral nervous tissues differ chemically, and this accounts for the specificity of MS for myelin of the central nervous system. Denuded foci along the nerve sheath create lesions that are characteristic of the disease and which are known as sclerotic plaques. These le-

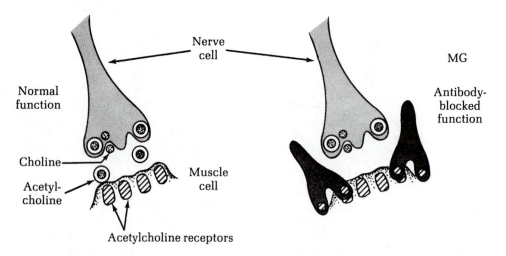

Fig. 21-6. At the normal neuromuscular junction *(left)* acetylcholine is released from the nerve cell and degraded by a cholinesterase in the acetylcholine receptor on the muscle cell. This causes the muscle to contract. This is prevented by antibody against the receptor in the person with MG *(right)*.

sions are associated with the neuromuscular symptoms of MS.

The basis for theories of a dietary cause of MS is based on modern diets that have a low content of polyunsaturated fatty acids, presumably leading to a defective lipid content of the myelin sheath. Evidence for a viral origin is more convincing and is based on epidemiologic studies and the reports of viruslike particles in early MS lesions.

Immunologic associations with MS include the identification of lymphocytes, plasma cells, monocytes, and macrophages in the plaques. Antibodies are present in serum and spinal fluid that react with the MBP. An increased content of IgG in the spinal fluid of MS patients is one of its most reliable clinical tests, being reported in up to 94% of the patients in some studies. Antibodies directed against the myelin-forming oligodendrocytes also may be present. Sera from MS patients are also toxic for myelinated cells in vitro, and the titer of these antibodies often correlates well with the severity of the disease. Although these facts indicate a potential immunoglobulin basis for MS, a loss of Ts cells could produce these same results. The immunologic basis of MS is still poorly defined.

The autoimmune basis of MS is indicated by its close association with HLA-B7 and HLA-Dw2. The incidence of the Dw2 antigen in MS patients is 70% versus 16% in healthy control subjects.

Numerous models of MS can be developed in laboratory animals. These demyelinating diseases include acute EAE, neurotropic virus infections, including visna in sheep, canine distemper, and encephalomyelitis virus infections in mice, and combinations of EAE with these viral infections. EAE is discussed previously with a full discussion of the MBP.

Poststreptococcal diseases

Rheumatic fever. Acute rheumatic fever has been recognized for some time as one of two important diseases that typically follow a group A streptococcal illness. Unlike poststreptococcal glomerulonephritis, poststreptococcal rheumatic heart disease may follow infection with any one of more than 50 types of group A streptococci. The latent period for the symptoms of the rheumatic heart disease coincides roughly with the time required for the development of high antistreptococcal titers. This has suggested an autoimmune origin of the illness, specifically, an involvement of circulating antibodies.

Among the immunopathologic changes that occur in rheumatic fever are elevated titers against streptolysin O, streptococcal DNAse B, and several other enzymes and toxins of group A streptococci. Inflammatory tissue changes in the heart include the aggregation of lymphocytes and macrophages around fibrinoid deposits to form Aschoff's bodies. These structures are almost pathognomonic of rheumatic fever. IgG and, to a lesser extent, IgM, IgA, and complement can be found deposited in the Aschoff body, in the perivascular connective tissue, and in the sarcolemma (Fig. 21-7). Many patients have antibody free in their blood plasma that is reactive with heart tissue.

Several potential mechanisms for poststreptococcal autoimmune heart disease have been suggested. The two most commonly discussed are the alteration of heart tissue by streptococci to create new hapten-antigen complexes, which initiate the formation of antiheart immunoglobulins, and the sharing of similar antigens by human heart and group A streptococci. Indirect support for the neoantigen hypothesis is supplied by the facts that streptolysin O does have a direct toxic effect on heart tissue and that streptococcal hyaluronidase, an enzyme, does solubilize the connective tissue ground substance. Attractive though the theory of a neoantigen cause for rheumatic fever may be, there is little factual support for a direct involvement of streptococcal toxins.

Most of the available information supports instead the cross-reacting antigen theory. The streptococcal groups, which are designated by the letters A, B, C, etc., are segregated according to the chemical and immunologic nature of the C carbohydrate in their cytoplasm. Within the group A organisms, serotyping is arranged on the basis of variations in the M protein. This protein is located on the cell surface, possibly in the fimbriae.

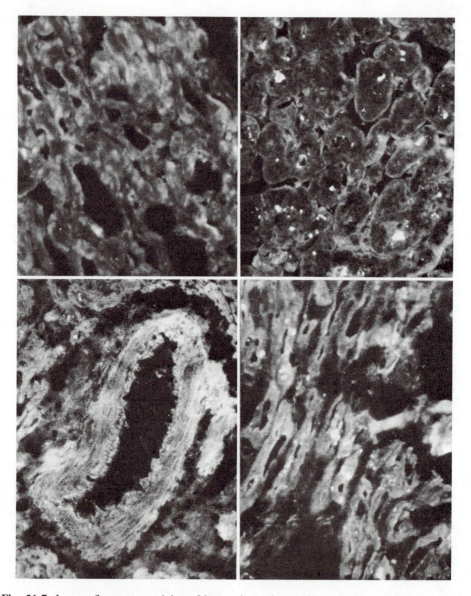

Fig. 21-7. Immunofluorescent staining of human heart tissue with antibody to group A strepto-coccus cell membrane; indirect fluorescent antibody procedure. (From Zabriskie, J.B.: Mimetic relationships between group A streptococci and mammalian tissues, Adv. Immunol. **7:**147, 1967.)

More than 60 different forms, or antigenic types (designated by numbers), of this M protein are known. This protein is associated with the virulence of the group A streptococci. Many of these infections, with little relationship to M protein type, precede rheumatic fever. These infections stimulate high antibody titers to the M protein and other streptococcal antigens, but the anti-M titer is higher in those who become rheumatic than in those with uncomplicated streptococcal infections. Antibody deposits on human cardiac myofibers can be identified in these rheumatic patients with fluorescent antihuman IgG. Complement component C3 also has been recognized in these deposits. The evidence now indicates that this antibody is specific for the M protein or another protein which is closely associated with the M protein. This streptococcal antigen is cross-reactive with human heart tissue. Rabbit antibody to group A streptococci will precipitate on human cardiac myofibers but not on fibers of the voluntary muscles. This can be prevented by adsorption of the antiserum either with bacterial cell wall preparations or extracts of human heart tissue.

Attempts to develop animal models of rheumatic fever have not been universally successful but tend to support the theory of a cross-reactive, immune complex origin of rheumatic fever.

Glomerulonephritis. Basically there are three forms of immune disease that involve the glomerulus. One is associated with antecedent group A streptococcal infection; a second is involved with heterologous antibodies versus glomerular basement membrane antigens (Masugi's nephritis); the third is based on immune complex formation with heteroantigens, as in serum sickness, or allo-antigens, as in LE.

Autoimmune glomerulonephritis, in which edema, hematuria, and other symptoms of kidney failure become manifest, is an immune complex disease in which globulins precipitate within the kidney. This may follow staphylococcal or pneumococcal infections or malaria, but in the United States it more commonly is considered the result of a prior group A streptococcal infection. Unlike rheumatic fever, which may follow virtually any group A streptococcal infection, poststreptococcal glomerulonephritis is limited to a few serologic types. These include types 12, 4, 5, 25, 49, 52, 55, and a few others. These nephritogenic cocci synthesize a lipoprotein molecule of about 120,000 mol wt that is a part of their cytoplasmic membrane. This antigenic lipoprotein is serologically cross-reactive with kidney tissue. Just as with rheumatic fever, when symptoms of the streptococcal infection begin to subside, some 10 to 14

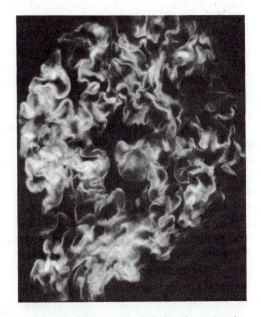

Fig. 21-8. Deposition of γ-globulin along the glomerular capillary walls in a human kidney of a patient with Goodpasture's disease; fluorescent antibody procedure. (From Lerner, R.A., Glascock, R.J., and Dixon, F.J.: The role of antiglomerular basement membrane antibody in the pathogenesis of human glomerulonephritis, J. Exp. Med. **126**:989, 1967.)

days after the initial infection, the symptoms of the autoimmune kidney disease begin to appear.

Fluorescent antibody and histologic studies of the kidney indicate that IgG (or sometimes IgA or IgM) and C3 are deposited in a granular distribution along the glomerular basement membrane (Fig. 21-8). Activation of the complement system generates chemotaxins, which cause the entrance of PMNs into the region. Infiltration of the PMNs into the tissues contributes to the disease.

Autoimmune and alloimmune duplicates of glomerulonephritis can be produced by preparing kidney homogenates with adjuvants and using these for immunization. The passive immunization of animals with heteroantisera developed against kidney antigens causes a form of nephritis known as Masugi's glomerulonephritis. Masugi's nephritis has been provoked in most experimental animal species. The pathologic manifestations of Masugi's autoimmune, and alloimmune nephritis will vary from one species to another and are close but not exact mimics of the poststreptococcal disease. They are useful models, since streptococcal infections are not reliable incitants of glomerulonephritis in animals.

Masugi's nephritis is a closer mimic of antiglomerular basement membrane nephritis seen after unsuccessful kidney grafts than it is of poststreptococcal disease. Goodpasture's syndrome and rapidly progressive nephritis are like the Masugi disease in that the γ-globulin and complement deposits are linear.

Autologous antibodies made against exogenous nonglomerular antigens will complex in the circulation and become trapped in the capillary vessel walls of the kidney. Since complement is fixed in the reaction, anaphylatoxins and chemotaxins are released. This leads to local tissue damage. This type of glomerulonephritis is produced in serum sickness and LE and during or after infections caused by the malarial parasite, streptococci, and certain viruses.

Autoimmune glomerulonephritis is observed in both the canine and mouse models of LE and in Aleutian mink disease. These mink, valued and bred for their unique pelt color, are infected by a virus (or cell-free agent) that promotes a sharp increase in the number of plasma cells and a hypergammaglobulinemia. The infective agent is transmitted easily to young mink, which die of glomerulonephritis within the first 6 months of life. The cause of renal failure is the accumulation of virus-antigen complexes with complement in the kidney.

A virus disease of horses is responsible for an equine form of autoimmune glomerulonephritis. This disease, like Aleutian mink disease, is characterized by an intense hypergammaglobulinemia and an accumulation of antibody-virus-complement complexes in the capillary bed of the glomeruli, causing a glomerulonephritis. A cardinal symptom of the disease is a hemolytic anemia, but the exact immunologic basis of this is uncertain.

The incrimination of chronic virus infections in Aleutian mink disease and equine hemolytic anemia plus the descriptions of chronic virus infections in subacute sclerosing panencephalitis, kuru, and Jakob-Creutzfeldt disease have heightened the interest in viruses as potential causative agents of human diabetes, SLE, rheumatoid arthritis, and other chronic, immunopathologic disorders.

Rheumatoid arthritis

Rheumatoid arthritis is an inflammatory disease of the joints and connective tissue; amyloid deposition in tissues and permanent deformity of the joints may result. Despite intensive study of the microbial flora of joint fluids, of the sex differences in susceptibilities, and of nutritional and genetic factors, the cause of the rheumatoid disease remains unknown. The induction of arthritis in rats by the injection of adjuvant and the known association of arthritis in certain lower animals with bacterial infection have done little to clarify the cause of human rheumatoid disease. Interest in this disease as a potential allergic disease was strengthened by the discovery that sera of rheumatoid patients would agglutinate erythrocytes coated with subagglutinating quantities of antibody. The agglutinating agent is known as rheumatoid factor (RF).

RF is a 19S immunoglobulin compatible in all respects with IgM. In the patient's sera RF may circulate as a 22S complex that, on dissociation, yields a molecule of IgM and one or perhaps as many as six molecules of IgG. RF is an unusual IgM antibody in only one respect—its relative lack of specificity for human IgG: it will react with rabbit IgG and that of other species. The original tests for RF depended on its ability to enhance erythrocyte agglutination with rabbit antibody; later erythrocytes or latex particles bearing pooled human IgG were used as the antigen. The sensitivities of these tests differ; in various study series between 50% and 95% of rheumatoid arthritic patients had positive RF tests. Such findings suggest that RF is an antibody to an altered form of IgG which usually is not found in the circulation.

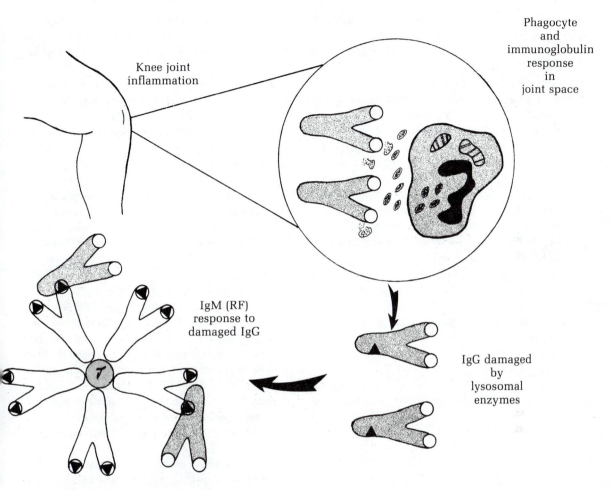

Fig. 21-9. One hypothesis for the origin of RF is related to formation of damaged IgG in infectious joint disease. RF attaches to the Fc section of the IgG molecule.

In tests for RF pooled human IgG is the usual antigen coated on erythrocytes or latex particles. If IgG from a specific individual is used as the antigen, many RF sera, positive according to the pooled antigen test, become negative. In a variation of the test based on inhibition of the agglutination reaction between RF and the pooled IgG antigen, the IgG from certain (but not all) individuals will inhibit the agglutination. This is the original method used to determine that all human IgG molecules are not antigenically identical; this test became the basis for the classification of the IgG-Gm allotypes. The reaction of RF with

the Gm determinants, which are in the Fc portion of IgG, may mean that RF reacts with polysaccharide determinants. This would account for its lack of specificity and IgM character.

Even though inflammatory cells, lymphocytes, and plasma cells are detectable in synovial tissue, and even though RF is present in sera, an autoimmune origin of rheumatic fever has been difficult to prove unequivocally. One conjectured mechanism is essentially as follows (Fig. 21-9). An initial joint inflammation possibly arises from some infectious agent. This stimulates an immunoglobulin response against the pathogen, and antibody of the IgG type is formed. The reaction of this immunoglobulin with the organisms releases (from the complement involved) chemotactic and anaphylatoxic reagents. These add to the inflammatory reaction with the release of lysosomal enzymes, which damage the IgG antibody and convert it to a neoantigen. This sparks an immune response of the IgM type, the product of which is RF. When RF reacts with the IgG, additional chemotactic and anaphylatoxic events occur that perpetuate the inflammation, the continued damage of IgG, and a continued recycling of these events. The theory seems quite logical, but unfortunately there is little evidence for or against it. If the facts do correspond with this theory, it will be confirmed that RF is not the direct cause of rheumatoid arthritis. Transfusion of blood with high levels of RF does not provoke rheumatoid arthritis, nor does the direct infusion of RF into joint fluid. RF is produced in the tissues of the joint, and RF-IgM-complement complexes can be detected in rheumatoid synovia. Whether these are the result or the cause of the joint disease is conjectural, but they most certainly are not the cause of other tissue aspects of rheumatoid arthritis, for example, subcutaneous nodules. There is no evidence as yet that cellular hypersensitivity contributes to this disease.

SLE

SLE or LE is a disease with a presumed immunologic cause. SLE is four times more common in women than in men, and many patients are HLA-B8 positive. The cardinal external sign of the disease is a red rash across the nose and upper cheeks, from which the disease gets its name (*lupus erythematosus,* the red wolf). More serious internal lesions involve the kidney, the blood vessels, the blood cells, and the heart. Several immunologic phenomena are associated with the disease, including hypergammaglobulinemia and hypocomplementemia.

One of the first immunologic changes noted was LE cell formation, first described in 1948. The LE cell is a neutrophil containing a large, pale

staining structure that often fills the cytoplasm of the phagocyte. Occasionally the LE body is not engulfed but can be seen free in stained blood films, often surrounded by neutrophils, whose dark staining nuclei produce a rosettelike arrangement. Microcinematography has revealed how these structures develop. If serum from an SLE patient is mixed with whole blood, it will be noted that the nucleus of certain white blood cells undergoes a sudden explosive swelling and loses its dark staining quality, becoming paler and spherical. Unaffected phagocytes approach the LE body, strip away its cytoplasm, and engulf it to become LE cells. Rosette formation results when the LE body is not engulfed but is surrounded by viable neutrophils, each of which apparently is competing with the others for phagocytosis of the deranged LE nucleus (Fig. 21-10).

The LE factor in serum responsible for these changes has been definitely identified as an anti-deoxyribonucleoprotein (anti-DNA) of the IgG isotype. This antibody will attach to nuclei from almost any source in agreement with the known nonspecificity of anti-DNA antibodies. LE cell formation is a useful diagnostic aid when positive, but many patients produce negative tests because of the difficulty in performing and interpreting LE cell tests. Consequently fluorescent antinuclear antibody (FANA) or other ANA tests have supplemented LE cell procedures. The human ANA, although usually an IgG, may be an IgM or IgA.

FANA in sera of SLE patients is identified by the indirect fluorescent antibody procedure. Yeast cells, calf thymus cells, or other mammalian cells are used as a source of DNA and prepared on a slide. This is developed with the patient's serum and then with a fluorescent antihuman γ-globulin. When whole cells are used, the pattern of staining will be distinctive from one patient to another. Staining of the perimeter of the nucleus indicates the serum is dominated by an anti-DNA antibody. A homogeneous staining of the nucleus indicates nucleoprotein (DNA-histone) staining. Fluorescence in the nucleolus is characteristic of an antibody specificity for RNA, and a speckled pat-

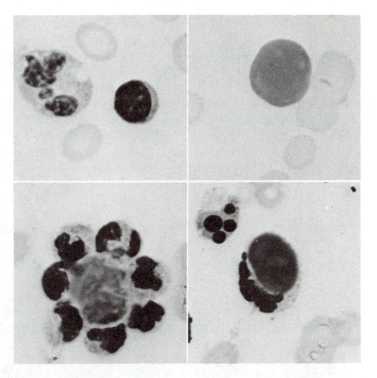

Fig. 21-10. LE cell test. Upper left quadrant, a normal neutrophil and lymphocyte; upper right, a free LE body; lower left, a rosette; and lower right, a single LE cell. (From Anderson, J.R., Buchanan, W.W., and Goudie, R.B.: Autoimmunity, Springfield, Ill., 1967, Charles C Thomas, Publisher.)

tern reflects the presence of an antibody to an extractable nuclear antigen (ENA).

ENA is not a single antigen; rather it is a mixture of perhaps as many as 20 antigens, which are acidic. Few of these have been characterized chemically other than for the presence of dsDNA, dsRNA, ssDNA, or ssRNA and of protein. Two ENAs that appear to have a high degree of specificity for SLE are the SM and MA antigens. SM is an acidic glycoprotein with a molecular weight of less than 150,000. Anti-SM is found in 24% of all SLE patients. Patients with severe SLE often have antibodies that react with the MA antigen.

Other antibodies found in SLE sera react with nRNP (nuclear ribonucleoprotein), PCNA (proliferating cell nuclear antigen), SS-A and SS-B (Sjögren's syndrome antigens A and B), H1, H3, and H4 (histone antigens), and others. Investigators are actively searching for an antigen or panel of antigens that will be of diagnostic significance for SLE.

In addition to the presence of antibodies to dsDNA, SLE patients have a high frequency (up to 90% in some studies) of circulating immune complexes. Removal of these in the kidney accounts for the glomerulonephritis characteristic of the disease (Fig. 21-11). About 75% of SLE patients will develop hypocomplementemia.

The success of immunosuppressive treatment of SLE with cyclophosphamide, azathioprine, and corticosteroids has underscored the immunologic nature of this disease. Although a viral origin is still possible (with viruses of the dsDNA type), current opinion is shifting to a loss of Ts cells

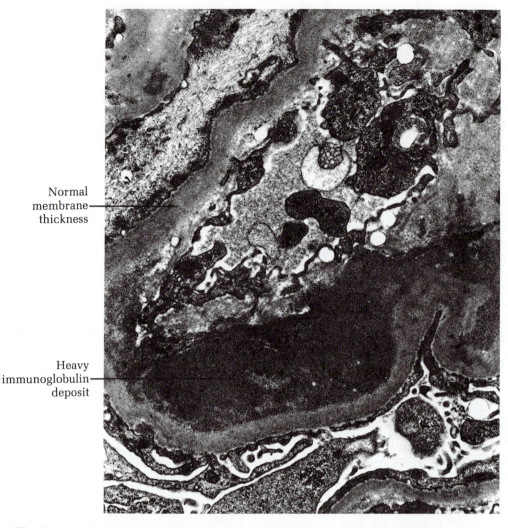

Normal
membrane
thickness

Heavy
immunoglobulin
deposit

Fig. 21-11. An immunoglobulin deposit in the basement membrane of a patient with SLE as seen by the electron microscope. (Courtesy Dr. E. Adelstein.)

as the basis for this disease. This hypothesis has received strong support from studies of murine SLE.

The best animal model of SLE is the NZB/NZW progeny that result from mating of New Zealand black (NZB) and New Zealand white (NZW) mice. These NZB/NZW hybrids develop antibodies versus dsDNA, ssDNA, dsRNA, ssRNA, and other ENA antigens. Virtually 100% of these mice develop and die of immune complex glomerulonephritis. In the first few months of life NZB/NZW mice appear completely normal, but this masks a gradual loss of Ts cell function, which ultimately explodes in the form of undesired B cell activities—the numerous autoantibodies (Fig. 21-12) and macroglobulinemia that precede death. The more recently described MLR mouse is also an excellent model of SLE, showing much the

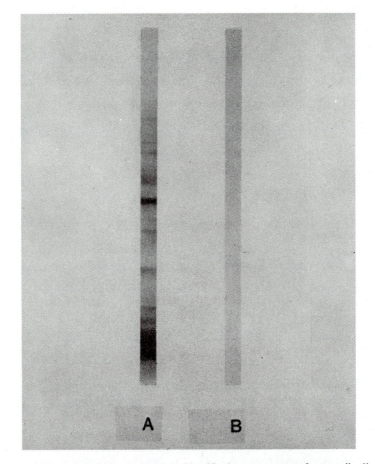

Fig. 21-12. An immunoperoxidase test used to identify the appearance of autoantibodies to RNP. The RNP antigen was separated by electrophoresis on both gels. Sera from an aged (**A**) and young MLR mouse (**B**) were incubated with the antigen on the electrophoretic strips. Then peroxidase-labeled antimouse globulin was used to localize the antibody in the aged mouse serum. The young mouse was negative in this test. (Courtesy Dr. K. Wise.)

same history as the New Zealand hybrids. These mice develop a thymotoxic antibody, an IgM, which reacts with 98% of mouse thymocytes and behaves like an anti-Thy serum. Such antibodies contribute to the loss of Ts cells and allow expression of undesired antibody responses.

Another excellent model for LE is the canine model, in which characteristics of SLE such as glomerulonephritis, positive LE cells, and antibodies to nuclear antigens and DNA are present.

These conditions are accompanied by a host of other physiologic abnormalities, including anemia, thrombocytopenia, polyarteritis, thyroiditis, and a chronic viral infection. A strong possibility exists that many of the symptoms of the autoimmune diseases in these dogs are the direct result of a viral infection or an indirect effect of a virus on lymphoid cells. Aleutian mink disease has a viral cause yet produces many of the immunopathologic aspects typical of SLE.

Drug-induced SLE has been associated with chemotherapy with several compounds, including hydralazine, penicillin, oral contraceptives, and procainamide. Although this form of LE may appear within a few weeks after therapy is initiated, a prodromal period of several months is more common. Anti-dsDNA is less common in drug-induced SLE than in the spontaneous disease.

Graves' disease

A thyroid disease more common than Hashimoto's disease is Graves' disease, a form of hyperthyroidism. The evidence, accumulated at a rapid pace after 1956, indicates that the hyperthyroidism associated with Graves' disease is caused by a long-acting thyroid stimulator (LATS), an immunoglobulin found in the sera of nearly 85% of all patients. Purified IgG that contains this LATS activity has been further analyzed with the discovery that the Fab and F(ab')$_2$ portions of the molecule contain the LATS activity. The LATS autoantibody is a type of enhancing antibody that operates at the cellular level, much like the thyroid stimulatory hormone, to stimulate thyroid hormone release and thyrotoxicosis.

Autoimmune skin diseases

Three serious diseases of the skin now are recognized to have a strong autoimmune component. These diseases are pemphigus vulgaris, bullous pemphigoid, and dermatitis herpetiformis. The first is characterized by a separation of the epidermis from the underlying intraepithelial cells and bullae (blister) formation. Fluorescent antibody staining for immunoglobulin and complement component C3 has revealed the presence of both in affected areas of the skin. In pemphigus vulgaris it is thought that the autoantibody, an IgG, may be specific for the intercellular cement substance and that fixation of complement results in chemotaxis and a self-destructive attack on the epidermis.

In the case of bullous pemphigoid, autoantibodies directed against the dermal epithelial junction of the skin can be found circulating in the blood and deposited in the skin. C3 also is demonstrable in the skin. Evidence for an activation of the alternate complement pathway is based on the presence of C3 proactivator and properdin in the dermal basement membranes.

The third skin disease, dermatitis herpetiformis, has many features that suggest an autoimmune origin, but these are inconsistent from patient to patient. Deposits of IgA at the dermal-epidermal junction are seen more frequently than are deposits of IgG and IgM. C3 is found frequently, but it is difficult to correlate it with the presence of IgA, which cannot fix complement. Circulating autoantibodies are not detectable in these patients.

Other diseases

Antibodies to tissue antigens have been recognized in a long list of human ailments, including Addison's disease (adrenal disease), Sjögren's syndrome (keratoconjunctivitis), Felty's syndrome (a characteristic type of leukopenia), pernicious anemia, gastrointestinal disease, celiac disease, diabetes, and cirrhosis of the liver. In certain of these diseases (for example, Hashimoto's disease) it is suspected that autoantibodies serve as a convenient diagnostic support when present, but this does not reflect any role of the autoantibody in the origin or continuation of the disease. For most of these conditions it simply is not possible to make any conclusions other than stating that autoantibodies often are associated with the disease.

BIBLIOGRAPHY

Aarli, J.A., and Tönder, O.: Immunological aspects of neurological diseases, Basel, 1980, S. Karger, AG, Medical and Scientific Publishers.

Albini, B., Brentjens, J.R., and Andres, G.A.: The immunopathology of the kidney, Chicago, 1979, Year Book Medical Publishers, Inc.

Asquith, P., editor: Immunology of the gastrointestinal tract, Edinburgh, 1979, Churchill Livingstone.

Behan, P.O., and Currie, S.: Clinical neuroimmunology, London, 1978, W.B. Saunders Co., Ltd.

Beutner, E., Chorzelski, T.P., and Bean, S.F., editors: Immunopathology of the skin, ed. 2, New York, 1979, John Wiley & Sons, Inc.

Christensen, P., Schalen, C., and Holm, S.E.: Re-evaluation of experiments intended to demonstrate immunological cross-reactions between mammalian tissues and streptococci, Prog. Allergy **26:**1, 1979.

Cohen, S., Ward, P.A., and McCluskey, R.T., editors: Mechanisms of immunopathology, New York, 1979, John Wiley & Sons, Inc.

Constantinides, P., and others, editors: Immunity and atherosclerosis, London, 1980, Academic Press, Inc. (London), Ltd.

Dau, P.C.: Plasmapheresis and the immunobiology of myasthenia gravis, New York, 1979, John Wiley & Sons, Inc.

Davison, A.N., and Cuzner, M.L., editors: The suppression of experimental allergic encephalomyelitis and multiple sclerosis, New York, 1980, Academic Press, Inc.

Day, E.D.: Myelin basic protein, Contemp. Top. Mol. Biol. **8:**1, 1981.

Dhindsa, D.S., and Schumacher, G.F.B., editors: Immunological aspects of infertility and fertility regulation, New York, 1980, Elsevier/North-Holland, Inc.

Eddleston, A.L.W.F., Weber, J.C.P., and Williams, R., editors: Immune reactions in liver disease, London, 1979, Pitman Medical Publishing Co., Ltd.

Fellner, M.J.: Immunology of skin diseases, New York, 1980, Elsevier/North-Holland, Inc.

Friedlaender, M.H.: Allergy and immunology of the eye, New York, 1979, Harper & Row Publishers, Inc.

Fukase, M., editor: Systemic lupus erythematosus, Baltimore, 1980, University Park Press.

Gell, P.G.H., Coombs, R.R.A., and Lachmann, P.J., editors: Clinical aspects of immunology, ed. 3, Oxford, 1974, Blackwell Scientific Publications, Ltd.

Hearn, J.P., editor: Immunologic aspects of reproduction and fertility control, Baltimore, 1980, University Park Press.

Krakauer, R.A., and Cathcart, M.K., editors: Immunoregulation and autoimmunity, New York, 1980, Elsevier/North-Holland, Inc.

McCluskey, R.T., and Andres, G.A., editors: Immunologically mediated renal disease, New York, 1978, Marcel Dekker, Inc.

McGiven, A.R.: Immunological investigation of renal disease, Edinburgh, 1980, Churchill Livingstone.

Miescher, P.A., and Müller-Eberhard, H.J., editors: Textbook of immunopathology, ed. 2, New York, 1976, Grune & Stratton, Inc.

Miescher, P.A., and others, editors: The Menarini series on immunopathology, vol. 1, New York, 1978, Springer-Verlag New York, Inc.

Neuwelt, E.A., and Clark, W.K.: Clinical aspects of neuroimmunology, Baltimore, 1978, Williams & Wilkins Co.

Okabayashi, A., and Kondo, Y., editors: Masugi nephritis and its immunopathologic implications, New York, 1980, Igaku-Shoin Medical Publishers, Inc.

Parker, C.W., editor: Clinical immunology, vols. 1 and 2, Philadelphia, 1980, W.B. Saunders Co.

Petz, L.D., and Garratty, G.: Acquired hemolytic anemias, New York, 1980, Churchill Livingstone, Inc.

Pinchera, A., and others, editors: Autoimmune aspects of endocrine disorders, London, 1980, Academic Press, Inc. (London), Ltd.

Porter, D.D., Larsen, A.E., and Porter, H.G.: Aleutian disease of mink, Adv. Immunol. **29:**261, 1980.

Read, S.E., and Zabriskie, J.B.: Streptococcal diseases and the immune response, New York, 1980, Academic Press, Inc.

Rose, N.R., Bigazzi, P.E., and Warner, N.L., editors: Genetic control of autoimmune disease, New York, 1978, Elsevier/North-Holland, Inc.

Shiokawa, Y., Abe, T., and Yamauchi, Y., editors: New horizons in rheumatoid arthritis, Amsterdam, 1981, Excerpta Medica.

Silverstein, A.M., and O'Connor, G.R., editors: Immunology and immunopathology of the eye, New York, 1979, Masson Publishing USA, Inc.

Steffen, C., and Ludwig, H., editors: Clinical immunology and allergology, Amsterdam, 1981, Elsevier/North Holland Biomedical Press.

Talal, N., editor: Autoimmunity; genetic, immunologic, virologic and clinical aspects, New York, 1978, Academic Press, Inc.

Weigle, W.O.: Analysis of autoimmunity through experimental models of thyroiditis and allergic encephalomyelitis, Adv. Immunol. **30:**159, 1980.

Wilson, C.B., Brenner, B.M., and Stein, J.H., editors: Immunologic mechanisms of renal disease, New York, 1979, Churchill Livingstone, Inc.

Wright, R.: Immunology of gastrointestinal and liver disease, London, 1977, Edward Arnold (Publishers), Ltd.

Zabriskie, J.B., Engle, M.A., and Villarreal, H., Jr.: Clinical immunology of the heart, New York, 1981, John Wiley & Sons, Inc.

SITUATION: LE AND COMPLEMENT

Steve is a 34-year-old assistant professor of microbiology whose specialty is pathogenic my-cology. His wife, Janice, has a B.S. degree in microbiology and volunteered to transfer Steve's fungus cultures for him while he was away for a week at the mycology society meetings. The transfer room was illuminated with both visible and ultraviolet light. Janice failed to turn off the ultraviolet light during the transfer and received a severe burn. Much of the burned area, including the eyes and hands, underwent normal healing, but the facial burn, especially across the cheeks and nose, persisted. On his return from the conference, her husband requested that she visit a local physician, who offered LE as a possible diagnosis.

Questions

1. What method(s) can be used to measure total complement activity in patient sera?
2. What would be the advantages in measuring certain specific components rather than total complement activity?
3. What method(s) can be used to measure the individual complement components?
4. What results would be anticipated from serum complement studies of this patient if LE actually were the diagnosis?

Solution

Total complement levels in sera are determined by hemolytic titrations. Other cytolytic tests could be used, since cytolysis requires the full cooperation of all nine complement components, but hemolytic titrations have obvious advantages. The erythrocyte membrane is very susceptible to complement lysis, technicians are generally familiar with the handling of erythrocytes in serologic tests, and hemolysis can be estimated visually or determined quantitatively by spectrophotometric means. Normally a suspension of sensitized erythrocytes is exposed to complement in a fluid system, but a radial diffusion system also can be used and is a semiquantitative method.

The reagents required for the hemolytic determination of complement are sheep erythrocytes sensitized with an optimal amount of anti–sheep red blood cell serum in a suitable buffer. This is known as hemolysin (or amboceptor). The buffer must contain free Mg^{2+}. Serum from the patient is used as the complement source in the test. Because of the sensitivity of complement to heat, special attention must be given to serum collection and storage. Blood should be allowed to clot for not more than 30 minutes at room temperature, followed by not more than 60 minutes at 4° C. The serum should be collected by centrifugation at 4° C and titrated immediately or stored at −70° C until evaluated.

For assay the serum in final dilutions ranging from 1:10 to 1:50 normally is added to the sensitized erythrocytes and evaluated against 100% lysis and normal cell (0% lysis) controls. The dilution of complement that will lyse 50% of the cells (the CH_{50} unit) is the basis for the expression of complement activity in the serum. Normal values range between 20 and 40 CH_{50}/ml.

In the radial diffusion test agarose containing sensitized sheep cells is poured onto a plate. Small wells are created in the gel film by removing agarose plugs. Samples of sera are added to the wells, and the plate is incubated for 1 hour at 37° C and overnight at room temperature. The hemolytic zone is graded only as normal, low, or absent based on comparison with standards.

Assays for total hemolytic activity do not reveal whether the alternate or classic pathway is responsible for lowered complement activity. Neither would this assist in the identification of a genetic deficiency or other loss of a specific component. Individual complement components can be measured in hemolytic assays using commercially available reagents. In general, these tests require sensitized erythrocytes and an excess of all the complement components except the one to be quantitated in the patient's serum. This method is not especially useful for measuring the amount of the components above C3 in the alternate pathway, for which quantitative radial immunodiffusion is the preferred method. (See Chapter 15.) This technique can be applied to C1 and its units, C4, C3, factor B, and properdin by using commercially produced reagents. Comparative assays for C4 and C3 are always of interest. If C4 remains high in the presence of depressed C3, then alternate pathway activation is indicated.

In the patient described the total complement and the C3 levels were depressed. The C4 level was also low. Radial immunodiffusion indicated a deficiency in factor B. These results are compatible with a diagnosis of LE. In one study total complement and C3 levels were lowered in 13 patients. Of these, 12 had a low C4 level, and 8 had a low factor B level, indicative of a complement depletion by both the alternate and classic pathways.

References

Frank, M.M., and Atkinson, J.P.: Complement in clinical medicine, Disease-A-Month, p. 1, January 1975.

Rose, N.R., and Friedman, H., editors: Manual of clinical immunology, ed. 2, Washington, D.C., 1980, American Society of Microbiology.

CHAPTER

22

IMMUNODEFICIENCY

GLOSSARY

ADA Adenosine deaminase.

agammaglobulinemia A condition in which all the immunoglobulins are absent from the serum.

ataxia telangiectasia A loss of muscle coordination accompanied by blood vessel dilation combined with deficits in IgA production and T lymphocytes.

Bruton's agammaglobulinemia A sex-linked congenital loss of B cells and hence immunoglobulins.

CGD Chronic granulomatous disease.

CHD Chédiak-Higashi disease.

Chédiak-Higashi disease A disease based on faulty phagocytic destruction of parasites, related to lysosomal abnormalities.

chronic granulomatous disease A sex-linked hereditary disease resulting in faulty phagocytic destruction of ingested parasites.

chronic mucocutaneous candidiasis A T cell deficiency disease resulting in a chronic *Candida* infection.

DiGeorge's syndrome A birth defect in the embryonic development of the thymus, resulting in losses of immune competence related to T lymphocytes.

dysgammaglobulinemia An imbalance from the normal concentration of the immunoglobulins or a malfunction of one or more immunoglobulins.

H chain disease A disease in which incomplete immunoglobulins consisting of H chains, or parts thereof, are synthesized.

HMP Hexose monophosphate.

hypogammaglobulinemia The opposite of hypergammaglobulinemia, or decreased levels of γ-globulin in plasma.

NBT Nitroblue tetrazolium.

neonatal hypogammaglobulinemia A transient hypogammaglobulinemia affecting all newborn infants.

nitroblue tetrazolium A dye used in a reductase test to measure the oxidative activity of phagocytes.

Nezelof's syndrome A genetic failure of T lymphocyte development and hence cell-mediated hypersensitivity.

PNP Purine nucleoside phosphorylase.

SCID Severe combined immunodeficiency disease.

severe combined immunodeficiency disease Immunodeficiency of both T and B cells.

Swiss-type agammaglobulinemia A genetic disease resulting in deficiencies in both T and B lymphocyte functions.

thymic aplasia DiGeorge's syndrome.

Wiskott-Aldrich syndrome A sex-linked genetic disease with combined losses of B and T lymphocytes and especially of IgM production.

Resistance to infectious disease is the expression of the body's natural and acquired defense forces to cope with internal and external antigenic threats to its well-being. Just as cuts and scratches of the skin can create a breach in the natural defense system and open the body to infection, so also can fissures in other parts of the defense system—phagocytosis, immunoglobulin synthesis, T cell activities, and the complement system—render the body susceptible to otherwise easily repelled organisms. Immunodeficiencies may arise from a genetic inability to produce a required cell or cell product (primary immunodeficiency), or they may be acquired, in which case the true cause of the condition may escape identification. Excessive proliferation of one kind of immunocompetent cell also may result in an increased susceptibility to disease, presumably by creating an imbalance in the defense system.

In the following discussion immunodeficiencies related to B lymphocytes, T lymphocytes, and the phagocytic cell system are considered separately and, in the case of the B and T cells, as severe combined immunodeficiencies (Table 22-1). This is not meant to minimize the interaction of these cell systems, which is necessary for a complete immune response. The participation of a healthy phagocytic system and T cell population for the perfect functioning of B cells, at least in regard to the T-dependent antigens, is well recognized and is discussed in Chapters 4 and 5.

IMMUNODEFICIENCIES INVOLVING LYMPHOCYTES
Immunodeficiencies involving B lymphocytes

Diagnosis. Assessment of B lymphocyte functioning is based on the past and present ability of the patient to produce immunoglobulins. Preexisting B cell functions are evaluated on the basis of the current serum immunoglobulin concentration by radial immunodiffusion tests for IgG, IgM, and IgA. Ordinary serum immunoelectrophoresis may be performed first as a screening method, but ultimately the individual globulins must be quantitated. A history of successful immunization against toxoids such as those from tetanus and diphtheria or of bacterial vaccines such as pertussis (but not BCG for tuberculosis) signifies a satis-

Table 22-1. Immunodeficiencies involving B and T lymphocytes*

Condition	Characteristics
B lymphocyte deficiencies	
Transient neonatal agammaglobulinemia	Does not involve IgG; normal; self-correcting
Congenital agammaglobulinemia	
Bruton's	Sex linked; involves all immunoglobulin classes
Common variable hypogammaglobulinemia	Involves one or more immunoglobulin classes
Acquired immunoglobulin deficiency	Often associated with RES malignancy
T lymphocyte deficiencies	
Nezelof's syndrome	True congenital failure in thymic embryogenesis
DiGeorge's syndrome	Nongenetic failure in thymic embryogenesis
Partial T cell loss	Present in leprosy, chronic mucocutaneous candidiasis, and other infections
Severe combined immunodeficiency disease (SCID)	
Sex-linked agammaglobulinemia	Not to be confused with Bruton's agammaglobulinemia
Swiss-type agammaglobulinemia	Not sex linked
Wiskott-Aldrich syndrome	Depressed IgM level
Ataxia telangiectasia	Lowered IgA and IgE levels

*WHO recognizes 17 forms of primary specific immunodeficiency (WHO Tech. Rep. Ser. **630:**5, 1978).

factory B cell system. Antibody titers should be determined by specific serologic tests. In the absence of an immunization record, past humoral immunity can be judged on the basis of normal levels of the anti-A or anti-B blood group hemagglutinins or antibodies to common bacteria or their products. *Escherichia coli* and streptolysin O are useful antigens in these tests.

The current status of the humoral immune system can be evaluated by the response to antigens not likely to be encountered in ordinary life. For this the rare bacteriophage ΦX174, bacterial flagellin, keyhole-limpet hemocyanin, or other antigens are used. Concurrent B cell evaluation should include an enumeration of circulating B cells, accomplished by identifying Fc receptors on lymphocytes or the presence of surface immunoglobulins by immunofluorescence. B cells also should be purified from the peripheral blood and examined for their capacity to respond to mitogens. PWM is one of the best activators of these cells, but PHA or other lectins can be selected.

B cell deficiency disease. The critical product of the B lymphocyte is ultimately immunoglobulin. Any interruption in cell differentiation and maturation from the level of the stem cells in the bone marrow to the mature functioning plasma cells of peripherally situated lymphoid tissues will affect immunoglobulin synthesis. The earlier the

rupture in the developmental pathway, the more extensive the loss in antibody-forming capacity. Although breaks in the maturation chain of the B lymphocytes clearly lead to immunoglobulin deficiencies, there is increasing evidence that T cells have a far broader regulatory role on the activities of B cells than previously suspected. Obviously losses of Th lymphocytes or an overabundance of Ts lymphocytes also could result in impaired immunoglobulin performance.

Although the term *agammaglobulinemia* is well entrenched in the immunologic literature, traces of γ-globulin, perhaps only 5 to 500 μg/ml, can be found in sera of agammaglobulinemic patients. Thus *hypogammaglobulinemia* is a more exact term, but the two are used interchangeably here (Table 22-1; Fig. 22-1).

Transient neonatal agammaglobulinemia. Transient hypogammaglobulinemia of the newborn infant is the culmination of the infant's inability to synthesize significant amounts of immunoglobulin until he or she has been challenged with antigen and the inability of IgA and IgM to pass the placental barrier from mother to fetus. The total amount of γ-globulin in the serum of the newborn infant is 1044 ± 201 mg/dl, or approximately two thirds the normal adult level of 1457 ± 353 mg/dl (Fig. 22-1). Since maternal IgG can pass the placenta, the IgG level in new-

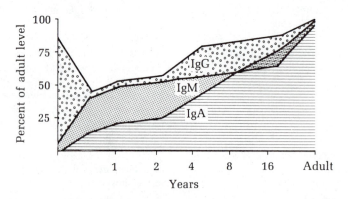

Fig. 22-1. Ontogeny of immunoglobulin formation in the human. IgG acquired by the infant transplacentally from the mother falls quickly in titer during the time that IgA and especially IgM levels are climbing. After 6 months all three immunoglobulins increase gradually toward the adult level.

born sera (1031 ± 200 mg/dl of serum) compares favorably with the adult level of 1158 ± 305 mg/dl. Neonatal levels of IgM and IgA average 11% and 1%, respectively, of the adult levels of 99 ± 27 mg/dl and 200 ± 61 mg/dl. IgD is difficult to detect in the sera of newborn infants, and IgE is found at approximately 15% of the adult level of 225 μg/ml.

After birth the infant's IgG level falls steadily for approximately 3 months. Between 3 and 6 months of age, when IgG is at its low ebb (300 to 600 mg/dl), the infant displays the greatest sensitivity to infectious disease. After the third month of life the IgG level increases steadily so that about 75% of the adult level is achieved by 3 years of age. IgM is synthesized earlier in infancy than IgG and increases in concentration so rapidly after birth that 50% of the adult level is reached within the first 6 months, whereas IgA does not achieve 50% of the adult level until the child is 1 year of age. At 5 years of age the IgD level is still one third that of adults, and the IgE level reaches approximately two thirds that of adults.

Congenital agammaglobulinemia. Congenital or genetic hypogammaglobulinemia results from a permanent inability to synthesize γ-globulins. The afflicted children suffer from repeated bouts of bacterial disease, often caused by feeble pathogens. If no accompanying disorder of the T cell system is involved, hypogammaglobulinemic children will contract and recover normally from the usual viral and fungal diseases of childhood. In the preantibiotic era these children died of bacterial septicemia before it could be recognized that they were hypogammaglobulinemic. In the 1950s the development and use of broad-spectrum antibiotics kept these children alive long enough for their congenital condition to be diagnosed. Now antibiotics and passive immunization with pooled human γ-globulin allow these individuals to lead a relatively normal life.

Bruton's agammaglobulinemia. A WHO committee has recommended that "infantile sex-linked agammaglobulinemia" be used as the official name of the disease commonly known as Bruton's agammaglobulinemia or Bruton's sex-linked agammaglobulinemia. As the new name indicates, this is a disease transmitted by the mother to her male children only. The disease does not become apparent until about 6 months of age, at which time the immunity the child derived from maternal IgG has waned. These young boys then begin what will invariably develop into a series of bacterial infections involving the usual pathogens of childhood, *Hemophilus, Streptococcus, Staphylococcus, Pseudomonas,* and other less pathogenic gram-negative bacilli. These primary bacterial infections do not result in immunity and the synthesis of immunoglobulins; instead they signal that recurrences of otitis media, conjunctivitis, pneumonia, meningitis, pyoderma, and septicemia will follow. The γ-globulin concentration in these children may fall below 25 mg/dl of serum. All classes of immunoglobulins are absent or extremely low. Lymphocyte counts in peripheral blood are within the normal range, but these are T cells, not B cells.

These children respond normally to most viral diseases of childhood (for example, measles, mumps, and chickenpox) and develop a lasting immunity. Their response to chemicals that provoke contact dermatitis is normal, also indicating that their T cell system is functioning suitably. Even after intensive stimulation with antigens, plasma cells rarely are found in lymphoid tissues. All the evidence suggests that infantile sex-linked agammaglobulinemia is a total incapacity to synthesize immunoglobulins concurrent with a normal T cell responsiveness. Since all the immunoglobulin classes are involved in the deficiency, the cellular fault occurs early, possibly in the bone marrow in the formation or early stages of development of prolymphocytes.

Common variable hypogammaglobulinemia. Far more common than generalized hypogammaglobulinemia is selective or variable hypogammaglobulinemia, in which only one or a combination of immunoglobulins is missing or present in much lower than normal concentrations. This condition also is known as dysgammaglobulinemia. Individuals with selective hypogammaglobulinemia cannot always be identified by a decrease in total γ-globulin levels, since a decrease in one class of immunoglobulin may be compensated by a disproportionate hypergammaglobulinemia of another class of immunoglobulin. For example, several patients deficient in IgG and IgA have been described, but they had sufficiently increased IgM levels to have a normal total γ-globulin level. Diagnosis of selective immunoglobulinemia is best made by quantitative radial immunodiffusion analysis for the separate immunoglobulin classes, although a first clue to the diagnosis is often an abnormal immunoelectrophoretic serum profile. An increased incidence of infectious diseases is an unreliable diagnostic criterion, since single deficiencies, except when IgG is the deficient immunoglobulin, do not always lead to an increased incidence of infectious disease. Patients with dysgammaglobulinemia often display a malabsorption syndrome with a noninfectious diarrhea of variable severity. When IgG is involved, its level is usually low, often less than 500 mg/dl, but not as low as in sex-linked agammaglobulinemia. IgG levels greater than 250 mg/dl are usually adequate for protection against most bacterial infections.

Virtually all mathematically possible forms of dysgammaglobulinemia have been detected, that is, those in which only one of the immunoglobulins is missing and all the possible combinations in which two, three, or more are missing. Of the selective hypogammaglobulinemias, the most frequently recognized is that involving a familial loss of IgA. The incidence of single IgA dysgammaglobulinemia has been estimated at 1 in 500 to 3,500 persons. Both serum and secretory IgA are diminished or absent, although SC is produced. There is frequently a corresponding increase in IgM. Patients with an isolated IgA loss commonly seek medical assistance because of the associated autoimmune disease. The diseases involved include rheumatoid arthritis, LE, and thyroiditis. IgA losses also are associated with sinopulmonary disease, a feature of the deficiency which indicates

that secretory IgA is important in protecting mucous membranes. A noninfectious diarrhea is also a common feature of IgA deficiency.

Recent evidence indicates that patients with common variable immunodeficiency have normal or near normal numbers of B lymphocytes, but these cells are unable to mature to plasma cells. The origin of the condition is found in the T cell compartment, in which there is an excessive number of Ts cells or an exaggerated activity of these cells. Cocultivation of B cells from persons who form normal amounts of the immunoglobulins with T cells from the immunodeficient person results in a failure of the normal cells to produce the expected immunoglobulins. This experiment clearly indicates that the immunologic fault resides in the patient's T cell population.

SC deficiency. As was expected, a case of genetic inability to form SC eventually was discovered. The consequence of this is an inability to form secretory IgA (and IgM). Heretofore all examples of IgA insufficiency involved both serum and secretory IgA, since the plasma cell was the absentee. Now, in SC deficiency, a required epithelial cell is missing, and a more restricted loss of only secretory IgA is the result.

Acquired immunoglobulin deficiency. Immunoglobulin deficiency associated with malignancies of the RES—thymoma, chronic lymphocytic leukemia, lymphoma, and lymphosarcoma—probably results from a combined loss of a lymphoid cell's capacity to synthesize a γ-globulin and its conversion to a neoplastic state. These conditions develop during the person's lifetime and are not genetic, at least in terms of the immunoglobulin loss. Multiple myeloma is the best known example of a neoplastic malignancy in which a hypogammaglobulinemia of one class of globulin develops.

Immunodeficiencies involving T lymphocytes

Diagnosis. A history of an effective cell-mediated arm of the immune system is judged by conducting skin tests with agents that provoke traditional delayed hypersensitive skin reactions in the majority of normal adults. Mumps vaccine, PPD or OT, trichophytin, candidin, or streptokinase-streptodornase can be used for this purpose. In certain geographic areas histoplasmin and coccidioidin were useful in the past. A history of a normal recovery from viral infections or BCG immunization is also helpful. Since smallpox vaccination is no longer required in the United States, this monitor cannot be used much longer, and a history of successful BCG vaccination is probably most applicable to foreign-born patients.

The contemporary status of T cells can be evaluated on the basis of T cell enumeration by the sheep erythrocyte rosette method and by the in vitro transformation of T cells exposed to Con A or in MLC. The latter is the more important of the two, since it reflects the functional capacity of the cells. The ability of a person to become dermally sensitized by a single exposure to 0.05 ml of 30% dinitrochlorobenzene should be determined. This will evoke a contact dermatitis in greater than 95% of T cell–sufficient persons. This is determined by the dermal application of 0.05 ml of a 0.1% solution of the chemical 14 days after the sensitizing exposure. Special enzyme studies for adenosine deaminase (ADA) or nucleoside phosphorylase also are useful diagnostic criteria.

T lymphocyte immunodeficiency disease. The contemporary interest in the T lymphocyte and its contribution to immunity is centered on those human illnesses associated with a loss of only the T lymphocyte. Until recently it was believed there were only two such examples: Nezelof's and DiGeorge's syndromes. More recently a series of acquired T cell defects has been encountered, including leprosy and chronic mucocutaneous candidiasis, which lack the proliferative aspects of Hodgkin's disease and the leukemias (Table 22-1; Fig. 22-2).

Nezelof's syndrome. Infants with Nezelof's syndrome are athymic by virtue of an autosomal

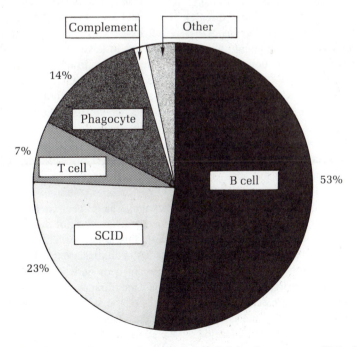

Fig. 22-2. This pie diagram illustrates that pure B cell deficiencies represent 53% of the human immunodeficiencies, T cells only 7%, SCIDs 23%, and phagocytic deficiencies 14%. Complement and undeciphered deficiencies represent less than 3%.

recessive trait whose inheritance prevents normal lymphoid development of the gland. Since the connective tissue of the gland is reasonably intact, the defect does not reside in embryogenesis of the thymus gland per se from the third and fourth pharyngeal pouches but in its fulfillment as a lymphoid organ. Consequently the block in cellular development resides in or near the stem cell level and its inability to generate the lymphocytes destined to become T cells. Children with Nezelof's syndrome generate typical germinal centers in the far cortical, or B cell, regions of their lymph nodes, produce plasma cells, and have a reasonably normal immunoglobulin response. However, the lymphoid development of the paracortical and medullary regions of lymph nodes, the T cell regions, is markedly restricted. This is demonstrated early in infancy by the development of infectious diseases that are resisted primarily by a suitable T cell activity: *Candida albicans* infections and those by other yeasts or fungi and severe, even fatal, chickenpox or a fatal outcome from smallpox vaccination. Respiratory disease caused by the feebly pathogenic *Pneumocystis carinii* and by bacteria is also prominent. A high incidence of malignancy also is noted in these unfortunate children.

Acquired T cell defects. Although Nezelof's syndrome is the sole example of an isolated T cell defect with a direct genetic origin, several forms of acquired T cell defects are known. One of these, the DiGeorge syndrome, closely mimics Nezelof's syndrome. Both are detectable in the very young infant; both are the result of aplasia of the lymphoid elements of the thymus and the effects that this has on the secondary lymphoid tissues. Infants with either disease respond normally to immunization with toxoids or killed bacterial vaccines and yet fail to resist viruses and fungi.

DiGeorge's syndrome. DiGeorge's syndrome is the result of an accidental failure in embryogenesis of the third and fourth branchial pouches and is not a familial, inherited disease like Nezelof's syndrome. In the DiGeorge form of congenital thymic hypoplasia, abnormalities of the aortic arch, the mandible, the ear, and the parathyroid may accompany those of the thymic gland, since all these tissues have a common embryonic origin. Of these accessory deficits, that of the parathyroid gland is the most important from a diagnostic viewpoint. The parathyroid gland is the regulatory organ for blood calcium. During fetal life the level of this mineral in fetal blood is regulated in part by the maternal parathyroid hormone. After birth, when this is no longer possible, the infant progresses toward a condition of hypocalcemia that is soon expressed as an involuntary rigid muscular contraction (tetany). Restoration of the blood calcium level by calcium or parathyroid hormone relieves this condition but of course can do nothing to restore thymic functioning. DiGeorge's syndrome is not a genetic disease; its cause is unknown. It may arise from an intrauterine infection. Presumably this infection would occur before the fourteenth week of gestation, when the development of the involved tissues ordinarily begins.

Chronic mucocutaneous candidiasis. Several conditions are known that involve only a partial T cell loss. One of the first infectious diseases recognized to have an attendant defect in the T cell system was chronic mucocutaneous candidiasis. The etiologic agent of this disease, a yeast, is a relatively feeble pathogen and a common part of the normal flora of the birth canal. As a consequence, neonates not infrequently develop mild infections with this yeast. Candidiasis (also known as moniliasis) also can be seen as an extensive and severe disease in persons with a thymus defect. Recurrent serious infections with *Candida albicans* have been noted in patients with DiGeorge's or Nezelof's syndrome and in patients with thymoma. Patients with chronic mucocutaneous candidiasis exhibit extensive destruction of the nail beds and persistent infections of the mucous membranes and the skin. The normal features of the skin may be almost totally obliterated by the serous exudate, crust, and granuloma formation of the affected regions. Patients with this disease do not respond to dermal injections of *Candida* organisms, and in vitro tests of lymphocytes from these patients reveal their inability to produce lymphokines. The cellular defect probably is not identical in all these patients; some may have a generalized T cell defect and others a specific *Candida* organism–related defect.

Leprosy. The cause of leprosy clearly is established as *Mycobacterium leprae,* and the disease is divided into two easily recognized clinical forms: lepromatous and tuberculoid leprosy. In the former the disease is progressive; the bacterial population is high and increases steadily with an associated increase in the necrotic destruction of tissue, and when untreated, it offers a bleak prognosis. On the other hand, tuberculoid leprosy has a better prognosis; there is less tissue destruction and a lower bacillary load. Diagnostic skin testing of persons with leprosy using lepromin, an extract of human tissue containing *M. leprae,* has revealed that those with the tuberculoid form of the disease give the typical delayed skin reaction, whereas those with lepromatous leprosy are more often than not unreactive to lepromin. Since bacteriologic and histologic evidence can confirm that both types of patients have leprosy, the unresponsiveness of those with the lepromatous disease requires an explanation.

This explanation recently has been discovered. Patients with lepromatous leprosy have depleted paracortical and medullary regions in their lymph nodes; their lymphocytes are unresponsive to mitogens such as PHA or *M. leprae* antigens in vitro and fail to produce lymphokines in culture. A recent study has revealed that the T cell population in the peripheral circulation of persons with lepromatous leprosy (but not those with tuberculoid leprosy) is depressed. The degree of this T cell loss is correlated directly with the bacillary load. It is tempting to conclude that the bacteria or products of the leprosy bacillus specifically destroy the T cells which might protect the patient against the disease, but more experimentation is needed before this can be proved. It is interesting that patients with lepromatous leprosy have about twice the B cell population of those with the tuberculoid disease, but since immunoglobulins contribute so little to protection and recovery from leprosy, this is of little benefit to them.

Severe combined immunodeficiency diseases (SCID)

Diagnosis. The diagnosis of severe combined immunodeficiency diseases (SCID) relies on the recognition of both B and T cell failures, as just described. SCIDs are those in which there is a decided loss in both B and T lymphocyte functions. As a consequence of this superimposed loss of humoral and cellular immunity, survival beyond infancy until recently was rare. Persons with combined immunodeficiency diseases have an extraordinarily high incidence of infectious disease and malignancy associated with an abbreviated life expectancy.

It is recognized now that there are many variants of this condition. In some only a partial loss of T cell functions can be identified; in others the loss appears almost total. Specific enzyme abnormalities may or may not be identified. Similar inconsistencies may be observed in the immunoglobulin patterns. In sex-linked agammaglobulinemia little, if any, immunoglobulin can be detected; in Wiskott-Aldrich syndrome IgM is the only significant absentee; and in ataxia telangiectasia both IgA and IgE are found in lowered quantities. It is also clear that some of the combined immunodeficiencies can be expressed in adulthood and are not so severe that they precipitate serious episodes of infectious disease (Table 22-1; Fig. 22-2).

Sex-linked agammaglobulinemia. Sex-linked agammaglobulinemia, in which there is a defect in cellular immune mechanisms associated with agammaglobulinemia, must not be confused with infantile sex-linked agammaglobulinemia of the Bruton type, in which no generalized loss of cellular immunity has ever been noted. In sex-linked agammaglobulinemia there is considerable variation in the immunoglobulin class that is deficient, and not all classes (as in Bruton's disease) may be involved. Likewise the extent of the immunoglobulin loss may not be as severe as in Bruton's disease. Losses in cellular immunity may not be absolute, but the thymus is small, weighing only about 1 g as compared with an expected weight of 4 g for the normal infant. The combination of B cell and T cell losses results in a life expectancy of only 2 years. The condition is seen only in boys and is inherited as a recessive characteristic.

Swiss-type agammaglobulinemia. A second disease embodying losses in both cellular and humoral immunity is Swiss-type agammaglobulinemia. Several dozen cases have been reported since the original description of this disease in 1950 by Glanzmann and Riniker, two Swiss pediatricians. The afflicted children, either boys or girls, since this disease is transmitted as an autosomal recessive disease, are vulnerable to severe diarrhea and severe pyogenic infections caused by the usual bacterial pathogens of childhood. More reflective of their severe immunologic handicap is the inability of these children to resist even feeble pathogens such as *E. coli, Pseudomonas aeruginosa,* and *Pneumocystis carinii.* Childhood viral and fungal diseases—measles, chickenpox, smallpox vaccination, and *Candida* infections— all can be fatal or contribute to fatality.

Autopsied tissues do not reveal plasma cells or germinal centers, and little, if any, immunoglobulin is present in the blood. The thymus exists as an epithelial structure without lymphoid elements. This is the key to the inability of these patients to resist viral or fungal pathogens or to respond to other T cell stimuli such as the contact sensitizers dinitrochlorobenzene and dinitrofluorobenzene.

Wiskott-Aldrich syndrome. The Wiskott-Aldrich syndrome is a sex-linked recessive disease whose victims suffer innumerable bacterial, viral, fungal, and protozoan infections as a result of their failure to generate a typical immunoglobulin or T cell response. In terms of the immunoglobulin aspects of their disease it has been noted that the total immunoglobulin level may be normal. This is because of elevated IgA and depressed IgM levels in the presence of an essentially normal or elevated level of IgG. The restriction of the immunoglobulin loss to IgM suggests that the B cell deficit is related primarily to polysaccharide antigens. The true locus of the defect may not be in the lymphocyte cell system at all but in the macrophages that process the polysaccharide antigens for the B cells. Further studies are needed to confirm the site of the metabolic error, but it is well known that patients with Wiskott-Aldrich syndrome respond poorly to *Salmonella* vaccines and have only low levels of hemagglutinins for red blood cells, both of which depend on polysaccharide antigens. The location of the defect in the T cell system is also obscure. The thymus itself is relatively normal; only peripheral lymphoid organs demonstrate losses in T cells. This appears to be a progressive condition associated with thrombocytopenia and eczema.

Ataxia telangiectasia. Ataxia telangiectasia is described as a disorder in which a progressive loss of muscle coordination (ataxia) is associated with a dilation of small blood vessels (telangiectasia), most notable in conjunctivae but also seen in the skin. It is transmitted as an autosomal recessive disease with an estimated incidence of 1.5 in 100,000 persons. There is a deficiency of both humoral and cellular immunity in homozygotes, which also can be demonstrated in heterozygotes with the condition. Most patients display an increased susceptibility to sinopulmonary infections and malignancy.

The cellular immune deficit is indicated by the finding that a third of the patients have lymphopenia. Virtually all patients have an aplastic or hypoplastic thymus with an unfulfilled T cell population. Repeated or serious viral infections are not as significant in patients with ataxia telangiectasia as in others with abnormal thymus development. Low-reactive skin tests or an absence of positive skin tests to normal antigens of fungal or mycotic origin is typical. It also has been difficult to sensitize these patients to dinitrochlorobenzene; 10 of 21 resisted sensitization in one study, and 12 of 16 did so in another. Malignancies, which develop in 10% of the victims, are further evidence of a T cell failure.

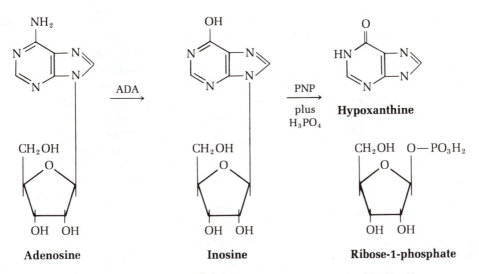

Fig. 22-3. The enzymes ADA and PNP are both present in healthy T cells.

In terms of the patient's humoral status the IgG levels are normal or exceed the normal as a result of repeated infections. IgE levels are depressed in 65% of the patients, but this is unrelated to the heightened incidence of upper respiratory tract infection. This is more certainly caused by loss of IgA, which is total or very nearly so in about 90% of the patients, and the presence of the abnormal 7S variety of IgM in about 78% of the patients. The low IgA levels may not reflect a loss of IgA lymphocytes but may be the result of faulty T cell–B cell interaction, since thymectomized laboratory animals also lose their serum IgA.

Combined immunodeficiency with abnormal purine enzymes. The importance of normal metabolic pathways for purines in lymphocytes has been exemplified by deficiencies of ADA and purine nucleoside phosphorylase (PNP) (Fig. 22-3). Almost 50% of the patients with severe combined immunodeficiency lack ADA. Among the several substrates this enzyme can use is adenosine, which is converted to inosine. When ADA is missing, adenosine accumulates in the blood. A rise in circulating adenosine also creates an increase in ATP and cAMP. An excess of the former disrupts energy metabolism, and an excess of the latter interferes with lymphocyte proliferation. The nucleoside phosphorylase deficiency appears closely related to the inability to form a lymphoid thymus. Both the ADA and PNP deficiencies are inherited as autosomal recessive conditions.

DEFICIENCIES OF THE PHAGOCYTIC SYSTEM

Deficiencies of the phagocytic system can result from several causes, among which those of congenital origin are perhaps the best understood (Table 22-2). Idiopathic, acquired conditions also may influence the behavior of phagocytes. Since the half-life of neutrophils in the blood may be as short as 6 hours and that of the monocytes only 1 to 2 days, the susceptibility of this cell population to transient damage is magnified. Many conditions ranging from the use of chemotherapeutic agents, the presence of kidney disease or cancer, autoimmune disease, and even infections themselves may produce a neutropenia. Cyclic neutropenia of all blood elements occurs in some individuals as the result of an inherited autosomal condition.

Table 22-2. Deficiencies in the phagocytic system

Condition	Characteristic
Chronic granulomatous disease (CGD)	Failure to form toxic forms of oxygen
G6PD deficiency	Failure of phagocyte to oxidize via shunt
Myeloperoxidase deficiency	Failure to use H_2O_2
Chédiak-Higashi disease (CHD)	Failure to release myeloperoxidase
Actin dysfunction	Granulocytes have reduced locomotion

Diagnosis

The evaluation of phagocytic cell defects is made from the clinical history and by in vitro tests to determine the oxidative and cell-killing capacity of the patient's white blood cells. The nitroblue tetrazolium (NBT) reductase test may be used but is not as popular as it once was. Intraphagocytic killing methods are not available in the usual clinical immunology laboratory. Reliance often must be placed on research scientists for a definite diagnosis of a phagocytic defect.

Chronic granulomatous disease (CGD)

Chronic granulomatous disease (CGD) is a sex-linked recessive disease of male infants that usually is recognized within the first few months of life. A second, less severe form of the disease is found in girls and probably is transmitted as an autosomal recessive trait. Differences in the exact nature of CGD in different patients also are reflected in their biochemistry. An inconsistency in the levels of G6PD from patient to patient is one example of this. Immunologic examination of infants with CGD has confirmed that they have a normal or even elevated immunoglobulin level, that they respond normally to vaccines, and that they have normal B and T lymphocyte functions and complement levels. Nevertheless

victims of CGD develop a series of infections early in infancy caused by bacterial pathogens such as *Klebsiella* species, *Proteus vulgaris, Staphylococcus epidermidis, E. coli, Enterobacter aerogenes, Serratia marcescens,* and the more virulent *Staphylococcus aureus.* Feebly virulent yeasts and fungi such as *Candida albicans* and *Aspergillus* species also may be involved in infections that are far more serious in these children than in the usual child. Surprisingly the pathogenic bacteria that cause the most serious diseases of childhood—*Neisseria meningitidis, Hemophilus influenzae, Streptococcus pyogenes,* and *Streptococcus (Diplococcus) pneumoniae*—are combated effectively.

As a result of these repeated infections, CGD patients typically have elevated immunoglobulin levels. Leukocytosis and granulomatous lymphadenitis are also hallmarks of the disease. Tissue biopsies will reveal granuloma formation in virtually every organ. Granulomas typically include tissue macrophages in various stages of digestion of bacterial cells, giant cells containing several nuclei, monocytes, and epithelioid cells. All parameters of the immune defense system function normally in these patients except for their intraphagocytic destruction of certain bacteria. Even the phagocytic cells of patients with CGD have normal chemotactic responses and are as active in engulfment as other phagocytes. Neutrophils of CGD patients kill engulfed bacteria at a reduced rate, and the recovery of 50% to 100% of ingested bacteria at a time when only 1% to 10% of bacteria can be recovered from normal leukocytes is typical (Fig. 22-4).

The biochemical lesion in neutrophils of CGD patients has been identified as a failure to accumulate H_2O_2 during phagocytosis. Prior to phagocytosis these cells use anaerobic glycolysis as their source of energy. During and after phagocytosis normal neutrophils demonstrate a burst in respiratory activity as they shift to the HMP shunt as their energy source. Use of the HMP pathway typically results in the formation of H_2O_2 as hydrogen is transferred by the nicotinamide-adenine

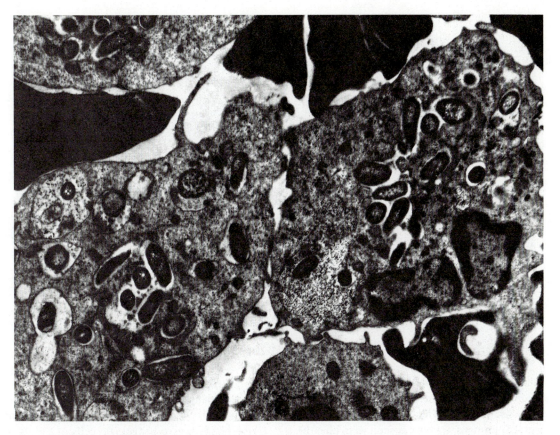

Fig. 22-4. Undigested bacteria are numerous within the phagosomes of these phagocytes taken from a patient with CGD. (Courtesy Dr. E. Adelstein.)

dinucleotide phosphate (NADP) system to oxygen. The resultant hydrogen peroxide functions in cooperation with lysosomal myeloperoxidase to iodinate and kill intracellular bacteria. This may be mediated by singlet oxygen, the superoxide radical, the hydroxyl radical, or other forms of oxygen derived from the hydrogen peroxide. Neutrophils of CGD patients do not make the shift to aerobic metabolism and therefore fail to accumulate H_2O_2 and to kill intracellular bacteria.

The role of H_2O_2 clearly is related to the type of pathogen that causes the most trouble for the CGD patient. Organisms such as *Hemophilus, Neisseria,* and *Streptococcus* species produce H_2O_2 but lack a catalase that can destroy it. Con-

sequently these bacteria develop a microenvironment just like that created in normal phagocytes, and this is suicidal. The feebler pathogens that so often are involved in CGD infections have a high level of catalase, an enzyme that converts H_2O_2 to water and oxygen. Neutrophils of the CGD patient simply do not produce enough H_2O_2 to overcome the bacterial catalase. The microorganisms that cause infections in CGD patients are typically those which do produce catalase, whereas bacteria that lack catalase but produce their own H_2O_2 are resisted by these patients.

The metabolic shift of normal phagocytes to oxidative metabolism can be determined easily by the NBT reductase test. In this test neutrophils

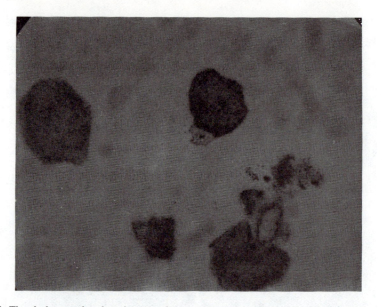

Fig. 22-5. The dark granulated perimeter of these unstained neutrophils are deposits of reduced NBT. The cell at the left is not as positive as the others.

in the act of phagocytosing latex spherules are incubated in a solution of NBT dye that serves as a hydrogen acceptor instead of oxygen as oxidative metabolism ensues. This reduces the dye to its insoluble formazan, which is seen as distinct blue intracytoplasmic granules (Fig. 22-5). Leukocytes of the CGD patient are not engaged in active oxidative metabolism and thus cannot reduce NBT. Female carriers of CGD have approximately a 50% loss in their ability to reduce NBT.

Chédiak-Higashi disease (CHD)

Chédiak-Higashi disease (CHD) is characterized by a pigmentary dilution of the eyes and skin (oculocutaneous albinism), extreme sensitivity to light (photophobia), rapid involuntary eye movements (nystagmus), and frequent pyogenic infections. Neutropenia, thrombocytopenia, and recurrent fever are also symptoms of the disease. The primary cellular defect noticed in victims of CHD is the presence of abnormally large granules in all phagocytic cells. Because of the recurrent infections, these persons have fever, lymphadenopathy,

and hepatosplenomegaly and a mean survival age of 6 years. In only 13 of 56 cases reported in one study did the patients live beyond 10 years of age.

In patients with CHD giant granules are found in the highly active phagocytic cells of the tissue and blood such as the tissue macrophages, alveolar macrophages and neutrophils, and other cells of the myeloid series. This makes diagnosis of the disease simple through the direct examination of stained blood films. An analysis of host defenses in CHD patients has revealed that immunoglobulin synthesis, CMI, and phagocytic endocytosis are all normal. The central defect is an inability to form normal primary granules in cells of the granulocytic series. Primary granules are the typical lysosomal granules that contain β-glucuronidase, myeloperoxidase, lysozyme, several hydrolases, etc. and can be compared with the secondary granules that contain alkaline phosphatase. Even though the engulfment by granulocytes in CHD patients is normal, bactericidal activity against *Staphylococcus aureus,* streptococci, pneumococci, and lesser pathogenic bacteria has proved to be deficient. Retarded intraphagocyte killing is not the result of depressed H_2O_2 formation, but it is associated with an ability of cells to degranulate normally and to deliver myeloperoxidase to the phagocytic vacuole. In CHD there is also an impaired chemotactic response, which would favor bacterial pathogens.

Job's syndrome

A specific phagocytic defect that permits *Staphylococcus aureus* to produce abscesses of the skin and subcutaneous tissue in the absence of any significant inflammatory response is known as Job's syndrome. Phagocytes from individuals with this disorder are normally active in endocytosis but are unable to kill the staphylococci, and the NBT test is negative. The location of the cellular defect has yet to be determined.

G6PD deficiency

An inability of neutrophils to destroy engulfed bacteria also has been associated with a deficiency in the enzyme G6PD. This enzyme is the first in the HMP shunt, where it diverts G6P from the glycolytic pathway. Accordingly, individuals who are devoid of this enzyme have a defective ability to generate H_2O_2; in fact it is estimated that their phagocytes produce only 25% of the normal level of hydrogen peroxide. *Staphylococcus, Escherichia,* and *Serratia* organisms survive inside these phagocytes, but H_2O_2-producing microbes do not.

Myeloperoxidase deficiency

Benzidine staining of granulocytes for myeloperoxidase activity has exposed a deficiency of this enzyme in certain patients with severe acute infections. During phagocytosis the shift of phagocytic metabolism to the oxygen-consuming pentose pathway occurs normally in these patients, which suggests that normal amounts of H_2O_2 are formed. Cell studies have revealed that little or no iodination of intracellular microbes occurs and that the killing rate is depressed. The similarity of myeloperoxidase deficiency to CGD is obvious; patients with the latter disease have myeloperoxidase but little H_2O_2, whereas patients with the former disease have H_2O_2 but no myeloperoxidase. Both are required for protection against many pyogenic bacteria. In this syndrome only PMNs are affected. Monocytes and eosinophils remain normal.

Dysfunction of neutrophil actin

At least one example of recurrent skin and intestinal infections with gram-negative and gram-positive bacteria has been attributed to a failure of actin in neutrophils to polymerize. In its rest state actin exists in a monomeric form but is converted to a polymeric or filamentous form during pseudopod formation and locomotion. Neutrophils unable to transform actin into its contractile state cannot respond properly to chemotactic stimuli, and this accounts for the failure of the patient to develop pus at the site of infections. Other metabolic functions of the neutrophils, including oxygen metabolism and degranulation, are normal, and the patient's monocytes function normally.

IMMUNOLOGIC RECONSTITUTION

Restoration of a suitable immune status to persons with uncomplicated agammaglobulinemia presents no novel problems; it is only necessary to provide them passive immunity by periodic injections of pooled human γ-globulin (Table 22-3). Since purification of γ-globulin often creates aggregates that will fix complement and produce anaphylactoid reactions, transfusions with plasma may be used to supplant injections of γ-globulin. When hepatitis-free donors are available, this is a safe and practical procedure.

Selective deficits in T cell responses also are subject to correction by a simple technical procedure (Table 22-3; Fig. 7-3). Nonviable T cell extracts or transfer factor prepared from the T cells of donors with a normal status of CMI can be injected into the T cell–deficient person to convert him or her to the immune condition of the donor. T cell extracts are not injected in their crude form. The lymphocytes of a donor with good T cell responses are subjected to several

Table 22-3. Immunologic reconstitution of immunodeficiency diseases

Condition	Method
B lymphocyte deficiencies	
Transient agammaglobulinemia	None needed; self-correcting
Bruton's agammaglobulinemia	Pooled human γ-globulin
Common variable hypogammaglobulinemia	Pooled human γ-globulin if IgG missing
T lymphocyte deficiencies	
Nezelof's syndrome	Thymus grafts ± bone marrow
DiGeorge's syndrome	Thymus grafts ± bone marrow
Leprosy, chronic mucocutaneous candidiasis	Transfer factor
Combined B and T lymphocyte deficiencies	
Sex-linked agammaglobulinemia	Transfer factor plus pooled human γ-globulin or bone marrow and thymus, depending on extent of T and B cell loss
Swiss-type agammaglobulinemia	
Wiskott-Aldrich syndrome	
Ataxia telangiectasia	
Phagocytic system deficiencies	Granulocyte transfusions (temporary value only)

freeze-thaw cycles. Cell fragments are removed by centrifugation, and high molecular weight molecules are trapped inside a dialysis membrane. The low molecular weight dialysate, the fraction originally described by Lawrence as transfer factor, is used. Human transfer factor is an antigen-specific low molecular weight oligonucleotide or peptide. Its mode of action in the recipient is unknown, but the recipient's lymphocytes are converted to a condition in which they will respond to foreign antigens in the typical way. This generally is determined externally by a skin test of the recipient with PPD, dermatophytin, coccidioidin, or some other preparation known to provoke a delayed skin reaction in the donor.

Transfer factor injections have been applied in the treatment of chronic mucocutaneous candidiasis, coccidioidomycosis, Swiss-type agammaglobulinemia, sex-linked agammaglobulinemia, ataxia telangiectasia, Wiskott-Aldrich syndrome, leprosy, and several forms of cancer. The results have been encouraging. Of seven patients with mucocutaneous candidiasis, four showed definite improvement; of 11 patients with Wiskott-Aldrich syndrome, six responded with a change in skin test results, five no longer have the eczema, and

four became free of infection; and some patients with coccidioidomycosis showed improvement after treatment with transfer factor.

Successful reconstitution of the immune status with transfer factor demands that the individual have a reasonably normal population of lymphocytes. Transfer factor merely triggers existing lymphocytes into activity; it does not generate lymphocytes. When these lymphocytes are not present or are present in extremely low numbers, transfer factor injections can be expected to fail. In these instances (Nezelof's and DiGeorge's syndromes and some cases of combined immunodeficiency disease) transplantation of bone marrow or thymus may be required to provide the needed T lymphocytes. Bone marrow transplants also would provide the B lymphocytes, but this usually is not the primary purpose of bone marrow transplants, since B cell products (immunoglobulins) are readily available. Bone marrow transplantation suffers the innate hazard of creating GVH reactions, since immunoresponsive cells are being transferred to an immunodeficient host. This problem is not met when the transplantation is between identical twins or between a histocompatible donor and recipient.

Since DiGeorge's and Nezelof's syndromes are characterized by the loss of only the cell-mediated arm of the immune response, marrow grafts to supply B cells are unnecessary, and thymus grafting alone is sufficient. Fetal thymus that has not yet reached immunologic maturity is the preferred tissue and has successfully reconstituted patients with Nezelof's or DiGeorge's syndrome. More recently it has been possible to transplant fragments of thymus cultured in vitro to patients with SCID and effect recovery from the condition. The fragments, which lose their lymphocytes during cultivation, are composed almost entirely of epithelium. Lymphocytes or prolymphocytes leaving the bone marrow of the transplant recipient repopulate the thymus fragments and are converted into functional T lymphocytes. This reveals the possibility that the thymic hormones required for T cell maturation are produced by the nonlymphoid portion of the thymus gland. One interesting aspect of this is that the thymus fragments can be successfully transplanted across the HLA barrier.

BIBLIOGRAPHY

Anonymous: Enzyme defects and immune dysfunction, Ciba Foundation Symposium, vol. 68, Amsterdam, 1979, Excerpta Medica.

Asherson, G.L., and Webster, A.D.B.: Diagnosis and treatment of immunodeficiency diseases, Oxford, 1980, Blackwell Scientific Publications, Ltd.

Barton, W.R., and Goldschneider, I.: Nucleotide-metabolizing enzymes and lymphocyte differentiation, Mol. Cell. Biochem. **28**:135, 1979.

Brody, N.: Laboratory tests to evaluate the immune system, Intern. J. Dermatol. **20**:301, 1981.

Dwyer, J.M.: Chronic mucocutaneous candidiasis, Annu. Rev. Med. **32**:491, 1981.

Gelfand, E.W., and Dosch, H.M., editors: Biological basis of immunodeficiency, New York, 1980, Raven Press.

Giblett, E.R., and Polmar, S.H.: Inherited immunodeficiency diseases: relationship to lymphocyte metabolic dysfunction, Prog. Med. Genet. **3**:177, 1979.

Godal, T.: Immunological status of leprosy—present status, Prog. Allergy **25**:211, 1978.

Güttler, F., Seakins, J.W.T., and Harkness, R.A.: Inborn errors of immunity and phagocytosis, Baltimore, 1979, University Park Press.

Hirschhorn, R.: Adenosine deaminase deficiency and immunodeficiency, Prog. Clin. Immunol. **3**:67, 1977.

Horowitz, S.D., and Hong, R., editors: The pathogenesis and treatment of immunodeficiency, Basel, 1977, S. Karger, AG, Medical and Scientific Publishers.

Jirsch, D.W., editor: Immunological engineering, Baltimore, 1978, University Park Press.

Pollara, B., and others, editors: Inborn errors of specific immunity, New York, 1979, Academic Press, Inc.

Polmar, S.H.: Metabolic aspects of immunodeficiency disease, Semin. Hematol. **17**:30, 1980.

Seligmann, M., and Hitzig, W.H., editors: Primary immunodeficiencies, Amsterdam, 1980, Elsevier/North Holland Biomedical Press.

Taubman, S.B.: Screening tests for cell-mediated immunodeficiency diseases, CRC Crit. Rev. Clin. Lab. Sci. **11**:207, 1979.

Verhoef, J., Peterson, P.K., and Quie, P.G., editors: Infections in the immunocompromised host—pathogenesis, prevention and therapy, Amsterdam, 1980, Elsevier/North Holland Biomedical Press.

Vyas, G.N., Stites, D.P., and Brecher, D.J., editors: Laboratory diagnosis of immunologic disorders, New York, 1975, Grune & Stratton, Inc.

SITUATION 1: SELECTIVE IgA DEFICIENCY

Karen, a 3-year-old girl, was referred to a regional hospital by her local physician in a small farming community because of recurrent respiratory tract infections. On admission she weighed 29 pounds, appeared thin and pale, had a temperature of 37.5° C, had a reddened throat, and had small white foci on her tonsils. The child's history indicated that she had had recurrent tonsillitis since 1½ years of age. Rarely were any significant pathogens isolated, but on one occasion *Streptococcus pyogenes* group A was recovered. Her present white blood cell count was moderately elevated, with a shift to the left. Throat cultures were taken, and blood was drawn for serum electrophoretic analysis.

Questions

1. Why is this child not considered to have agammaglobulinemia?
2. What is the status of secretory IgA in the serum IgA–deficient person?
3. What diseases are associated with IgA dysgammaglobulinemia?
4. Is IgA antigenic for the patient with IgA dysgammaglobulinemia?

Solution

It is the general experience that, even though many IgA-deficient individuals are asymptomatic, recurrent infections are also common. Recognized infectious diseases include tonsillitis, otitis media, febrile disease with cough, nasal discharge, and other upper respiratory tract diseases not further identified. In older children and adults asthmatic episodes are triggered by these infections, which suggests an allergic disposition toward the pathogens. This is not the case in hereditary telangiectasia, where an IgE deficiency accompanies the IgA loss. Since this child had not had a life-threatening illness in the first years of her life, combined immunodeficiency disease was not considered. Because the child was female, Bruton's agammaglobulinemia was discounted.

Individuals deficient in serum IgA are likewise deficient in secretory IgA. Since the patient with IgA dysgammaglobulinemia has never experienced any self-contact with IgA, it is recognized as a foreign antigen. The immune response to external IgA in plasma or blood transfusions could result in anaphylaxis if a prior exposure induced sufficient antibody formation.

References

Rockey, J.H., and others: Beta-2A aglobulinemia in two healthy men, J. Lab. Clin. Med. **63**:205, 1964.

Tomasi, T.B., and Grey, H.M.: Structure and function of immunoglobulin A, Prog. Allergy **16**:81, 1972.

West, C.D., Hong, R., and Holland, N.H.: Immunoglobulin levels from the newborn period to adulthood and in immunoglobulin deficiency states, J. Clin. Invest. **41**:2054, 1962.

SITUATION 2: LEUKOCYTE FUNCTION—CGD

Mark, a 3-year-old boy, entered the hospital for the sixth time in the past 2½ years. His admission was for a fever of unknown origin. His white blood cell count was 18,500 per mm³, of which 46% were PMNs. His temperature was 38.8° C, and the liver and spleen were enlarged. Blood cultures were taken and reported to be positive for *E. coli*. On previous hospitalizations for septicemia, boils, cervical lymphadenopathy, and pneumonia, bacterial cultures had been positive for *E. coli* and/or *Klebsiella* organisms and coagulase-positive staphylococci. A diagnosis of CGD was considered, and the following laboratory tests were ordered: total γ-globulin, NBT reductase test, and bactericidal killing test.

Questions

1. What is CGD, and what are the hallmarks of leukocyte function in this disease?
2. What is the importance of the four special laboratory procedures, and what are the normal values of these tests?
3. How is CGD treated?

Solution

CGD is typified by repeated, slow-healing infections caused by ordinarily feeble infectious organisms. The disease is seen only in young boys because of its sex-linked inheritance, although similar diseases are seen in girls. Granulomatous deposits in visceral organs, especially the lungs, facilitate radiologic diagnosis; however, deficits in neutrophil function with normal T and B lymphocyte functions are instrumental in confirming the diagnosis.

Patients with CGD, because of the high incidence of bacterial infections, have higher γ-globulin levels than normal, and this was seen in the case of Mark, who had a total γ-globulin level of 1,400 mg/dl. The presence of such high levels of immunoglobulins promotes phagocytosis of bacteria but does not necessarily accelerate the intraphagocytic death of the ingested bacteria. For this reason a bactericidal killing test is performed. The buffy coat of heparinized blood from the patient is adjusted to a suitable neutrophil cell count rather than to some specific dilution. Cell counts are necessary because of the fluctuation in granulocyte counts in such patients. Generally 10^6 white blood cells per milliliter and 10^6 bacteria per milliliter are attained in the final mixture, which is contained in a tissue culture fluid supplemented with normal serum to the extent of 10%. After incubation of the mixture at 37° C for 30 minutes and at 30-minute intervals thereafter penicillin and streptomycin are added to kill extracellular bacteria. (Penicillin-sensitive *Staphylococcus aureus* is used in the test.) The centrifuged pellet is subjected to total plate counts for surviving bacteria. The normal control uses white blood cells from a healthy subject.

Normal leukocytes kill staphylococci and most other bacteria rapidly, with a 1% viable remainder being typical after 2 hours of incubation. Patients with CGD may have as much as 95% bacterial survival in the same test, although 70% survival would be more typical. PMNs from Mark reduced the staphylococcal population from 10^6 to only 8×10^5. Examination of white blood cell smears revealed that adequate ingestion had occurred.

Because the bactericidal killing test is cumbersome and time consuming, the NBT reductase test often is used to evaluate neutrophil performance instead. The test is based on the knowledge that phagocytosis is accompanied by a burst in respiratory metabolism that can be detected by the ability of white blood cells to transfer hydrogen to the NBT dye. This reduces the dye and causes the appearance of dark blue dye granules inside the neutrophils. Neutrophils from patients with CGD are genetically incapable of leaving their glycolytic energy-deriving system for the oxidative pathways associated with intraphagocytic killing. In the NBT reductase test latex spherules are used as the phagocytic subject for white blood cells incubated with NBT. About 50% of the neutrophils will have phagocytosed at least five latex beads and be positive. Patients with CGD have decidedly lower scores, as do some other restricted patient categories and neonates. Mark had a score of 5%, which was definitely below the normal and compatible with the diagnosis.

There is no suitable therapy for CGD other than treatment of the bacterial infections as they occur. For this reason the average life expectancy of such patients is only 10 years.

References

Baehner, R.L., and Nathan, G.: Quantitative nitroblue tetrazolium test in chronic granulomatous disease, N. Engl. J. Med. **278:**971, 1968.

Holmes, B., and others: Fatal granulomatous disease of childhood; an inborn abnormality of phagocytic function, Lancet **1:**1225, 1966.

Park, B.H.: The use and limitations of the nitroblue tetrazolium test as a diagnostic aid, J. Pediatr. **78:**376, 1971.

Quie, P.G., and Hill, H.R.: Granulocytopathies, Disease-A-Month, p. 1, August 1973.

READINGS IN IMMUNOLOGY

The inclusion of these readings in immunology is intended to serve at least three instructional purposes. It will be seen immediately that several of the readings have been chosen for their historical significance—the reporting of important firsts in immunology. The articles chosen for this purpose are from the recent rather than the early historical records so that the modern language used and the possibility of current applications of the information reported will give additional appeal to the reading lesson. Even so, the student will note in the earlier papers that briefly written reports based on unsophisticated procedures can be as vital to the development of a science as the longer, more complex reports so common in the present literature. A second purpose of these readings is to support the summary views in the body of the text with specific selections from the scientific literature, with the intent to exemplify the exact procedures and terminology used. It is not possible to present samples corresponding to each chapter in the text; nevertheless those presented do introduce cause and effect relationships and other aspects of the scientific method that are applicable to diverse subtopics in immunology. A third purpose, embodied especially in the recent selections, is to provide an opportunity for students to gain confidence in their mastery of immunology by realizing that, from the base of classroom lectures and text assignments, they in fact have learned enough immunology to comprehend current scientific writings.

No foreign language readings have been included in order that the intended purpose of this volume—instruction of beginning students of immunology—might be achieved.

Reading 1

One of the perplexing questions that recur in biology is, how does the cell that produces a poisonous or toxic substance protect itself against the toxin? How does the tissue producing a proteolytic enzyme protect itself against self-digestion? How does the electric eel keep from shocking itself? How does the phagocyte keep from oxidizing and digesting itself? Insight into the solution of the last problem is presented in this discussion from *Infection and Immunity* **12**:252-256, 1975.

In this report the high intracellular content of ascorbic acid in phagocytes is noted to be divided between ascorbate and dehydroascorbate. Phagocytic studies with ascorbic acid–deficient guinea pigs indicated that dietary vitamin C did not influence the capacity of the cells to kill *Staphylococcus aureus* or to produce H_2O_2. During phagocytosis by human PMNs, dehydroascorbate in the cells increased, with an increase in reduced ascorbate. This suggests that the PMNs use the ascorbate-dehydroascorbate system as an oxidation reduction balance during phagocytosis.

ASCORBATE AND PHAGOCYTE FUNCTION

LIBUSE STANKOVA, NANCY B. GERHARDT, LARRY NAGEL, and ROBERT H. BIGLEY*

Scorbutic guinea pig neutrophils (PMN) were found to produce H_2O_2 and kill Staphylococcus aureus as well as control PMN, suggesting that ascorbate does not contribute significantly to phagocyte H_2O_2 production or bacterial killing. Total and reduced ascorbate contents of human PMN were observed to fall upon phagocytosis, whereas dehydroascorbate increased to a lesser extent. These observations are consistent with the view

*Department of Medicine and Department of Microbiology and Immunology, University of Oregon Health Sciences Center, Portland, Oregon 97201.

that ascorbate constitutes a functional part of the PMN's redox-active components and may thus function to protect cell constituents from denaturation by the oxidants produced during phagocytosis.

In a previous study (5), we found that human neutrophil leukocytes have impressive capacity for reducing dehydroascorbate and thus for regenerating their content of reduced ascorbate upon oxidation. This property of neutrophils (PMN), along with their relatively high ascorbate content, suggests that ascorbate may play an important role in PMN function. Phagocyte ascorbate might promote oxidative denaturation of bacterial components and thus potentiate bacterial killing, as proposed by Miller (18) and by Drath and Karnofsky (10). Ascorbate also might function to preserve cell integrity by inactivating free radicals and oxidants (8, 9, 26) produced during phagocytosis (2, 3, 14).

To determine whether physiological concentrations of ascorbate are critical for optimal phagocytosis and bacterial killing, we assayed H_2O_2 production and bactericidal activity in scorbutic guinea pig PMN. To examine the possibility that ascorbate is a redox-active component of oxidant-producing cells, we have measured changes in human PMN ascorbate contents during phagocytosis.

Materials and methods

Ascorbate contents. Ascorbate contents of tissues and cell preparations were measured by the method of Roe et al. (22). This method quantitatively distinguishes reduced ascorbate, dehydroascorbate, and diketogulonate from each other and from other organic compounds. Dehydroascorbate, the oxidized derivative of ascorbic acid, is reducible to ascorbate in most mammalian tissues. Diketogulonate, the hydrated derivative of dehydroascorbate, is not converted to dehydroascorbate in mammalian tissues.

Guinea pig experiments. Two-month-old guinea pigs weighing 325 to 375 g were divided into two groups. Both groups were fed for 18 days with an ascorbic acid–deficient diet (Nutritional Biochemicals Co., Cleveland, Ohio). Control animals were also fed by gavage 1 mg of ascorbate per g of body weight daily. Single experiments utilized pairs of animals, one scor-

butic and one control. The order of harvest of control and scorbutic cells was alternated in successive experiments.

Guinea pig peritoneal PMN were harvested 12 h after intraperitoneal injection of 15 ml of 20% autoclaved sodium caseinate. Cells were suspended in calcium-free Krebs-Ringer phosphate buffer (KRP), pH 7.4. After 2 volumes of 0.87% ammonium chloride was added to lyse contaminating erythrocytes, leukocytes were collected by centrifugation for 10 min at $150 \times g$, washed twice in KRP, counted in a hemocytometer, and diluted with KRP to an approximate concentration of 100×10^6 phagocytes (PMN plus macrophages)/ml. Final suspensions contained 74 to 95% neutrophils, 3 to 25% macrophages, 0 to 8% lymphocytes, and 0 to 2% eosinophils.

H_2O_2 production was measured continuously as the rate of $^{14}CO_2$ production from $[1\text{-}^{14}C]$formate (1, 14) (New England Nuclear Corp., Boston, Mass.), using the gas flow-ionization chamber system of Davidson and Tanaka (7). This technique converts charge accumulated in an ionization chamber to a mullivolt signal. Unstimulated reaction mixtures (1 ml) containing 20×10^6 to 40×10^6 leukocytes, 0.7 μmol of sodium formate including 0.86 μCi of $[^{14}C]$formate, and 5.6 μmol of glucose in KRP were incubated in 20-ml flat-bottomed glass vials in a Dubnoff shaking incubator (Precision Scientific Co., Chicago, Ill.) at 37 C, 80 oscillations/min. Phagocytosing signals were recorded after the addition of approximately 2×10^9 thrice-washed polystyrene latex spheres (0.81 μm in diameter; Bacto-Latex, Difco Laboratories, Detroit, Mich.) in 0.2 ml of KRP. The depth of the reaction mixtures was 2 mm and the surface area was 5 cm². Vials were gassed with 5% CO_2 in air, flowing at 73 ml/min. Nanomoles of formate oxidized were calculated from the millivolt signal, using factors derived from calibrations previously reported (5).

Bacterial killing by guinea pig peritoneal PMN was measured using a modification of the method of Pincus and Klebanoff (21), within 2 to 4 h of cell collection. Assay mixtures (1 ml) contained 30×10^6 phagocytes, 5×10^6 colony-forming units of *Staphylococcus aureus* 502A (kindly supplied by G. Mandell), 0.1 ml of serum separated from blood obtained by cardiac puncture at the time of cell harvest, 10 μmol of glucose, and KRP. These were incubated at 37 C in stoppered siliconized glass tubes (12 by 75 mm), which were rotated on a model 150 Multi-Purpose Rotator (Scientific Industries,

Inc.) at 24 rpm. At intervals noted in Fig. 1, 0.1-ml aliquants were removed, diluted in distilled water, vortexed heavily to disrupt PMN, and plated in duplicate in Trypticase soy broth containing 15% agar. Colonies were counted after 44 to 48 h of culture at 37 C.

Human experiments. Human PMN were separated from peripheral blood as previously described (5). These preparations contained 85% neutrophils, 5 to 15% monocytes, 0 to 8% lymphocytes, and 0 to 5% eosinophils.

Ascorbate contents of resting and phagocytosing PMN were measured by using the entire 1.5-ml reaction mixtures: 0.7×10^8 to 1.2×10^8 phagocytes, with or without approximately 2×10^9 latex particles, suspended in KRP containing 8.25 μmol of glucose. Samples were incubated in the shaking incubator at 80 oscillations/min at 37 C for the times indicated in the tables.

Results

The ascorbate contents of scorbutic guinea pig peritoneal PMN, whole blood, liver, and kidney were about 15% of normal (Table 1). These values agree well with published data for comparably treated animals (20).

Scorbutic guinea pig leukocytes produced normal amounts of H_2O_2 during phagocytosis (Table 2). Four of thirteen scorbutic peritoneal exudates were grossly bloody. PMN in those samples were packed with ingested erythrocytes and exhibited high resting H_2O_2 production (mean, 1.69 nmol of formate oxidized/10 min per 10^8 PMN), which did not increase upon addition of latex particles. Giemsa-stained smears showed that less than 1% of these cells had ingested latex spheres. These findings were reproduced in PMN from a control

Table 1. Total ascorbate content of scorbutic and control guinea pig tissues

Tissue	Total ascorbate		Ratio (scorbutic/control)
	Control	Scorbutic	
Peritoneal PMN[a]	42.4 (34.8-51.0)	4.5 (3.2-5.5)	0.11
Blood[b]	4.9 ± 0.3	0.6 ± 0.17	0.12
Liver[c]	126.7 ± 23.8	18.8 ± 1.7	0.15
Kidney[c]	68.8 ± 10.7	10.8 ± 2.8	0.16

[a] $n = 3$ control, 3 scorbutic; expressed as nmol/10^8 cells; mean (range).
[b] $n = 6$ control, 6 scorbutic; expressed as nmol/0.1 ml; mean ± standard deviation.
[c] $n = 6$ control, 6 scorbutic; nmol/100 mg of tissue; mean ± standard deviation.

Table 2. H_2O_2 production by scorbutic and control guinea pig PMN without and with latex particles

PMN	Formate oxidation[a]		Ratio (phagocytosing/unstimulated)
	Unstimulated	Phagocytosing	
Control[b]	0.532 ± 0.206	1.480 ± 0.552	2.8 ± 0.3
Scorbutic[c]	0.575 ± 0.294	1.401 ± 0.367	2.7 ± 0.7

[a] Expressed as nmol of formate oxidized/10 min per 10^8 PMN; mean ± standard deviation.
[b] $n = 10$.
[c] $n = 9$.

guinea pig given isologous whole blood intraperitoneally 12 h before PMN harvest. Such bloody samples were excluded from this study.

Scorbutic PMN killed *S. aureus* as efficiently as did control guinea pig cells (Fig. 1). It can also be inferred from Fig. 1 that normal and scorbutic sera supported opsonization equally well, since phagocytosis-dependent bacterial killing did not vary significantly with serum source.

The total ascorbate content of phagocytosing human peripheral blood PMN decreased during the 60 min after phagocytosis and then remained stable (Table 3). Table 4 shows that total ascorbate decreased by an average of 12% in phagocytosing normal human PMN but did not change during phagocytosis in cells from two patients with chronic granulomatous disease. The decrease in total ascorbate content of phagocytosing normal

cells was accompanied by a marked decrease in reduced ascorbate which was not accounted for by a moderate increase in dehydroascorbate. Only trace amounts of diketogulonate were detectable in both resting and phagocytosing samples.

Discussion

The present study shows that PMN obtained from scorbutic guinea pigs produce H_2O_2 and kill *S. aureus* as well as do control cells, at least briefly after phagocytosis. Since these functions depend on phagocytosis, our results argue against the conclusion of Nungester and Ames that phagocytosis is impaired in scorbutic guinea pig phagocytes (19). The discrepancy is best explained by the fact that the peritoneal exudates in the study of Nungester and Ames were hemorrhagic, as often occurs with advanced ascorbate deficiency. As we have demonstrated, erythrophagocytosis interferes with further particle ingestion and therefore with enhanced H_2O_2 production upon incubation with latex spheres. Experiments using bloody exudates were excluded from the present study.

The observations that H_2O_2 production and bacterial killing are unimpaired in scorbutic PMN imply that these activities are not sensitive to changes in ascorbate concentration over the range studied here. The 15% of normal ascorbate residual in scorbutic cells might suffice to support H_2O_2 production, since neutrophils possess ef-

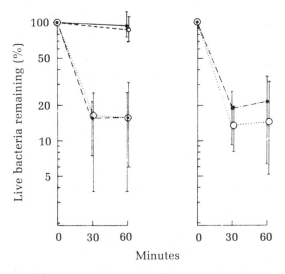

Fig. 1. In vitro killing of *S. aureus* 502A by scorbutic and control guinea pig PMN. n = 3 for scorbutic PMN plus control serum; n = 4 for the other groups; mean values and ranges are indicated. Symbols for left-hand panel: ○ − − − ○, Scorbutic serum; ● − · − ●, control PMN plus serum; ● — ●, control serum; ○ · · · · ○, scorbutic PMN plus serum. Symbols for right-hand panel: ●, Control PMN plus scorbutic serum; ○, scorbutic PMN plus control serum.

Table 3. Total ascorbate content of human PMN; effect of time of incubation without and with latex particles[a]

Incubation time (min)	Unstimulated	Phagocytosing
0	73	73
40	73	68
60	71	65
90	74	66
120	72	66

[a]Expressed as nmol of ascorbate/10^8 PMN.

454 Readings in immunology

Table 4. Ascorbate contents of human PMN after 60-min incubation without and with latex particles[a]

PMN	Ascorbate content (nmol/10^8 cells)		
	Total	Reduced	Dehydroascorbate
Normal[a]			
Unstimulated	78.1 ± 8.3	54.9 ± 10.3	23.2 ± 8.9
Phagocytosing	68.6 ± 4.8	40.0 ± 7.4	28.6 ± 7.6
Difference	(−)9.5 ± 4.6[b]	(−)14.9 ± 4.4[b]	(+)5.4 ± 4.6[c]
Chronic granulomatous disease[d]			
Unstimulated	54.7 52.9	46.8 44.6	7.8 8.3
Phagocytosing	54.7 53.5	41.2 43.4	13.4 10.2
Difference	0.0 (+)0.6	(−)5.6 (−)1.2	(+)5.6 (+)1.9

[a]$n = 10$; mean ± standard deviation.
[b]$P < 0.001$ by paired t test.
[c]$P < 0.005$ by paired t test.
[d]$n = 2$; recorded separately.

ficient dehydroascorbate reducing activity (5). However, it would be unusual for a biological reaction to be insensitive to a decrease in substrate concentration to less than one-fifth of the physiological level. Therefore, we doubt that ascorbate participates directly in phagocyte H_2O_2 production or bacterial killing.

Upon phagocytosis, human PMN oxygen consumption increases by 100 to 300 nmol/10^8 cells per min (13, 15). Measurements of the H_2O_2 and activated oxygen species produced during phagocytosis account for up to 80% of the increment in oxygen consumption (4, 6, 12, 13, 15, 28). Despite exposure to these potent and largely diffusible denaturants, PMN survive and function at least briefly (23) and do not accumulate lipid peroxides (17) after phagocytosis. Catalase, myeloperoxidase, and glutathione peroxidase catalyze destruction of H_2O_2; glutathione peroxidase also catalyzes lipid peroxide reduction (16). Ascorbate and other small molecules, including reduced glutathione and α-tocopherol, are effective antioxidants and free radical scavengers (8, 9, 26). Human leukocytes (10^8) contain 107 to 205 nmol of reduced glutathione (11), 3.2 ± 0.2 nmol of oxidized nicotinamide adenine dinucleotide

(NAD^+), 2.5 ± 0.2 nmol NADH, 0.8 ± 0.2 nmol of $NADP^+$, and 2.4 ± 0.4 nmol of NADPH (24). The cell contents of these redox-active molecules are comparable to the ascorbate contents measured in the present study (Table 4). Human PMN can reduce more than 200 nmol of dehydroascorbate/10^8 cells per min (5). This activity would appear sufficient to maintain ascorbate in reduced form, able to act as a significant part of the PMN's capacity for inactivating free radicals and oxidants and thus for preventing denaturation of cell constituents.

Chronic granulomatous disease neutrophils phagocytose normally (25), but their ability to produce H_2O_2 and activated oxygen species is markedly impaired (4, 6). In the studies reported here, ascorbate levels were stable during phagocytosis in chronic granulomatous disease phagocytes but fell significantly in normal phagocytes. The latter observation probably reflects degradation of ascorbate, mediated by oxidants produced during phagocytosis, to compounds other than those assayable as total ascorbate. The degraded ascorbate may be sequestered from the cell's dehydroascorbate reducing activity, perhaps in phagolysosomes.

The ratio of NADP$^+$ to NADPH in PMN was observed to increase from 0.11 to 0.31 during phagocytosis (27). This has been interpreted to reflect NADPH oxidation in the process of H_2O_2 production (27) or the oxidation of reduced glutathione by H_2O_2 (4). Neutrophil-unsaturated membrane lipid, an easily oxidized cell component, is not detectably oxidized after phagocytosis (17). This suggests that extensive oxidation of cell constituents is not a general phenomenon in phagocytosing PMN. The present study demonstrates that ascorbate is oxidized during phagocytosis. This observation is consistent with the view that ascorbate is a functional part of the cell's redox-active components.

Acknowledgments

This work was supported by Public Health Service grant no. AM 13173 from the National Institute of Arthritis, Metabolism, and Digestive Diseases and Medical Research Foundation grant no. 7412.

The expert technical assistance of John Niedra, Department of Microbiology and Immunology, is gratefully acknowledged.

LITERATURE CITED

1. Aebi, H. 1963. Detection and fixation of radiation-produced peroxide by enzymes. Radiat. Res. **3**(Suppl.):130-152.
2. Allen, R.C., R.L. Stjernholm, and R.H. Steele. 1972. Evidence for the generation of an electronic excitation state(s) in human polymorphonuclear leukocytes and its participation in bacterial activity. Biochem. Biophys. Res. Commun. **47**:679-684.
3. Babior, B.M., R.S. Kipnes, and J.T. Curnutte. 1973. The production by leukocytes of superoxide, a potential bactericidal agent. J. Clin. Invest. **52**:741-754.
4. Baehner, R.L., N. Gilman, and M.L. Karnofsky. 1970. Respiration and glucose oxidation in human and guinea pig leukocytes: comparative studies. J. Clin. Invest. **49**:692-699.
5. Bigley, R.H., and L. Stankova. 1974. Uptake and reduction of oxidized and reduced ascorbate by human leukocytes. J. Exp. Med. **139**:1084-92.
6. Curnutte, J.T., D.M. Whitten, and B.M. Babior. 1974. Defective superoxide production by granulocytes from patients with chronic granulomatous disease. N. Engl. J. Med. **290**:593-597.
7. Davidson, W.D., and K.R. Tanaka. 1969. Continuous measurement of pentose phosphate pathway activity in erythrocytes. An ionization chamber method. J. Lab. Clin. Med. **73**:173-180.
8. Demopoulos, H.B. 1973. Control of free radicals in biologic systems. Fed. Proc. **32**:1903-1908.
9. DiLuzio, N.R. 1973. Antioxidants, lipid peroxidation and chemical-induced liver injury. Fed. Proc. **32**:1875-1881.
10. Drath, D.B., and M.L. Karnofsky. 1974. Bactericidal activity of metal-mediated peroxide-ascorbate systems. Infect. Immun. **10**:1077-1083.
11. Hardin, B., W.N. Valentine, J.H. Follette, and J.S. Lawrence. 1954. Studies on the sulfhydryl content of human leukocytes and erythrocytes. Am. J. Med. Sci. **228**:73-82.
12. Holmes, B., A.R. Page, and R.A. Good. 1967. Studies of the metabolic activity of leukocytes from patients with a genetic abnormality of phagocyte function. J. Clin. Invest. **46**:1422-1432.
13. Homan-Muller, J.W.T., T.S. Weening, and D. Roos. 1975. Production of hydrogen peroxide by phagocytosing human granulocytes. J. Lab. Clin. Med. **85**:198-207.
14. Iyer, G.Y.N., D.M.F. Islam, and J.H. Quastel. 1961. Biochemical aspects of phagocytosis. Nature (London) **192**:535-541.
15. Klebanoff, S.J., and C.B. Hamon. 1972. Role of myeloperoxidase-mediated antimicrobial systems in intact leukocytes. RES J. Reticuloendothel. Soc. **12**:170-196.
16. Little, C., and P.J. Obrien. 1968. An intracellular GSH-peroxidase with a lipid peroxide substrate. Biochem. Biophys. Res. Commun. **31**:145-150.
17. Mason, R.J., T.P. Stossel, and M. Vaughn. 1972. Lipids of alveolar macrophages, polymorphonuclear leukocytes, and their phagocytic vesicles. J. Clin. Invest. **51**:2399-2407.
18. Miller, T.E. 1969. Killing and lysis of gram-negative bacteria through the synergistic effect of hydrogen peroxide, ascorbic acid, and lysozyme. J. Bacteriol. **98**:949-955.
19. Nungester, W.J., and A.M. Ames. 1948. The relationship between ascorbic acid and phagocytic activity. J. Infect. Dis. **83**:50-59.
20. Penney, J.R., and S.S. Zilva. 1945. The fixation and retention of ascorbic acid by the guinea-pig. Biochem. J. **40**:695-706.
21. Pincus, S.H., and S.J. Klebanoff. 1971. Quantitative leukocyte iodination. N. Engl. J. Med. **284**:744-750.
22. Roe, J.H., M.B. Milles, M.J. Osterling, and C.M. Damron. 1948. The detection of diketo-1-gulonic acid, dehydro-1-ascorbic acid and 1-ascorbic acid in the same tissue extract by the 2,4-dinitrophenylhydrazine method. J. Biol. Chem. **174**:201-208.
23. Rosner, F., I. Valmont, P.J. Kozinn, and L. Caroline. 1970. Leukocyte function in patients with leukemia. Cancer **25**:835-842.

24. Silber, R., and B. Gabrio. 1962. Studies on normal and leukemic leukocytes. III. Pyridine nucleotides. J. Clin. Invest. **41:**230-234.
25. Stossel, T.P., R.K. Root, and M. Vaughan. 1972. Phagocytosis in chronic granulomatous disease and the Chediak-Higashi syndrome. N. Engl. J. Med. **286:**120-123.
26. Tappel, A.L. 1973. Lipid peroxidation damage to cell components. Fed. Proc. **32:**1870-1874.
27. Zatti, M., and F. Rossi. 1965. Early changes of hexose monophosphate pathway activity and of NADPH oxidation in phagocytosing leucocytes. Biochim. Biophys. Acta **99:**557-561.
28. Zatti, M., F. Rossi, and P. Patriarca. 1968. The H_2O_2 production by polymorphonuclear leucocytes during phagocytosis. Experientia **24:**669-670.

Reading 2

This reading, entitled "The Bursa of Fabricius and Antibody Production," is taken from *Poultry Science* **35:**224-225, 1956 (copyright 1956, *Poultry Science*). This succinct report attributed for the first time a dependence of immunoglobulin production by chickens to a cloacal organ known as the bursa of Fabricius. Even though this paper was published in 1956, it is still possible to consider it as a paper of historical interest because of the important first that it describes. The evidence for the conclusion drawn is presented in the form of a single table, which needs no statistical interpretation.

This article inaugurated two major types of investigation: the search for similar immunoglobulin-dependent tissues in higher animals and a search for the basis (either cellular or humoral) for the bursa's contribution to birds. Regrettably neither of these has been finally determined; however, this in no way detracts from the keystone position of this paper to the phylogenetic basis of comparative immunology.

THE BURSA OF FABRICIUS AND ANTIBODY PRODUCTION

BRUCE GLICK, TIMOTHY S. CHANG, and R. GEORGE JAAP*

The bursa of Fabricius is a structure peculiar to *Aves*. It is a blind sac connected by a small duct to the dorsal part of the cloaca. Often nicknamed "cloacal thymus," the function of the bursa is believed to be similar to that of the thymus (Riddle,

---

*The Ohio Agricultural Experiment Station, Columbus, Ohio.

1928; Taibel, 1938). There is no question that the bursa of Fabricius functions as a lymph gland during the first two to three months after the chicken hatches (Jolly, 1914; Calhoun, 1933; Glick, 1955). Like the thymus, the bursa in birds is believed to have some endocrine function in relation to growth and sexual development (Riddle, 1928; Woodward, 1931; and others).

Although reticular cells of lymph glands and lymphocytes may participate in globulin and antibody synthesis (Raffel, 1953), suspicion regarding the importance of the bursa in antibody production arose in the following accidental manner. A source of chicken blood possessing a high titre of antibody for antigen O of *Salmonella typhimurium* was desired for other experiments. Seventeen and one-half milliliters of a 48 hour, heat inactivated, broth culture (Kauffmann, 1950) were injected intravenously during a 20 day period. Surplus 6 month old females from an experiment designed to study the effect of bursectomy were used. To our surprise six females which had been bursectomized at 12 days of age died as a result of the injections. Three survived but produced no antibodies. The non-bursectomized females seemed unaffected and built up normal titres of antibodies in their blood.

To test whether the bursa of Fabricius was involved in antibody production, 85 out of 168 male and female chickens were bursectomized at two weeks of age. Twenty of these White Leghorns received 8.5 ml of *S. typhimurium* antigen per bird in six intramuscular injections at four day intervals between the 3rd and 6th week after hatching. Blood samples taken one week after the last injection were tested by the homologous antigen-antibody reaction test at 1:25 dilution. Out of ten bursectomized birds antibodies to *S. typhimurium* were present in three individuals while eight of the ten normal controls developed antibodies.

The larger group composed of 74 White Leghorns and 74 Rhode Island Reds were each injected with 17.5 ml of the suspension of *S. typhimurium* in six intramuscular injections at four-day intervals from the 13th to the 16th week after hatching. Their reaction to the test for antibodies

Table 1. Number of chickens and antibody production resulting from injections of O antigen *(S. typhimurium)* between the 13th and 17th week after hatching

	Bursectomized		Controls	
	Posi-tive	Nega-tive	Posi-tive	Nega-tive
Rhode Island Red	5	33	35	1
White Leghorn	3	34	28	9
Total	8	67	63	10

at 17 weeks of age is given in the accompanying table.

Antibody titres were demonstrated for 63 out of 73 controls. This is considered to be a normal result with the typhimurium antigen. Only 8 of the 75 bursectomized birds developed antibodies. These results demonstrate that the bursa of Fabricius plays a vital role in the production of antibodies to *S. typhimurium*. No information is available concerning the possible role of the bursa in the production of antibodies for other antigens.

The bursa of Fabricius reaches its maximum size as early as 4 to 5 weeks in White Leghorns and as late as 9 to 10 weeks in Rhode Island Reds (Glick, 1955). This rapid growth period for the bursa coincides with the period when chickens attain the ability to develop many antibodies to foreign proteins (Wolfe and Dilks, 1948). Once the bird has developed the ability to produce antibodies this ability is maintained throughout life.

The bursae of White Leghorns begin to atrophy about seven weeks after hatching. In Rhode Island Reds atrophy of the bursa begins later, about the 13th week (Glick, 1955). It is unlikely that the atrophic bursae of chickens between the 13th and 17th week after hatching could have a direct influence on antibody production. To determine where and how the bursa is involved in antibody production should prove promising for further research.

The White Leghorn breed has a greater resistance to *S. pullorum* then Rhode Island Reds during the first two weeks after hatching (Hutt and Scholes, 1941). The more rapid growth rate and larger mature size of the bursa in White Leghorns has been demonstrated. Disease resistance in general may be associated with rate of growth and size of the bursa during the period when the bird first develops the capacity to produce many of its antibodies.

REFERENCES

Calhoun, M.L., 1933. Microscopic anatomy of the digestive tract of *Gallus domesticus*. Iowa State College J. Sci. **7:** 261-382.

Glick, B., 1955. Growth and function of the Bursa of Fabricius in the domestic fowl. Ph.D. dissertation, Ohio State University.

Hutt, F.B., and J.C. Scholes, 1941. Genetics of the fowl. 13, Breed differences in susceptibility to *Salmonella pullorum*. Poultry Sci. **20:**342-352.

Jolly, J., 1914. La bourse de Fabricius. Et les organes lymphoepithéliauz. Arch. d'Anat. Micr. **16:**316-546.

Kauffmann, F., 1950. The Diagnosis of *Salmonella* types. Charles C Thomas, Illinois.

Raffel, S., 1953. Immunity. Appleton-Century-Crofts, Inc., New York.

Riddle, O., 1928. Growth of the gonads and bursa of Fabricius in doves and pigeons with data for body growth and age at maturity. Amer. J. Physiol. **86:**243-265.

Taibel, A.M., 1938. Effetto della bursectomia sul timo in *Gallus domesticus*. Riv. Biol. **24:**364-372.

Wolfe, H.R., and E. Dilks, 1948. Precipitin production in the chicken. III: Variation in antibody response as correlated with age of animal. J. Immunology **58:**245-250.

Woodward, M., 1931. Studies in bursectomized and thymectomized chicken. M.S. thesis, Kansas State College.

Reading 3

The article "Thymus-Marrow Immunocompetence. III. The Requirement for Living Thymus Cells" often is quoted as among the first articles to clearly substantiate the importance of the interaction between thymus cells and bone marrow cells in the formation of immunoglobulins. As indicated in the title, this is actually the third of a series of articles from this group of experimenters on essentially the same subject. The importance of this particular article is its proof that the thymus-marrow (currently referred to as the T cell–B cell) interaction is clearly synergistic and depends on living thymus cells. Irradiated or sonic-treated thymus cells improved the response slightly compared with animals that did not receive any type of thymus stimulant, and this type of data often has been presented as evidence of the thymus hormone. Note that the authors emphasize the contribution of living syngeneic thymus tissue, since the response is so much greater than with dead or foreign thymus tissue, which could have low activity merely as a nonspecific adjuvant effect. Note also that the numbers appear more meaningful when expressed as plaque-forming centers rather than as the titer of the antisera.

This article is reprinted from the *Proceedings of the Society of Experimental Biology and Medicine* **127**:462-466, 1968.

THYMUS-MARROW IMMUNOCOMPETENCE. III. THE REQUIREMENT FOR LIVING THYMUS CELLS* (32715)

HENRY N. CLAMAN, EDWARD A. CHAPERON,[1] and JOHN C. SELNER[2]

The immunocompetence of thymus-marrow cell suspensions has been demonstrated (1, 2). Suspensions containing both thymus and marrow cells produced more antibody to sheep erythrocytes (SRBC) when transferred to irradiated syngeneic hosts and stimulated with antigen than could be accounted for by the summation of the activities of thymus or marrow cell suspensions considered singly. Thymus-marrow interaction has also been demonstrated in other systems (3-6).

The nature of the thymus-marrow interaction is obscure. The purpose of these experiments was to investigate the system using the Jerne plaque assay method and to determine whether isologous living thymus cells could be replaced by irradiated cells, cell sonicates, or heterologous cells. The importance of the recipient thymus was also investigated.

*This work was supported by USPHS grants, 5 TI AI 13, AM-10145, AM-07529, AI-04152, and AI-33165.
[1]Postdoctoral Fellow, USPHS grant AM-33525.
[2]Departments of Medicine and Pediatrics, University of Colorado Medical Center, Denver, Colorado 80220.

Materials and methods

LAF_1 mice were used and the description of the mice, method of cell suspension preparation and hemolysin assay have already been published (1, 2). Immunization was with 0.2 ml of 10% washed SRBC. Rat thymus cell suspensions were made from freshly sacrificed young adult Sprague-Dawley Rats (Simonson Laboratories). Fetal liver cell suspensions were made by passing fetal LAF_1 livers through a graded series of needles as was done with marrow. "Minced" thymus preparations each consisted of a pair of thymic lobes cut into 8-12 pieces with scissors; these pieces were injected ip through a 20-gauge needle. Chilled thymus cells suspensions were disrupted by sonication for 5 min. Thymectomy was done under secobarbital anesthesia one week before irradiation and cell transfer. The sternum was split, the fascia incised, and the thymus aspirated. Sham thymectomies were done similarly except that aspiration was omitted.

Irradiation was carried out either with a 250 kV_p GE Maxitron or a 220 kV_p Westinghouse therapy unit. HVT for both units was 1.57 mm Cu. Radiation was delivered at 26r/min.

In most of the experiments the recipient mice were irradiated on day 0 and cells from normal donors together with SRBC were injected iv several hours later. On day 4 recipients were given an additional ip injection of SRBC. At sacrifice on day 8 the mice were bled and the sera from each group were pooled for hemolysin titrations. The recipient spleens were removed and passed through a stainless steel screen to make a single cell suspension. Plates were made according to the method of Jerne *et al.* (7) as described in detail elsewhere (8). Plaques were counted with an image amplifier and the geometric mean number of plaque-forming cells (PFC) per spleen for each group was calculated together with the 95% confidence limits.

Histological examination of tissues was made by fixation in Zenker-formalin, imbedding in methyl methacrylate, sectioning and staining with hematoxylin-eosin-azure.

Results

Tables 1 and 3 show that the enhanced effect of thymus-plus-marrow combinations over the sum of thymus and marrow taken singly may be demonstrated using the Jerne plaque-assay method. The importance of the route of injection of cells is shown by comparing groups A, B, and C in Table 1. If marrow was given iv thymus cells were effective if given either iv (A) or ip (C). If marrow was given ip, however, thymus cells iv were ineffective in augmenting the PFC in host spleens (B). The hemolysin titer of group B, on the other hand, was as great as A or C. We interpret this to indicate that antibody-producing cells were present in the body outside the spleen (see *Discussion*).

Table 2 shows that the sonicated cells of one

Table 1. Immunocompetence of thymus-marrow cell combinations

Group	No. of animals	Cells received on day 0[a]	Results day 8 PFC/spleen ($\pm$95% limits)	Log$_2$ hemolysins
A	5	Thymus iv + marrow iv + SRBC iv	892 (276-2233)	4
B	5	Thymus iv + marrow ip + SRBC iv	13 (3-68)	5
C	5	Thymus ip + marrow iv + SRBC iv	468 (86-2570)	4
D	4	Thymus iv + SRBC iv	11 (1-125)	0
E	4	Marrow iv + SRBC iv	110 (19-624)	2
F	4	SRBC iv	2 (1-5)	0

[a]All recipients were given 855r 250 kV_p X-rays on day 0 prior to injection of cells, and on day 4 were given SRBC ip. Doses of cells were: thymus (5.1×10^7) and marrow (3.6×10^7).

Table 2. Effects of suspensions of whole and sonicated mouse thymus cells

Group	No. of animals[a]	Cells received on day 0	Daily	Results day 8 PFC/spleen ($\pm$95% limits)	Log$_2$ hemolysins
A	5	Mouse thymus (3×10^7) iv Marrow (9.1×10^6) + SRBC iv		383 (180-812)	3
B	6	Marrow (9.1×10^6) + SRBC iv	Sonicated thymus ip[b]	90 (33-249)	0
C	5	Marrow (9.1×10^6) + SRBC iv		76 (15-375)	0
D	4	SRBC iv	Sonicated thymus ip[b]	3 (1-17)	0

[a]All recipient mice received 855r on day 0.
[b]Each mouse in Groups B and D received the cells of one thymus, sonicated ip daily.

Table 3. Effects of rat thymus cell suspensions

| | | | | Results day 8 | |
				PFC/spleen ($\pm$95% limits)	Log$_2$ hemolysins
Group	No. of animals[a]	Cells received on day 0	Daily		
A	4	Mouse thymus (5×10^7) iv Marrow (10^7) + SRBC iv		404 (107-962)	4
B	5	Rat thymus (3×10^7) iv Marrow (10^7) + SRBC iv	Rat thymus ip[b]	42 (14-131)	0
C	3	Mouse thymus (5×10^7) + SRBC iv		12 (3-55)	0
D	5	Mouse (10^7) + SRBC iv		16 (6-38)	0
E	5	Rat thymus (3×10^7) + SRBC iv	Rat thymus ip[b]	8 (1-45)	0
F	5	SRBC iv		2 (1-3)	0

[a] All recipients given 855r irradiation and SRBC as in Table 1.
[b] Each mouse in Groups B and E received 1/12 fresh rat thymus suspension ip daily, days 1-7.

thymus per day injected ip daily into each mouse for 8 days did not interact with iv marrow, while 3×10^7 iv thymus cells given once only on day 0 with iv marrow did result in production of significant antibody.

Table 3 shows that daily injections of suspensions of rat thymus cells ip were unable to substitute for a single iv injection of mouse thymus cells.

Other workers have shown that the immunocompetence of thymus cells was resistant to 500r *in vitro* and may be associated with the radioresistant thymic epithelial and reticular cells rather than the radiosensitive thymic small lymphocyte (9). Our previous experiments, on the contrary, showed that the immunocompetence of the thymus component in this thymus-marrow system was abolished by 500r *in vivo* (2). One possible explanation for this discrepancy is that in using screened suspensions of thymus cells prepared after irradiation, a selected population of epithelial and reticular cells adhered to the stroma during preparation and was not passed through the screen nor injected into the recipient. To test this, minced

whole thymus preparations, presumably containing all the cells of the thymus, were injected ip. While these minced preparations showed immunocompetence when injected with iv marrow (Table 4, A), similar minced thymus preparations from irradiated donors (530r) showed very little antibody production (B) when injected with iv marrow.

Thymectomy 1 week prior to the injection of cells (Table 5) had no significant effect on the antibody-forming potential of transfused thymus-marrow suspensions. Histological examination of tissue from the anterior mediastinum showed no thymic remnants in the thymectomized group.

Other experiments have shown that fetal liver may substitute for marrow since fetal liver-plus-thymus combinations were more immunogenic than the sum of both cell suspensions alone. Fetal liver suspensions were about half as effective as suspensions containing equal numbers of marrow cells.

Discussion

These data clearly demonstrate that the phenomenon of thymus-marrow "synergism" may be seen

Table 4. Effects of minced normal or irradiated mouse thymus preparations

			Results day 8	
Group	No. of animals	Cells received on day 0[a]	PFC/spleen ($\pm$95% limits)	Log$_2$ hemolysins
A	11	1 Normal thymus (minced) ip Marrow + SRBC iv	1006[b] (550-1756)	4.5[b]
B	8	1 Irradiated thymus (minced) ip Marrow + SRBC iv	209[b] (98-448)	1[b]
C	5	1 Normal thymus (minced) ip SRBC iv	15 (15-45)	0
D	5	Marrow + SRBC iv	69 (17-276)	0
E	3	SRBC iv	10 (2-47)	0

[a]All recipients were given 742-795r on day 0 prior to injection of cells, and on day 4 were given SRBC ip. Marrow dosage was 7.4-10.0 $\times$ 10^6. Group-B recipients received minced thymus from donors which had received 530r 2-3 hours before transfer of cells.
[b]Groups A and B are pooled from two experiments.

Table 5. Effect of thymectomy of hosts

			Results day 8	
No. of animals	Treatment	Cells received on day 0[a]	PFC/spleen ($\pm$95% limits)	Log$_2$ hemolysins
7	Thymectomy	Thymus + marrow + SRBC	1810 (920-3557)	4
6	Sham thymectomy	Thymus + marrow + SRBC	1566 (926-2650)	4
3	None	SRBC	11 (2-48)	0

[a]Hosts were thymectomized or sham thymectomized on day 7. On day 0 hosts received 742r and then were given 5 $\times$ 10^7 thymus cells plus 10^7 marrow cells plus SRBC iv.

using the Jerne plaque assay on recipient spleens. This technique is more readily quantitated than the previously used technique of Playfair *et al*. (9). A drawback of the Jerne technique, as used here and in other experimental systems, is that it measures antibody production only in the tissue sampled, e.g., spleen in these experiments. Serum-antibody titers probably reflect antibody production in the *whole* animal to a greater degree than do spleen PFC. On the other hand, it is known that the antibody response of mice to iv SRBC is concentrated in the spleen. These factors, together with the known migration of antibody-forming cells between tissues (8), complicate the interpretation of the numbers of spleen PFC. This is particularly obvious in Group B of Table 1 where the discrepancy between spleen PFC and serum hemolysins is large. We interpret this discrepancy to indicate that antibody is being formed by thymus- or marrow-cell descendants in tissues other than the spleen. Since this discrepancy was seen only with iv thymus and ip marrow, the route of injection of marrow becomes crucial. These data suggest that the marrow cells must be present within the spleen in order to get PFC in that organ while the thymus cells probably do not appear in the spleen in significant numbers. This conclusion is based on the findings that iv marrow is more effective in thymus-marrow interaction than ip marrow, and that dividing cells from iv marrow "home" to the spleen in 8 days (11). Marrow cells given ip "home" to the spleen in much less efficient manner. Dividing thymus cells given iv do not appear in the recipient spleen in significant numbers (11), and in our experiments, both ip thymus cells and ip minced thymus were effective in thymus-marrow synergism.

These data show that the thymus component of the "synergistic" combination must consist of living cells. Thymic cell suspensions from irradiated donors and thymic cell sonicates are ineffective. In view of the large amount of sonicated thymic tissue given (Groups B and D in Table 2 received approximately 10 times more thymus tissue than did Group A), it is unlikely that a "humoral factor" is involved. The absence of activity following large daily doses of living rat thymus cells indicates a need for genetically related thymus cells. Recent experiments in our laboratory have shown that allogeneic (parental) thymus cells are less effective than are syngeneic cells (12).

The failure of recipient thymectomy to alter the thymus-marrow synergism indicates that this synergism does not depend on the presence of recipient's thymus during the period following irradiation and cell transfer. The mechanism of the phenomenon of thymus-marrow interaction remains obscure. ·

Summary

The enhanced immunocompetence of transferred thymus–marrow cell combinations was demonstrated using the Jerne plaque assay method. Suspensions containing both thymus and marrow cells produced more antibody to sheep erythrocytes when transferred to irradiated syngeneic hosts and stimulated with antigen than could be accounted for by the summation of thymus- or marrow-cell activities considered singly. Living homologous thymus cells were required, since the following materials were incapable of interacting with isologous marrow cells: sonicated or irradiated (530r) mouse thymus cells or living rat thymus cells. The thymus of the host was not necessary for demonstrating thymus-marrow immunocompetence.

We are grateful to Jean Baughman for excellent technical assistance and to the Department of Radiology for aid in irradiating the mice.

1. Claman, H.N., Chaperon, E.A., and Triplett, R.F., Proc. Soc. Exptl. Biol. Med. **122**, 1167 (1966).
2. Claman, H.N., Chaperon, E.A., and Triplett, R.F., J. Immunol. **97**, 828 (1966).
3. Miller, J.F.A.P., Leuchars, E., Cross, A.M., and Dukor, P., Ann. N.Y. Acad. Sci. **120**, 205 (1964).
4. Globerson, A., and Auerbach, R., J. Exptl. Med. **126**, 223 (1967).
5. Cheng, V., and Trentin, J.J., Federation Proc. **26**, 641 (1967).
6. Davies, A.J.S., Leuchars, E., Wallis, V., Marchant, R., and Elliott, E.V., Transplantation **5**, 222 (1967).
7. Jerne, N.K., and Nordin, A.A., Science **140**, 405 (1955).
8. Chaperon, E.A., Selner, J.C., and Claman, H.N., Immunology **14**, 553 (1968).
9. Miller, J.F.A.P., DeBurgh, P.M., Dukor, P., Grant, G., Allman, V., and House, W., Clin. Exptl. Immunol. **1**, 61 (1966).
10. Playfair, J.H.L., Papermaster, B.W., and Cole, L.J., Science **149**, 998 (1965).
11. Micklem, H.S., Ford, C.E., Evans, E.P., and Gray, J., Proc. Royal Soc. Ser. B. **165**, 78 (1966).
12. Chaperon, E.A., and Claman, H.N., Federation Proc. **26**, 640 (1967).

Reading 4

This reading indicates some of the known facts and future possibilities about interferon. Drs. Norris and Loh in their article "Coxsackievirus Myocarditis: Prophylaxis and Therapy with an Interferon Stimulator," from *Proceedings of the Society of Experimental Biology and Medicine* **142**:133-136, 1973, utilized double-stranded polyinosinic acid–polycytidylic acid (poly I · C) as an interferon inducer in mice. This complex is one of the most commonly used inducers, and the prevention of cytopathic effects of vesicular stomatitis virus in tissue culture, which these authors also used, is a common indicator for interferon. After establishing that the degree of pathology resulting from Coxsackie virus injection in young mice was related to the virus dose (except for large doses of virus), the authors present data to illustrate the protective effect of a single dose of poly I · C given prior to and as late as 1 day after virus injection but not if given later. Interferon levels were determined at various intervals after injection of the inducer. The results indicate high levels of interferon were present in blood within 4 hours and began to wane by 48 hours, as expected. Application of this type of information to domestic animals prior to exposure to certain disease agents, as in shipping fever in cattle, is a real possibility, although poly I · C is perhaps too toxic a compound for human use.

COXSACKIEVIRUS MYOCARDITIS: PROPHYLAXIS AND THERAPY WITH AN INTERFERON STIMULATOR[1] (36975)

DAVID NORRIS and PHILIP C. LOH*

It is becoming increasingly evident that viral infections play a significant role in the etiology of heart diseases (1-3). Coxsackie B viruses, which have been implicated as responsible agents in fatal myocarditis in the newborn (4-6) as well as adult myocarditis and pericarditis (3, 7-9), are currently thought to be the commonest cause of virus-induced heart illness in man (3, 9). The susceptibility of weanling mice to myocarditis in a nonlethal, experimental coxsackievirus B-3 infection (10) has provided us with a host-virus model which imitates the coxsackievirus-human relationship.

Numerous studies have demonstrated that interferon (IF) and interferon inducers are highly effective when used prophylactically in a variety of experimental viral infections (11-14). The present investigation was conducted to determine the effect of treatment with an IF inducer polyinosinic · polycytidylic acid (poly I · poly C) on myocarditis produced during an experimental coxsackievirus B-3 infection of mice.

[1]Supported in part by a Biomedical Sciences Grant from the University Research Council.
* Virus Laboratory, Department of Microbiology, University of Hawaii, Honolulu, Hawaii 96822.

Materials and methods

Mice. Thirteen-day-old general purpose Swiss mice obtained from the Animal Colony, University of Hawaii, were used in all experiments.

Virus. Coxsackievirus B-3 was obtained from the Department of Health, State of Hawaii, and was passed three times in suckling mice (<72 hr) by the intraperitoneal route (ip). A stock 20% carcass suspension was prepared after the final passage and yielded a LD_{50} of $10^{-5 \cdot 3}$/ml in 1-day-old mice inoculated ip.

Histological examination and scoring of lesions. The hearts were removed and examined microscopically. They were then fresh frozen and cut into 8 μm sections. Each 30th section was mounted and stained with haematoxylin and eosin. The severity of microscopic lesions was scored as described by Grodums and Dempster (15) with 1+ = lesions involving <25% of the myocardium, 2+ = lesions involving 50% of the myocardium, 3+ = lesions involving 75% of the myocardium, and 4+ = most of the myocardium has undergone pathological change. Susceptibility of each experimental group was graded on a percentile basis using "cumulative lesion score," divided by "maximum possible score" as described by Rytel and Kilbourne (16).

Interferon inducer. A commercial sterile preparation of double-stranded poly I · poly C obtained from Microbiology Associates, Bethesda, MD, was used for interferon induction.

Interferon assay. Serum IF concentrations were determined by the viral plaque reduction method (17) employing vesicular stomatitis virus (VSV) and mouse L cells.

Results and discussion

Testing host-virus system and determination of virus dose. To establish the degree of myocarditis to be expected, and to determine the appropriate virus challenge dose to be used in interferon studies, groups of 4-6 mice were inoculated ip with 0.5 ml of varying dilutions of the stock virus suspension. After 7 days, the mice were sacrificed and the hearts were examined. The affected hearts with gross damage exhibited yellow-white streaks or patches on the ventricular surface. Microscopic examination revealed focal areas of necrosis and degeneration of the myocardium with a mononuclear cell infiltrate. The results of histological examination of a representative experiment are shown in Table 1.

All of the mice challenged with virus dilutions to 10^{-3} developed myocarditis with the most severe damage occurring when the 10^{-2} dilution was used. However, animals inoculated with the higher concentration of virus (10^{-1} or undiluted) showed less damage. The reason for the decreased severity of damage with the lower dilutions is unknown. It can be speculated that at these dilutions the virus suspension contains a factor(s) which either passively inhibited the viral infection or induced a host response which interfered with the infectious process. This "factor(s)," which could be either IF in the inoculum or IF-induction by the large virus inoculum, is no longer effective at the higher dilutions. Also, it is possible that inoculation of high concentrations of virus may induce early antibody formation which may play a role here (21).

Table 1. Degree of myocarditis in mice inoculated intraperitoneally with (0.5 ml) varying dilutions of virus

Dilution of stock virus suspension	Frequency and severity[a] of histological lesions					
	−	1+	2+	3+	4+	Score %[b]
Undiluted	0	0	4	2	0	58
10^{-1}	0	0	1	0	3	87
10^{-2}	0	0	0	1	3	94
10^{-3}	0	0	2	3	0	65
10^{-4}	2	2	0	1	0	25

[a]Severity is graded as follows: 1+ = lesions involving <25% of the myocardium, 2+ = lesions involving 50% of the myocardium, 3+ = lesions involving 75% of the myocardium, 4+ = most of the myocardium involved.
[b]The score percentage was calculated according to the method of Rytel and Kilbourne (16).

Effect of poly I · C on virus induced myocarditis. To determine the prophylactic and therapeutic effect of poly I · C on coxsackievirus B-3–induced myocarditis, groups of 4-6 mice were given a single 150 μg dose of the interferon inducer ip at intervals from 48 hr prior to, to 96 hr after virus challenge. The challenge dose consisted of 0.5 ml of a 10^{-2} dilution of the stock virus suspension administered by the ip route. Seven days after challenge the mice were sacrificed and the frequency and severity of histological lesions of the hearts were examined.

The results of a representative experiment shown in Fig. 1 indicate that significant protection was provided when the poly I · C was given between 48 hr prior to, and 24 hr after challenge. Protection was almost complete when poly I · C was given 12 hr prior to challenge. In contrast no protection was observed when the inducer was given on the second or fourth day after challenge.

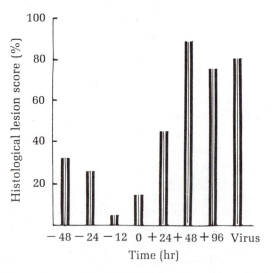

Fig. 1. Comparison of lesion severity in mice inoculated ip with 150 μg of poly I · C at intervals from 48 hr prior to, to 96 hr after challenge with 0.5 ml of 10^{-2} dilution of the stock coxsackievirus B-3 (ip). Histological lesions were graded as described in the text. Score percentage for each experimental group was calculated according to the method of Rytel and Kilbourne (16.)

When serum IF concentrations were determined at different times after poly I · C inoculation, maximal production was obtained 12 hr after induction (Table 2). This time period coincided with the period when the animals exhibited maximal protection to challenge with coxsackievirus. The protection decreased with increasing intervals between induction and challenge.

Previous studies have shown that poly I · C induces high levels of serum IF in mice within a few hours of inoculation (13, 18). Numerous studies have also demonstrated that IF provides resistance to a variety of experimental viral infections (12-14). The inhibition of myocarditis by poly I · C in the present study can therefore also be attributed to be due to the induction of IF. The fact that the inducer no longer provides protection when administered 48 hr after challenge indicated that by this time the infectious process may have either progressed to the point that IF was ineffective in preventing damage, or the protective effect of the single induction of IF may have waned. Rytel and Kilbourne (16) have shown that in experimental infection of mice with coxsackievirus B-3, the severity of cardiac lesions begins to increase rapidly after 24 hr postchallenge attaining almost maximum severity by 72 hr. Furthermore, the present results show that the protective effect induced by poly I · C decreases as a function of

time when it is given 24 hr or more before the challenge. This is in agreement with the reported kinetics of IF induction and duration (16, 19, 20).

Since a single dose of poly I · C in the present experiment provided a significant degree of therapeutic effect, it would be interesting to examine the effect of a multiple dose schedule on coxsackievirus-induced myocarditis. Daily treatments of Semliki Forest virus–infected mice with 100 μg of poly I · C (ip) have been reported to be most effective in reducing mortality compared to other dose schedules tested (22).

Summary

A single dose of the synthetic double-stranded polynucleotide poly I · C inoculated intraperitoneally into mice 12 to 48 hr before challenge with coxsackievirus B-3 resulted in almost complete protection from virus-induced myocarditis. Protection was related to the presence of high titers of circulating IF in the serum. Significant protection was also obtained even when poly I · C was given 24 hr after challenge with coxsackievirus.

Table 2. Serum interferon response in mice at different times after poly I · C inoculation[a]

Poly I · C time (hr)	Log_{10} IF/ml
None	<1.0
4	3.6
12	4.3
24	3.6
48	3.3

[a]A single dose of 150 μg of poly I · C/animal was injected intraperitoneally in mice. The animals were sacrificed at different times after inoculation and their serum interferon levels were determined by the 50% VSV plaque reduction technique (17).

1. Woodward, T.E., Togo, Y., Lee, Y., and Hornick, R.B., Arch. Intern. Med. **120,** 279 (1967).
2. Smith, W.G., Amer. Heart J. **73,** 439 (1967).
3. Smith, W.G., Amer. Heart J. **80,** 34 (1970).
4. Javett, S.N., Heymann, S., Mundel, B., Pepler, W.J., Lurie, H.I., Gear, J., Measroch, V., and Kirsch, Z., J. Pediat. **48,** 1 (1956).
5. Sussman, K.L., Strauss, L., and Hodes, H.L., AMA J. Dis. Child. **97,** 483 (1959).
6. Burch, G.E., Sun, S-C., Chu, K-C., Sohal, R.S., and Colcolough, H.L., J. Amer. Med. Ass. **203,** 1 (1968).
7. Fletcher, E., and Brennan, C.F., Lancet **1,** 913 (1957).
8. Burch, G.E., and Colcolough, H.L., Ann. Intern. Med. **71,** (5), 963 (1969).
9. Grist, N.R., and Bell, E.J., Amer. Heart J. **77,** 295 (1969).
10. Grodums, E.I., and Dempster, G., Can. J. Microbiol. **5,** 605 (1959).
11. Field, A.K., Tyrell, A.A., Lampson, G.P., and Hilleman, M.R., Proc. Nat. Acad. Sci. USA **58,** 1004 (1967).
12. Gresser, L., Bourali, C., Thouas, M.T., and Falcoff, E., Proc. Soc. Exp. Biol. Med. **127,** 491 (1968).
13. Catalano, L.W., and Baron, S., Proc. Soc. Exp. Biol. Med. **133,** 684 (1970).

14. Richmond, J.Y., and Hamilton, L.D., Proc. Nat. Acad. Sci. USA **64,** 81 (1969).
15. Grodums, E.I., and Dempster, G., Can. J. Microbiol. **5,** 595 (1959).
16. Rytel, M.W., and Kilbourne, E.D., Proc. Soc. Exp. Biol. Med. **137,** 443 (1971).
17. Wagner, R.R., Virology **13,** 323 (1961).
18. Youngner, J.S., and Hallum, J.V., Virology **35,** 177 (1968).
19. DuBuy, H.G., Johnson, M.O., Buckler, C.E., and Baron, S., Proc. Soc. Exp. Biol. Med. **135,** 349 (1970).
20. Buckler, C.E., DuBuy, H.G., Johnson, M.L., and Baron, S., Proc. Soc. Exp. Biol. Med. **136,** 394 (1971).
21. Murphy, E.R., and Glasgow, L.A., J. Exp. Med. **127,** 1035 (1968).
22. Worthington, M., and Baron, S., Proc. Soc. Exp. Biol. Med. **136,** 323 (1971).

Reading 5

This reading (from *Science* 102:400-401, 1945) by Ray D. Owen, entitled "Immunogenetic Consequences of Vascular Anastomoses Between Bovine Twins," has been selected, as was the second reading, for its historical import. In this brief communication Professor Owen combines information that he retrieved from the scientific literature of the previous 30 years with the then unexplainable observations about blood group patterns in twin calves. The scientific harvest from this article was not simply the solution of this blood grouping problem but also the opening of new vistas in immunotolerance and immunogenetics. Today immunologists are actively involved in research on the subjects of skin and tissue grafting, histocompatibility testing, fetal immune tolerance, and the ontogeny of the immune response, any one of which would be an adequate reason for the inclusion of this article here.

IMMUNOGENETIC CONSEQUENCES OF VASCULAR ANASTOMOSES BETWEEN BOVINE TWINS[1]

RAY D. OWEN

Almost thirty years have passed since Lillie[2] used the demonstrated union of the circulatory systems of twin bovine embryos of opposite sex to explain, on an endocrine basis, the frequent reproductive abnormalities of the female twin. Since the appearance of Lillie's paper, the freemartin, as the modified female is called, has become an important example of the effects of hormones on sex-differentiation and sexual development in mammals.[3] Consequences other than endocrinological of nature's experiment in parabiosis have, however, received little attention.

Estimates of the frequency of identical as compared with fraternal twinning indicate that the former is relatively rare in cattle.[4] Tests for inherited cellular antigens in the blood of more than eighty pairs of bovine twins show, however, that in the majority of these pairs the twins have identical blood types. Identity of blood types between full sibs not twins is infrequent, as might be expected from the large number of different, genetically controlled antigens[5,6] (now approximately 40) identified in the tests. If, therefore, the frequent identity of blood types in twin pairs can be explained neither as the result of monozygotic twinning nor as chance identity between fraternal twins, nor as the sum of these two factors, it is evident that some mechanism is operating to produce frequent phenotypic identity of blood types in genetically dissimilar twins. The vascular anastomosis between bovine twins, known to be a common occurrence,[2] provides an explanation.

Three additional, independent sources of evidence help to define the action of this mechanism. (1) One twin sire failed to transmit to any of his twenty progeny certain of the antigens found in his blood. In other words, the genotype of this bull

[1]From the Departments of Genetics (No. 346) and Veterinary Science, University of Wisconsin, in cooperation with the Bureau of Animal Industry, U.S. Department of Agriculture. This is part of a program aided by grants from the American Guernsey Cattle Club, the Holstein-Friesian Association of America, the Rockefeller Foundation and the Wisconsin Alumni Research Foundation. Appreciated contributions to various phases of the investigation have been made by Professor M.R. Irwin, C.J. Stormont and Mary W. Ycas. This study has been possible only through the generous cooperation of workers at many state experiment stations and of numerous private breeders of cattle.
[2]F.R. Lillie, *Science*, 43:611-613, 1916.
[3]See "Sex and Internal Secretions," edited by Edgar Allen (Williams and Wilkins, Baltimore, 1939), for general discussions of and references to the literature on the freemartin.
[4]D. Sanders, *Zeit. fur Zuchtung B*, **32**:223-268, 1935.
[5]L.C. Ferguson, *Jour. Immunol.*, **40**:213-242, 1940.
[6]L.C. Ferguson, C. Stormont and M.R. Irwin, *Jour. Immunol.*, **44**:147-164, 1942.

as determined from his progeny appeared to lack factors responsible for some of the antigens found in his phenotype. Tests showed that cells containing these antigens could have been derived from his twin, whose genotype did contain the necessary factors. (2) In a case of superfecundation in cattle, involving twins of opposite sex and by different sires,[7] the twins had identical blood types, each possessing two antigens the genetic factors for which could not have come from his own sire or from the dam. Cells containing those critical antigens could in each case have been derived from the co-twin. (3) It has been demonstrated, by a simple immunological technique developed for this purpose, that there is a mixture of two distinct types of erythrocytes in certain twins.

These facts are consistent with the conclusion that an interchange of cells between bovine twin embryos occurred as a result of vascular anastomoses. Since many of the twins in this study were adults when they were tested, and since the interchange of formed erythrocytes alone between embryos occurs as a result of vascular anastomosient modification of the variety of circulating cells, it is further indicated that the critical interchange is of embryonal cells ancestral to the erythrocytes of the adult animal.[8] These cells are apparently capable of becoming established in the hemapoietic tissues of their co-twin hosts and continuing to provide a source of blood cells distinct from those of the host, presumably throughout his life.

Several interesting problems in the fields of genetics, immunology and development are suggested by these observations. Most of them are still largely speculative and will not be considered here. An application that may be mentioned is the tool now provided by the blood tests for selecting, with a high degree of reliability, those heifers, born twin with bulls, that are potentially not freemartins but normal, fertile individuals. A heifer whose blood type is the same as her twin brother's will very probably be a freemartin, while a difference in even a single antigen between twins of opposite sex may indicate that vascular anastomosis did not occur, and therefore that the heifer will be normal. Thus clinical observations on the heifer alone, probably not always reliable when the heifer is young, can be supplemented by an objective laboratory test applicable as soon as the twins are born. Possible limitations of this application, as well as a more complete presentation of the data and further discussion of the implications of the present study, will be included in another paper.

Reading 6

The importance of complement in nonhemolytic reactions, in company with the unraveling of its structural complexities, has been the center of research with complement over the past decade. During this same period considerable debate has existed as to how lymphoid cells and monocytes participated with antibody and complement in ADCC reactions. In this report from *Science* **192**:563-565, 1976 (copyright 1976, the American Association for the Advancement of Science), a system of ADCC attack on sheep red blood cells, which could be blocked by normal IgG, is released from this block by coating the target cells with complement and antibody. Thus the complement receptor of the ADCC effector cells, in an as yet unidentified fashion, generates with C3b a lytic attack that can overcome the normal antibody blockade. This may be important in the interpretation of some aspects of transplantation and tumor immunity as well as the area of autoimmune disease.

COMPLEMENT-DEPENDENT IMMUNOGLOBULIN G RECEPTOR FUNCTION IN LYMPHOID CELLS

JUAN CARLOS SCORNICK*

Abstract. Lymphoid cells are unable to lyse antibody-coated target cells in the presence of normal immu-

---

[7]A description and discussion of this case will be published elsewhere by Mr. B.H. Roche, who called it to our attention and provided us with blood samples from the animals involved.

[8]Cf. H.E. Jordan, *Physiol. Rev.*, **22**:375-384, 1942.

*Hematology Section, Department of Clinical Chemistry and Laboratory Medicine, University of Texas System Cancer Center, M.D. Anderson Hospital and Tumor Institute, Houston, Texas 77025. Present address: Department of Pathology, University of Florida College of Medicine, Gainesville, Fla. 32610.

noglobulin G (IgG), presumably because their surface receptors for IgG are blocked. However, when target cells are sensitized with antibodies and complement, IgG receptors are unblocked and cytotoxicity occurs even in the presence of normal IgG. Thus, IgG receptors may function in vivo despite the relatively high concentrations of IgG in serum and interstitial fluid.

Cell-mediated cytotoxicity induced by immunoglobulin G (IgG) antibodies to target cell (antibody-dependent cell-mediated cytotoxicity, ADCC) has been advocated as a possible mechanism involved in allograft rejection *(1)*, viral infections *(2)*, tumor immunity *(3)*, and autoimmune diseases *(4)*. However, no direct evidence of its participation in vivo has been obtained. Furthermore, ADCC is inhibited by normal IgG *(5)* at concentrations below those in normal serum or interstitial fluid *(6)*. I now report an in vitro model in which ADCC is induced even in the presence of inhibitory concentrations of IgG, providing an experimental basis for a possible in vivo function of the IgG receptors.

Effector cells were obtained from spleens surgically removed from patients undergoing staging laparotomies *(7)*. A cell suspension was prepared and mononuclear cells were concentrated by Ficoll-Hypaque centrifugation *(8)*. Sheep red blood cells (SRBC), used as target cells, were labeled with 100 μc of ^{51}Cr ($Na_2^{51}CrO_4$, New England Nuclear) *(9)* and treated with different antibody preparations. The following groups of sensitized target cells were prepared: EA-G, SRBC coated with IgG antibodies *(10)*; EA-M, SRBC sensitized with IgM antibodies; EAC-M and EAC-G, SRBC sensitized with IgM or IgG antibodies and complement (C); EA-M-G, SRBC sensitized with IgM first and subsequently with IgG; EAC-M-G, SRBC sensitized with IgM and C and subsequently with IgG.

Effector cells (30×10^6) and target cells (2×10^6) were placed in plastic petri dishes (35 by 10 mm; Falcon Plastics) in 1 ml of Ham's F-10 medium (Grand Island) supplemented with 20 percent fetal calf serum and 50 μg of gentamicin (Schering) per milliliter. Inhibitors were added prior to

the addition of the target cells. The cell mixtures were incubated (on a rocking platform) in an atmosphere of 5 percent CO_2 at 37° C for 18 hours and the percentage of cytotoxicity was determined *(11)*. Values were expressed as specific cytotoxicity after subtraction of nonspecific lysis obtained in the absence of spleen cells. Nonspecific lysis was determined for each type of target cell (EA-G, EAC-G, EAC-M, and others).

Lymphoid cells carry on their surface receptors for the third component of complement (C3), which enable them to bind SRBC coated with C *(12)*. However, such a binding does not induce lysis of the target cell, an observation that has led to the suggestion that the C3 receptor does not have a major role in ADCC *(13)*. The following results indicate that the C3 receptor does have a major role since it allows the induction of ADCC in the presence of inhibitory concentrations of serum IgG. Lysis of EA-G is inhibited by human serum at dilutions of 10^{-2} and 10^{-1}. However,

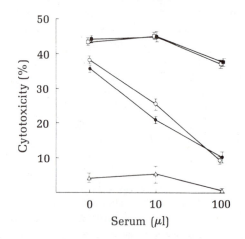

Fig. 1. Inhibition of cytotoxicity by human serum. Human serum, obtained from normal donors, was pooled, inactivated by heat, and absorbed with SRBC. Cytotoxicity was induced by human spleen lymphoid cells against SRBC sensitized in different ways. △, EA-M; ●, EA-G; ○, EA-M-G; ■, EAC-G; □, EAC-M-G. The total volume of the cell mixture was 1 ml. The bars correspond to the range of duplicate determinations.

lysis of EAC-G is inhibited to a much lesser extent, and a significant degree of cytotoxicity is still observed at the higher concentrations of serum (Fig. 1). The same effect is observed when C is bound to the erythrocyte by IgM antibody, and IgG antibody is added later (EAC-M-G); the lysis of EA-G is not affected by the simultaneous presence of IgM (EA-M-G). Similar results were obtained in four independent experiments *(14)*.

An excess of free molecules of serum IgG may block the IgG receptors but not the C3 receptors. However, since the binding through C3 receptors does not trigger lysis of the target cells, an explanation must be offered for the cytotoxicity of EAC-G (but not of EA-G) obtained in the presence of serum IgG. Taking into account that the IgG antibody must be present on the target cell for the induction of cytotoxicity and that the binding of free monomeric IgG molecules to the IgG receptors is weak *(15)*, then it can be postulated that the

intimate contact between effector and target cell, brought about through the C3 receptor, promotes the displacement of the free IgG from the lymphocyte receptor by the IgG antibody bound to the target cell, making possible the occurrence of ADCC. If this hypothesis is correct, blocking of the IgG receptors with soluble antigen-antibody complexes, whose binding with the IgG receptor is stronger than that of free IgG (and more difficult to displace), should lead to a pronounced inhibition of the lysis of EAC-G.

The following experiments support this possibility. Serum from a rabbit immunized against *Candida albicans* antigens *(16)* produced significant inhibition of cytotoxicity of EA-G, but little effect on the lysis of EAC-G (Fig. 2, *A*). However, when the antigen was also added to the cell mixture, cytotoxicity for both EA-G and EAC-G was inhibited (Fig. 2, *B*). Antigen alone did not inhibit cytotoxicity. In other experiments, antigen-

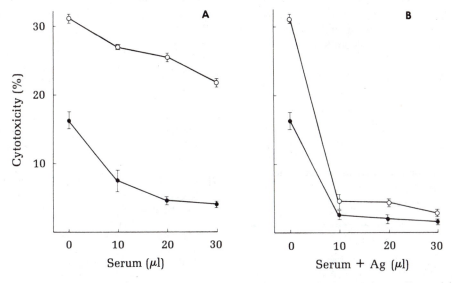

Fig. 2. Inhibition of cytotoxicity by rabbit serum and antigen-antibody complexes. Cytotoxicity was induced by human spleen lymphoid cells in a total volume of 1 ml. The target cells used were as follows: ●, EA-G; ○, EAC-G. Lysis of EAC-M was 2.2 percent. **A,** Effect of increasing concentrations of rabbit antiserum to *Candida albicans* antigens. **B,** Effect of the rabbit antiserum plus equal volume of *Candida albicans* antigen. No inhibition of cytoxicity was observed with 10, 20, or 30 µl of the antigen preparation in the absence of the rabbit antiserum. The bars correspond to the range of duplicate determinations.

antibody complexes did not inhibit binding of EAC-G *(17).*

The foregoing results suggest that the antigen-antibody complexes do not block the C3 receptors, and hence binding of EAC-G ensues unaffected. Antigen-antibody complexes do not block IgG receptors, in a reaction not easily reversible; and lysis of target cells does not occur in their presence. Thus, the lysis of EAC-G obtained in the presence of monomeric serum IgG represents an induction of the classical ADCC, generated through the IgG receptors.

Most cells that carry IgG receptors (B lymphocytes, granulocytes, monocytes, macrophages), which are efficient effector cells for ADCC *(11, 18),* also carry C receptors *(12).* This may be a structural arrangement designed for a cooperative function of C and IgG receptors *(19).*

In conclusion, the classical mechanism of ADCC may operate in the presence of normal IgG, provided that both IgG antibody and C are present on the target cell. The function of the C3 receptor is to promote the binding of effector and target cells, generating favorable conditions for the interaction of the IgG antibody and the lymphocyte receptor, and overcoming the inhibitory effect of normal IgG.

The occurrence of IgG antibodies and the presence of C on target cells or tissues are features frequently found in some autoimmune diseases *(4)* and in allograft reactions *(20).* Consequently, the above results suggest that the participation of ADCC in those situations is not only possible but is also likely to occur.

REFERENCES AND NOTES

1. T.B. Strom, N.L. Tilney, C.B. Carpenter, G.J. Busch, *N. Engl. J. Med.* **292,** 1257 (1975); A. Ting and P.I. Terasaki, *Transplantation* **18,** 371 (1974).

2. S.L. Shore, A.J. Nahmias, S.E. Starr, P.A. Wood, D.E. McFarlin, *Nature (London)* **251,** 350 (1974).

3. M.O. Landazuri, E. Kedar, J.L. Fahey, *J. Natl. Cancer Inst.* **52,** 147 (1974).

4. R.W. Steblay and U. Rudofsky, *Science* **180,** 966 (1973); U.H. Rudofsky, R.W. Steblay, B. Pollara, *Clin. Immunol. Immunopathol.* **3,** 396 (1975).

5. I.C.M. MacLennan, *Clin. Exp. Immunol.* **10,** 275 (1972); G. Holm, E. Engwall, S. Hammarström, J. B. Natvig, *Scand. J. Immunol.* **3,** 173 (1974); J.C. Scornik, H. Cosenza, W. Lee, H. Köhler, D.A. Rowley, *J. Immunol.* **113,** 1510 (1974); J.C. Scornik, M.C. Salinas, B. Drewinko, *ibid.* **115,** 901 (1975).

6. H.L. Poulsen, *Scand. J. Clin. Lab. Invest.* **34,** 119 (1974). Poulsen reported an IgG concentration of approximately 10 mg/ml in serum and 6 mg/ml in interstitial fluid.

7. Nine spleens were used in this study, all from patients with Hodgkin's disease of the nodular sclerosing or mixed cellularity type. Six spleens were macroscopically and microscopically normal. In three cases the spleen was involved, and areas without macroscopic nodules were used to prepare the cell suspensions. Two patients received radiotherapy 1 month before splenectomy; the remaining patients were untreated at the time of the study. Experiments were also done with mouse spleen cells as effector cells; the results were similar to those obtained with human cells.

8. A. Böyum, *Scand. J. Clin. Lab. Invest.* **21** (Suppl. 97), 1 (1968). The cells collected at the interphase were washed three times with Hanks solution before use. Viability was 85 to 90 percent, and the cell population comprised more than 90 percent lymphoid cells, the rest being mainly monocytes and granulocytes.

9. P. Perlmann and H. Perlmann, *Cell. Immunol.* **1,** 300 (1970).

10. Packed SRBC (50 μl) were incubated with 0.5 ml of the appropriate dilution of antibodies for 15 minutes at 37° C and then washed three times. The IgG (7S) fraction of a rabbit antibody to SRBC was used at 1:400 dilution, whereas a rabbit antibody to SRBC stromata [the immunoglobulin M (IgM) fraction] was used at a 1:120 dilution. Both preparations were obtained from Cordis (Miami, Florida). A 1:5 dilution of mouse serum in Hanks solution, which was the source of complement, was added for 30 minutes at 37° C to the sensitized RBC for the preparation of EAC.

11. J.C. Scornik and H. Cosenza, *J. Immunol.* **113,** 1527 (1974). The content (1 ml total volume) of each petri dish was placed in a tube (tube A), and the saline (1 ml) used to rinse the petri dish was added. The tube was centrifuged, and the supernatant was placed in another tube (tube B). The cells remaining in the petri dishes were removed with 2 ml of distilled water and placed in tube A. The radioactivity in both tubes was counted in a well-type gamma counter and the percentage of cytotoxicity was calculated by dividing the radioactivity of tube B by the total radioactivity (tube A + tube B) and multiplying by 100.

12. V. Nussenzweig, *Adv. Immunol.* **19,** 217 (1974).

13. J.A. Van Boxel, W.E. Paul, I. Green, M.M. Frank, *J. Immunol.* **112,** 398 (1974); P. Perlmann, H. Perlmann, H.J. Müller-Eberhard, *J. Exp. Med.* **141,** 287 (1975).

14. Experiments where the human serum concentrations were

more than 50 percent are not reported because they produced agglutination of SRBC (despite repeated absorptions). However, purified human IgG at 4 mg/ml produced complete inhibition of lysis of EA-G but not of EAC-G.

15. J.C. Cerottini and K.T. Brunner, *Adv. Immunol.* **18**, 67 (1974).

16. Antigen and antiserum were provided by Dr. Roy Hopfer. Soluble *Candida albicans* antigens were prepared by mechanically disrupting the organisms and discarding insoluble particles by centrifugation and filtration through a 0.22-μm Millipore filter. Rabbit antiserum was obtained after repeated immunizations with the antigen preparation in complete Freund's adjuvant. The rabbit antiserum was inactivated by heat and absorbed with SRBC before use. The antigen preparation was used at a 1:20 dilution, which was optimal for obtaining precipitation lines in counterelectrophoresis.

17. Spleen cells attached to plastic petri dishes treated with poly-L-lysine [J.C. Kennedy and M.A. Axelrod, *Immunology* **20**, 253 (1971)] were incubated with ^{51}Cr-labeled target cells (E, EA-G, EA-M, EAC-M, EAC-G) for 1 hour at 37° C in a rocking platform. Each petri dish was then washed three times with saline and immersed three more times in a beaker with saline. The target cells that remained attached to the spleen cells were lysed with distilled water, and radioactivity was measured in a well-type gamma counter [J.C. Scornik and B. Drewinko, *J. Immunol.* **115**, 1223 (1975)].

18. J.A. Van Boxel, W.E. Paul, M.M. Frank, I. Green, *J. Immunol.* **110**, 1027 (1973); R.R. Gale and J. Zighelboim, *ibid.* **113**, 1793 (1974); G. Holm, E. Engwall, W. Hammarström, J.B. Natvig, *Scand. J. Immunol.* **3**, 173 (1974).

19. A similar cooperative effect has been described in the phagocytosis of erythrocytes by human monocytes [H. Huber, M.J. Polley, W.D. Linscott, H.H. Fudenberg, H.J. Müller-Eberhard, *Science* **162**, 1281 (1968)] and mouse polymorphonuclear leukocytes [B. Mantovani, *J. Immunol.* **115**, 15 (1975)].

20. A.J. D'Apice and P.J. Morris, *Transplantation* **18**, 20 (1974); K.A. Porter, *Transpl. Proc.* **6** (Suppl. 1), 79 (1974).

21. I thank B. Drewinko for his support for this work and A. Gage for technical assistance. Supported by NIH grant CA 17072-01.

22. August 1975; revised 16 January 1976.

Reading 7

One of the many services provided by WHO to immunologists is the assembly and debate of expert committees on unsettled topics in their science. These committees consist of acknowledged authorities on the specific subject they consider, be it the need for better typhoid vaccines, the status of immunity in malaria or schistosomiasis, the mode of action of adjuvants, or systems of standard nomenclature for immunoglobulins or complement. This report on nomenclature for the HLA system was prepared by a committee of geneticists and immunologists and was published in the *Bulletin of the World Health Organization* **52**:261-265, 1975.

A new HLA classification scheme has been published (in French in the *Bulletin of the World Health Organization* **59**:159-162, 1981; an English version is forthcoming). However, since the reading enclosed here contains historically important facts not presented in the text (FOUR locus, for example), it has been retained.

NOMENCLATURE FOR FACTORS OF THE HLA SYSTEM*

A Nomenclature Committee composed of geneticists and immunologists, including specialists in tissue typing, has met after each of the Histocompatibility Workshops beginning with the Third Workship in 1967. The Committee, in part under the auspices of the World Health Organization and the International Union of Immunological Societies (WHO/IUIS), met after the Sixth Workshop in Aarhus in July 1975. The expanding knowledge of the genetics of the major histocompatibility system of man has necessitated a revision of the terminology for the HLA region following the principles established in previous reports. This has been done with as few changes as possible.

It has been realized for a number of years that in man there is a major histocompatibility system of great complexity, homologous to those of other mammalian species and composed of a series of many closely-linked genes. The original serologically-defined specificities of the HLA system were assigned to two separate series (first or LA, and second or FOUR) corresponding to two linked foci with multiple alleles. These loci have been assigned to chromosome 6, both by family studies and by genetic analysis with somatic cell hybrids. Recent studies, especially in mouse and man, have shown that the genetic region identified by these

---

*This Terminology Note was drafted by the signatories listed on pp. 476-477. A French version will be published in a future issue of the *Bulletin*.

two loci also contains many other genes controlling cell surface determinants, immune response differences, some components of the complement system and, perhaps, other related functions. The purpose of the revised nomenclature is to take account of this increasing complexity.

The genetic region encompassing this large series of interrelated loci will be called HLA (the hyphen previously used in the designation of the HLA system is being dropped in order to minimize the increasing number of symbols needed to define loci and specificities belonging to the system). Genetic loci belonging to the system will be designated by one or more letters following the HLA. Individual alleles of each locus, and the corresponding specificities, will be designated by numbers following the locus symbols. Provisionally identified specificities will, as before, carry the additional letter W(w), which will now be inserted between the locus letter(s) and the allele and specificity number. Although many computer outputs contain only capital letters, nevertheless it is suggested that in writing and printing a lower case "w" should be used.

The general notational scheme is therefore as follows:

HLA: region or system designation.

A, B, C, D, etc.: locus symbols.

W(w): symbol to indicate a provisional specificity (may later be dropped when specificity is confirmed).

1, 2, etc.: number identifying specificities belonging to each locus.

Detailed examples of this system of notation are given later.

The decision as to whether a locus belongs to the HLA system will, as discussed in previous reports, be based at least on genetic mapping data, on evidence as to function and chemical structure, and on population data showing evidence of significant population associations (linkage disequilibrium). By these criteria, for example, a human analogue of the mouse T1a locus would most probably be assigned to the HLA system. The loci controlling complement components C2, C4, and properdin factor B (GBG, Bf, etc.), as well as those controlling the Chido and Rogers blood groups, should probably also be assigned to HLA. In this report, however, we shall confine our attention to the serologically-defined determinants found mainly on lymphocytes, other nucleated cells, and also platelets, and to the determinants recently identified by MLC-typing (mixed lymphocyte cultures).

The loci previously called LA (or first and FOUR (or second) will now be designated by the letters A and B, respectively. The complete locus symbols will therefore be HLA-A for the LA (or first), and HLA-B for the FOUR (or second) loci. For historical reasons the specificities determined by the alleles of these two loci are numbered jointly, so that apart from W5 and W10 (see below), there is no overlap in numbers between them. For example, specificities 1, 2, 3, 9, 10, 11, etc. belong to the HLA-A locus while 5, 7, 8, 12, 13, etc. belong to the HLA-B locus. This joint numbering scheme will be continued for these first two loci, and in local use the prefixes A and B may be optional. For other loci (C, D, etc.) the numbering of specificities will start in sequence from 1, separately for each locus, so that the prefix locus letter will be an essential part of the notation for a specificity. It is expected that, in most cases, a specificity will first receive a provisional w designation, but may later be upgraded by omitting the w, while keeping the same number.

The locus designated by the prefix C corresponds to that previously known as the AJ or third locus, and the locus designated D corresponds to what has variously been called MLR-S1, LD-1, MLC-1, etc.

The Committee recognized that many new specificities are being detected on lymphoid subpopulations such as B cells, T cells, lymphoblastoid lines, and chronic lymphatic leukaemia cells. Some of these specificities can also be detected on, for example, macrophages, endothelial cells, and sperm. It is probable that more than one locus is represented, as is the case for the corresponding specificities in the mouse, and as may also prove to be the case for lymphocyte-stimulating activities now provisionally assigned to locus D. Since the knowledge concerning these newer serological specificities is very recent and incomplete, it was felt that the assignment of one or more loci to them was premature.

An approach will be made to the Committee, at an appropriate future date, concerning the symbols to be used for the loci in the HLA region controlling or regulating some complement components.

The Committee considered the status of the existing W specificities and agreed that a number of them could now be upgraded from their provisional status. In considering the state of definition of a specificity, the previous criteria was somewhat modified. A specificity formerly designated W was upgraded to full HLA status provided it could be clearly and reproducibly recognized by several generally available antisera, which were represented at one or more workshops. The antigens so considered had all been tested for segregation in informative families and, generally, for their con-

sistent behaviour in different populations.[a] Absorptions are, in general, required but it was felt that absorption had less significance than had previously been thought because of the quantitative difficulties associated with varying degrees of cross-reactivity. Absorption is, however, still considered important and especially useful in the preliminary identification of new specificities. To this aim co-capping and stripping are other important serological tools. The upgraded specificities and newly designated w specificities, together with their previous equivalents, are listed in Table 1.

The new provisional Cw and Dw specificities, together with their previous equivalents, are given in Table 2.

The specificities W5 and W10 have, for historical reasons, been the only designations that overlap other numbered specificities (HLA-B5 and HLA-A10). In order to correct this anomaly, it is

[a]*Bulletin of the World Health Organization*, **47**:659-662 (1972).

Table 1. New designations for specificities of the HLA-A and HLA-B loci

New HLA nomenclature	Old nomenclature	Representative equivalents where applicable
HLA-B14	W14	
HLA-B18	W18	
HLA-B27	W27	
HLA-A28	W28	
HLA-A29	W29	
HLA-Aw33	W19.6	Including Fe55, 10.4, Bar 3, Malay 1
HLA-Aw34[a]		Malay 2, HL-A10-3, F26
HLA-Bw35	W5	
HLA-Aw36[a]		Mo*, LT
HLA-Bw37		TY
HLA-Bw38	W16.1	W16, W4, Da31
HLA-Bw39	W16.2	W16, W6, W16,382
HLA-Bw40	W10	
HLA-Bw41		Sabell, LK, Da34
HLA-Bw42[a]		MWA
HLA-Aw43[a]		BK

[a] Some of the new specificities are most frequently identified in certain population groups. Examples are Aw36, Bw42, and Aw43, which are most frequently found in certain African groups. HLA-Aw34 (HLA-10 related antigen) is frequently observed in some Orientals and in some Blacks from Africa and America.

Table 2. New designations for specificities of the HLA-C and HLA-D loci[a]

New HLA-C nomenclature	Representative equivalents	New HLA-D nomenclature
HLA-Cw1	T1-AJ	HLA-Dw1
HLA-Cw2	T2-Sa532	HLA-Dw2
HLA-Cw3	T3-UPS	HLA-Dw3
HLA-Cw4	T4-RH315	HLA-Dw4
HLA-Cw5	T5	HLA-Dw5
		HLA-Dw6

[a]For a more complete listing of Dw equivalents see Table 4.

proposed to renumber the W5 specificity Bw35 and the W10 specificity Bw40, as indicated in Table 1. The 'local' HLA-B specificities, TT* (HLA-B12 related), 407*, KSO (=JA), HR, and HS (=SIN 2) are still under consideration for upgrading.

A complete listing of all recognized HLA specificities is given in Table 3, together with the most common of the previously used symbols. A more comprehensive list of equivalents for the HLA-D specificities is given in Table 4.

Many additional specificities were considered as candidates for w classification. Those not included in Tables 1 and 2 were withheld pending further clarification by WHO collaborating laboratories. The specificities HLA-Aw32, Aw33, Bw17, Bw21, B5 (previously HL-A5), Bw35, HR,

Table 3. Complete listing of recognized HLA specificities[a]

New	Previous[b]	New	Previous	New	Previous	New	Previous
HLA-A1	HL-A1	HLA-B5	HL-A5	HLA-Cw1	T1	HLA-Dw1	LD 101
HLA-A2	HL-A2	HLA-B7	HL-A7	HLA-Cw2	T2	HLA-Dw2	LD 102
HLA-A3	HL-A3	HLA-B8	HL-A8	HLA-Cw3	T3	HLA-Dw3	LD 103
HLA-A9	HL-A9	HLA-B12	HL-A12	HLA-Cw4	T4	HLA-Dw4	LD 104
HLA-A10	HL-A10	HLA-B13	HL-A13	HLA-Cw5	T5	HLA-Dw5	LD 105
HLA-A11	HL-A11	HLA-B14	W14			HLA-Dw6	LD 106
HLA-A28	W28	HLA-B18	W18				
HLA-A29	W29	HLA-B27	W27				
HLA-Aw19	Li[c]	HLA-Bw15	W15				
HLA-Aw23	W23	HLA-Bw16	W16				
HLA-Aw24	W24	HLA-Bw17	W17				
HLA-Aw25	W25	HLA-Bw21	W21				
HLA-Aw26	W26	HLA-Bw22	W22				
HLA-Aw30	W30	HLA-Bw35	W5				
HLA-Aw31	W31	HLA-Bw37	TY				
HLA-Aw32	W32	HLA-Bw38	W16.1				
HLA-Aw33	W19.6	HLA-Bw39	W16.2				
HLA-Aw34	Malay 2	HLA-Bw40	W10				
HLA-Aw36	Mo*	HLA-Bw41	Sabell				
HLA-Aw43	BK	HLA-Bw42	MWA				

[a]The previously reserved specificities W4 (4a) and W6 (4b) remain w4 and w6. These specificities are closely associated with the B locus.

[b]For a more comprehensive listing of equivalents see Table 1 and the 'table of equivalent nomenclature' in: Dausset, J., & Colombani J., ed. Histocompatibility testing. Copenhagen, Munksgaard, 1972, p. 7.

[c]HLA-Aw19 includes at least HLA-A29, Aw30, Aw31, Aw32, Aw33, and Aw34 (?).

Table 4. List of equivalent HLA-D antigen designations

Nomenclature		Laboratory no.[a]											
WHO	Workshop	1	2	3	6	7	8	9	11	12	13	14	15
Dw1	LD 101	MLR-S W5a			Theis Lad27a Fes 1	LD-W5a	Tasz	TB1	LD-W5a	LD-W5a	'J'	PF	LD-XVII
Dw2	LD 102	MLR-S 7a	LD-7a	LD-7a	Fes 2	LD-7a		TB3	LD-7a	LD-7a	'S'	PI(BA)	LD-V
Dw3	LD 103	MLR-S 8a	LD-8a LD-8b	LD-8ab		LD-8a	Plock	TB4	LD-8a	LD-8a		SR	LD-XI
Dw4	LD 104	R LD-12a		LD-12a LD-W15a		LD-12a		TB5	LD-W15a	LD-W15a	'L'		LD-XVIII
Dw5	LD 105			SFN1				TB2	LD-'W16a'	Sa1			LD-IV
Dw6	LD 106		LD-12b		Fes 3	LD-W15a	Krej	TB6	LD-pm	PR			LD-XIV
	LD 107								LD-12a	LD-12a			LD-XII
	LD 108								LD-ae	LD-W10a			

[a] The investigators belonging to the individual laboratories will appear in the list of LD laboratories and in the LD-reports from these laboratories published in: Kiss-meyer-Nielsen, F., ed. Histocompatibility testing. Copenhagen, Munksgaard, 1975.

Bw38, Bw39, TT*, 407*, and KSO (JA) are under consideration for upgrading or further clarification. For these purposes the collaborating laboratories will solicit additional antisera from other investigators and will exchange sera and, where practicable, informative cells with other groups. Absorption, family, and population studies will be carried out, following the principles set out in this and previous reports, and revision of status will then be further considered by the Committee. A list of the WHO collaborating laboratories is given in the Annex.

Some typical examples of the usage of the new terminology will now be given. An individual carrying the specificities A1, A3, B7, B8 might, for example, also carry the specificities Cw1, Cw2. The phenotype would be given as HLA-A1, 3; B7, 8; Cw1, w2. Note that in writing the phenotype, serological specificities controlled by the same locus are separated by commas, while products of different loci are separated by semicolons. This avoids repetition of the locus symbols and also makes it easy to incorporate cross-reacting and subtypic specificities (e.g., HLA-A9, 10, w23, w25; Bw16, w37; C . . .). The genotype would be written in terms of the two haplotypes as HLA-A1, B8, Cw1/A3, B7, Cw2. Other possible phenotypes would, for example, be HLA-A1, w32; Bw22, w35; Cw1, w3, or HLA-A1, 28; B7, w37; Cw1; Dw2. The presence of only a single specificity for a locus implies a phenotypic blank with respect to the specificities being tested for. A blank in a genotype, established by a family study, could be written, for example, as HLA-A1, Bw35, C—, Dw2/A28, B7, Cw1, D—. When w4 (4a) and w6 (4b) are designated in a pheno- or genotype, they can be inserted after the B locus specificities, e.g., HLA-Ax, y; B7, 12, w4, w6; Cx, y. Following a convention widely accepted in genetics, genetic symbols, such as for loci, alleles, haplotypes, or genotypes, should be italicized in print and underlined in manuscripts and typed scripts, while antigens, serological specificities, etc. should be written and printed in normal type (e.g., A1 is the antigen; *A1* or A1 is the corre-

sponding allele). The loci in the haplotype are written in alphabetical order and so do not represent the relative map position on the chromosome.

There may often be no need to include the system prefix, HLA, when it is clear from the context that loci of this system are being referred to.

In its revision of nomenclature, the Committee considered and unanimously rejected various alternative suggestions, including the possibility of designating the lymphocyte activating determinants and lymphocyte subclass specificities HL-B, HL-C, etc. Attention is drawn to a previous statement on this point, to the effect that the major designations be reserved for other genetic systems not closely linked to or part of the HLA region. The pre-emption of formal symbols such as HLB (or HL-B), HLA-E, etc. before their use has been formally considered by this nomenclature committee, is to be strongly discouraged as being detrimental to a clear development of a systematic classification.

We realize that no system of notation can be guaranteed to cope with all future developments. In particular if, as seems likely, the D-locus is split, its specificities may have to be reassigned. We do, however, believe that the system proposed here has considerable flexibility and can be adopted with minimal changes to present usage.

D.B. Amos, Duke Medical Center, Durham, NC, USA *(Chairman)*.

R. Batchelor, The East Grinstead Research Trust, Blond Laboratories, Queen Victoria Hospital, East Grinstead, England.

W.F. Bodmer, University of Oxford, Oxford, England *(Rapporteur)*.

R. Ceppellini, Institute for Immunology, Basle, Switzerland.

J. Dausset, Institut de Recherches sur les Maladies du Sang, Hôpital Saint-Louis, Paris, France.

F. Kissmeyer-Nielsen, The University Hospital, Aarhus, Denmark.

P. Morris, Nuffield Department of Surgery, University of Oxford, Oxford, England.

Rose Payne, Stanford University School of Medicine, Stanford, CA, USA.

J.J. van Rood, University of Leiden, Leiden, Netherlands.

P.I. Terasaki, University of California School of Medicine, Los Angeles, CA, USA.

Z. Trnka, Institute for Immunology, Basle, Switzerland *(Secretary)*.

R.L. Walford, University of California School of Medicine, Los Angeles, CA, USA.

Acknowledgments

The contributions of Dr Julia Bodmer, Dr Sergio Curtoni, Dr Alberto Piazza, and Dr Erik Thorsby to this report are gratefully acknowledged.

COLLABORATING LABORATORIES FOR LEUCOCYTE ANTIGEN TESTING

Department of Microbiology and Immunology, Duke University Medical Center, Durham NC, USA (D.B. Amos & F.E. Ward).

McIndoe Memorial Research Unit, Blond Laboratories, Queen Victoria Hospital, East Grinstead, Sussex, England (R. Batchelor).

Genetics Laboratory, Department of Biochemistry, University of Oxford, Oxford, England (W.F. Bodmer & J.G. Bodmer).

Central CNR per l'Immunogenetica e l'Istocompatibilità, c/o Istituto di Genetica Medica dell'Università di Torino, Torino, Italy (R. Ceppellini & S.E. Curtoni).

Institut de Recherches sur les Maladies du Sang, Hôpital Saint-Louis, Paris, France (J. Dausset & J. Colombani).

Central Laboratory, Netherlands Red Cross Blood Transfusion Service, Amsterdam, Netherlands (C.P. Engelfriet & Ella van den Berg-Loonen).

Institute of Experimental Biology and Genetics, Czechoslovak Academy of Sciences, Prague, Czechoslovakia (P. Ivanyi).

Histocompatibility Laboratory, Geneva, Switzerland (M. Jeannet).

Tissue Typing Laboratory, University Hospital, Aarhus, Denmark (F. Kissmeyer-Nielsen).

Department of Medicine (Hematology), Stanford University School of Medicine, Palo Alto, CA, USA (Rose Payne).

Department of Immunohaematology, University of Leiden, Leiden, Netherlands (J.J. van Rood).

Department of Surgery, University of California School of Medicine, Los Angeles, CA, USA (P.I. Terasaki).

University of California School of Medicine, Los Angeles, CA, USA (R.L. Walford & G. Smith).

Reading 8

The opinion that sensitized T lymphocytes exert their major cytotoxic effects only by cell-cell contact with the target cell is an idea which has by now totally collapsed, despite its long history as a basic tenet of CMI. In this article, reprinted from *Science* 172:729-731, 1972 (copyright 1972, the American Association for the Advancement of Science), the investigators have exposed PPD-sensitive lymphocytes to PPD, to medium lacking antigen, and to a heterologous antigen. This latter type of control with an unrelated antigen now is becoming standard in studies of cellular immunity, although it has been a traditional part of serologic studies for years. Only recently, in comparison, have cellular immunologists guarded themselves against nonspecific stimulatory effects by incorporating additional controls. Purified supernatant fluids, with potent MIF activity, and fluids from the control systems were tested in vivo for their ability to impair tumor growth, and only the experimental MIF material was active. This material was inactive on distantly placed tumors (thereby possibly limiting its potential therapeutic use). Nonetheless an antitumor product is released by cells that are not specifically sensitized to the tumor, and this material can be purified easily. The article reveals the type of experiments and data being accumulated and published currently in the area of tumor immunology.

TUMOR IMMUNITY: TUMOR SUPPRESSION IN VIVO INITIATED BY SOLUBLE PRODUCTS OF SPECIFICALLY STIMULATED LYMPHOCYTES

IRWIN D. BERNSTEIN, DANIEL E. THOR, BERTON ZBAR, and HERBERT J. RAPP*

Abstract. *Supernatant fluids of specifically stimulated lymphocyte cultures were purified. Fractions containing migration inhibition factor when injected intradermally into strain-2 guinea pigs produced a reaction similar in appearance to delayed cutaneous hypersensitivity. There was an accumulation of mononuclear cells at the injection sites and the growth of syngenetic tumor grafts at the sites was suppressed.*

The immunologic rejection of tumors in syngeneic animals is mediated by specifically sensitized lymphoid cells *(1)*. Delayed hypersensitivity has been associated with the rejection of some syngeneic hepatomas induced by diethylnitrosamine *(2)*. However, hepatomas that do not provoke a delayed hypersensitivity reaction can be in-

*Biology Branch, National Cancer Institute and Laboratory of Virology and Rickettsiology, Division of Biologics Standards, Bethesda, Maryland 20014.

hibited at the site of a delayed hypersensitivity reaction initiated by an unrelated antigen. Delayed hypersensitivity reactions consist of the specific recognition of an antigen by a relatively small number of sensitized lymphocytes followed by the accumulation of a relatively large number of mononuclear cells (3). We have found that macrophages from unimmunized animals, but not neutrophils or lymphocytes, can inhibit the growth of one of these tumors in vivo and in vitro (4). Cell-mediated tumor immunity, therefore, requires at least two distinct reactions: (i) specific interaction of sensitized lymphocytes and tumor cell antigen, and (ii) the local accumulation of mononuclear cells that prevent the growth of tumor cells at that site.

Lymphocytes incubated in vitro with the specific antigen to which they were sensitized produce substances that (i) inhibit the migration of macrophages from capillary tubes (5), (ii) are cytotoxic in vitro (6), (iii) are leukotactic (7), and (iv) can give skin reactions similar to delayed hypersensitivity (8). Tumor cell antigens have been shown to cause the release of macrophage migration inhibition factor (MIF) (9). We have been able to obtain inhibition of tumor growth at sites of inflammatory reactions produced by the intradermal injections of crude supernatants of specifically stimulated lymphocyte cultures (10). In this report we show that intradermal injection of tissue culture fluids containing MIF is followed by the accumulation of mononuclear cells and an inflammatory response at the site of injection. The growth of tumors at these sites is inhibited.

Age-matched, adult, Sewall-Wright NIH inbred strain-2 guinea pigs were used. Induction of primary hepatomas by the administration of diethylnitrosamine in the drinking water and the formation of an ascites variant have been described (11). Ascites cells from the sixth generation of a transplantable hepatoma (line 10) were prepared (12). In all experiments 10^6 tumor cells mixed with the appropriate reagent were injected intradermally in a volume of 0.1 ml. Each result given is the mean for three animals.

Inbred strain-2 guinea pigs were immunized by the injection of heat-killed *Mycobacterium tuberculosis* (0.1 ml, H37Rv strain 2 mg/ml in a 1:1 mixture of 0.15M NaCl and 15 percent Arlacel A in Bayol F) into each footpad and posterior nuchal area (five injections). Fourteen to 18 days later the animals were killed, the lymph nodes collected, and cell suspensions made as previously described (13). The cells were washed with Hanks balanced salt solution and resuspended in RPMI-1640 tissue culture medium to contain 3 to 4 × 10^6 viable cells per milliliter (1.2 to 1.6 × 10^7 per 4-ml of culture). The medium contained fresh frozen glutamine (15 mg/liter) and Ampicillin (100 μg/ml at 288 milliosmoles, pH 7.4). Cultures for MIF production contained PPD-S antigen (10 μg/ml) without preservation. Two control cultures were included: one without antigen (control A) and one with coccidioidin, an antigen unrelated to tubercle bacilli (control D). The supernatants, after 36 hours, were harvested, dialyzed against distilled water, lyophilized, and kept frozen at $-70°$ C. Lyophilized samples were reconstituted with distilled water, and fractionated by gel filtration on Sephadex columns; the peak of biologic activity was located by testing the fractions for capillary migration inhibition (13). Sephadex G-75 was eluted with 0.01M borate buffer, pH 8, and the fraction having a molecular weight of 30,000 to 40,000 was collected and found to contain the MIF activity by the indirect assay. Pooled fractions of this peak were lyophilized and redissolved in 0.01M tris buffer, pH 8.7, and fractionated further by electrophoresis on polyacrylamide gel. With a 10 percent gel, separation pH 10.2, concentration pH 9.65, on a 1 by 20 cm column, electrophoresis was performed at 4° C (200 volts, 5 to 10 ma). The active MIF fraction migrated ahead of albumin. In the stained gel there was no visible band in the area containing active MIF. Active MIF could be eluted from the gel either by extraction of minced sections of gel in distilled water or by continued electrophoresis from individual sections into dialysis bags. The purified MIF fraction was dissolved in a volume of medium equal to the volume of the original supernatant fluid obtained from the lymphocyte cultures. MIF activity was present at this final concentration. Corresponding fractions of control A from Sephadex and poly-acrylamide gels were used. An additional control consisting of supernatant fluid from unstimulated lymphocyte cultures and an amount of PPD-S equivalent to the maximal possible amount in the purified material had shown neither inflammatory nor tumor-inhibiting activity.

Fluids containing MIF and control fluids were injected intradermally. Skin reactions to fluids containing MIF were present at 3 to 4 hours and reached maximal size between 12 and 24 hours; there was no reaction to the intradermal injection of control fluids. Histologic sections of reaction sites taken at 24 hours revealed a typical picture of tuberculin hypersensitivity reaction. There was a preponderance (70 to 80 percent) of mononucle-

ar cells. Supernatants incubated with tumor cells were injected intradermally. The results of this experiment are shown in Table 1. It can be seen that fluids containing MIF inhibit tumor growth and control fluids do not.

We next tested whether tumor rejection initiated by MIF at one intradermal site would affect tumor growth at another intradermal site. The design and results of this experiment are given in Table 2. It can be seen that a tumor adjacent to a rejected tumor was unaffected. This observation opposes the view that tumor rejection initiated by MIF was due to a systemic adjuvant effect.

It is possible that supernatants containing MIF exert a direct cytotoxic effect on tumor cells. In order to test this possibility, tumor cells were inoculated into skin sites where MIF or control supernatants had been injected 24 hours earlier. Tumor cell growth was inhibited (see Table 3) at sites

Table 1. Inhibition of tumor growth in vivo by tissue culture fluids containing MIF

Supernatant injected*	Delayed hypersensitivity skin reactions at 24 hours† (mm²)	Size of intradermal tumor papule on day 14† (mm²)
Control A	0	15 ± 1.0
Supernatant containing MIF	15.6 ± 2.5	0
Control D	0	9.3 ± 0.7
Medium 199	0	6.0 ± 1.0

*10^7 Tumor cells per milliliter of supernatant were incubated at 37° C for 10 minutes; 0.1 ml of the mixture was injected intra-dermally at each site.
†Results are expressed as means of the average radius squared (mm²) ± standard error of the mean.

Table 2. Tumor growth in vivo at a site adjacent to MIF-mediated rejection of tumor cells

Supernatant injected*	Growth of tumor cells inoculated in medium 199: size of papule on day 14†	Growth of tumor cells inoculated in MIF or control supernatants: size of papule on day 14†
Control A	19.9 ± 1.0	20 ± 2.3
Supernatant containing MIF	17.7 ± 3.0	0
Control D	16.2 ± 2.3	18.1 ± 1.2

*10^7 Tumor cells per milliliter of supernatant or medium 199 were incubated at 37° C for 10 minutes; 0.1 ml of the mixture was in-jected intradermally at each site. The distance between sites of tumor rejection and adjacent tumor sites was 1.5 to 2.0 cm.
†Results are expressed as mean of the average radius squared (mm²) ± standard error of the mean.

Table 3. Inhibition of tumor growth at sites of skin reactions to MIF

Supernatant injected*	Size of skin reaction at 24 hours† (mm^2)	Size of tumor papule at 14 days† (mm^2)
Control A	0	7.1 ± 2.6
Supernatant containing MIF	16.4 ± 1.2	0.2 ± 0.2
Control D	0	5.9 ± 3.2

*0.1 ml of each supernatant was injected intradermally 24 hours prior to the injection of 10^6 tumor cells in a volume of 0.1 ml into each site.

†Results are expressed as mean of the average radius squared (mm^2) ± standard error of the mean.

where an inflammatory reaction was present before tumor cells were injected. This observation favors the view that tumor rejection was due to host cells rather than to a direct effect by MIF.

These experiments support the concept that animals immunized to a given tumor contain lymphocytes capable of specific immunologic interaction with that tumor and that following this interaction, the lymphocytes elaborate substances that cause the accumulation of mononuclear cells; these mononuclear cells are then responsible for the rejection of tumor grafts. Present evidence indicates that this activity of the mononuclear cells is immunologically nonspecific, and, therefore, tumor rejection by these cells does not require their specific recognition of tumor antigen.

REFERENCES

1. L.J. Old, E.A. Boyse, D.A. Clarke, E.A. Carswell, *Ann. N.Y. Acad. Sci.* **101**, 80 (1962-63); G. Klein, H.O. Sjögren, E. Klein, K.E. Hellström, *Cancer Res.* **20**, 1561 (1960).
2. B. Zbar, H.T. Wepsic, H.J. Rapp, T. Borsos, B.S Kronman, W.H. Churchill, Jr., *J. Nat. Cancer Inst.* **43**, 833 (1969); B. Zbar, H.T. Wepsic, T. Borsos, H.J. Rapp, *ibid.* **44**, 473 (1970).
3. R.T. McCluskey, B. Benacerraf, J.W. McCluskey, *J. Immunol.* **90**, 466 (1963).
4. B. Zbar, I.D. Bernstein, H.T. Wepsic, L. Stewart, T. Borsos, H.J. Rapp, in preparation: J. Oppenheim, B. Zbar, H.J. Rapp, *Proc. Nat. Acad. Sci. U.S.* **66**, 119 (1970).
5. B.R. Bloom and B. Bennett, *Science* **153**, 80 (1966); B. Bennett and B.R. Bloom, *Proc. Nat. Acad. Sci. U.S.* **59**, 759 (1968); B.R. Bloom and B. Bennett, *Ann. N.Y. Acad.*

Sci. **169**, 258 (1970); J.R. David, in *Mediators of Cellular Immunity,* M. Landy and H.S. Lawrence, Eds. (Academic Press, New York, 1969); J.R. David, *Proc. Nat. Acad. Sci. U.S.* **56**, 72 (1966); D. Thor, R.E. Jureziz, S.R. Veach, E. Miller, S. Dray, *Nature* **219**, 5155 (1968); D. Thor, in *Mediators of Cellular Immunity,* M. Landy and H.S. Lawrence, Eds. (Academic Press, New York, 1969).
6. N.H. Ruddle and B.H. Waksman, *Science* **157**, 1060 (1967); *J. Exp. Med.* **128**, 1267 (1968); G.A. Granger and W.P. Kolb, *J. Immunol.* **101**, 111 (1968); G.A. Granger, in *Mediators of Cellular Immunity,* M. Landy and H.S. Lawrence, Eds. (Academic Press, New York, 1969).
7. P.A. Ward, H.G. Remold, J.R. David, *Science* **163**, 1081 (1969).
8. B. Bennett and B.R. Bloom, *Proc. Nat. Acad. Sci. U.S.* **59**, 756 (1968); E. Pick, J. Krevci, K. Coch, J.L. Turk, *Immunology* **17**, 741 (1969); J.L. Turk, in *Mediators of Cellular Immunity,* M. Landy and H.S. Lawrence, Eds. (Academic Press, New York, 1969).
9. B.S. Kronman, H.T. Wepsic, W.H. Churchill, Jr., B. Zbar, T. Borsos, H.J. Rapp, *Science* **165**, 296 (1969); B.R. Bloom, B. Bennett, H.F. Oettgen, E.P. McLean, L.J. Old, *Proc. Nat. Acad. Sci. U.S.* **64**, 1176 (1969).
10. I.D. Bernstein, D.E. Thor, B. Zbar, H.J. Rapp, unpublished observations.
11. H.J. Rapp, W.H. Churchill, Jr., B.S. Kronman, R.T. Rolley, W.G. Hammond, T. Borsos, *J. Nat. Cancer Inst.* **41**, 1 (1968).
12. W.H. Churchill, Jr., H.J. Rapp, B.S. Kronman, T. Borsos, *ibid.,* p. 13.
13. D.E. Thor and S. Dray, *J. Immunol.* **101**, 51 (1968); D.E. Thor, in *In vitro Methods of Cellular Immunity,* B. Bloom and P. Glade, Eds. (Academic Press, New York, 1971).

Reading 9

"Barbiturates: Radioimmunoassay" by Sydney Spector and Edward J. Flynn is an article that reveals the simplicity by which immunoassays of great sensitivity can be developed for low molecular weight compounds of biologic importance. This article illustrates by chemical formulas how modification of the barbituric acid compound was necessary before it could be coupled to a carrier protein by carbodiimide conjugation and used as a hapten-antigen conjugate for the production of antisera. Fig. 2 presents the data for the determinations that were necessary preludes to the development of the radioassay itself, that is, the titrations of antiserum and of hapten against varying concentrations of hapten and antiserum, respectively. The data precisely fit the theoretic curves. In the complete test some variance from a straight line was observed in determining the concentration of barbiturates in biologic fluids, but this is not greater than observed by other methods or in other RIAs. The results reveal that the test is 20 to 200 times more sensitive than other procedures.

This article is reprinted from *Science* **174**:1036-1038, 1971 (copyright 1971, the American Association for the Advancement of Science).

BARBITURATES: RADIOIMMUNOASSAY
SYDNEY SPECTOR AND EDWARD J. FLYNN*

Abstract. The development of a radioimmunoassay for barbiturate is described. The barbiturate is made antigenic by coupling it to a protein, bovine gamma globulin. The radioimmunoassay can measure as little as 5 nanograms of barbiturate.

For the study of the metabolism of barbiturates, quantitative assays that are rapid, sensitive, specific, and reliable even for small amounts of barbiturates would be most advantageous. Methods now available are suited for qualitative and quantitative analysis only if an adequate sample of biological tissue, 1 to 5 ml, is available *(1)*. In addition, these methods require solvent extraction *(1)* and, in some instances, filtration and evaporation *(2)*. Gas chromatography and spectrophotometry are sensitive to 10 μg/ml but require solvent extraction *(3)*. Immunologic methods for assaying polypeptides, hormones, and drugs have been reported *(4)*. We have conjugated a barbiturate to bovine gamma globulin (BGG), produced antibodies against the barbiturate hapten, and developed a radioimmunoassay capable of measuring nanogram levels of barbiturates.

Antibodies were induced by immunization of rabbits with a barbiturate-protein conjugate. The barbiturate, 5-allyl-5-(1-carboxyisopropyl) barbituric acid, was converted to 5-allyl-5-(1-*p*-nitrophenyloxycarbonylisopropyl) barbituric acid by reacting the free base (10 mg) with *p*-nitrophenol (12 mg) in *N,-N*-dimethylformamide for 24 hours at 4° C. The 5-allyl-5-(1-*p*-nitrophenyloxycarbonylisopropyl) barbituric acid was coupled to BGG (10 mg) in a glycerin-water solution (1:1, by volume) in the presence of dicyclohexylcarbodiimide (5 mg) *(5)*. The mixture was incubated overnight at 4° C, and the protein-hapten complex was dialyzed against distilled water. Conjugation of the barbiturate to the protein carrier was confirmed by the increase in absorbance at 202 nm of the barbiturate-BGG conjugate as compared to control BGG solutions. From the molar extinction coefficient of the barbiturate ($E_m = 19,500$), the degree of substitution was estimated to be 2 to 3 moles of barbiturate per mole of protein. New Zealand albino rabbits were immunized with 1 mg of barbiturate-BGG (Fig. 1). The immunogen (100 μg) in phosphate-buffered saline, *p*H 7.2, was emulsified with an equal volume of complete Freund's adjuvant. The initial dose was 1.6 ml, 0.4 ml injected into each footpad. A booster injection of 100 μg of antigen in adjuvant was given every 6 to 8 weeks, 25 μg in each of the footpads. Blood was collected 5 to 7 days after booster injections and the serum was examined for antibodies to barbiturates.

Various dilutions of antiserums were incubated with 8×10^{-4} μc of [^{14}C]pentobarbital sodium (New England Nuclear, 4.13 mc/mmole), approximately 1000 count/min, at 4° C overnight. After incubation, a neutral saturated ammonium sulfate solution (volume equal to incubation medium) was added to all tubes. The precipitate, containing pentobarbital bound to antibody, was washed two times with an equal volume of 50 percent saturated ammonium sulfate and then dis-

*Department of Physiological Chemistry, Pharmacology Section, Roche Institute of Molecular Biology, Nutley, New Jersey 07110.

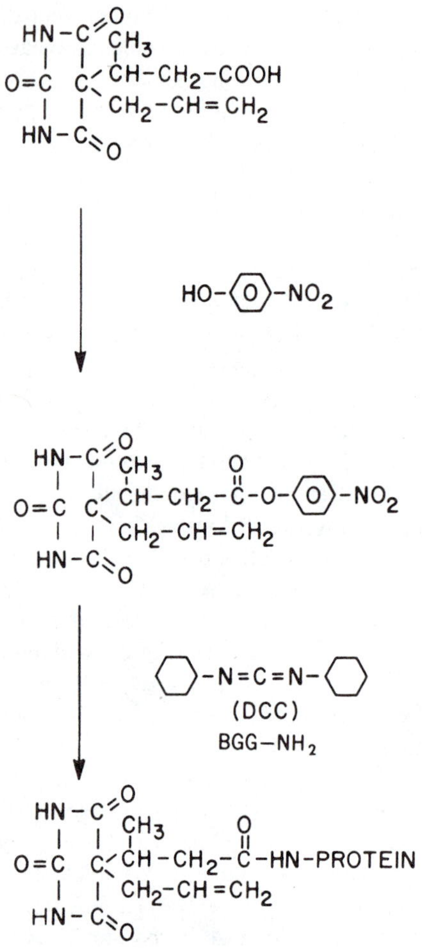

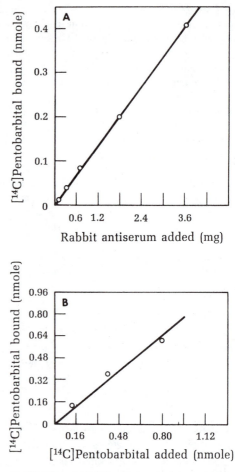

Fig. 1. Synthesis of the barbiturate antigen. *DCC,* Dicyclohexylcarbodiimide; *BGG,* bovine gamma globulin.

Fig. 2. Binding of [^{14}C]pentobarbital by rabbit antiserum. In **A,** varying amounts of antiserum (milligrams of protein per reaction tube) were added to a constant amount of [^{14}C]pentobarbital (0.8 nmole). In **B,** varying amounts of [^{14}C]pentobarbital were added to a constant amount of rabbit antiserum (3.5 mg of protein per reaction tube).

solved in 0.5 ml of Nuclear-Chicago Solubilizer *(6),* and the radioactivity was counted in a liquid scintillation spectrometer (Packard Tri-Carb). While normal rabbit serum failed to bind labeled pentobarbital, the serum from immunized rabbits bound 75 to 80 percent of the added labeled pentobarbital, and there was a linear relationship between bound [^{14}C]pentobarbital and the concentration of added antibody (Fig. 2, *A*). When variable amounts of [^{14}C]pentobarbital were added

to a constant amount of antibody, there was a linear relationship between added and bound [^{14}C]pentobarbital (Fig. 2, *B*).

The radioimmunoassay depends on competition between unlabeled pentobarbital and a standard of [^{14}C]pentobarbital for combination with barbiturate antibodies in rabbit antisera. A tube that con-

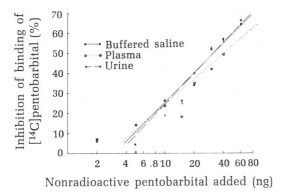

Y-axis: Inhibition of binding of [^{14}C]pentobarbital (%)

X-axis: Nonradioactive pentobarbital added (ng)

Legend: •—• Buffered saline / o · · o Plasma / X—X Urine

Fig. 3. Inhibition of binding of [^{14}C]pentobarbital to rabbit antiserum by nonradioactive pentobarbital in buffered saline (•—•), plasma (o · · · o), or urine (X——X). Incubation medium consisted of 0.10 ml of normal rabbit serum, 0.10 ml of rabbit antiserum (0.4 mg of protein), 0.01 ml of [^{14}C]pentobarbital (0.1 nmole), and 0.01 ml of either standard unlabeled pentobarbital (1 to 100 ng) or unknown sample and sufficient phosphate-buffered saline (0.01M phosphate, pH 7.4) to make a final volume of 0.50 ml. Lines of regression were calculated by the method of least squares.

tained radioactive pentobarbital and antiserum, but no unlabeled pentobarbital, measured maximum radioactivity bound to antibody. The addition of increasing amounts of unlabeled pentobarbital to fixed amounts of [^{14}C]pentobarbital and antiserum resulted in competitive inhibition of binding of labeled pentobarbital by antibody (Fig. 3). The similarity of the standard curves obtained when pentobarbital was added in plasma, urine, or buffered saline indicates that there are no interfering substances in the two body fluids. In addition, the data demonstrate the sensitivity of the method. Pentobarbital (5 ng) in a sample volume of 10 μl caused a 20 percent inhibition of binding of the labeled compound. The same amount of pentobarbital can be assayed in a larger sample volume (200 μl), which increases the sensitivity 20-fold.

The antibody bound barbital, pentobarbital and phenobarbital equally well. These three compounds differ only by the substituents on the C-5 position. Since BGG was conjugated to the bar-

bituric acid moiety at C-5 it is understandable that the antibody fails to differentiate between these barbituric acids. In contrast, at equimolar concentration of hexobarbital or thiopental the antibody bound these compounds to a lesser degree. These compounds have different substituents at either position 2 or 3 in the barbituric acid ring. Thus, the urea portion of the ring may be critical in determining antibody specificity.

The barbiturate-BGG antigen was effective in eliciting antibodies against barbituric acid derivatives. We believe that this is the first report of the experimental production of antibodies capable of recognizing barbiturates. The radioimmunoassay technique reported here is rapid and extremely sensitive, and should be useful for the determination of barbiturate concentrations in biological tissues and fluids. Theoretically, since metabolic products with changes at the C-5 position may also be detected by the antibody, our procedure, coupled with a solvent extraction, could measure both total concentration of barbiturate and its hydroxylated metabolites. Antibodies directed against steroid haptens *(7)* and digitalis *(8)* have been reported to modify the physiological actions of these agents, and it would be interesting to determine whether antibodies against barbiturates interfere with the pharmacological effects of barbiturates.

REFERENCES AND NOTES

1. T. Koppanyi, J.M. Dille, W.S. Murphy, S. Krop, *J. Amer. Pharm. Ass.* **23**, 1074 (1934); J.W. Jailer and L.R. Goldbaum, *J. Lab. Clin. Med.* **31**, 1344 (1946); R. Deininger, *Arzneim. Forsch.* **5**, 472, (1955).
2. K.D. Parker and P.L. Kirk, *Anal. Chem.* **33**, 1378 (1961); H.F. Martin and J.L. Driscoll, *ibid.* **38**, 345 (1966).
3. M.W. Anders, *ibid.* **38**, 1945 (1966); J.T. Walker, R.S. Fisher, J.J. McHugh, *Amer. J. Clin. Pathol.* **18**, 451 (1948); L.B. Hellman, L.B. Shettles, H. Strau, *J. Biol. Chem.* **148**, 293 (1943); L.R. Goldbaum, *J. Pharmacol. Exp. Ther.* **94**, 68 (1948).
4. R.S. Yalow, S.M. Glick, J. Roth, S.A. Berson, *J. Clin. Endocrinol. Metab.* **24**, 1219 (1964); R.D. Utiger, *J. Clin. Invest.* **44**, 1277 (1965); S.A. Berson and R.S. Yalow, *ibid.* **38**, 1966 (1959); M.B. Vallotton, L.B. Page, E.

Haber, *Nature* **215,** 714 (1967); S. Spector and C.W. Parker, *Science* **168,** 1347 (1970).

5. Ott Chemical Company, Muskegan, Michigan.

6. Amersham/Searle.

7. L. Goodfriend and A.H. Sehon, *Can. J. Biochem. Physiol.* **39,** 941 (1961); R.O. Neri, S. Tolksdorf, S.M. Belser, F. Erlanger, J. Agate, S. Lieberman, *Endocrinology* **74,** 593 (1964).

8. V.P. Butler, *N. Engl. J. Med.* **283,** 1150 (1970).

9. Supported by a postdoctoral fellowship (E.J.F.) from Hoffmann-La Roche Inc.

INDEX

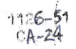